Receptors and Hormone Action

VOLUME II

Contributors

THOMAS C. ALLEN
NORMAN S. ANDERSON, III
C. WAYNE BARDIN
JOHN D. BAXTER
LESLIE P. BULLOCK
BETSY D. CARLTON
GARY C. CHAMNESS
TONG J. CHEN
FRANK CHYTIL
JAMES H. CLARK
PAUL D. COLMAN
YUNG S. DO
HAKAN ERIKSSON
DARRELL D. FANESTIL
PHILIP FEIGELSON
FRANK S. FRENCH
J. GORSKI
JAMES W. HARDIN
J. N. HARRIS
KATHRYN B. HORWITZ
ROBERT D. IVARIE
SAMSON T. JACOB
OSCAR A. LEA
WENDELL W. LEAVITT
TEHMING LIANG
SHUTSUNG LIAO
YEN-CHIU LIN
BRUCE S. McEWEN
WILLIAM L. McGUIRE
W. I. P. MAINWARING
E. MILGROM
NATHANIEL C. MILLS
ANTHONY W. NORMAN
ANGELO C. NOTIDES
BERT W. O'MALLEY
DAVID E. ONG
ERNEST J. PECK, JR.
LEELAVATI RAMANARAYANAN-MURTHY
GORDON M. RINGOLD
WILLIAM T. SCHRADER
F. STORMSHAK
JOHN T. TYMOCZKO
WAYNE R. WECKSLER
ULRICH WESTPHAL
ELIZABETH M. WILSON
KEITH R. YAMAMOTO
DAVID T. ZAVA

Receptors and Hormone Action

VOLUME II

Edited by

Bert W. O'Malley
Lutz Birnbaumer

Department of Cell Biology
Baylor College of Medicine
Houston, Texas

Academic Press New York San Francisco London 1978
A Subsidiary of Harcourt Brace Jovanovich, Publishers

COPYRIGHT © 1978, BY ACADEMIC PRESS, INC.
ALL RIGHTS RESERVED.
NO PART OF THIS PUBLICATION MAY BE REPRODUCED OR
TRANSMITTED IN ANY FORM OR BY ANY MEANS, ELECTRONIC
OR MECHANICAL, INCLUDING PHOTOCOPY, RECORDING, OR ANY
INFORMATION STORAGE AND RETRIEVAL SYSTEM, WITHOUT
PERMISSION IN WRITING FROM THE PUBLISHER.

ACADEMIC PRESS, INC.
111 Fifth Avenue, New York, New York 10003

United Kingdom Edition published by
ACADEMIC PRESS, INC. (LONDON) LTD.
24/28 Oval Road, London NW1 7DX

Library of Congress Cataloging in Publication Data
Main entry under title:

Receptors and hormone action.

    1. Hormones.   2. Hormone receptors.   I. O'Malley,
Bert W.   II. Birnbaumer, Lutz.
QP571.R4   591.1'42   77-74060
ISBN 0-12-526302-3

PRINTED IN THE UNITED STATES OF AMERICA

Contents

List of Contributors — xi

Preface — xv

1 The Biology and Pharmacology of Estrogen Receptor Binding: Relationship to Uterine Growth
JAMES H. CLARK, ERNEST J. PECK, JR., JAMES W. HARDIN, and HAKAN ERIKSSON

I.	Introduction	1
II.	Relationship between Receptor Binding and Uterine Growth	2
III.	Nuclear Receptor Binding and RNA Polymerase Activity	4
IV.	Nuclear Retention and the Agonistic-Antagonistic Properties of Estriol	11
V.	Nuclear Retention and Replenishment of Estrogen Receptor and Hormone Antagonism	18
VI.	Long-Term Nuclear Retention and Acceptor Sites	24
VII.	Conclusion	28
	References	29

2 Conformational Forms of the Estrogen Receptor
ANGELO C. NOTIDES

I.	Introduction	33
II.	Transformation of the Rat Uterine Estrogen Receptor	35
III.	Kinetic Analysis of the Relationship of the 4 S to the 5 S Estrogen Receptor	41
IV.	Molecular Properties of the Estrogen Receptor from the Human Uterus	47
V.	Conformational Models of the Estrogen Receptor	54
VI.	Conclusion	58
	References	59

3 Nuclear Estrogen Receptor and DNA Synthesis
F. STORMSHAK, J. N. HARRIS, and J. GORSKI

I.	Introduction	63
II.	Estrogen and the Cell Cycle	64

	III.	Dynamics of DNA Synthesis in Response to Sequential Injections of Estrogen	73
	IV.	Antimitotic Effects of Estrogen	78
	V.	Conclusions	79
		References	79

4 The Role of Receptors in the Anabolic Action of Androgens
C. WAYNE BARDIN, LESLIE P. BULLOCK, NATHANIEL C. MILLS, YEN-CHIU LIN, and SAMSON T. JACOB

I.	Introduction	83
II.	Metabolism of Androgens by Mouse Kidney	85
III.	Androgen Receptors in Mouse Kidney	87
IV.	Androgen Receptors in Mice with Testicular Feminization (tfm)	90
V.	Effects of Androgen Receptors on RNA Polymerase and Chromatin Template Activation	92
VI.	Role of Androgen Receptors in the Action of Progestins on Mouse Kidney	94
VII.	Effects of Androgens on Kidney Growth	97
VIII.	Summary and Conclusions	100
	References	101

5 Androgen Receptors and Biologic Responses: A Survey
W. I. P. MAINWARING

I.	Introduction	105
II.	General Model for the Mechanism of Action of Androgens	106
III.	Desirable Trends in Future Research	111
IV.	Summary	117
	References	117

6 Androgen Receptor Interactions in Target Cells: Biochemical Evaluation
JOHN L. TYMOCZKO, TEHMING LIANG, and SHUTSUNG LIAO

I.	Evidence for Existence of Androgen Receptors	122
II.	Identification and Characterization of Androgen Receptors	123
III.	Specificities in Androgen–Receptor Interactions	130
IV.	Cell Nucleus and Chromatin Binding of Androgen Receptor	136
V.	Interaction of Androgen Receptors with Other Cellular Components	144
VI.	Concluding Remarks	148
	References	153

7 Biology of Progesterone Receptors
WENDELL W. LEAVITT, TONG J. CHEN, YUNG S. DO, BETSY D. CARLTON, and THOMAS C. ALLEN

I.	Introduction	157
II.	Progesterone Action in the Hamster	159

III.	Progesterone Uptake *in Vivo*	160
IV.	Methods for Cytosol Progesterone Receptor	161
V.	Progesterone Receptor Distribution in Different Tissues	169
VI.	Regulation of Progesterone Receptor Levels	173
VII.	Progesterone Receptor Synthesis *in Vitro*	184
	References	186

8 Molecular Structure and Analysis of Progesterone Receptors
WILLIAM T. SCHRADER and BERT W. O'MALLEY

I.	Introduction	189
II.	The Progesterone Receptor Protein	193
III.	Effects of Progesterone *in Vivo* on Chromatin Gene Transcription	207
IV.	Effects of Purified Progesterone-Receptor Complexes *in Vitro* on Chromatin Gene Transcription	210
V.	A Proposed Model for Steroid Hormone Regulation of Gene Transcription	218
	References	222

9 Studies on the Cytoplasmic Glucocorticoid Receptor and Its Nuclear Interaction in Mediating Induction of Tryptophan Oxygenase Messenger RNA in Liver and Hepatoma
PHILIP FEIGELSON, LEELAVATI RAMANARAYANAN-MURTHY, and PAUL D. COLMAN

I.	Introduction	226
II.	Glucocorticoid Receptor	227
III.	Metabolic Effects of Glucocorticoids	238
IV.	Control of Specific Species of mRNA by Glucocorticoids	238
V.	Glucocorticoidal Control of the mRNA for Tryptophan Oxygenase in Hepatomas	243
VI.	Interaction of the Receptor with Nuclear Components	246
VII.	Conclusions	247
	References	248

10 Regulation of Gene Expression by Glucocorticoid Hormones: Studies of Receptors and Responses in Cultured Cells
JOHN D. BAXTER and ROBERT D. IVARIE

I.	Introduction	252
II.	Glucocorticoid Hormone Receptors	254
III.	The Domain of Response to Glucocorticoid Hormones	258
IV.	Agonists, Partial Agonists, and Antagonists: Comparisons of Actions in Various Systems	262
V.	Structure-Activity Relations: Nature of the Receptor-Binding Site	263
VI.	Mechanism of Agonist and Antagonist Steroid Action: Allosteric Model for Steroid Hormone Action	265

VII.	Activation of the Receptor–Glucocorticoid Complex	268
VIII.	Return of the Receptor to the Cytosol: The First Step in Deinduction	270
IX.	Nuclear Binding of Receptor–Glucocorticoid Complexes	271
X.	Genetic Approaches to the Study of Glucocorticoid Hormone Action	279
XI.	Regulation of mRNA by Glucocorticoid Hormones	283
XII.	Deinduction of the Glucocorticoid Response: Posttranscriptional Control of Tyrosine Aminotransferase	287
XIII.	Mechanism of Glucocorticoid Receptor Action: Parallels with Cyclic AMP Action in Bacteria	288
XIV.	Summary	290
	References	292

11 Glucocorticoid Regulation of Mammary Tumor Virus Gene Expression
KEITH R. YAMAMOTO and GORDON M. RINGOLD

I.	Introduction: Defining the Problems	298
II.	Mammary Tumor Virus Genes in Murine Cells	300
III.	MTV RNA Induction Is a Receptor-Mediated Primary Hormone Response	302
IV.	Dexamethasone Stimulates the Rate of MTV RNA Synthesis	304
V.	Glucocorticoid-Responsive MTV Genes Are Mobile	307
VI.	MTV-Infected HTC Cells Contain Unintegrated Viral DNA	311
VII.	MTV Infection Alters Host Gene Response to Glucocorticoids	315
VIII.	Discussion	316
	References	319

12 Biology of Mineralocorticoid Receptors
NORMAN S. ANDERSON, III, and DARRELL D. FANESTIL

I.	Introduction	323
II.	General Presence of [^{3}H]Aldosterone in Target Cells	324
III.	Properties of the Cytosol Aldosterone Receptor	329
IV.	Properties of the Nuclear Aldosterone Receptor	339
V.	Evidence for a Receptor-Mediated Response	342
	References	349

13 Gonadal Steroid Receptors in Neuroendocrine Tissues
BRUCE S. McEWEN

I.	Introduction	354
II.	Estradiol	355
III.	Testosterone	369
IV.	Progesterone	379
V.	Steroid Receptors and Sexual Differentiation of the Brain	384
VI.	Conclusion	391
	References	393

14 Hormones and Their Receptors in Breast Cancer
WILLIAM L. McGUIRE, GARY C. CHAMNESS,
KATHRYN B. HORWITZ, and DAVID T. ZAVA

I.	Introduction	402
II.	Prolactin	403
III.	Estrogen	409
IV.	Progesterone	417
V.	Glucocorticoids	425
VI.	Androgens	427
VII.	Summary and Conclusions	431
	References	431

15 Steroid-Binding Serum Globulins: Recent Results
ULRICH WESTPHAL

I.	Introduction	443
II.	Progesterone-Binding Globulin of the Pregnant Guinea Pig	445
III.	Kinetics of Steroid-Protein Interactions	458
IV.	On the Chemical Nature of the Binding Site	464
	References	471

16 Progesterone-Binding Proteins in Plasma and the Reproductive Tract
E. MILGROM

I.	Progesterone-Binding Plasma Proteins	474
II.	Progesterone Receptors	476
III.	Female Genital Tract Secretory Proteins	485
IV.	Discussion	488
	References	489

17 Androgen-Binding Proteins of the Male Rat Reproductive Tract
ELIZABETH M. WILSON, OSCAR A. LEA, and FRANK S. FRENCH

I.	Introduction	492
II.	Androgen-Binding Protein (ABP)	492
III.	9 S Androgen- and Progesterone-Binding Protein	501
IV.	Androgen Receptor	507
V.	Concluding Remarks	525
	References	528

18 Vitamin D Receptors and Biologic Responses
ANTHONY W. NORMAN and WAYNE R. WECKSLER

I.	Introduction	533
II.	Receptors for Vitamin D	541
III.	Receptors for 25-(OH)D	545
IV.	Receptors for 1,25-$(OH)_2D_3$	553
V.	Summary	567
	References	568

19 Cellular-Binding Protein for Compounds with Vitamin A Activity
FRANK CHYTIL and DAVID E. ONG

I.	Introduction	573
II.	The Vitamin A-Deficient Animal	574
III.	Vitamin A Acid (Retinoic Acid)	576
IV.	Fate of Vitamin A-Active Compounds *in Vivo*	577
V.	Vitamin A and Cellular Differentiation	578
VI.	Cellular Retinol-Binding Protein (CRBP)	579
VII.	Cellular Retinoic Acid-Binding Protein (CRABP)	580
VIII.	Properties of the Cellular-Binding Proteins	581
IX.	Other Vitamin A-Binding Proteins	587
X.	Cellular-Binding Proteins and Cancer	587
XI.	Conclusions	589
	References	590

Index 593

List of Contributors

Numbers in parentheses indicate the pages on which the authors' contributions begin.

THOMAS C. ALLEN (157), Department of Physiology, College of Medicine, University of Cincinnati, Cincinnati, Ohio

NORMAN S. ANDERSON, III (323), Department of Medicine, School of Medicine, University of California at San Diego, La Jolla, California

C. WAYNE BARDIN (83), Department of Medicine, Division of Endocrinology, The Milton S. Hershey Medical Center, Pennsylvania State University, Hershey, Pennsylvania

JOHN D. BAXTER (252), Departments of Medicine, Biochemistry, and Biophysics, and the Metabolic Research Unit, University of California, San Francisco, California

LESLIE P. BULLOCK (83), Department of Medicine, Division of Endocrinology, The Milton S. Hershey Medical Center, Pennsylvania State University, Hershey, Pennsylvania

BETSY D. CARLTON (157), Department of Physiology, College of Medicine, University of Cincinnati, Cincinnati, Ohio

GARY C. CHAMNESS (402), Department of Medicine, University of Texas, San Antonio, Texas

TONG J. CHEN (157), Department of Physiology, College of Medicine, University of Cincinnati, Cincinnati, Ohio

FRANK CHYTIL (573), Department of Biochemistry, Vanderbilt School of Medicine, Vanderbilt University, Nashville, Tennessee

JAMES H. CLARK (1), Department of Cell Biology, Baylor College of Medicine, Houston, Texas

PAUL D. COLMAN (226), Institute of Cancer Research, and the Department of Biochemistry, College of Physicians and Surgeons of Columbia University, New York, New York

List of Contributors

YUNG S. DO (157), Department of Physiology, College of Medicine, University of Cincinnati, Cincinnati, Ohio

HAKAN ERIKSSON* (1), Department of Cell Biology, Baylor College of Medicine, Houston, Texas

DARRELL D. FANESTIL (323), Division of Nephrology, Department of Medicine, University of California at San Diego, La Jolla, California

PHILIP FEIGELSON (226), Institute of Cancer Research, and Department of Biochemistry, College of Physicians and Surgeons, Columbia University, New York, New York

FRANK S. FRENCH (492), Department of Pediatrics, University of North Carolina, Chapel Hill, North Carolina

J. GORSKI (63), Department of Biochemistry, University of Wisconsin, Madison, Wisconsin

JAMES W. HARDIN (1), Department of Cell Biology, Baylor College of Medicine, Houston, Texas

J. N. HARRIS† (63), Department of Biochemistry, University of Wisconsin, Madison, Wisconsin

KATHRYN B. HORWITZ (402), Department of Medicine, University of Texas, San Antonio, Texas

ROBERT D. IVARIE (252), Departments of Medicine, Biochemistry, and Biophysics, and the Metabolic Research Unit, University of California, San Francisco, California

SAMSON T. JACOB (83), Department of Pharmacology, The Milton S. Hershey Medical Center, Pennsylvania State University, Hershey, Pennsylvania

OSCAR A. LEA (492), Department of Pediatrics, University of North Carolina, Chapel, Hill, North Carolina

WENDELL W. LEAVITT§ (157), Department of Physiology, College of Medicine, University of Cincinnati, Cincinnati, Ohio

TEHMING LIANG (122), The Ben May Laboratory for Cancer Research, and Department of Biochemistry, The University of Chicago, Chicago, Illinois

SHUTSUNG LIAO (122), The Ben May Laboratory for Cancer Research, and Department of Biochemistry, The University of Chicago, Chicago, Illinois

YEN-CHIU LIN (83), Department of Medicine, Division of Endocrinology, The Milton S. Hershey Medical Center, Pennsylvania State University, Hershey, Pennsylvania

* Present address: Kemiska Institutionen 1, Karolinska Institutet, 104 01 Stockholm 60, Sweden.

† Present address: Department of Pathology, School of Medicine, Temple University, Philadelphia, Pennsylvania.

§ Present address: Worcester Foundation for Experimental Biology, Shrewsbury, Massachusetts.

List of Contributors

BRUCE S. McEWEN (354), Department of Neurobiology, The Rockefeller University, New York, New York

WILLIAM L. McGUIRE (402), Department of Medicine, University of Texas, San Antonio, Texas

W. I. P. MAINWARING (105), Androgen Physiology Department, Imperial Cancer Research Fund, London, England

E. MILGROM (474), Groupe de Recherches sur la Biochimie Endocrinienne et la Reproduction, Faculté de Médecine de Bicêtre, Université Paris, Paris, France

NATHANIEL C. MILLS (83), Department of Medicine, Division of Endocrinology, The Milton S. Hershey Medical Center, Pennsylvania State University, Hershey, Pennsylvania

ANTHONY W. NORMAN (533), Department of Biochemistry, University of California, Riverside, California

ANGELO C. NOTIDES (33), Department of Pharmacology, School of Medicine and Dentistry, University of Rochester, Rochester, New York

BERT W. O'MALLEY (189), Department of Cell Biology, Baylor College of Medicine, Houston, Texas

DAVID E. ONG (573), Department of Biochemistry, Vanderbilt School of Medicine, Vanderbilt University, Nashville, Tennessee

ERNEST J. PECK, JR. (1), Department of Cell Biology, Baylor College of Medicine, Houston, Texas

LEELAVATI RAMANARAYANAN-MURTHY (226), Institute of Cancer Research, and Department of Biochemistry, College of Physicians and Surgeons, Columbia University, New York, New York

GORDON M. RINGOLD (298), Department of Biochemistry and Biophysics, University of California, San Francisco, California

WILLIAM T. SCHRADER (189), Department of Cell Biology, Baylor College of Medicine, Houston, Texas

F. STORMSHAK* (63), Department of Biochemistry, University of Wisconsin, Madison, Wisconsin

JOHN T. TYMOCZKO† (122), The Ben May Laboratory for Cancer Research, and Department of Biochemistry, The University of Chicago, Chicago, Illinois

WAYNE R. WECKSLER (533), Department of Biochemistry, University of California, Riverside, California

ULRICH WESTPHAL (443), Biochemistry Department, School of Medicine, University of Louisville, Louisville, Kentucky

---

* Present address: Department of Animal Science, Oregon State University, Corvallis, Oregon.

† Present address: Biology Department, Carleton College, Northfield, Minnesota.

ELIZABETH M. WILSON (492), Department of Pediatrics, University of North Carolina, Chapel Hill, North Carolina

KEITH R. YAMAMOTO (298), Department of Biochemistry and Biophysics, University of California, San Francisco, California

DAVID T. ZAVA (402), Department of Medicine, University of Texas, San Antonio, Texas

Preface

The field of hormone action is undoubtedly one of the fastest growing areas of biological science. A rough assessment of the rate of growth of this field as determined from an evaluation of journal articles and programs of national meetings leads us to the surprising conclusion that an approximate tenfold expansion of this field has occurred over the last decade. Research in hormone action not only has grown into a dominant effort in endocrinology and reproductive biology, but also has captured a large share of the more general disciplines of biochemistry, cell biology, and molecular biology. This development has occurred because of the dynamic aspects of the field and the increasing interest inherent to the new discipline of regulatory biology.

The creation of a series of volumes summarizing the advances in the field of hormone action has been a major undertaking. Nevertheless, the investment of time required for this project on the part of the contributors and editors appears to be justified since the compilation of a series of volumes on receptors and hormone action should prove useful to those interested in studying the regulatory biology of the eukaryotic cell. The articles contained in these books are oriented toward a description of basic methodologies and model systems used in the exploration of the molecular bases of hormone action and are aimed at a broad spectrum of readers including those who have not yet worked in the field as well as those who have considerable expertise in one or another aspect of hormone action. In the initial three volumes we therefore compiled articles that present not only a rather extensive description of hormone receptors and their properties, but also basic aspects of structure and function of chromatin and membranes, the sites at which hormones and their receptors exert their action. The receptors discussed include soluble cytoplasmic and nuclear receptors for steroid hormones and vitamins, membrane-bound receptors for protein hormones and biogenic amines, and nuclear receptors for thyroid hormones. It seemed appropriate to cover receptor types, in view of the large body of literature accumulated recently dealing with the various functions of these fascinating but elusive molecules. Thus, while steroid hormone receptors have been isolated and purified, this has not yet been possible for other types of hormone receptors, a fact that clearly highlights a hiatus in our knowledge and demarcates an area for intense future work. We hope that the background and recent advancements presented here will stimulate further experimentation. Future volumes will deal more with the detailed molecular and biochemical processes regulated by these hormones.

Certain omissions have inevitably occurred in the compilation of these initial volumes. Some are due to the fact that certain authors were overcommitted or unable to meet the present deadlines. Other omissions were due to editorial oversight. Nevertheless, we hope that the completion of future volumes will permit this series to stand as a reference of the complete works of the major laboratories working in the field of receptors and hormone action.

Bert W. O'Malley
Lutz Birmbaumer

1

The Biology and Pharmacology of Estrogen Receptor Binding: Relationship to Uterine Growth

JAMES H. CLARK, ERNEST J. PECK, JR.,
JAMES W. HARDIN, AND HAKAN ERIKSSON

I.	Introduction	1
II.	Relationship between Receptor Binding and Uterine Growth	2
III.	Nuclear Receptor Binding and RNA Polymerase Activity	4
IV.	Nuclear Retention and the Agonistic–Antagonistic Properties of Estriol	11
V.	Nuclear Retention and Replenishment of Estrogen Receptor and Hormone Antagonism	18
VI.	Long-Term Nuclear Retention and Acceptor Sites	24
VII.	Conclusion	28
	References	29

I. INTRODUCTION

The relationship between steroid hormone–receptor binding and biologic response is of great interest because the elucidation of this relationship should add much to our knowledge of the mechanism of hormone action. One of the basic criteria that defines a receptor is a cause-and-effect relationship between hormone receptor binding and biologic response. This correlation is difficult and complex to demonstrate; however, recent successes with the integration of endocrinology and molecular biology have allowed progress in the elucidation of these relationships.

II. RELATIONSHIP BETWEEN RECEPTOR BINDING AND UTERINE GROWTH

It is generally accepted that steroid hormones bind to cytoplasmic receptor molecules and undergo translocation to nuclear sites. The nuclear binding of these receptor-steroid complexes is considered to be an important step in the stimulation of nuclear-mediated events that result in the biologic response. These interactions have been studied extensively in the rat uterus, and a general picture of estrogen receptor binding has emerged. Cells of the immature rat uterus contain approximately 15,000–20,000 cytoplasmic receptor sites for estrogen (R_c). These sites undergo translocation to the nucleus to form receptor-estrogen complexes (R_nE) when estrogen is injected or when the blood levels of endogenous estrogen are elevated (Anderson et al., 1972a,b, 1975; Clark et al., 1972; Clark and Peck, 1976). An injection of hyperphysiological doses of estradiol will cause the nuclear translocation of essentially all R_c sites, whereas low or more physiological quantities of estradiol cause the translocation of only 2000–3000 sites. Regardless of the initial number of R_nE complexes in the nucleus after estrogen treatment, only 2000–3000 are retained by the nucleus for longer than 4–6 hours. Since maximal uterine growth correlates with the number of R_nE sites that undergo long-term nuclear retention, we have proposed that retained R_nE complexes may be associated with nuclear acceptor sites (Clark and Peck, 1976). Thus, the binding of R_nE complexes probably involves at least two kinds of nuclear sites (Fig. 1): (a) nonacceptor sites which are in large number and serve to maximize the probability that nuclear binding of the R_nE complex will occur, and (b) acceptor sites which are in small number and involved with the long-term retention of the R_nE complex and the subsequent stimulation of true uterine growth (Fig. 1).

To test the concept that long-term nuclear retention of the R_nE complex is necessary for the stimulation of uterine growth, we have used the differential effects of various estrogens on nuclear binding and uterine growth. It has been known for many years that estrogens vary in their ability to stimulate true uterine growth, i.e., to stimulate cellular hypertrophy plus hyperplasia. It has been demonstrated that estriol (E_3) was as potent as estradiol (E_2) in stimulating early uterotropic responses, i.e., those responses that occur within 1–6 hours after hormone treatment, but was essentially ineffective in causing significant increases in uterine weight at 24–48 hours (Hisaw et al., 1953; Hisaw, 1959). We have confirmed and extended these observations of Hisaw (Figs. 2 and 3) and, in addition, have shown that E_2 and E_3 are of equal potency with regard to nuclear accumulation and short-term retention of the R_nE complex. Thus, it is expected that they should have equal effects in stimulating early uterotropic responses. However,

1. Estrogen Receptor Binding

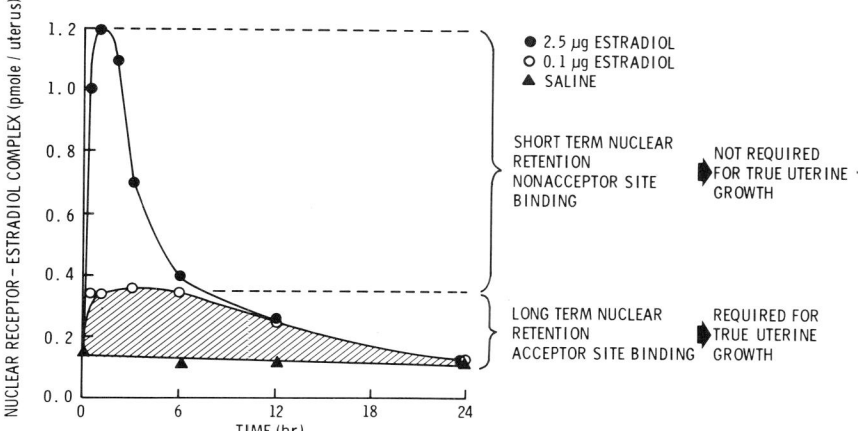

Fig. 1. Relationship between nuclear retention of the estrogen receptor and uterine growth. Immature rats 21–23 days of age were injected with either 0.1 or 2.5 μg of estradiol, and the accumulation and retention of the estrogen receptor by the uterine nuclear fraction was examined by the [^{3}H]estradiol exchange assay. Uterine growth responses (DNA, RNA, and protein content; wet and dry weight) were measured at 24–48 hours after injection (data not shown), and were found to be maximally stimulated by 0.1 μg of estradiol. Therefore, we have concluded that 0.1–0.2 pmoles of receptor/uterus are required for the stimulation of true uterine growth.

unlike R_nE_2, R_nE_3 complexes do not undergo significant long-term nuclear retention, which correlates with the inability of E_3 to stimulate true uterine growth. Therefore, it is likely that R_nE_3 complexes bind to nuclear acceptor sites and stimulate initial cellular events. However, because the complexes are not retained for a sufficient length of time, the complex fails to sustain the stimulation of the appropriate events which culminate in true uterine growth.

In contrast to the short nuclear residency of the R_nE_3 complex, we have shown that nafoxidine and other triphenylethylene derivatives cause nuclear retention of the receptor for long periods of time (Fig. 3). This long-term retention of the R_nN complex correlates with the extended stimulation of true uterine growth by nafoxidine. This stimulation is equal to that of E_2 in magnitude and superior to that of E_2 in the length of time of growth stimulation (Fig. 3). Thus, the R_nN complex undergoes long-term nuclear retention which is correlated with sustained uterotropic stimulation. In the immature rat, this phenomenon of nuclear retention for very long periods of time with accompanying prolonged uterotropic stimulation can last for weeks (Clark *et al.*, 1973, 1974). Therefore, nafoxidine is representative of a class of compounds which cause anomalous behavior with respect to both nuclear retention and uterine growth stimulation. As a consequence, nafoxi-

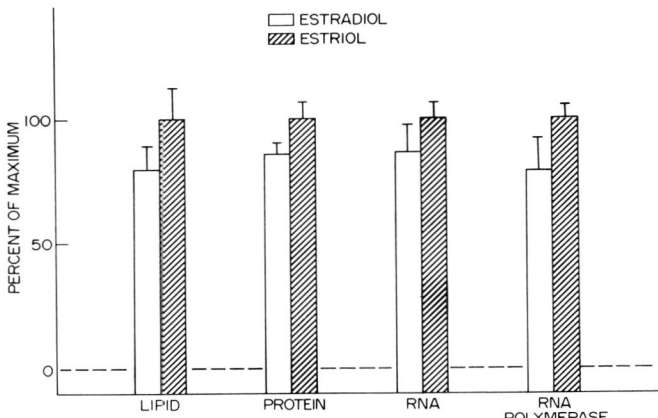

Fig. 2. Effects of estradiol and estriol on short-term uterine responses. Rats were killed at 3 hours after the injection of saline, estradiol (1 μg), or estriol (1 μg). The mean SEM conversion of [^{14}C]glucose to [^{14}C]lipid, [^{14}C]protein, and [^{14}C]RNA was calculated from four determinations with two uteri per determination. RNA polymerase activity, expressed as dpm of [^{3}H]-UMP incorporated into RNA per 100 μg of RNA, was determined by procedures described by Gorski (1964).

dine is very useful in comparative studies with E_2 and E_3 for the detection of the important response profiles that are associated with the stimulation of true growth.

III. NUCLEAR RECEPTOR BINDING AND RNA POLYMERASE ACTIVITY

As pointed out above, estrogens stimulate many early uterotropic responses; however, the most important of these probably involve the augmentation of RNA synthesis. It is well known that estrogen administration to either immature or ovariectomized animals increases RNA synthesis in the uterus (Hamilton, 1968; O'Malley and Means, 1974; Katzenellenbogen and Gorski, 1975). Quantitatively, these changes have been most marked in rRNA and are measurable within 4–6 hours following hormone administration (Hamilton, 1968; Hamilton *et al.*, 1968; Billing *et al.*, 1968). Recently, several groups have reported an early increase in very high molecular weight RNA (DNA-like), and have suggested that the marked increase in total RNA which follows may be dependent on this early appearance of mRNA (Knowler and Smellie, 1971; Luck and Hamilton, 1972; Borthwick and Smellie, 1975). Complementary to these results on high molecular weight RNA, E treatment also results in an early increase in endogenous

1. Estrogen Receptor Binding

nuclear RNA polymerase II activity. This initial surge of polymerase II activity is followed at later times (2-4 hours) by an increase in the activity of RNA polymerase I and a second rise in RNA polymerase II activity (Glasser *et al.*, 1972; Borthwick and Smellie, 1975). These findings suggest that RNA polymerase activity could be used as one end point for the detection of important differences between the receptor binding and uterotropic stimulation by E_2, E_3, and nafoxidine. Therefore, we have examined the RNA polymerase response profiles induced by these compounds and compared them to their ability to cause long-term retention of the R_n complex by the nucleus (Hardin *et al.*, 1976).

A single injection of E_2, E_3, or N causes a transient rise in endogenous nuclear RNA polymerase II activity which reaches a peak 1 hour after hor-

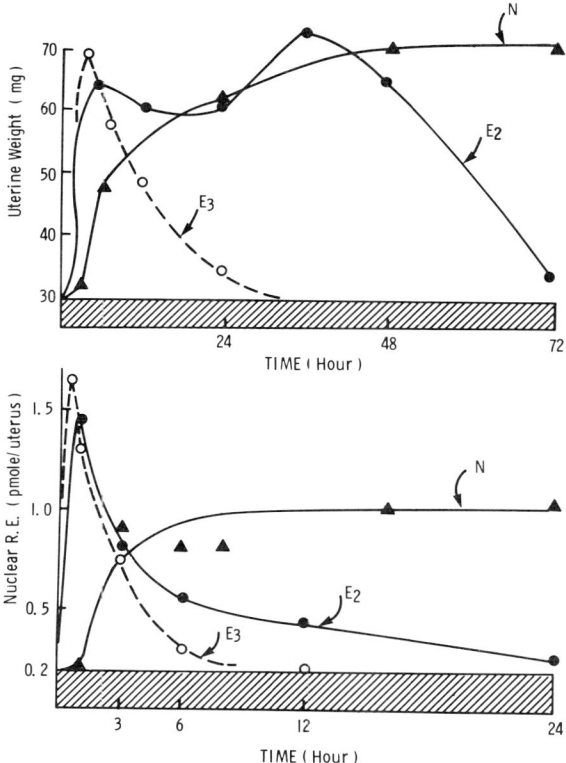

Fig. 3. Effect of estradiol, estriol, and nafoxidine on uterine growth and nuclear retention of the receptor–hormone complex. Immature rats were injected at zero time with estradiol (●), estriol (○), or nafoxidine (▲), and the uterine wet weight and nuclear estrogen receptor content were determined at various times after the injection.

mone treatment (Figs. 4–6). The greatest response at this time is elicited by estradiol and estriol, either of which cause a significant increase in enzymatic activity as early as 30 minutes after hormone treatment. Nafoxidine has little, if any, effect at this very early time and evokes less response at 1 hour than do the other two compounds. This decreased response is correlated with the slower rate of nuclear accumulation of the nafoxidine–receptor complex (Fig. 6).

The activity of polymerase II declines dramatically by 2 hours after injection in all three groups. This decline is followed by a second elevation in activity in estradiol-treated animals which reaches a maximum by 4 hours

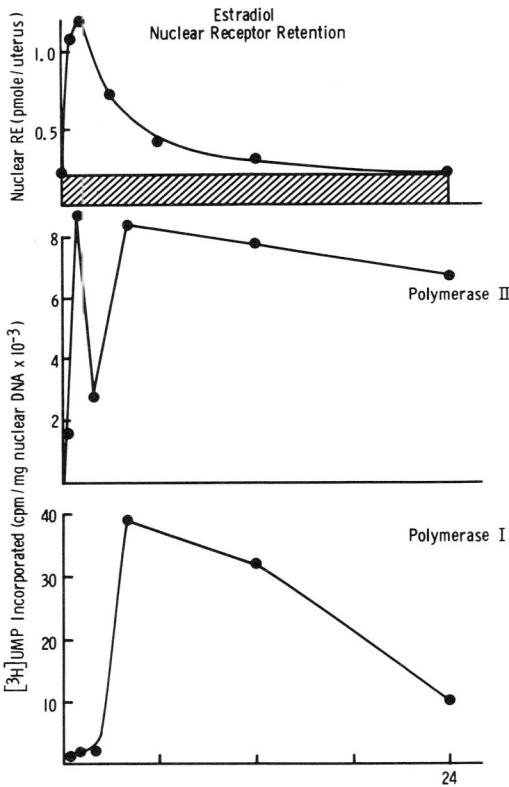

Fig. 4. Relationship between nuclear retention of the receptor–estradiol complex and RNA polymerase activity in the rat uterus. Immature rats were injected with estradiol and the quantity of estrogen receptor in the nuclear fraction was determined by [^{3}H]estradiol exchange assay (Anderson et al., 1972a). RNA polymerase activities were determined as described in Hardin et al. (1976).

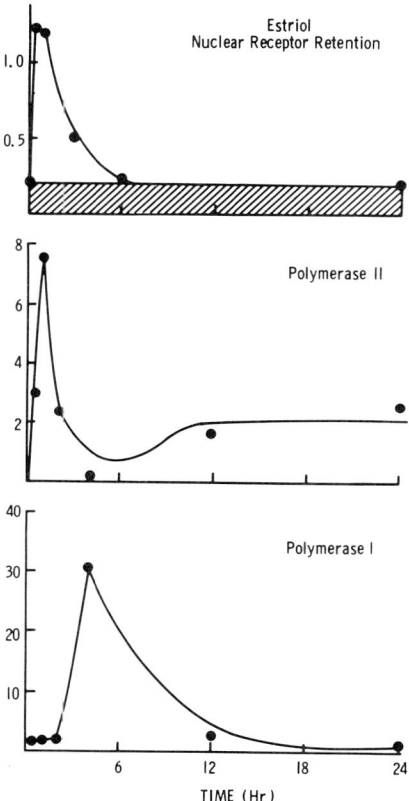

Fig. 5. Relationship between nuclear retention of the receptor–estriol complex and RNA polymerase activity in the rat uterus. For description of methods see Fig. 4.

(Fig. 4). A similar elevation in polymerase II activity in nafoxidine-treated animals is followed by another large late increase which occurs between 12 and 24 hours after the injection (Fig. 6). A second elevation in enzyme activity was not observed in the estriol-treated animals, and the activity of polymerase II remained low between 4 and 24 hours (Fig. 5).

Following the early transient increase in uterine nuclear RNA polymerase II activity, an increase in RNA polymerase I activity occurred in all hormone groups by 4 hours (Figs. 4–6). Estriol caused a transient rise in this activity which was characterized by a regression phase between 4 and 12 hours (Fig. 5). Estradiol treatment results in a marked elevation in RNA polymerase I activity by 4 hours. This rise is followed by a slow decline in activity; however, values remain significantly above those of the control at

TABLE 1
Classification of Estrogen Agonists and Antagonists[a]

Class	Examples	Nuclear retention	Pharmacologic characteristics	Uterotropic properties[b]
1. Short acting	Estriol, dimethylstilbestrol, 16-oxoestradiol	Short (1–4 hours)	Partial agonist/antagonist when injected Agonist when implanted	Early responses[c]
2. Long acting	A. Estradiol, diethylstilbestrol	Intermediate (6–24 hours)	Agonist	Early and late responses
	B. Triphenylethylene derivatives (e.g., nafoxidine, CI-628, Tamoxifin)	Long (greater than 24–48 hours)	Agonist—one injection Antagonist—multiple injections	Early and late responses

[a] This classification is based on events that occur after a single injection of the compound, except where noted otherwise.
[b] Early responses include water imbibition, hyperemia, amino acid, and nucleotide uptake, activation of RNA polymerase I and II, stimulation of induce protein.
[c] Late responses include cellular hypertrophy and hyperplasia, sustained RNA polymerase I and II activity.

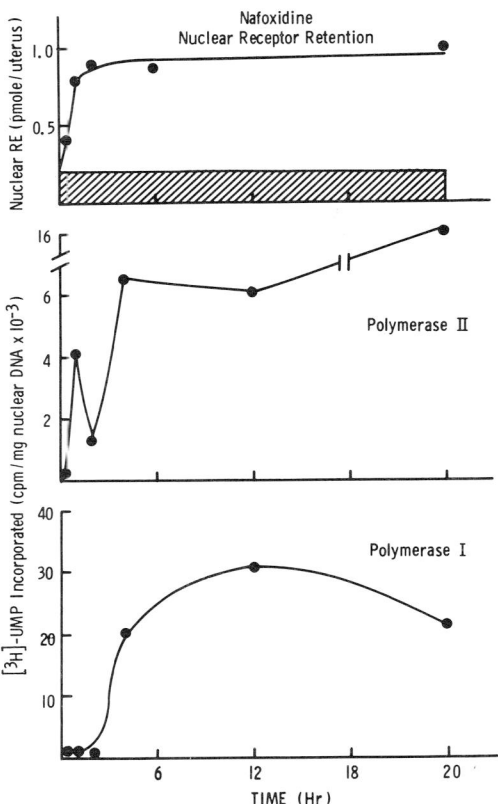

Fig. 6. Relationship between nuclear retention of the receptor–nafoxidine complex and RNA polymerase activity in the rat uterus. For description of methods see Fig. 4.

24 hours (Fig. 4). Nafoxidine treatment results in a similar elevation of endogenous RNA polymerase I activity by 4 hours, which is maintained at levels as high or higher than those induced by estradiol (Fig. 6).

The correlations made earlier in this chapter between nuclear retention of the receptor and estrogenic potency are also apparent in the polymerase experiments. The greatest increase in early polymerase II activity (Figs. 4 and 5) occurred in response to estradiol and estriol, the compounds that cause the most rapid accumulation of receptor by the nucleus. On the other hand, nafoxidine, which accumulates more slowly as R_nN, produces a peak of polymerase II activity, which is approximately 50% less than that produced by either estradiol or estriol at early times after hormone administration. The second elevation of polymerase II activity, which was observed by 4 hours in estradiol and nafoxidine-treated animals, but not in estriol-treated animals, may be dependent upon long-term retention of the receptor by the nucleus (Figs. 4 and 6). The failure of estriol to stimulate this second rise in activity may be one of the factors involved in the inability of this estrogen to stimulate true uterine growth.

The elevation of polymerase I activity, which was stimulated by all three compounds, was maintained for much longer periods of time by treatment with estradiol and nafoxidine. The rapid decline in polymerase I activity in the estriol-treated animals may result from the short-term residency of the R_nE_3 complex in the nucleus (Fig. 5). These data demonstrate that the secondary rise in polymerase II activity, as well as the duration and magnitude of the increase in polymerase I activity, correlate with the nuclear retention of receptor–estrogen complexes.

The early (30 minutes) estrogen-dependent rise in uterine endogenous nuclear RNA polymerase II activity was first measured directly by Glasser et al. (1972) in the mature ovariectomized rat and subsequently confirmed in the immature rat (these data) and immature rabbit (Borthwick and Smellie, 1975). The initial rise in polymerase II activity was blocked by the prior in vivo administration of α-amanitin (Glasser et al., 1972) and actinomycin D, but not by cycloheximide (Means and Hamilton, 1966; Glasser and Spelsberg, 1973). From these data, the suggestion was first derived that estradiol evokes an early increase in polymerase II activity. This early stimulation of putative mRNA synthesis (Knowler and Smellie, 1971; Glasser et al., 1972; Borthwick and Smellie, 1975) may be involved in the synthesis of uterine proteins which, in turn, are involved in later increases of both polymerases, as well as other proliferative changes characteristic of estrogen's uterotropic action. A similar suggestion was made by Raynaud-Jammet et al. (1972), who found an RNA product, the synthesis of which was sensitive to α-amanitin and which also appeared necessary for the increase in RNA polymerase I activity that followed estradiol administration. Our present results would indicate, however, that the action of estrogen on RNA synthesis may be more complex and difficult to interpret than simply relating an early effect in RNA polymerase II activity to the synthesis of a product that modulates the later increases in the activities of both polymerases. Thus, an injection of E_3 to immature rats, which evokes as great an increase in polymerase II activity at 30–60 minutes, as does E_2 (Figs. 4 and 5), fails to produce the secondary increase in polymerase II activity and evokes only a transient increase in RNA polymerase I activity (Fig. 5B). The failure of estriol to continue to stimulate RNA synthesis is reflected in both the disappearance of the receptor–estriol complex from the nucleus and the failure of the hormone to stimulate true uterine growth.

Nafoxidine, in comparison, causes only a small early increase in polymerase II activity, but produces a substantial and sustained increase in polymerase I and a large secondary stimulation in polymerase II activity, as well as true uterine growth. The highly elevated activity of RNA polymerase II in nafoxidine-treated animals may mean that many gene sites are "turned on" and remain in the "on" position. This seems even more likely when one considers the large number of R_nN complexes that are present in the nucleus. Approximately 10,000 R_nN complexes remain in the nucleus for long periods of time. This quantity exceeds the number of R_nE complexes required to maximize uterine growth by a factor of 5 and leads to the speculation that R_nN complexes are binding to secondary and tertiary nuclear sites that control RNA synthesis. If this is the case, these binding interactions might lead to the stimulation of many uterine gene sites that would not normally be turned on and, thus, could account for the highly elevated RNA polymerase II activity. This anomalous nuclear-binding behavior may also be linked to the antiestrogenicity of these compounds. One can envision the possibility that either inappropriate genes are turned on or that they are activated in the incorrect temporal sequence. Therefore, it is possible that the activation of such "right" and "wrong" genes might result in the inhibition of growth. This is particularly relevant when one considers that estrogens act in concert with other hormones to produce the biochemical changes that occur during the estrous cycle of the rat. These changes involve both synthetic and degradative enzymatic activities, and account for the fluctuations in uterine size and morphology during the cycle. Thus, the uterus is programmed for both anabolic and catabolic events, and any compound which alters the proper sequence of these events could result in the anomalous growth state, as observed with nafoxidine.

The precise mechanisms by which long-term nuclear retention of receptor–estrogen complexes stimulates both RNA synthesis and uterine growth are not clear. However, results from other steroid hormone systems would suggest that the most likely possibility is some modification of chromatin by the steroid receptor–hormone complex. Thus, it was shown recently that estrogen stimulation of the chick oviduct brings about an increase in the number of RNA polymerase initiation sites present in oviduct chromatin (Schwartz *et al.*, 1975).

In summary, the stimulation of true uterine growth is not characteristic of every estrogen. Of the varied multiple effects that characterize the biologic action of each estrogen, only certain correlated sets of events stimulate true uterine growth. Of prime importance, the estrogen receptor must be retained in the nucleus for some critical period in order to effect true uterine growth. Retention of the receptor correlates with a secondary increase and sustained activation in RNA polymerase II activity and a sustained elevation in RNA polymerase I activity. These effects on RNA polymerase I and II appear necessary for true uterine growth.

IV. NUCLEAR RETENTION AND THE AGONISTIC–ANTAGONISTIC PROPERTIES OF ESTRIOL

In preceding sections, we have shown that estriol (E_3) is a weak estrogen when injected because it does not promote long-term retention of the R_nE_3 complex in the nucleus. Estriol, however, is usually present in the blood at relatively high constant levels for periods of hours or days, not as a pulse as produced by an injection. Under these conditions, estriol could cause long-term receptor occupancy in the nucleus of target cells and, thereby, exhibit a high level of estrogenicity. In fact, multiple and frequent injections of estriol do cause uterine growth comparable to that observed with estradiol, leading us to suggest that this growth is the result of long-term receptor occupancy in the nucleus of target cells (Anderson *et al.*, 1975).

To examine these relationships further and to evaluate the agonist–antagonist properties of E_3, we have studied the effects of estradiol (E_2), estriol (E_3), and $E_2 + E_3$ on cytoplasmic content of estrogen receptor, nuclear retention of receptor–estrogen complexes, and uterine growth in rats that received these estrogens either by injection or by implant.

An injection of E_2 or E_3 causes a rapid accumulation of receptor in the nucleus and a concomitant depletion of receptor in the cytoplasm. Both hormones share equal potency in this regard, establishing that the antagonistic effect of estriol cannot lie at this level (Anderson *et al.*, 1972b; 1973, 1975). However, the depletion of cytoplasmic receptor (R_c) by E_2 injection is followed by the gradual replenishment of this receptor species, suggesting that E_3 could act as a partial agonist–antagonist by failing to stimulate the replenishment of R_c. Such a failure to replenish R_c would decrease the receptor sites available for estrogen binding and produce a uterus relatively insensitive to subsequent estrogen treatments. This possibility was examined by injecting immature rats with E_2, E_3, or $E_2 + E_3$, as described in Fig. 7, and by measuring both the quantity of uterine cytoplasmic receptor and uterine weight 24 and 48 hours after injection.

Estriol clearly antagonized the effect of E_2 on uterine weight and cytoplasmic receptor (Fig. 7; compare E_2 with $E_2 + E_3$). Estriol was also clearly a partial agonist, since it stimulated uterine growth as well as increased the cytoplasmic receptor level (Fig. 7; compare saline and E_3). Although cytoplasmic receptor levels in the E_3 group are low, compared to E_2 alone, the levels in the E_3 or $E_2 + E_3$ groups were above control, and, thus, receptor

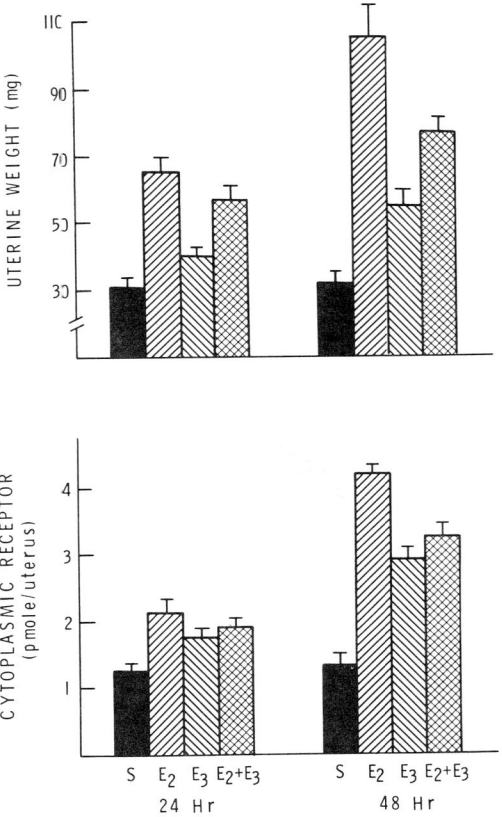

Fig. 7. Antagonism of estriol when administered by injection. Immature rats were injected with saline, 1.0 μg estriol, 0.1 μg estradiol, or a combination of these two hormones (E_2, 0.1, and E_3, 1.0 μg). Rats were either killed 24 hours after treatment, or were reinjected at 24 hours and killed at 48 hours. The uteri were weighed, and the quantity of cytoplasmic estrogen receptor was determined by the [^{3}H]estradiol exchange assay.

number was not likely to be the source of antagonism. In the experiment shown in Fig. 7, rats were injected with 0.1 μg E_2, 1.0 μg E_3, or a combination of those hormone doses. Similar experiments in which E_2 and E_3 were injected at identical dose levels (0.1 μg) produced similar patterns of uterine growth and R_c levels.

As discussed earlier in this chapter, the retention of receptor estradiol complexes by uterine nuclei appears to be an obligatory step in the stimulation of true growth (Anderson *et al.*, 1975; Clark *et al.*, 1977). Thus, any process which interferes with long-term nuclear retention would result in estrogen antagonism. We have previously shown that E_3 does not promote long-term nuclear retention and, therefore, have suggested that R_nE_3 complexes might compete with R_nE_2 complexes for nuclear retention sites. To test this proposal, immature rats were injected as described in Fig. 8, and the quantity of receptor in the uterine nuclear fraction was assessed as a function of time. Both estrogens caused a rapid accumulation of receptor by the nucleus (Fig. 8). As in Fig. 8, E_3 was injected as a 1 μg dose, while E_2 was injected at the 0.1 μg level. This difference in dose accounts for the greater initial nuclear accumulation of receptor following E_3 treatment. These two hormones are not significantly different with respect to initial nuclear accumulation when administered at the same dose (Fig. 3). E_2 treatment resulted in long-term nuclear retention of the receptor, while a rapid decline in nuclear-bound receptor was observed following E_3 treatment. With E_3 treatment, nuclear-bound receptor returned to control levels within 6 hours (Fig. 8). When E_2 and E_3 were administered simultaneously, the quantity of receptor that exhibited long-term retention was reduced (Fig. 8). A similar reduction in the quantity of nuclear-bound receptor at 6 hours was also noted in rats that were injected with identical dose levels (0.1 or 1.0 μg—data not shown).

From the results above and from our previous work, which demonstrated that E_3 promotes significant uterine growth when injected every 3 hours (Anderson et al., 1975), one can predict that E_3 would not act as an estrogen antagonist if it were present in a continuous fashion. To examine this proposal, immature intact or ovariectomized rats received paraffin implants of E_2, E_3, or $E_2 + E_3$, as described in Fig. 9. Each hormone treat-

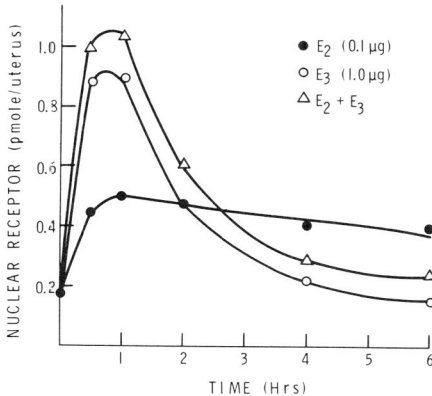

Fig. 8. Nuclear retention of the receptor–estrogen complex after treatment with estradiol, estriol, or a combination of the hormones. Immature rats were injected with estradiol (●), estriol (○), or a combination of the two steroids (△), and the quantity of receptor–estrogen complex was measured in the nucleus at various times.

ment produced identical increases in uterine weight, and no antagonism by E_3 was noted (Fig. 9). Likewise, no differences were observed in the effects of these treatments on the compartmentalization or quantities of the various estrogen receptor species (Fig. 10). Each hormone or combination of hormones caused an accumulation and maintenance of nuclear R_nE at relatively high levels (0.8–1.2 pmoles/uterus). This accumulation and retention of nuclear R_nE was accompanied by a depletion of R_c, which gradually increased to very high levels by 48–72 hours (Fig. 10).

These results demonstrate that E_3 is neither a weak estrogen nor an estrogen antagonist when present in a continuous or chronic fashion (Figs. 9 and 10). However, E_3 does manifest these properties when injected (Fig. 7). This paradox relates to the concept, previously suggested by Martin (1969) and Miller (1969), that weak estrogenicity correlates with short-term receptor occupancy. What is clear from the present results is that weak estrogenicity in the case of E_3 arises from competition between RE_2 and RE_3 complexes for nuclear retention sites (Fig. 8) and from the rapid clearance of E_3 from uterine tissue (Jensen *et al.*, 1966). Thus, E_2 and E_3 promote the translocation of cytoplasmic receptors to the nuclear compartment where RE_3 complexes compete with RE_2 complexes for those nuclear sites which are involved in long-term retention and promotion of uterotropic responses (Anderson *et al.*, 1972b, 1973, 1975). Since E_3 is cleared rapidly and because RE_3 is in equilibrium with R and E_3, the competition between RE_2 and RE_3 reduces the number of receptor–estrogen complexes retained in the nuclear compartment. Since long-term retention may be casually related to the stimulation of true uterine growth, this reduction in the number of effec-

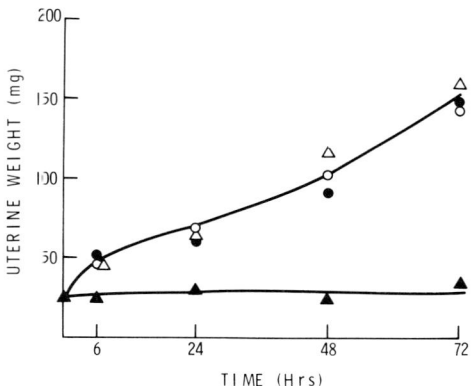

Fig. 9. Failure of estriol to antagonize uterine growth induced by estradiol. Immature rats were implanted with paraffin pellets that contained estradiol (●), estriol (○), estradiol + estriol (△), or no hormone (▲). The animals were killed at various time intervals, and the uterine weights were determined.

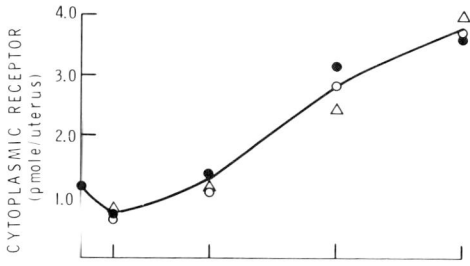
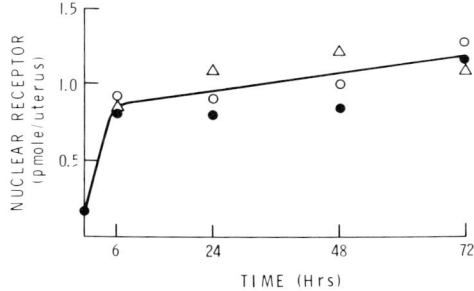

Fig. 10. Effects of estrogen implants on cytoplasmic and nuclear–estrogen receptors in the uterus. Immature rats were implanted with paraffin pellets as described in Fig. 9. The quantities of cytoplasmic and nuclear–estrogen receptor were determined by the [^{3}H]estradiol exchange assay.

tive receptor–estrogen complexes could account for the observed antagonism. However, when E_3 is present in a continuous fashion, as in the pellet implant experiments presented here, E_3 promotes long-term nuclear retention and true uterine growth equivalent to that of E_2 (Figs. 9 and 10). Since long-term retention of the receptor–estrogen complex by the nucleus appears to cause true growth, regardless of the estrogen which occupies the receptor, E_3 acts as an estrogen agonist under these conditions.

The clarification of this apparent paradox and the establishment of E_3 as a potent estrogen when present under steady-state conditions has important implications with respect to certain hypotheses on the role of E_3 in physiology and pathology. Estriol is present at high levels in the blood during pregnancy in the human (Hobkirk and Nilsen, 1962), and it is the major estrogen present during the menstrual cycle (Goebelsmann et al., 1969). Therefore, E_3 is likely to be a major contributor to the total estrogen state of the human. Its role in this capacity needs reappraisal in light of the present results.

A protective role has been ascribed to E_3 in breast cancer. This suggestion is based on the observation that Oriental women, who have a high (estriol)/(estradiol + estrone) ratio in blood, also have a low incidence of breast cancer (Wotiz et al., 1968; Goebelsman et al., 1969; Cole and MacMahon, 1969; Lemon et al., 1971). This hypothesis was formulated on the assumption that E_3 was a weak estrogen under all circumstances and that, during each menstrual cycle, E_3 would act to reduce the "carcinogenic potential" of the more potent E_2. Our results indicate that this theory is suspect and, in light of recent evidence which shows that E_3 and E_2 are of equal potential in facilitating the onset of mammary tumors in mice (Rudali et al., 1975), we suggest that the E_3 theory of mammary cancer protection is untenable.

Based on the work of our laboratory and others, we propose the classification of estrogens shown in Table I. We propose that E_3 be classified as a short-acting estrogen, rather than a weak or impeded estrogen. The terms "weak" and "impeded" imply that E_3 is less effective under all circumstances. Since this is not the case, the classification of E_3 as a short-acting estrogen provides a functional definition that applies in all cases. In this scheme, dimethylstilbestrol, *meso*-butoestrol, and 16-oxoestradiol are similar to estriol and, thus, may be classified together (Martin, 1969; Terenius, 1970). These compounds have in common the ability to stimulate early uterotropic responses as shown in Table I; however, they fail to significantly influence the long-term responses that promote uterine growth when given as an injection.

Estradiol promotes both early and late growth responses in the uterus and manifests nuclear retention of the receptor–estrogen complex for significantly longer periods of time than do the short-acting estrogens. Diethylstilbestrol is similar to estradiol, and the two are classified as long-acting, subclass A. Long-acting estrogens are divided into two classes because the triphenylethylene derivatives, subclass B (e.g., nafoxidine, CI-628, and clomiphene) caused growth stimulation and nuclear retention of the receptor, which exceeds that induced by estradiol (Clark et al., 1973, 1974; Rochefort et al., 1972). It is difficult to explain the mode of action of the long-acting compounds of class B. They act as estrogen agonists after one injection and manifest antagonistic properties after two or more injections (Clark et al., 1972, 1973). The agonistic properties result from their ability to produce initial nuclear binding and uterotropic response patterns that resemble E_2 (Clark et al., 1972). Since these compounds are cleared slowly from the body, they cause nuclear retention of the receptor for much longer periods than E_2 or DES, and, thus, show no antagonistic properties after a single injection (Clark et al., 1972, 1973). However, compounds of this group do not promote rapid replenishment of R_c and, therefore, may decrease the ability of the uterus to respond to subsequent estrogen exposure (Clark *et al.,* 1972, 1973; Rochefort *et al.,* 1972; Capony and Rochefort, 1975).

In summary, we have shown that estriol is neither a weak nor an impeded estrogen. Rather, it appears that estriol–receptor complexes, both nuclear and cytoplasmic, are short-lived, due to rapid tissue clearance of estriol. On the basis of these observations, we have proposed a new system for the classification of estrogens, which relates their functional activity to the retention of receptor by the nucleus of target cells. This classification avoids the complexities and vagaries introduced by the words "weak" and "impeded."

V. NUCLEAR RETENTION AND REPLENISHMENT OF ESTROGEN RECEPTOR AND HORMONE ANTAGONISM

In Section III, we demonstrated that nafoxidine causes long-term nuclear retention of the estrogen receptor (R_n) and stimulates RNA polymerase activity and uterine growth. These observations are paradoxical, since nonsteroidal antiestrogens, such as nafoxidine, are generally considered to antagonize the effects of estrogen on uterine growth, vaginal cornification, and ovulation (Emmens, 1970). It has been proposed by others that the mechanism of action of estrogen antagonists resides in their ability to compete with estrogens for cytoplasmic receptors, thereby reducing the number of receptor–estrogen complexes in the cytoplasm of estrogen target tissues (Jensen *et al.,* 1966; Terenius, 1971; Rochefort *et al.,* 1972). With subsequent translocation to nuclear sites considered the primary event in the mechanism of estrogen action, this reduction in receptor–estradiol complex would lead to decreased physiological responses. Implicit in this hypothesis is that the receptor antagonist complex should have a lower intrinsic biologic activity than that of the receptor–estradiol complex. That is, the ability of the receptor–antagonist complex to stimulate estrogenic responses should be less than that of the receptor–estradiol complex.

Based on these assumptions, one would predict that estrogen antagonism should be observed following a single injection of estrogen and the antagonists; however, as is shown in Fig. 11, this is not the case. Immature rats, 21–22 days old, were injected with 2.5 µg estradiol, 100 µg nafoxidine hydrochloride, or a combination of the two compounds, and uterine dry weights were determined 24 or 48 hours later. The increases in uterine dry weight following a single injection of estradiol, nafoxidine, or estradiol plus nafoxidine are identical at 24 hours after the injection. By 48 hours, treatment with nafoxidine or estradiol plus nafoxidine is superior to that with

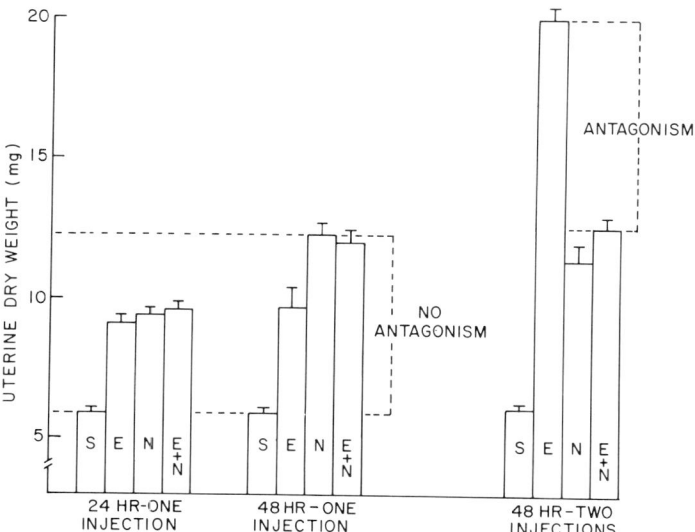

Fig. 11. The agonistic and antagonistic effects of nafoxidine on uterine growth. Immature female rats were injected with saline (S), 2.5 µg of estradiol (E), 100 µg of nafoxidine (N), or estradiol plus nafoxidine (E + N) according to the following design. Two groups received one injection, and uterine weights were determined 24 or 48 hours later. A third group received two injections 24 hours apart, and uterine weights were determined 24 hours after the second injection.

estradiol alone in the stimulation of uterine growth (Fig. 11). Therefore, following a single injection of estradiol plus nafoxidine, there is no antagonism; indeed, nafoxidine is clearly acting as an estrogen. This is also true for CI-628 and clomiphene. However, the antagonistic properties of nafoxidine can be observed when the compounds are administered at 24-hour intervals, and the uterine weights are determined at 48 hours (Fig. 11). Serial injections (3–8 in number) at 24-hour intervals have been used routinely by many investigators, and it is well established that estrogen antagonism can be observed under these conditions (Fig. 11, two injections; Emmens, 1970; Dorfman, 1962; Lerner, 1964; Callantine et al., 1966). The routine application of this method has resulted in the failure to recognize the significance of the agonist properties of these compounds after a single injection. It should be noted that we have used much lower doses of these compounds with similar results; i.e., doses of 1–10 µg display both agonistic and antagonistic properties, depending on the injection scheme.

Antiestrogens stimulate cellular hypertrophy, thereby increasing uterine weight, but fail to stimulate uterine hyperplasia. In such a case, the number of cells capable of responding to subsequent estrogen treatment would be reduced, and this reduction would result in diminished uterotropic responses when compared to estrogen treatment alone. This does not appear to be the case, since both estradiol and nafoxidine increase DNA content by 48 hours, and no differences are apparent in the capacity of these compounds to elicit uterine hyperplasia (Clark *et al.*, 1974).

We have proposed that antiestrogens antagonize estrogen-induced uterine growth as a result of their failure to stimulate the replenishment of the cytoplasmic estrogen receptor (Clark *et al.*, 1973, 1974). As previously described, nafoxidine causes accumulation and long-term retention of the R_n ligand complex; however, this retention is not accompanied by the usual replenishment of the cytoplasmic receptor (R_c), as is the case after estradiol

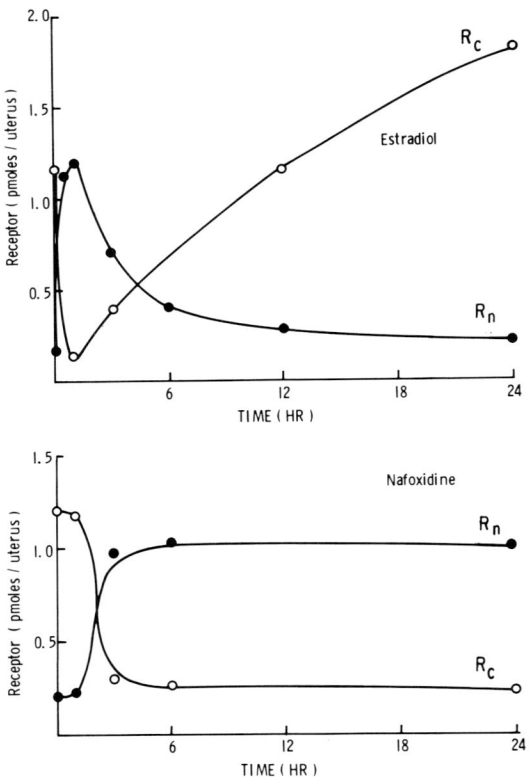

Fig. 12. Effect of estradiol and nafoxidine on nuclear retention and cytoplasmic replenishment of the estrogen receptor. Immature rats were injected with estradiol or nafoxidine, and the quantities of estrogen receptor in the nuclear (R_n) and cytoplasmic (R_c) fractions were determined.

1. Estrogen Receptor Binding

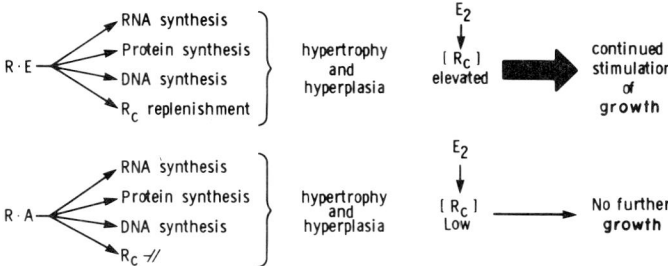

Fig. 13. Mechanism of action of nonsteroidal estrogen antagonists. For discussion of this model see text.

treatment (Fig. 12). This failure to stimulate the replenishment of R_c may render the uterus insensitive to subsequent injection of estrogen, and, therefore, antagonism can be observed. These mechanisms can be visualized according to the model presented in Fig. 13. Receptor–estrogen complexes (RE) and receptor–antagonists complexes (RA) stimulate cellular hypertrophy and hyperplasia. Thus, uterine growth is observed in both cases after a single injection of the compound. However, the RA complex fails to cause the replenishment of R_c, whereas the RE complex has stimulated full replenishment by 24 hours. When the animal receives a second injection of estrogen at this time, the uterus is nonresponsive in the animals that received the antagonist and highly responsive in the estrogen-treated animals. Therefore, the uterus continues to grow in the estrogen-treated rat and remains unstimulated in the antagonist-treated animal. Although this reasoning appears logical, it fails to offer a complete explanation. One must explain how antagonism is expressed when large quantities of receptor–estrogen complexes are being retained for long periods of time in the nucleus as RA complexes. This should cause continued stimulation of uterine growth; instead, nafoxidine, either as a single dose or as multiple injections, causes the uterus to double in size and to remain at this level for long periods of time (Fig. 14). In contrast, serial injection of E_2 causes continued stimulation of uterine growth, which produces a uterus five times as large as the control.

We have already suggested that the RA complex may stimulate uterine genes in an anomalous manner, perhaps causing self-limiting processes to be set in motion. However, the recycling of receptor to the cytoplasmic compartment may also play an important role in the overall receptor–hormone–gene stimulation reaction. To test this idea, we injected rats with a large dose of estradiol 24 hours after they received an injection of nafoxidine. At this time, the quantity of R_c is low, and the uterus is nonresponsive

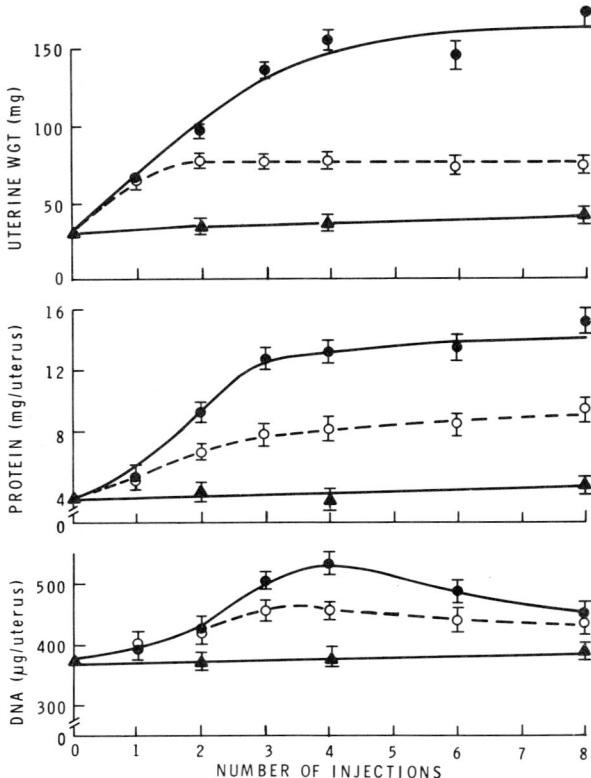

Fig. 14. Effect of serial injections of estradiol or nafoxidine on uterine growth. Immature rats were injected daily with estradiol (●), nafoxidine (○), or saline (controls) (▲), and the uterine weight, protein, and DNA content were determined 24 hours after the last injection.

to an injection of E_2 (Fig. 15). The rationale for this experiment was that we should be able to bring about *in vivo* exchange of E_2 for nafoxidine and form R_nE_2 complexes. The work of Katzenellenbogen and Ferguson (1975) indicated that this might be possible. If *in vivo* exchange were to occur, then the normal nuclear replenishment processes should take place, and some R_c should appear in the cytoplasm. As shown in Fig. 15, the quantity of R_c was elevated by 48 hours (24 hours after the E_2 injection). An injection of either E_2 or Nafoxidine at this time causes significant uterine growth by 72 hours (Fig. 15B). Thus, it appears that replenishment or recycling of R_c may be an important component in the array of complex interactions that stimulate the uterus to grow. These conclusions are shown in summary form in Fig. 16. The binding of the R_nE complex to nuclear sites causes uterotropic stimulation and replenishment (possibly via recycling and resynthesis) of R_c. The replenished R_c is then free to interact with estrogen to form receptor–hormone complexes which bind to nuclear sites and cause a second cycle of uterine growth stimulation. On the other hand, the R_nA complex, although capable of causing one cycle of uterotropic stimulation, is unable to effect replenishment of R_c, and, hence, multiple cycles of nuclear binding and stimulation are not possible.

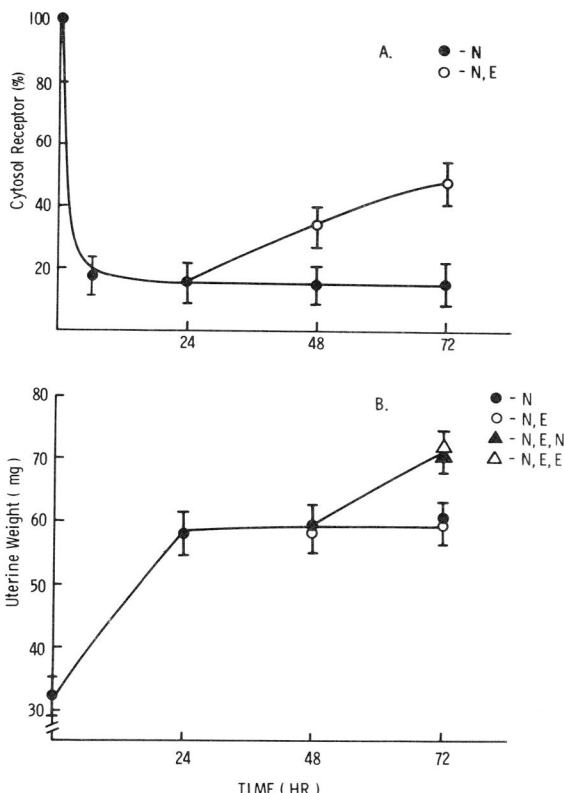

Fig. 15. Effect of estradiol on the replenishment of cytoplasmic estrogen receptors in nafoxidine-treated rats. Immature rats were injected with 50 μg of nafoxidine (●) at time zero. Twenty-four hours later they were injected with 10 μg of estradiol (○), and the quantity of cytoplasmic receptor was determined (upper panel). Forty-eight hours after the nafoxidine injection (24 hours after the first estradiol injection), the animals either received no further treatment (●,○) or were injected with nafoxidine (▲) or estradiol (△). Uterine weight was measured at each time interval.

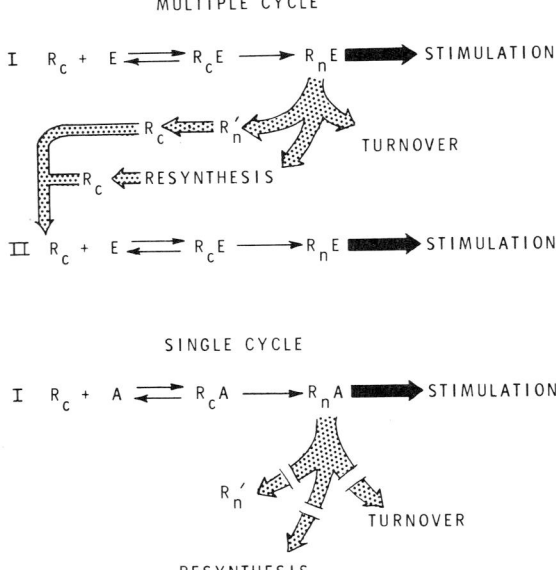

Fig. 16. Nuclear binding and replenishment of the estrogen receptor: relation to uterine growth stimulation. See text for discussion.

VI. LONG-TERM NUCLEAR RETENTION AND ACCEPTOR SITES

In this chapter, we have suggested that long-term nuclear retention of the R_nE complex results from their interaction with specific nuclear acceptor sites. Our evidence derives from *in vivo* experiments in which we have demonstrated that the long-term retention of 1000–3000 R_nE complexes per cell is a requirement for uterine growth. Most investigators have used *in vitro* systems in an attempt to demonstrate nuclear acceptor activity. The character of these binding sites in the nucleus is still a matter of some controversy. While some investigators have shown that nuclear binding of receptor–steroid complexes is a saturatable phenomenon (Alberga *et al.*, 1971; Fang and Liao, 1971; Mainwaring and Peterken, 1971; King and Gordon, 1972; O'Malley *et al.*, 1972; Higgins *et al.*, 1973; Kalimi *et al.*, 1973; Buller *et al.*, 1975), others claim that limited numbers of specific nuclear sites do not exist (Chamness *et al.*, 1973, 1974; André and Rochefort, 1975). Some authors claim that the acceptor sites are located on DNA (Yamamoto and Alberts, 1975), while others find them mainly on nonhistone proteins (O'Malley *et al.*, 1972). Much of this conflict probably stems from the difficulty inherent in the detection of a low number of specific binding sites (Yamamoto and Alberts, 1975). Thus, studies of the binding of receptor–estrogen complexes to nuclei, chromatin, and/or DNA under cell-free conditions are susceptible to the error introduced by the masking effect of nonspecific binding. However, despite the problem with *in vitro* binding systems, it is possible to show that a limited number of nuclear binding sites must be involved in the events leading to maximal uterine growth in the rat and to suggest that these nuclear sites may represent nuclear acceptor sites.

To test this hypothesis further, we have used extraction of uterine nuclei to examine for differential extractability of receptor–estrogen complexes. The rationale for this approach was based on the observation by several investigators that extraction of nuclei with 0.3–0.4 M KCl does not remove all of the nuclear-bound estrogen (Puca and Bresciani, 1969; DeHertogh *et al.*, 1973; Mester and Baulieu, 1975).

Figure 17 outlines results obtained by differential salt extraction of nuclear-bound receptor–estrogen complexes from uteri of immature rats treated with either 0.1 µg or 2.5 µg of estradiol 1 hour prior to sacrifice. The nuclear fraction from rats that received 2.5 µg of estradiol contains a large number of receptor sites that are extractable with KCl at concentrations lower than 0.4 M (R_n-extractable). The quantity of receptor remaining in the nuclear fraction (R_n-resistant) after exposure to KCl concentrations of 0.4 M or higher is approximately 0.1 pmoles/uterus. This small number of R_n-resistant complexes could repesent those receptors which exhibit

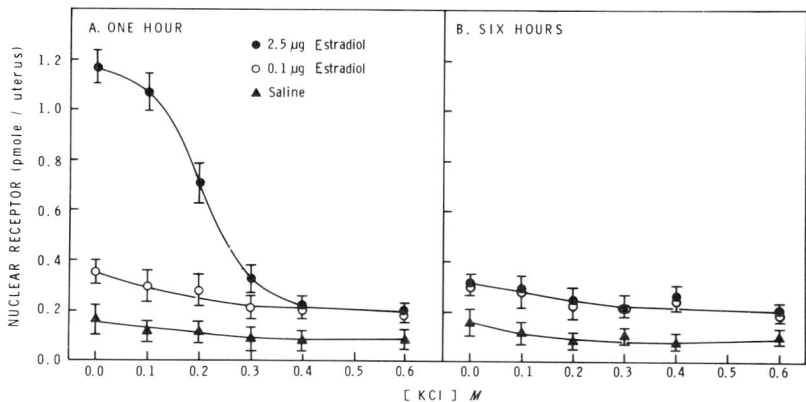

Fig. 17. Differential salt extraction of nuclear-bound estrogen receptor. Immature rats were injected with estradiol and uterine nuclear fractions were prepared (A) 1 and (B) 6 hours after the injection, and differential KCl extraction was performed as previously described (Clark and Peck, 1976). After extraction, the quantity of receptor which remained in the nuclear fraction was measured by the [³H]estradiol exchange assay.

long-term nuclear retention (Figs. 1 and 3). Animals receiving the high dose of hormone have the same number of R_n-resistant sites as those receiving the low dose, an observation which is in good agreement with the finding that both high and low doses produce the long-term retention of the same number of receptor complexes (Fig. 2). Furthermore, the number of R_n-resistant complexes are equal 6 hours after an injection of either dose of estrogen. Thus, the number of hormone–receptor complexes remaining in the nucleus after 0.4 M KCl extraction seems to correlate with the number of complexes that exhibit long-term nuclear retention.

The relationship between the disappearance of receptor–estrogen complexes from the cytosol and the appearance of $R_n E_2$-extractable and $R_n E_2$-resistant complexes in the nucleus as a function of time after exposure of immature rat uteri to estradiol *in vitro* or *in vivo* is shown in Fig. 18. Under *in vitro* conditions, R_c concentration declined rapidly during the first 60 minutes of incubation, with a concomitant increase in the quantity of R_n-extractable complexes, reaching a maximum by 60 minutes. This was followed by a gradual increase in the quantity of R_n-resistant complexes which reached a peak by 150 minutes. This "transformation process" of R_n-extractable to R_n-resistant complexes was more rapid *in vivo* (Fig. 19). R_c decreased to a minimum by 30 minutes, R_n-extractable complexes increased rapidly during the same time period and then dropped to control levels over the following 150 minutes, whereas R_n-resistant complexes increased slowly reaching a maximum after 60 minutes and then declined slowly during the subsequent 120 minutes. These data support the concept

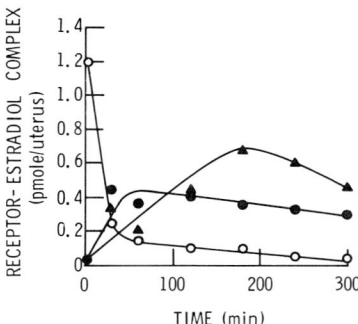

Fig. 18. Effect of estradiol on KCl-extractable and KCl-resistant nuclear receptor–estrogen complexes *in vitro*. Uteri from immature rats were incubated in Eagle's medium at 37°C in the presence of 20 nM [^{3}H]estradiol plus or minus a 100-fold excess of nonlabeled DES. The tissue was removed at various times, and the quantities of cytoplasmic receptor (○) and nuclear receptor, KCl extractable (●), were determined by the hydroxylapatite assay, and the nuclear receptor, KCl resistant (▲), was determined by ethanol extraction of the nuclear pellet (Clark *et al.*, 1976).

1. Estrogen Receptor Binding

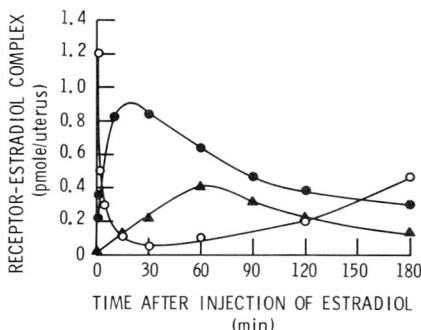

Fig. 19. Effect of estradiol on KCl-extractable and KCl-resistant nuclear receptor–estrogen complexes *in vivo*. Immature rats were injected with 2.5 µg of estradiol, and the quantities of various receptor forms were determined by [^{3}H]estradiol exchange (Clark *et al.*, 1976) at different times after the injection. For symbols, see Fig. 18.

of a time-dependent shift of nuclear estrogen–receptor complexes from R_n-extractable to R_n-resistant binding sites, both *in vitro* and *in vivo*.

When chromatin from immature rat uteri, which were incubated *in vitro* with [^{3}H]estradiol at 37°C, was subjected to 0.4 M KCl extraction, about 60% of the nuclear-bound radioactivity remained bound to the chromatin pellet. About 70% of this KCl-resistant radioactivity could be released by treatment with pronase, trypsin, or proteinase K, whereas deoxyribonuclease digestion liberated only a small amount of the bound radioactivity (data not shown).

The steroid-binding specificity of the three different states of the estrogen receptor in rat uteri is shown in Fig. 20. As can be seen, the specificity is not dramatically changed during the transformation process: $R_c \rightarrow R_n$-extractable $\rightarrow R_n$-resistant. When the kinetics of dissociation for the three forms of receptor–estrogen complex were measured by the addition of a 200-fold molar excess of nonlabeled estradiol to the receptor [^{3}H]estradiol preparation, the half-lives of the receptor–steroid complexes were approximately the same (280–300 minutes at 4°C), corresponding to a dissociation rate of 3.7×10^{-5} sec^{-1}. These data indicate that the specificity of the receptor bound to nuclear acceptor sites has not been changed.

In addition to the rat uterus, R_n-resistant complexes have also been demonstrated in other target organs for estrogens, namely, the rat pituitary and liver (Clark *et al.*, 1976) and in the chicken liver (H. Eriksson, J. Hardin, and J. Clark, unpublished observation).

Thus, accumulating data support the hypothesis that nuclear hormone receptors are one protein that exists in two different states due to the localization of the receptor—an extractable form which is loosely bound to chro-

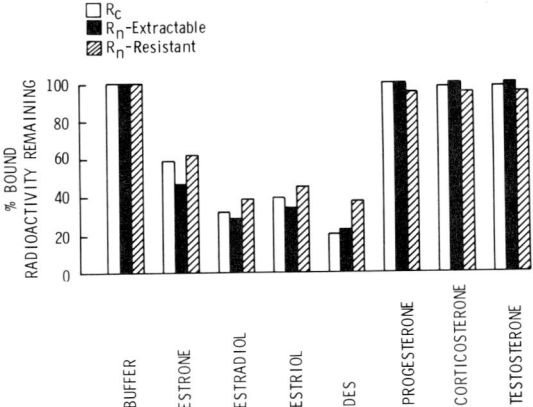

Fig. 20. Hormone specificity of the KCl-extractable and KCl-resistant forms of the nuclear-bound receptor–estrogen complex. Cytoplasmic receptor proteins were prepared from uteri of untreated immature rats; KCl-extractable and KCl-resistant nuclear receptor–steroid complexes were prepared from uteri of immature rats treated with 2.5 µg of unlabeled estradiol 1 hour prior to sacrifice. The receptor preparations were incubated with 20 nM [^{3}H]estradiol + 100-fold excess of the listed unlabeled steroids (R_c: at 2°C/60 minutes in a competition assay; R_n^e and R_n^r at 37°C/30 minutes in displacement assays). After incubation, the amount of labeled estradiol still bound in a receptor–steroid complex was determined.

matin and/or located in a hydrophilic environment and a resistant form which is much more strongly attached to chromatin and/or located in a hydrophobic environment. The resistant receptor species seems to be of biologic importance in the processes by which estrogens express their action in responsive tissues.

VII. CONCLUSION

In this chapter, we have demonstrated that the accumulation of the RE complex by the nucleus is not sufficient to elicit true growth of the uterus. Even though this initial accumulation is correlated with the stimulation of early uterotropic events, true uterine growth results only when the RE complex remains bound in the nucleus for 6 hours or longer. This long-term nuclear retention of the RE complex is accompanied by the stimulation of a second elevation in RNA polymerase II activity and a sustained stimulation of RNA polymerase I activity. These responses may be characteristic of the obligatory response profile that is associated with true uterine growth. The concept of long-term nuclear retention as a requisite for true growth provides new insight into the apparent paradox of the so-called weak or impeded estrogens. These compounds, such as estriol, are weak only when injected as a result of their inability to promote long-term retention of the receptor complex by the nucleus. If estriol blood levels are maintained, as under physiological conditions or when given as an implant, long-term nuclear retention and true uterine growth occur. These findings and concepts have led to the proposal that estriol, and compounds similar to it, be classified as short-acting, rather than weak or impeded estrogens.

We have also shown that long-term nuclear retention may result from two different binding states of the RE complex in the nucleus: one form tightly bound to chromatin which we call KCl resistant and another more loosely bound form which we call KCl extractable. These two forms show quantitative and temporal relationships that suggest that the KCl-resistant form is derived from the KCl-extractable form. It appears likely the KCl-resistant RE complexes represent those which undergo long-term nuclear retention and which are involved in mediating the nuclear events responsible for true uterine growth.

ACKNOWLEDGMENT

This work is supported by USPHS Grants HD-04985 and HD-08389 and Grant BD-92 from The American Cancer Society.

REFERENCES

Alberga, A., Massol, N., Raynaud, J. P., and Baulieu, E. E. (1971). *Biochemistry* **10,** 3835–3843.
Anderson, J. N., Clark, J. H., and Peck, E. J., Jr. (1972a). *Biochem. J.* **126,** 561–567.
Anderson, J. N., Clark, J. H., and Peck, E. J., Jr. (1972b). *Biochem. Biophys. Res. Commun.* **48,** 1460–1467.
Anderson, J. N., Peck, E. J., Jr., and Clark, J. H. (1973). *Endocrinology* **92,** 1488–1495.
Anderson, J. N., Peck, E. J., Jr., and Clark, J. H. (1975). *Endocrinology* **96,** 160–167.
André, J., and Rochefort, H. (1975). *FEBS Lett.* **50,** 319–323.
Billing, R. J. Barbiroli, B., and Smellie, R. M. S. (1968). *Biochem. J.* **109,** 705–713.
Borthwick, N. M., and Smellie, R. M. S. (1975). *Biochem. J.* **147,** 91–101.
Buller, R. E., Schrader, W. T., and O'Malley, B. W. (1975). *J. Biol. Chem.* **250,** 809–818.
Callantine, M. R., Humphrey, R. R., Lee, S. L., Windsor, B. L., Schottin, N. H., and O'Brien, O. P. (1966). *Endocrinology* **79,** 153.
Capony, F., and Rochefort, H. (1975). *Mol. Cell. Endocrinol.* **3,** 233–251.
Chamness, G. C., Jennings, A. W., and McGuire, W. L. (1973). *Nature (London)* **241,** 458–460.
Chamness, G. C., Jennings, A. W., and McGuire, W. L. (1974). *Biochemistry* **13,** 327–331.
Clark, J. H., and Peck, E. J., Jr. (1976). *Nature (London)* **260,** 635–636.
Clark, J. H., Anderson, J. N., and Peck, E. J., Jr. (1972). *Science* **176,** 528–530.

Clark, J. H., Anderson, J. N., and Peck, E. J., Jr. (1973). *Steroids* **22**, 707–718.
Clark, J. H., Anderson, J. N., and Peck, E. J., Jr. (1974). *Nature (London)* **251**, 446–448.
Clark, J. H., Peck, E. J., Jr., and Glasser, S. R. (1977). In "Reproduction in Domestic Animals," (H. H. Cole and P. T. Cupps, eds.), 3rd ed., pp. 143–173, Academic Press, New York.
Clark, J. H., Eriksson, H. A., and Hardin, J. W. (1976). *J. Steroid Biochem.* **7**, 1039–1043.
Cole, P., and MacMahon, B. (1969). *Lancet* **1**, 604–606.
De Hertogh, R., Ekka, E., Vanderheyden, J., and Hoet, J. J. (1973). *J. Steroid Biochem.* **4**, 313–320.
Dorfman, R. I. (1962). *Methods Horm. Res.* **2**, 113–126.
Emmens, C. W. (1970). *Ann. Rev. Pharmacol.* **4**, 237–254.
Fang, S., and Liao, S. (1971). *J. Biol. Chem.* **246**, 16–24.
Glasser, S. R., and Spelsberg, T. C. (1973). *Proc. 55th Annu. Meet. Am. Endocr. Soc.* p. A88.
Glasser, S. R., Chytil, F., and Spelsberg, T. C. (1972). *Biochem. J.* **130**, 947–957.
Goebelsmann, W., Midgley, A. R., Jr., and Jaffe, R. B. (1969). *J. Clin. Endocrinol. Metab.* **29**, 1222–1228.
Gorski, J. (1964). *J. Biol. Chem.* **239**, 889–896.
Hamilton, T. H. (1968). *Science* **161**, 649–661.
Hamilton, T. H., Teng, C. S., and Means, A. R. (1968). *Proc. Natl. Acad. Sci. U.S.A.* **59**, 1265–1268.
Hardin, J. W., Clark, J. H., Glasser, S. R., and Peck, E. J., Jr. (1976). *Biochemistry* **15**, 1370–1374.
Higgins, S. J., Rousseau, G. G., Baxter, J. D., and Tomkins, G. M. (1973). *J. Biol. Chem.* **248**, 5873–5879.
Hisaw, F. L., Jr. (1959). *Endocrinology* **64**, 276–289.
Hisaw, F. L., Jr., Velardo, J. T., and Goolsby, C. M. (1953). *Fed. Proc., Fed. Am. Soc. Exp. Biol.* **12**, 68.
Hobkirk, R., and Nilsen, M. (1962). *J. Clin. Endocrinol. Metab.* **22**, 134–141.
Jensen, E. V., Jacobson, H. I., Flesher, J. W., Saha, N. N., Gupta, G., Smith, S., Colucci, V., Shiplacoff, D., Neumann, H. G., and De Sombre, G. R. (1966). *Steroid Dyn., Proc. Symp., 1965*, pp. 133–157.
Kalimi, M., Beato, M., and Feigelson, P. (1973). *Biochemistry* **12**, 3365–3371.
Katzenellenbogen, B. S., and Ferguson, E. R. (1975). *Endocrinology* **97**, 1–12.
Katzenellenbogen, B. S., and Gorski, J. (1975). *Biochem. Actions Horm.* **3**, 187–243.
King, R. J. B., and Gordon, J. (1972). *Nature (London), New Biol.* **240**, 185–187.
Knowler, J. T., and Smellie, R. M. S. (1971). *Biochem. J.* **125**, 605–614.
Lemon, H. M., Miller, D. M., and Foley, J. F. (1971). *Natl. Cancer Inst., Monogr.* **34**, 77–86.
Lerner, L. J. (1964). *Recent Prog. Horm. Res.* **20**, 119–123.
Luck, D. N., and Hamilton, T. H. (1972). *Proc. Natl. Acad. Sci. U.S.A.* **69**, 157–161.
Mainwaring, W. I. P., and Peterken, B. M. (1971). *Biochem. J.* **125**, 285–295.
Martin, L. (1969). *Steroids* **13**, 1–10.
Means, A. R., and Hamilton, T. H. (1966). *Proc. Natl. Acad. Sci. U.S.A.* **56**, 686–689.
Mester, J., and Baulieu, E. E. (1975). *Biochem. J.* **146**, 617–627.
Miller, B. G. (1969). *J. Endocrinol.* **43**, 563–570.
O'Malley, B. W., and Means, A. R. (1974). *Science* **183**, 610–620.
O'Malley, B. W., Spelsberg, T. C., Schrader, W. T., Chytil, F., and Steggles, A. W. (1972). *Nature (London)* **235**, 141–144.
Puca, G. A., and Bresciani, F. (1969). *Nature (London)* **218**, 962–969.
Raynaud-Jammet, C., Cattelli, M. G., and Baulieu, E. E. (1972). *FEBS Lett.* **22**, 93–95.

Rochefort, H., Lignon, F., and Capony, F. (1972). *Biochem. Biophys. Res. Commun.* **47**, 662–668.

Rudali, G., Apiou, F., and Mael, B. (1975). *Eur. J. Cancer* **11**, 39–41.

Schwartz, R. J., Tsai, M. J., Tsai, S. Y., and O'Malley, B. W. (1975). *J. Biol. Chem.* **250**, 5175–5182.

Terenius, L. (1970). *Acta Endocrinol.* (*Copenhagen*) **61**, 47–58.

Terenius, L. (1971). *Acta Endocrinol.* (*Copenhagen*) **66**, 431–447.

Wotiz, H. H., Shane, J. A., Vigersky, R., and Brecher, P. I. (1968). *In* "Prognostic Factors in Breast Cancer" (A. P. M. Forrest and P. B. Kunkler, eds.), pp. 368–382. Livingstone, Edinburgh.

Yamamoto, K. R., and Alberts, B. (1975). *Cell* **4**, 301–310.

2

Conformational Forms of the Estrogen Receptor

ANGELO C. NOTIDES

I.	Introduction	33
II.	Transformation of the Rat Uterine Estrogen Receptor	35
	A. *In Vitro* Receptor Transformation, Temperature-Induced	35
	B. *In Vitro* Receptor Transformation, Salt-Induced	36
	C. The Effect of Urea on the Conformation of the Receptor	38
	D. The Molecular Weight of the Estrogen Receptor	39
III.	Kinetic Analysis of the Relationship of the 4 S to the 5 S Estrogen Receptor	41
	A. Formation of the 5 S Estrogen Receptor	41
	B. Dissociation of the 5 S Estrogen Receptor	46
IV.	Molecular Properties of the Estrogen Receptor from the Human Uterus	47
	A. Cytoplasmic Forms of the Estrogen Receptor	47
	B. The Relationship between Uterine Proteases and the Estrogen Receptor	49
	C. Nuclear and Conformational Forms of the Human Estrogen Receptor	51
V.	Conformational Models of the Estrogen Receptor	54
	A. The 4 S EBP as the Activated Receptor	55
	B. The 5 S EBP as the Activated Receptor	57
VI.	Conclusion	58
	References	59

I. INTRODUCTION

In the past few years there has been substantial evidence that estradiol initiates its biologic action by forming a complex with an estrogen-binding protein (EBP), referred to as an estrogen receptor (Jensen and De Sombre, 1973; Jensen et al., 1974; Gorski et al., 1968; Gorski and Gannon, 1976). It is recognized that not only estrogen-responsive tissues, but all steroid-dependent tissues, contain a corresponding specific steroid-binding protein or receptor (O'Malley et al., 1973; Liao, 1975; Baulieu et al., 1971; Edelman, 1975). The stereospecific estrogen receptor, initially found in the cytoplasmic fraction, was detected with sucrose-gradient centrifugation analysis (Toft and Gorski, 1966; Toft et al., 1967; Erdos, 1968). The uterine estrogen receptor from the cytoplasmic fraction sediments as an 8 S EBP in sucrose gradients without KCl, while in the presence of 0.4 M KCl the receptor dissociates into a 4 S EBP (Korenman and Rao, 1968; Jensen et al., 1969).

The transformation or activation of the estrogen receptor is an estradiol- and temperature-dependent conformational change modifying the receptor's intrinsic activity and its sedimentation characteristics. Autoradiographic and cell fraction studies demonstrated that uterine tissue incubated at 4°C with [^{3}H]-estradiol had more than 70% of the estrogen in the cytoplasmic fraction, while in tissue incubated at 37°C 80–90% of the estrogen receptor was associated with the nuclear fraction (Jensen et al., 1968). Sucrose-gradient analyses established that, during in vivo estradiol treatment or in vitro tissue incubation, the concentration of the estrogen receptor diminishes in the cytosol and concomitantly increases in the nuclear fraction. Coincident with nuclear uptake of the estrogen receptor, the sedimentation coefficient of the receptor increases from 4 S to 5 S in salt-containing gradients (Jensen et al., 1969; Shyamala and Gorski, 1969; Giannopoulos and Gorski, 1971). Incubation of the uterine cytosol with estradiol at 25°–37°C, but not at 0°C, yields the 4 S to 5 S EBP transformation, while incubation of the uterine nuclei or nuclear extract with estradiol does not yield any estrogen receptor (Jensen et al., 1971). Potent estrogens such as estradiol, diethylstilbestrol, hexestrol, and ethynylestradiol can promote the 4 S to 5 S transformation (Jensen et al., 1971), as can higher concentrations of estrone, a weaker estrogen (Ruh et al., 1973). The 5 S, but not the 4 S, EBP shows a high affinity for uterine nuclei (De Sombre et al., 1972) and is capable of increasing RNA polymerase activity (Raynaud-Jammet and Baulieu, 1969; Mohla et al., 1972). The activated receptor interacts with "acceptor" components of the cell's nuclear structure (Spelsberg et al., 1972; Buller and O'Malley, 1976), or enzymatically alters or supplements a nuclear biochemical activity (Lohmar and Toft, 1975; Jensen and De Sombre, 1973).

Thus, the 4 S to 5 S EBP transformation is associated with receptor activation and provides a convenient biochemical basis for measuring and investigating the activation process. A number of laboratories have provided essential data and molecular models for the estrogen receptor (Yamamoto and Alberts, 1972; Little et al., 1975; Puca et al., 1972; Mueller et al., 1972; Gorski and Gannon, 1976; Baulieu et al., 1971; Jensen and De Sombre, 1973). From our kinetic and molecular analyses of the 4 S to 5 S estrogen receptor transformation, a monomer–dimer model of the receptor structure and activation process will be presented here. The nomenclature of Frieden (1971) has been adopted; therefore, the 4 S EBP can be considered a monomer whose activity is regulated by an oligomerization process. The 4 S EBP by an estradiol- and temperature-dependent process associates to form a dimer, the 5 S EBP, that has enhanced activity. The monomers that constitute the dimer may not necessarily be identical. The monomer, in turn, may be composed of more than one subunit. The dissociation of a monomer into its subunits (by 8 M urea, 6 M guanidine HCl, sodium dodecyl sulfate, or acid pH) results in a loss of its biologic activity.

II. TRANSFORMATION OF THE RAT UTERINE ESTROGEN RECEPTOR

The estrogen-induced transformation of the receptor may be attributed to a change in one or more of the following properties of the 4 S estrogen-binding protein: (a) shape, producing a form with hydrodynamic properties that permit faster sedimentation; (b) partial specific volume or density, e.g., by phosphorylation or by dissociation of a lipid moiety; or (c) mass, by association with another macromolecule. A change in any of these properties could be provoked by the binding of estradiol to the 4 S form of the receptor, in association with or independent of the action of an enzyme. Measurements of the sedimentation coefficient by sucrose-gradient analysis and the molecular Stokes radius by gel filtration with Sephadex G-200, under identical buffer conditions, provide an accurate estimation of the molecular parameters and molecular weights of the 4 S EBP and the transformed receptor, the 5 S EBP (Siegel and Monty, 1966); these measurements provide sufficient data to exclude the first two alternatives. The 5 S activated or transformed receptor is formed by the association of the 4 S protein with another macromolecule, independently of the action of an enzyme (Notides and Nielsen, 1974, 1975; Notides et al., 1975).

A. *In Vitro* Receptor Transformation, Temperature-Induced

Our studies confirm the original reports of Jensen and his associates (1971) that the conversion of the cytoplasmic 4 S estrogen receptor to the 5

S form, which is indistinguishable from the 5 S receptor isolated from nuclei of estrogen-treated animals, can be produced by incubating uterine cytosol, at any temperature between 10° and 37°C, in the presence of estradiol. The *in vitro* transformation is enhanced when uterine tissue is homogenized in buffer containing 40 mM Tris, 1 mM dithiothreitol, and 100 mM KCl at pH 7.5, rather than 10 mM Tris buffer, pH 7.5 (Notides *et al.*, 1975). Following equilibration of the cytosol with [³H]estradiol, the sample was made 1 M with respect to urea, and aliquots were then incubated, at a temperature between 10° and 37°C, without loss of estradiol-binding activity. The presence of 1 M urea is not necessary, but yields more reproducible results, without causing aggregation of the receptor. Urea assists in forming the 5 S EBP dimer, possibly by retarding nonspecific macromolecular associations, by aiding in the dissociation of the 4 S EBP from other inhibitory complexes or associations, or by promoting specific conformation changes.

A species variation of the *in vitro* 4 S to 5 S receptor transformation has been observed. The amount of 5 S EBP formed under identical conditions appears to be greatest using the estrogen receptor from the calf, moderate using receptor from the rat uterus or the anterior pituitary (A. C. Notides, unpublished observation), and least with the estrogen receptor from the human uterus; there is less of the 5 S formed because of a qualitative difference in its molecular behavior (Section IV,B).

B. *In Vitro* Receptor Transformation, Salt-Induced

Although *in vitro* studies have indicated an estradiol- and temperature-dependent nuclear uptake of the estrogen receptor, it is not surprising to find processes other than temperature that can provoke conformational changes in the estrogen receptor, resulting in the formation of the 5 S EBP and activation. The observations of Milgrom *et al.* (1973), Giannopoulos (1975), and Higgins *et al.* (1973) that nuclear binding of the glucocorticoid or estrogen receptor can be substantially enhanced by pretreatment with 0.4 M KCl at 4°C, by ammonium sulfate precipitation, or by dilution of the cytosol suggest that receptor activation is essentially a salt-induced conformational change that does not require formation of the 5 S EBP dimer. This explanation is inconsistent with sucrose-gradient analysis which demonstrates, at least for the estrogen receptor, that perturbation of the ionic environment can produce an *in vitro* 4 S to 5 S transformation as effectively as temperature. Rat or calf uterine cytosol containing [³H]estradiol, when incubated with 0.3–0.4 M KCl for 1 hour at 0°C, showed predominantly a 4 S sedimenting protein; when the KCl concentration was

2. Conformational Forms of the Estrogen Receptor

reduced to 0.05 M by the addition of dilute Tris buffer, centrifugation analysis indicated that the sedimentation coefficient of the receptor had increased to 5 S. The addition of an equal volume of buffer containing 0.4 M KCl, or reduction of the KCl concentration to 0.15 M, failed to induce the formation of the 5 S receptor (Fig. 1).

Apparently, the 4 S EBP in the absence of salt, or even in 0.1 M KCl, forms weak associations with itself or other macromolecules. These weak associations may be reflected in the propensity of the estrogen receptor, as well as all other steroid hormone receptors, to form an 8 S sedimenting protein in the absence of KCl (Toft and Gorski, 1966). A high-salt environment (0.4 M KCl) leads to the dissociation of the 4 S EBP from weak associations that are counterproductive to 5 S receptor formation. When a high-salt environment is followed by a rapid desalting, such as by dilution, an increase in macromolecular interaction between the released 4 S EBP and its complementary monomer takes place, leading to the formation of the 5 S dimer and activation of the receptor. It should be noted that the *in vitro* nuclear-binding assay of the salt-activated receptor is not performed in 0.4 M KCl, but only after desalting or dilution to reduce the salt concentration below 0.1 M KCl (Milgrom *et al.*, 1973).

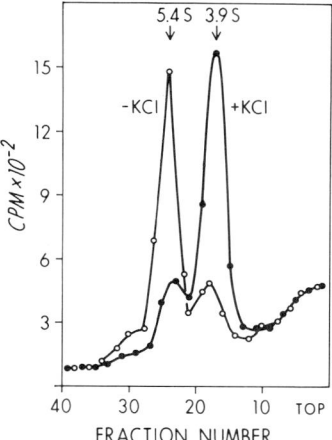

Fig. 1. Salt-induced transformation of the rat estrogen receptor. Uterine cytosol was equilibrated with [³H]estradiol for 1 hour at 0°C, then made 0.4 M with respect to KCl for 2 hours at 0°C. To 1 aliquot, dilute Tris buffer was added so that the final KCl concentration was 0.05 M KCl (○); to a second aliquot, an equal volume of Tris buffer containing 0.4 M KCl was added (●). Centrifugation analysis was performed in sucrose gradients containing 0.4 M KCl (A. C. Notides, unpublished observation.)

C. The Effect of Urea on the Conformation of the Receptor

The estrogen receptor is a protein with a significant degree of conformational mobility, as demonstrated by changes in its hydrodynamic properties when measured in the presence of urea. In Tris buffer, pH 7.5, containing 0.4 M KCl and 3 M urea at 0°C, the 4 S and 5 S receptors show a decrease in their sedimentation coefficients and an increase in their molecular Stokes radii, indicating either an expansion of the receptor's structure, e.g., by an increased hydration of the protein, or an unfolding of its polypeptide structure. Under the same conditions, [^{3}H]estradiol-binding activity of the receptor was not significantly reduced by 3 M urea; in 4 M urea, binding activity was still 86% of the control value. This would suggest that 1–4 M urea at 0°C does not significantly perturb the estradiol-binding site; if urea induces a macromolecular unfolding, it does not extend to the binding site of the protein (Notides and Nielsen, 1974).

The 4 S and 5 S forms of the receptor show an inverse relationship between their molecular Stokes radii and their sedimentation coefficients; as the molecular radius increases under the influence of urea, the sedimentation coefficient decreases, indicating changes in conformation (Fig. 2). The molecular Stokes radii of the 4 S EBP and the 5 S EBP were measured by comparing the elution parameters on Sephadex G-200 with those of other proteins whose molecular Stokes radii are known. The 4 S EBP has a molecular Stokes radius of 44 Å in the absence of and 54 Å in

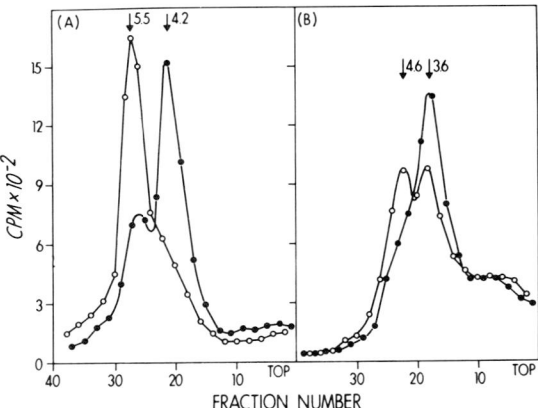

Fig. 2. The decrease in the sedimentation rate of the 4 S and 5 S EBP with 3 M urea. Aliquots of uterine cytosol equilibrated with [^{3}H]estradiol at 0°C were incubated for an additional 30 minutes at 0°C (●, untransformed receptor); or 28°C (○, transformed). Aliquots were centrifuged in buffer containing 0.4 M KCl (A), or in buffer containing 0.4 M KCl and 3 M urea (B). Reproduced from Notides and Nielsen (1974).

2. Conformational Forms of the Estrogen Receptor

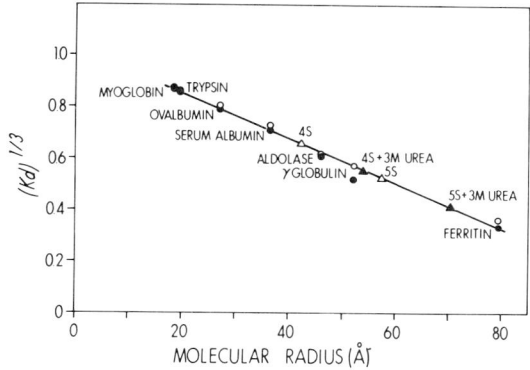

Fig. 3. The increase in the molecular radius of the 4 S EBP and the 5 S EPB with 3 M urea. Sephadex G-200 columns were equilibrated with Tris buffer containing 0.4 M KCl (○), or 0.4 M KCl and 3 M urea (●), and standardized with proteins of known molecular Stokes radii. The molecular Stokes radii of the 4 S (△) and 5 S (△) measured in 0.4 M KCl; the 4 S (▲) and 5 S (▲) measured in 0.4 M KCl and 3 M urea. Reproduced from Notides and Nielsen (1974).

the presence of urea, while the 5 S EBP has a molecular Stokes radius of 59 Å, which expands to 71 Å in urea (Fig. 3). Following Sephadex G-200 chromatography with buffer containing 3 M urea, the 4 S EBP, and the 5 S EBP were eluted as separate proteins, and the 3 M urea was removed by dialysis. Upon removal of the urea, the 4 S and 5 S receptors resumed their original molecular parameters, strongly indicating that urea has induced marked conformational changes in the receptor (Notides and Nielsen, 1974, 1975). The biochemical significance of the estrogen receptor's capacity for such marked conformational fluctuation is unclear. It may reflect conformational changes that the receptor undergoes during its activation, or during performance of its nuclear biochemical action.

D. The Molecular Weight of the Estrogen Receptor

The molecular weight (MW) of the 4 S EBP is 70,000–80,000 daltons, while that of the 5 S form of the receptor is approximately double, 130,000–140,000 daltons. The molecular weights of the 4 S EBP and 5 S EBP remain unaltered in the presence of urea, although marked conformational changes have been provoked: compare the sedimentation coefficient and molecular Stokes radius values in buffers with or without 3 M urea (Table I). Whether the 5 S EBP is extracted from uterine nuclei of estrogen-treated rats, or induced by warming a uterine cytosol–estradiol mixture, there is no significant difference in the molecular Stokes radius or in the sedimentation coefficient.

TABLE I

Molecular Parameters of the Estrogen Receptor from Gel Chromatography and Sucrose Gradient Analysis[a,b]

Buffer	Sedimentation coefficient (S)	Molecular Stokes radius (Å)	Molecular weight	Frictional ratio (f/f_0)
Untransformed receptor				
TEK	4.2 ± 0.04	44.0 ± 0.4	76,200 ± 4200	1.45
TEK + 3 M urea	3.6 ± 0.04	53.8 ± 0.9	79,900 ± 3400	1.75
Transformed receptor				
TEK	5.5 ± 0.02	58.5 ± 0.5	132,700 ± 5100	1.60
TEK + 3 M urea	4.6 ± 0.09	70.6 ± 1.0	133,900 ± 8200	1.93

[a] (Reproduced from Notides and Nielsen, 1974).
[b] The TEK buffer used was 40 mM Tris, 2 mM EDTA, and 400 mM KCl at pH 7.4. The molecular weight was estimated using the relationship MW = $6 \pi n$N ÅS/1 $- \bar{v}p$, where n is the viscosity, N is Avogadro's number, Å is the molecular Stokes radius, S is the sedimentation coefficient, $\bar{v}$; the partial specific volume is assumed to be 0.725 cm^3 g^{-1}, and p is the solvent density. The values are the mean ± SEM.

Other investigators (Jensen et al., 1973) have reported a small but reproducible difference between the sedimentation coefficients (5.2 S versus 5.5 S) of the 5 S EBP's generated in vivo and in vitro. Whether this difference reflects macromolecular interactions of the 5 S EBP with the milieu of the cytosol as opposed to interactions in the nuclear extract or reflects changes in conformation or mass, remains to be resolved by more precise techniques.

Theoretical considerations and experimental data indicate that it is highly improbable that the differences in the results from the sedimentation and chromatography analyses of the two receptor forms can be attributed to differences in those molecular parameters which contribute to their partial specific volume, such as lipid or nucleotide content, phosphorylation, acetylation, or hydration. The sedimentation rates of the 4 S EBP and 5 S EBP in very dense sucrose gradients for 20, 60, or 90 hours showed no change with time, compared with each other or with the protein standards. This indicates similar densities for the 4 S and 5 S EBP. For the apparent increase in mass of the 5 S EBP to be solely caused by a change in specific volume during the transformation process, one must assume a 20–30% change in the partial specific volume. Such a change extends beyond the range of values known for proteins: the partial specific volume of the lipoproteins is about 0.78 cm^3/g, whereas the denser glycoproteins may have a value as low as 0.69 cm^3/g (Sober, 1968). The partial specific volume of the

4 S EBP and 5 S EBP was assumed to be 0.725 cm^3/g (Notides and Nielsen, 1974).

The frictional ratio of the estrogen receptor, an index of the shape and solvation for a protein, was 1.45 for the 4 S EBP. Following receptor transformation, the asymmetry of the 5 S receptor was increased to 1.60. The frictional ratio of most globular proteins falls within the range of 1.1–1.3 (Sober, 1968). The molecular analysis of the two forms of the receptor in 3 M urea showed that the frictional ratio of each had increased as a result of either a change in shape or an alteration of the receptor's hydration (Table I).

The increase in sedimentation value, indicative of receptor activation, is a consequence of estradiol- and temperature-generated dimerization; the 4 S EBP interacts with a second macromolecule to form the 5 S EBP, a dimer. The increase in the sedimentation coefficient of the estrogen receptor is not due to changes in conformation (i.e., shape) or partial specific volume (i.e., density) of the 4 S EBP. Undoubtedly, changes in protein hydration, conformation, and intramacromolecular rearrangement of the receptor also take place, but more sophisticated techniques will be required to assess the contributions of these secondary molecular changes.

III. KINETIC ANALYSIS OF THE RELATIONSHIP OF THE 4 S TO THE 5 S ESTROGEN RECEPTOR

A. Formation of the 5 S Estrogen Receptor

Notides *et al.* (1975) have shown that the estradiol- and temperature-dependent formation of the 5 S EBP under specific *in vitro* conditions is a bimolecular reaction, supporting the molecular model in which the 4 S EBP interacts with a second macromolecule to form the 5 S EBP, a dimer. Under *in vitro* conditions, the transformation of the receptor–estradiol complex from the 4 S to the 5 S form proceeds at elevated temperatures. The transformation is effectively halted by cooling the receptor–estradiol complex to 0°C and is analogous to the temperature dependence shown during nuclear uptake of the estrogen receptor (Jensen *et al.*, 1968; Shyamalä and Gorski, 1969; Williams and Gorski, 1973). Notides *et al.* monitored the rate of receptor activation by sucrose-gradient centrifugation resolution of the 4 S and 5 S EBP. This was followed by measurements of the radioactivity associated with each of the EBP's, using a curve-resolving computer (Fig. 4).

The association rate of the 4 S EBP with its complementary monomer can be calculated from the amount of 5 S EBP generated. From our

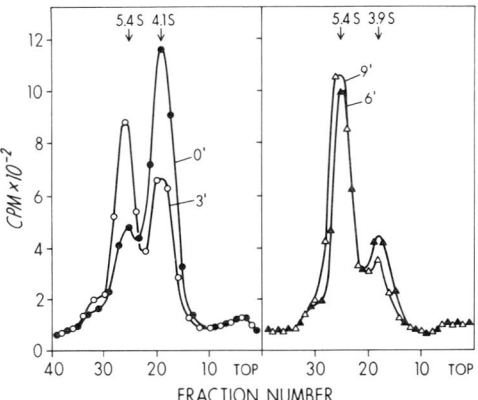

Fig. 4. The rate of 4 S to 5 S EBP transformation at 35°C. Uterine cytosol was equilibrated with 10 nM [³H]estradiol at 0°C for 1 hour. Urea (1 M) was added; then the aliquots were incubated for the times noted. The reaction was stopped by cooling to 0°C, and the excess [³H]estradiol was adsorbed to charcoal. Reproduced from Notides et al. (1975).

molecular characterization of the 5 S EBP, we are able to conclude that the composition of the 5 S EBP must be either a dimer of two identical 4 S EBP's or a dimer of a 4 S EBP with a second dissimilar macromolecule (E-?) which may or may not bind estradiol (Fig. 5a,b). The macromolecule associating with the 4 S EBP to form the 5 S EBP has identical or very similar properties to those of the 4 S EBP, since this putative macromolecule cofractionates with the 4 S EBP during standard protein isolation procedures (Nielsen and Notides, 1975). If we assume that the second macromolecular component (E-?) is present at a concentration equal to that of the 4 S EBP (Fig. 5c), then the kinetic analyses for the two alternative models for the composition of the 5 S EBP have identical solutions (Fig. 5a,b). The reaction is second order, and the rate of the 5 S EBP formation is proportional to the square of the 4 S EBP concentration (Fig. 5d). As indicated by the integrated rate equation (Fig. 5e), a plot of the inverse of the 4 S EBP concentration versus time yields a linear relationship with the intercept being equal to the inverse of the initial 4 S concentration, and the slope, k_a, is the second order rate constant in M^{-1} min^{-1} (Notides et al., 1975).

If the above assumptions are valid, the kinetic analysis will conform to a second-order reaction, allowing us to exclude several models proposed by other investigators: (a) the 4 S to 5 S EBP transformation as a conformational change (i.e., an isomerization reaction) with the appearance of a first-order reaction (Jensen and De Sombre, 1973); (b) the 4 S EBP as a non-

2. Conformational Forms of the Estrogen Receptor

specific association with other uterine proteins with the appearance of a pseudo first-order reaction (Stancel et al., 1973a); (c) estrogen receptor activation as dependent upon a proteolytic step, which would show complex kinetics and be essentially irreversible (Puca et al., 1972). The kinetics of the *in vitro* formation of the 5 S EBP indicate that the estrogen receptor transformation is a bimolecular reaction in which two identical 4 S EBP's dimerize with one another, or in which a 4 S EBP associates with a second, dissimilar monomer (E-?). The complementary unit with which the 4 S EBP associates must be present at approximately the same concentration; i.e., it cannot be greater than four- to sixfold above the 4 S EBP concentration and still maintain the appearance of second-order kinetics.

During equilibration with estradiol and high salt, the estrogen receptor forms an estradiol complex, and, at the same time, the 4 S monomer units, which may have been weakly associated, are dissociated from each other or from other proteins. As a consequence of a heat-promoted conformational change, the propensity of the 4 S EBP's to dimerize is enhanced. The second-order rate constant of the 5 S EBP formation at 28°C, in the presence of 0.4 M KCl, was 2×10^{-7} M^{-1} min^{-1} and is independent of the initial 4 S EBP concentration (Fig. 6A). The 4 S monomer in a high ionic strength environment behaves as a single independent component in a bimolecular reaction (Fig. 7A).

In the absence of salt or near physiological salt concentrations (0.1–0.15 M KCl), the molecular interactions of the 5 S EBP indicate a complex second-order reaction. This complex interaction of the 4 S EBP may reflect a molecular mechanism for modulating receptor activity *in vivo* (Section, V,B).

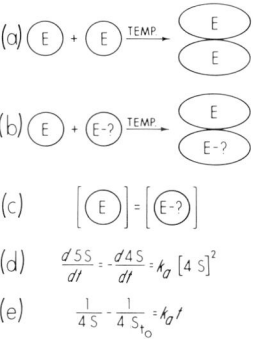

Fig. 5. Kinetic assumption for the analysis of the *in vitro* 4 S to 5 S EBP transformation promoted by temperature. Estradiol, E, is present in excess and occupies all available binding sites of the 4 S EBP; E-? represents the complementary monomer, of unknown identity, that associates with the 4 S EBP.

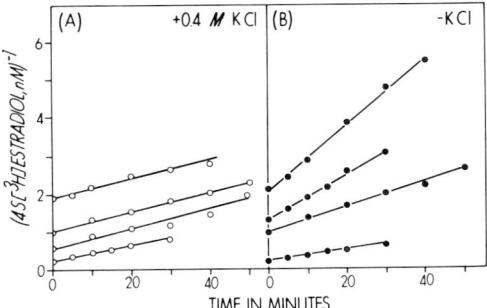

Fig. 6. The rate of 4 S to 5 S EBP transformation plotted as a second-order function. Receptor transformation measured in 40 mM Tris, 1 mM dithiothreitol, pH 7.4, with 0.4 M KCl at 28°C was 2×10^{-7} M^{-1} min^{-1}, independent of the initial 4 S EBP concentration, indicating a simple second-order reaction (A). The rate of receptor transformation in the absence of KCl indicates the presence of a complex second-order reaction mechanism (B). Reproduced from Notides and Nielsen (1975).

The apparent second-order rate constant of the 5 S EBP formation increases 6-fold when there is a 10-fold decrease in the initial 4 S EBP concentration (Fig. 6B). This implies, based on the Le Chatelier principle, that cytosol dilution leads to a shift in the equilibrium of the 4 S EBP (or the complementary monomer, E-?) with another molecule, possibly an inhibitor, Y, so that a larger fraction of the 4 S EBP is present in the dissociated state. Consequently, the temperature-promoted formation of the 5 S EBP is modulated by the fraction of 4 S EBP joined in a weak inhibitory complex with the presumed inhibitor, Y. The inhibitor, Y, is more likely to be a macromolecule than a low molecular weight substance, since the complex second-order kinetics of the 5 S EBP formation is not eliminated by ammonium sulfate fractionation or Sephadex G-25 filtration of the uterine cytosol (Fig. 7B). The rate of 5 S EBP dimer formation is changed by a secondary effect of ionic strength on the macromolecular reactants, which is unrelated to the bimolecular reaction mechanism. The rate of 5 S EBP formation is maximal at 0.1–0.15 M KCl and minimal in the absence of KCl or in the presence of 0.4 M KCl (Notides *et al.*, 1975). For example, in the absence of KCl, the 4 S EBP could be preferentially associated with the inhibitor Y, while in the high salt environment the ionic interaction of the 4 S EBP with its complementary monomer during dimerization might be retarded. Thus, ionic strength conditions higher or lower than physiological may retard 5 S EBP formation by two different salt effects on the kinetics of the reaction.

The rate of formation of the 5 S EBP dimer is highly temperature-dependent, increasing 200-fold when the rate at 35°C is compared with that

2. Conformational Forms of the Estrogen Receptor

at 0°C. The Arrhenius energy of activation was approximately 20 kcal mole^{-1} when measured in buffer with or without 0.4 M KCl (Fig. 8). This high energy of activation suggests that marked conformational changes must accompany the conversion of the receptor from an inactive to an active protein. The identity of the energy of activation for the formation of the 5 S receptor, in the presence or absence of 0.4 M KCl, suggests that the receptor activation process in 0.4 M KCl (in which the receptor is completely dissociated into the 4 S EBP monomer) is similar to that occurring in the absence of KCl. An equilibrium of 4 S EBP–protein interaction is present; i.e., with the macromolecular inhibitor, Y (Fig. 7B). Thus, the dissociation of the 4 S EBP from the inhibitor Y (Fig. 7; compare A with B) is not a step contributing to the energy required for receptor activation. Rather, receptor activation must include estradiol-binding by the 4 S EBP and the subsequent conformation changes, followed by dimerization with its complementary monomer. Although dissociation of the 4 S EBP from any inhibitor protein interaction may be necessary, dissociation alone is insufficient for receptor activation. The 4 S EBP–macromolecular inhibitory complex indicated by the kinetic data may be reflected in the sedimentation characteristics of the estrogen receptor; in the absence of KCl, the 4 S EBP has a propensity to either self-associate or associate with other proteins to form the 8 S EBP oligomer or aggregate.

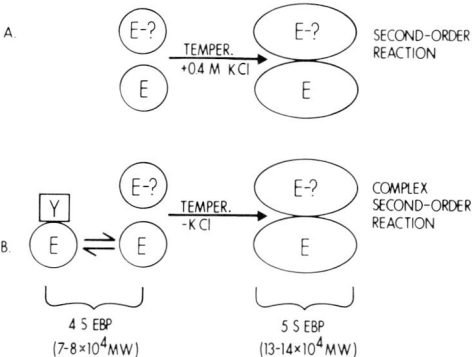

Fig. 7. The interactions of the estrogen-binding proteins during transformation. In the presence of 0.4 M KCl, the 4 S EBP in the monomeric state dimerizes, unimpeded, with a second macromolecule (E-?) which may or may not be identical. The reaction is a simple second-order reaction (A). In buffers without, or with, 0.1 M KCl, the second-order rate constant increases with dilution, indicating a preequilibrium of the 4 S EBP with another macromolecule(s) Y (B). The weak association of the 4 S EBP with Y is broken up by sucrose-gradient analysis in 0.4 M KCl, although the transformed 4 S EBP is not dissociated from its complementary monomeric unit (E-?) and appears as a 5 S EBP dimer. Reproduced from Notides and Nielsen (1975).

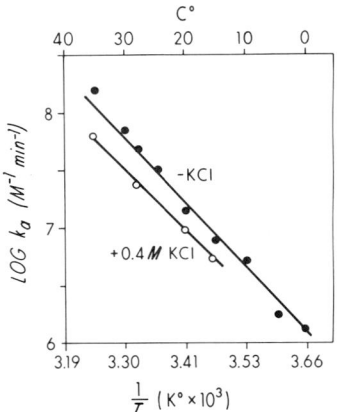

Fig. 8. The Arrhenius plot of the second-order rate constants for receptor transformation. The energy of activation for the 4 S EBP transformation in the absence of KCl was 21.3 kcal mole^{-1}, and in buffer containing 0.4 M KCl was 19.1 kcal mole^{-1}. Reproduced from Notides *et al.* (1975).

The energy of activation of the formation of the 5 S EBP is in good agreement with the comparable *in vivo* measurement by Williams and Gorski (1973). These investigators measured the specific estrogen-binding sites formed in uterine cell suspensions incubated at temperatures ranging from 0° to 37°C, and estimated that the energy of activation for this process was 20.7 kcal mole^{-1}. Based upon reports that 80–90% of the specific estradiol-binding sites in the rat uterine cell are nuclear (Williams and Gorski, 1971, 1972), we can assume by correlation that the measurements of Williams and Gorski reflect the energy of activation required to form the nuclear form of the estrogen receptor, the 5 S dimer.

B. Dissociation of the 5 S Estrogen Receptor

The dissociation of the 5 S EBP dimer to the 4 S EBP monomers suggests a reversible relationship between the 4 S and 5 S EBP's under the appropriate conditions, e.g., pH, ionic strength, and temperature. The first-order kinetics indicates a simple macromolecular dissociation process without the involvement of enzymes.

The dissociation of the 5 S EBP to a 4 S EBP with molecular parameters (molecular Stokes radius and sedimentation coefficient) similar to the original 4 S can be effectively produced by carrying out the incubation in a buffer that causes dissociation, one containing 40 mM HEPES, 400 mM

KCl, and 3 M urea, pH 6.8, at 0°C. The rate of dissociation of the 5 S receptor is first-order with a half-time of 5–6 hours (Fig. 9). The total estradiol-binding activity is not significantly decreased by incubation in the "dissociating buffer" containing an excess of estradiol (Notides and Nielsen, 1974). Stancel *et al.* (1973b) reported that a buffer containing 4 M urea, 1 M KCl, 50 mM β-mercaptoethanol, 50 mM sodium bisulfite, and 50 mM Tris, pH 7.4, can effectively dissociate the nuclear estrogen receptor to a form indistinguishable from the cytoplasmic 4 S EBP.

IV. MOLECULAR PROPERTIES OF THE ESTROGEN RECEPTOR FROM THE HUMAN UTERUS

A. Cytoplasmic Forms of the Estrogen Receptor

Analyses of the estrogen receptor from the human uterus are greatly facilitated by adaptation of the methodology and molecular models derived from studies using experimental animals. The differences in the molecular structure or interactions of the estrogen receptors found in different species aid in elucidating the molecular basis of the receptor's regulatory function. The estrogen receptor from the human uterus compared with that of the rat or calf shows a distinct difference in its sedimentation behavior. A comparative analysis demonstrates the existence of a protease in the human uterus, active at neutral pH and 0°C (Notides *et al.*, 1972, 1973). Sucrose-gradient analyses in the absence of KCl reveals a variety of [³H]estradiol-

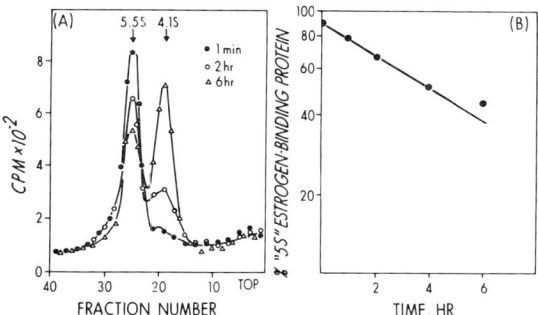

Fig. 9. The rate of dissociation of the 5 S EBP to the 4 S EBP. The receptor was incubated with 40 mM HEPES, 0.4 M KCl, and 3 M urea at pH 6.8, for the time noted, prior to centrifugation in sucrose gradients containing 40 mM Tris, 2 mM EDTA, and 0.4 M KCl at pH 7.4 (A). The log of the percent of 5 S EBP remaining, with time and incubation in the dissociation buffer (B). Reproduced from Notides and Nielsen (1974).

binding proteins in the human uterine cytosol. The endometrial cytosol contains primarily an 8 S sedimenting estrogen receptor and a trace of a 3–4 S form which sediments more slowly than serum albumin, 4.3–4.6 S (Fig. 10A). The myometrial cytosol contains primarily the 3–4 S form of the receptor, serum albumin, and occasionally the 8 S form of the receptor (Fig. 10B). In contrast, the receptor from calf or immature rat uteri sediments clearly as a single 8 S peak in the absence of KCl.

This variety of specific estrogen-binding proteins observed in the human uterus is more apparent than real, since it is due to the action of a trypsin-like enzyme on the 8 S receptor complex, which reduces the receptor's mass, but not its ability to bind the estrogen. Diisopropyl fluorophosphate (DFP), an inhibitor of serine proteases, inhibits the appearance of the 3–4 S receptor fragment while maintaining the 8 S form of the receptor intact (Fig. 11). The 3–4 S receptor fragment, following ammonium sulfate purification, sediments as a 3.1 S EBP with a molecular Stokes radius of 27 Å and an MW of 30,000–40,000. The 3–4 S EBP has a dissociation constant for estradiol of 1 nM and retains its estrogenic specificity (Notides et al., 1972). The salt-dissociated form of the human estrogen receptor has a molecular radius of 38–40 Å, a sedimentation coefficient of 3.8 S, and an MW of 60,000–70,000 (Notides et al., 1976). Based solely upon sucrose-gradient analyses, unfamiliar sedimentation forms of the steroid receptor cannot *a priori* be assumed to be dissociated subunits, new conformational forms, or nuclear forms (Wyss et al., 1968; Sherman et al., 1974; Vonderhaar et al., 1970).

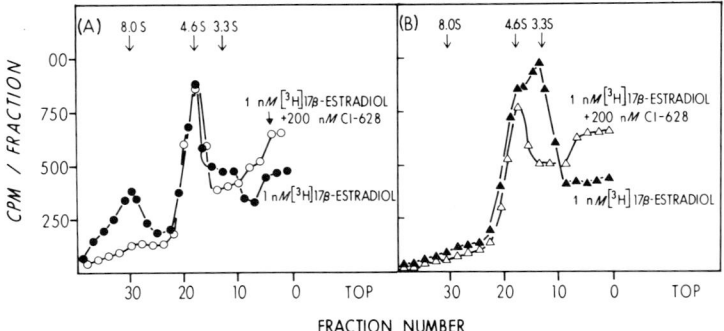

Fig. 10. Sucrose-gradient centrifugation analysis of the estrogen-binding proteins of the human uterus. Endometrial cytosol (A) and myometrial cytosol (B) were incubated with [³H]estradiol or [³H]estradiol plus CI-628, an estrogen antagonist. Sucrose gradients were prepared in 40 mM Tris and 2 mM EDTA buffer at pH 7.4. The nonspecific 4.6 S is serum albumin, while the 8 S and 3.3 S [³H]estradiol peaks are components of the specific estrogen receptor. Reproduced from Notides *et al.* (1972).

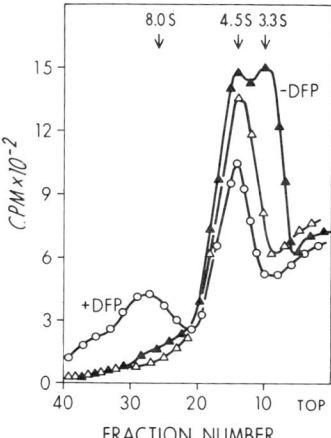

Fig. 11. Sucrose-gradient centrifugation analysis of human myometrial cytosol prepared with or without diisopropyl fluorophosphate (DFP). Myometrial tissue was homogenized in 40 mM Tris and 2 mM EDTA; the cytosol was equilibrated with 1 nM [^{3}H]estradiol (▲) or 1 nM [^{3}H]estradiol plus 200 nM CI-528 (△); the 8 S peak is absent, and a 3.3 S specific estradiol-binding peak is present. Cytosol prepared with buffer containing 5 mM DFP was equilibrated with 1 nM [^{3}H]estradiol (○); the 8 S peak is present. Sucrose gradients were prepared with 40 mM Tris and 2 mM EDTA, pH 7.4 buffer. Reproduced from Notides et al. (1972).

B. The Relationship between Uterine Proteases and the Estrogen Receptor

A comparison of the proteases from the human, calf, and rat uteri, which are active at neutral pH, indicates distinctive differences in their biochemical properties. The heterogeneity in the types of proteases present, and the lack of any significant amount of protease activity in the immature rat uterus, negates the view (Puca et al., 1972; Bresciani et al., 1973) that the action of a protease on the estrogen receptor is a common or essential step of receptor activation.

The hydrolysis of tritium-labeled hemoglobin at pH 7.5 was used as a sensitive indicator of general protease activity in the uterine cytosol (Table II). Among those species assayed, the human uterine cytosol had the highest capacity to digest denatured hemoglobin. This activity was inhibited by DFP, but not by EDTA or p-chloromercuribenzoate. The proteolytic activity of cytosol from the calf uterus was inhibited by EDTA or p-chloromercuribenzoate, but not by DFP. The cytosol from the immature rat uterus has minimal or no ability to hydrolyze the hemoglobin substrate.

Human uterine protease hydrolyzes trypsin substrates, such as benzoyl-arginine-p-nitroanilide and tosylarginine methyl ester. This activity was

TABLE II
Inhibition of Uterine Protease Activity Using [³H]Acetylated Hemoglobin as the Substrate[a,b]

Source of uterine cytosol	Proteolytic activity (cpm/hour/5 mg uterine cytosol)			
	Additions			
	None	1 mM DFP	1 mM EDTA	1 mM p-Chloromercuribenzoate
Human	3710	25	2895	2915
Calf	1876	1910	656	20
Rat	108	105	120	65

[a] (A. C. Notides and D. E. Hamilton, unpublished data.)
[b] Denatured bovine hemoglobin was labeled with [³H]acetic anhydride by the method of Hille *et al.* (1970). The uterine cytosols were incubated with the [³H]hemoglobin for 1 hour at 37°C in Tris buffer, pH 7.5. The reaction was stopped with trichloroacetic acid; the protease activity is equivalent to the trichloroacetic acid-soluble [³H]peptides remaining in solution minus the radioactivity in control tubes containing buffer only.

completely inhibited by DFP and weakly inhibited by phenylmethylsulfonyl fluoride, but was not affected by EDTA, p-chloromercuribenzoate, or trypsin soy bean inhibitor. The uterine protease does not hydrolyze the substrates of chymotrypsin carboxypeptidase, leucine aminopeptidase, collagenase, or elastase (Notides *et al.*, 1973).

The protease from the human uterus was partially purified by ammonium sulfate fractionation and Sephadex G-200 filtration, and its action on the estrogen receptor from the rat uterus was measured. The protease is active at 0°C without Ca^{2+} and converts the 8 S sedimenting protein to a 4.5 S EBP. The 4.5 S EBP has an MW of 61,000 and sediments as the 4.5 S EBP in gradients without KCl (Notides *et al.*, 1973). Thus, the human protease produces, by limited proteolysis of the rat estrogen receptor, a product that is larger than the 3 S EBP fragment of the human estrogen receptor. An interesting manifestation of the protease from the human is its preferential ability to act on the receptor when the receptor is complexed with estradiol (Fig. 12). This is in accord with the observation that conformational changes brought about by ligand-binding affect the susceptibility of a number of proteins to proteolysis (Zito *et al.*, 1964; Markus, 1965).

In contrast to the human uterine protease, the calf uterine protease is activated by Ca^{2+}, is not inhibited by DFP, and converts the calf uterine receptor to a 4.5 S EBP with an MW of 61,000 (Puca *et al.*, 1972). A calcium-mediated reduction in the molecular weight of the chick oviduct

2. Conformational Forms of the Estrogen Receptor

progesterone receptor, presumably caused by protease activation, has also been described (Sherman *et al.,* 1974, 1976). The steroid receptor modified by protease is not capable of binding to the nucleus under *in vitro* assay conditions (Notides *et al.,* 1976; André and Rochefort, 1973). Nevertheless, these enzymes, particularly the human protease with its specificity for the estrogen–receptor complex, may serve *in vivo* as a mechanism for inactivating the receptor, a more plausible role than that of a component of the receptor-activating mechanism.

C. Nuclear and Conformational Forms of the Human Estrogen Receptor

Human myometrial tissue slices were incubated at 37°C in medium containing [^{3}H]estradiol and DFP to translocate the estrogen receptor into the nucleus and simultaneously inhibit the serine proteases. The receptor, isolated from the nuclear fraction, sediments as a 4 S receptor in high salt-

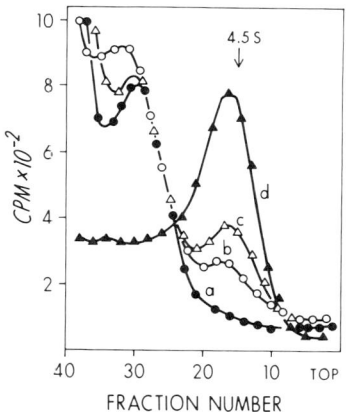

Fig. 12. The preferential action of the human uterine protease on the estrogen receptor when the receptor is complexed with estradiol. The receptor from the rat uterus, equilibrated with estradiol at 0°C, shows an 8 S, but not a 4.5 S estradiol-binding protein (a). When the cytosol–estradiol sample was incubated for 30 minutes at 25°C, a small quantity of the receptor is observed in the 4.5 S region, suggesting some endogenous proteaselike activity in the rat cytosol (b). The receptor without estradiol was incubated with the partially purified human uterine protease for 30 minutes at 25°C, followed by 5 mM DFP for 1 hour at 0°C (to inhibit the protease); then, estradiol for 1 hour at 0°C (c). The receptor with estradiol was incubated with the partially purified human uterine protease for 30 minutes at 25°C followed by 5 mM DFP for 1 hour at 0°C (d). There is a greater quantity of the 4.5 S receptor fragment generated in (d) than in (c). The partially purified human uterine protease does not show estradiol-binding activity. Reproduced from Notides *et al.* (1973).

sucrose gradients, clearly slower than the 5 S receptor from rat or calf nuclei (Notides et al., 1976). Thus, the human estrogen receptor shows a sedimentation characteristic similar to that of other steroid receptors: whether isolated from nuclei or the cytoplasm, they cosediment as a 4 S steroid-binding protein (Liao, 1975). Several observations suggest that the nuclear 4 S EBP from the human tissue is not a proteolytic fragment of the receptor. The estrogen receptor isolated from the uterine nuclei has a sedimentation coefficient of 3.7–4.0 S, a molecular Stokes radius of 37–40 Å, and an MW of 60,000–70,000 (not to be confused with the 30,000–40,000 MW fragment of the receptor, which sediments as a 3–4 S EBP.

The estrogen receptor from human uterine cytosol, prepared rapidly in buffer containing DFP at 0°C, did not show an *in vitro* 4 S to 5 S transformation when the cytosol–estrogen mixture was incubated at 28°C for 30 minutes; these conditions successfully produce a 5 S EBP receptor using rat or calf uterine cytosol. This suggests that the 4 S receptor from the uterine nuclei of tissue slices incubated at 37°C was not produced by the uterine protease. Although the cytosol prepared in DFP does not show a 4 S to 5 S receptor transformation, it is capable of a temperature-provoked activation, as indicated by the receptor's enhanced *in vitro* nuclear-binding activity. The receptor prepared in the absence of DFP sedimented as a 3.1–3.3 S protein which did not bind to the purified nuclear fraction at 0°C or after incubating at 28°C (Table III). The DFP preserves the integrity of the receptor and its nuclear-binding activity, even though sucrose gradient analysis (at least under the experimental conditions used with the rat or calf estrogen receptor) did not show those conformation changes usually associated with receptor activation and formation of the 5 S EBP.

The monomer–dimer interconversion observed between the 4 S and 5 S forms of the EBP from calf or rat uterus (Sections II and III) implies that the dimerization reaction has a very large equilibrium constant, under the specific conditions used for the analysis of the receptor transformation: buffers containing sucrose and 0.4 M KCl at 0°C for 16–20 hours. The human estrogen receptor may also undergo a monomer–dimer interconversion, but the customary sucrose-gradient analysis in high salt at 0°C for 16–20 hours shifts the reaction to produce the 4 S EBP monomer. The estrogen receptor from the human may have a lower equilibrium constant for dimerization than the rat or calf receptor under identical conditions.

At physiological salt concentrations (0.15 M KCl), 20°C, sedimentation of the human estrogen receptor in sucrose gradients showed that the 5 S EBP dimer, not the 4 S EBP, is the preferred conformation of the receptor. Human uterine cytosol prepared in buffers containing DFP, and partially purified by ammonium sulfate fractionation, showed a single 3.9 S [³H]estra-

2. Conformational Forms of the Estrogen Receptor

TABLE III

In Vitro Nuclear Binding of the Estrogen Receptor from Human Uterine Extract in Buffers with and without DFP[a,b]

Cytosol	[³H]Estradiol bound (cpm/0.5 ml)	Nuclear binding (cpm/0.5 ml)	
		Cytosol preincubation at	
		0°C	28°C
With DFP	12,918	3790	9360
Without DFP	16,090	166	113

[a] (Notides *et al.*, 1976).

[b] Human myometrial tissue was homogenized, 1 g/5 ml in 40 mM Tris plus 1 mM dithiothreitol, pH 7.5, with or without 5 mM DFP. The cytosol fractions of the homogenates were equilibrated with 0.2–10 nM [³H]-estradiol for 2 hours at 0°C. To determine the nonspecifically bound estradiol, parallel incubations were performed with the addition of a 100-fold excess of unlabeled diethylstilbestrol to the cytosols. The Scatchard plot indicates that the cytosol prepared with or without DFP contained an EBP with a dissociation constant of 1–3 nM, and a binding capacity of 0.4 nM and 0.6 nM [³H]estradiol for the cytosol with and without the DFP, respectively. Aliquots of the cytosols equilibrated with 5 nM [³H]estradiol, with and without DFP, were made 1 M with respect to urea and incubated 30 minutes at 28°C. Human myometrial nuclei were isolated by the method of Buller *et al.* (1975). Cytosol and nuclei were incubated for 1 hour at 0°C; then the nuclei were washed twice with buffer and counted. The data are the means of duplicate determinations minus the nonspecific binding.

diol-binding peak in gradients with 0.15 M KCl centrifugation at 0°C. As the temperature at which the centrifugation was carried out increased, the [³H]estradiol-binding peak, representing the average sedimentation behavior of the mixed population of monomers and dimers, shifted gradually until at 20°C the 5 S dimer was the major constituent (Fig. 13). The appearance of a single distinct peak for each sedimentation value is typical of proteins which show a rapid association–dissociation equilibrium relative to the time of centrifugation (Notides *et al.*, 1976). The sedimentation behavior of associating systems has been described previously; for general reviews, see Van Holde (1975), Klotz *et al.* (1975), and Roark and Yphantis (1969). Isolation of the human estrogen receptor in buffers without DFP yielded the 3 S EBP, which cannot undergo a temperature-promoted association reaction to form a dimer (Fig. 13). The 3 S EBP is a protein fragment that has retained its ability to bind estradiol, but which has lost its ability to oligomerize.

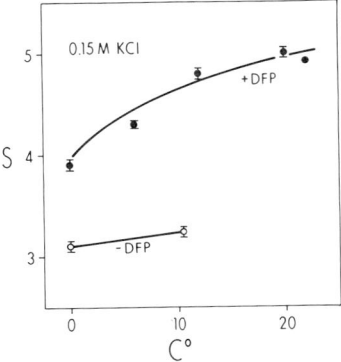

Fig. 13. The temperature-dependent dimerization of the human estrogen receptor. Human myometrial tissue was homogenized in 40 mM Tris, 1 mM dithiothreitol, and 0.15 M KCl, pH 7.5, with 5 mM DFP (●) and without DFP (○). The cytosols were equilibrated with 5 mM [³H]estradiol, then made 30% saturated with respect to ammonium sulfate. The precipitate was dissolved and dialyzed against the same buffer. Sucrose gradients were centrifuged at the temperatures noted. The 4 S EBP is capable of dimerizing during centrifugation, while the 3 S EBP proteolytic fragment is not (Notides et al., 1976).

V. CONFORMATIONAL MODELS OF THE ESTROGEN RECEPTOR

The estrogen receptor is an oligomeric protein, which sediments as an 8 S protein in gradients without salt, and is present at the 4 S or 5 S sedimenting protein in gradients with 0.15–0.4 M KCl. The oligomeric state of the receptor appears to correlate with its biochemical activity. Because the 4 S [³H]estradiol-binding monomer may interact with other essential nonestrogen binding components of the receptor (e.g., the complementary monomer that may not bind estradiol), these analyses were performed without extensive purification of the receptor to avoid their loss. Our analyses of the receptor reveal that the 4 S EBP is involved in two significant macromolecular interactions, each of which may indicate the existence of a separate macromolecule that does not necessarily bind [³H]estradiol. The first, referred to as Y protein, forms a weak inhibitory or dead-end conformation with the 4 S EBP. The second macromolecule is the complementary monomer (E-?) with which the 4 S EBP must associate to form the 5 S EBP dimer.

The molecular interactions of the 4 S EBP and 5 S EBP reveal a number of structural and conformation characteristics, which may have functional and regulatory consequences when viewed as possible models operating *in vivo*.

A. The 4 S EBP as the Activated Receptor

The 4 S EBP may be transformed to the active form of the receptor by an estradiol and temperature-induced conformational change without requiring dissociation from a macromolecular inhibitor or dimerization. This model of receptor activation is analogous to the allosteric enzyme model of Monod *et al.* (1965) or the model of Koshland *et al.* (1966), and is favored by a number of investigators, principally on the basis of studies of the glucocorticoid receptor (Giannopoulous, 1975; Baulieu, 1975; Samuels and Tomkins, 1970). Although such a model has merit and should be seriously considered, several observations and theoretical considerations suggest that receptor activation may involve more complex macromolecular interactions.

A basic requirement of an allosteric regulatory protein, whether evoking the concerted model of Monod or the sequential model of Koshland, is that it possess a quaternary structure composed of a number of subunits whose relationship to one another is altered by the binding of an allosteric ligand (e.g., estradiol) to produce modulation of the receptor's catalytic or "nuclear acceptor-binding site." The 4 S estrogen or progesterone-binding protein appears to be a monomer composed of a single peptide chain, which is inconsistent with the multisubunit structure of allosteric regulatory proteins. The molecular weight measured under denaturing conditions with 6 M guanidine–HCl on a Sepharose 6 B column indicates that the 4 S EBP and the 5 S EBP, when renatured, bound [^{3}H]estradiol in the 60,000-dalton fraction (Erdos and Fries, 1974). Presumably, under these denaturing conditions, the 4 S EBP and 5 S EBP would have denatured and dissociated into their subunit components. These data are consistent with the estimations of the molecular weight (60,000–80,000 daltons) of the 4 S EBP by a number of investigators (Notides and Nielsen, 1974; Gorell *et al.*, 1974; Puca *et al.*, 1971). The observation of Erdos and Fries (1974) also suggests that the 6 M guanidine–HCl dissociated the nuclear 5 S form into an estradiol-binding protein indistinguishable from the 4 S EBP, in agreement with other reports (Stancel *et al.*, 1973b; Notides and Nielsen, 1974). The successful isolation of two 4 S progesterone-binding proteins from the chick oviduct (Schrader and O'Malley, 1972; Kuhn *et al.*, 1975), referred to as the A and B receptors or subunits, reveals that they are each a single peptide chain with an MW of 110,000 and 117,000 daltons, respectively, which is clearly inconsistent with the multisubunit structures of allosteric regulatory proteins.

To attribute a structure and mechanism analogous to that of allosteric enzymes (i.e., estradiol- and temperature-induced conformational transition within the 4 S EBP, which modulates a second "nuclear-binding site" on the 4 S EBP) to the structure and regulatory mechanism of the estrogen receptor may be erroneous.

We believe that estrogen receptor activation is better described by a complex monomer–dimer equilibrium, with the 4 S EBP as a participant. This model is based upon the kinetics of the 5 S EBP formation: the 4 S EBP is joined in an inhibitory association with a macromolecule Y, from which the 4 S EBP must dissociate before it can form the 5 S EBP dimer (Section IV). The salt-induced activation of the estrogen receptor is consistent with this molecular mechanism of receptor activation (Section II,A). Although some investigators favor the view that salt-induced receptor activation provokes an allosteric transition (Milgrom et al., 1973; Giannopoulous, 1975; Higgins et al., 1973), others suggest that salt-induced receptor activation may involve the dissociation of the macromolecule, functioning as an inhibitor, from the receptor (Chamness et al., 1974; Notides et al., 1975; Simons et al., 1976). Sucrose gradient analysis fails to precisely identify the inhibitor Y; nevertheless, the propensity of the 4 S EBP to associate with itself or with other proteins to form the 8 S EBP in a low-salt environment may be indicative of the inhibitory complex.

The impressive kinetic and equilibrium studies of Williams and Gorski (1972, 1974) using isolated uteri or a uterine cell suspension have demonstrated that estradiol binding by the receptor has a Hill coefficient of 1.03, indicating the absence of allosteric interactions between estradiol-binding sites. These investigators concluded that a rapid and reversible equilibrium of the receptor between cytoplasmic and nuclear compartments is occurring with a first-order reaction for nuclear translocation of the receptor. Williams and Gorski propose a model in which there is an excess of "nuclear acceptor sites" in the uterine cell, and that the receptor moving into the nucleus contains a single estradiol-binding site.

The kinetic studies of Williams and Gorski suggest that the 4 S EBP may be the active form of the receptor. A number of other models are consistent with these kinetic analyses, including that of the 5 S EBP dimer as the active form of the receptor with a noncooperative monomer–dimer equilibrium. Possibly, for example, in vivo the 4 S EBP is associated with its complementary monomer, which does not bind estradiol; then, upon estradiol binding, a conformational change in the receptor occurs, transforming it to the activated 5 S EBP form, which subsequently moves into the nucleus. This reaction would appear to be first order. This model indicates that the 5

2. Conformational Forms of the Estrogen Receptor

S EBP cannot be dissociated by high salt at 0°C, while the "inactive 5 S" conformation can be dissociated. Another model consistent with the first-order *in vivo* kinetics of Williams and Gorski, while retaining a second-order reaction mechanism for the 5 S EBP formation, assumes that the 4 S EBP monomer moves into the nucleus independently, and that formation of the 5 S EBP occurs in the nucleus. If the *in vivo* 5 S EBP formation follows a complex second-order reaction, as observed during *in vitro* receptor transformation in the absence of KCl or in 0.1 M KCl (Section III,A), then more molecular models consistent with the *in vivo* kinetic studies of Williams and Gorski and the 5 S EBP dimer as the active nuclear form of the receptor are possible.

The observation of Siiteri *et al.* (1973) that the appearance of the 4 S receptor in sucrose-purified nuclei from estrogen-treated animals precedes the appearance of the 5 S EBP suggests that receptor translocation occurs before transformation. The data of Jensen and De Sombre (1973) indicate that the transformation of the receptor precedes its translocation into the nucleus.

Possibly as a consequence of the limitations of the analytical methods available, there has been no evidence presented for the existence of two forms of the 4 S estrogen receptor based upon an assumed conformational change, other than the 5 S EBP dimer with an enhanced biochemical activity.

B. The 5 S EBP as the Active Form of the Receptor

If the monomeric species of the EBP cannot function as an allosteric regulatory protein, can the 5 S or 8 S EBP function *in vivo* as a multi-subunit allosteric protein? Based solely upon structural requirements expected of an allosteric regulatory protein, the oligomeric nature of the 5 S or 8 S EBP would meet these requirements. Nevertheless, several experimental observations and biologic considerations place obstacles against the acceptance of the estrogen receptor as a regulatory protein operating by a simple subunit–subunit interaction mechanism. The structure and kinetic behavior of the estrogen receptor reflect the properties of a protein whose biologic activity is regulated by a monomer–dimer (4 S $\rightleftharpoons$ 5 S) equilibrium, mediated by estradiol and strongly influenced by temperature, in which dimerization is a necessary step for receptor activation. This regulatory process is clearly different from the subunit–subunit interactions of the allosteric regulatory enzyme model developed by Monod *et al.* (1965).

Enzymes whose activity is modulated by ligand binding and a temperature-dependent oligomerization show a number of structural and functional properties that are strikingly similar to the characteristics of the estrogen receptor. The activity of aspartokinase shows a dependency on lysine and temperature, correlated with a monomer to dimer association process (Funkhouser et al., 1974). Threonine dehydrase undergoes an AMP-dependent dimerization and, consequently, an increase in activity (Gerlt et al., 1973). Hexokinase undergoes a concentration-dependent dimerization in the presence of its regulator, glucose 6-phosphate (Chakrabarti and Kenkare, 1974). The properties of enzymes whose activities are regulated by ligand-induced oligomerization have been reviewed by Frieden (1971), Phillips (1974), and Dunne and Wood (1975).

Interestingly, many of the regulatory enzymes which show ligand-induced oligomerization are cold labile proteins; i.e., exposure to 0°–4°C destabilizes their structure, leading to dissociation of the oligomeric proteins and inactivation (see Dunne and Wood, 1975, for specific details). The inactive 4 S monomer and the active 5 S dimer, whose structure is dependent on estradiol and temperature, are analogous in their molecular behavior to the oligomerizing enzymes, whose structure and biochemical activity are also ligand mediated and temperature dependent. Our results on the behavior of the human estrogen receptor emphasize the necessity to centrifuge at elevated temperatures in order to prevent the cold-induced dissociation of its dimer structure (Section IV,C).

The kinetics of a ligand-modulated oligomerization reaction can be more complex than that from an allosteric model of enzyme regulation. A protein whose activity is dependent upon an equilibrium between a monomer and a dimer also has activity dependent upon the total enzyme or receptor concentration, in the absence and presence of the ligand. Presumably, dimer formation serves to stabilize the activated conformation, having a buffering effect on the activation process, to provide a more linear response with ligand concentration.

VI. CONCLUSION

We propose the following *in vivo* regulating model for receptor activation. Three separate molecular interactions are present, each with an equilibrium that influences the final product: the formation of the 5 S EBP dimer (Fig. 14). The 4 S EBP is associated with a macromolecular inhibitor Y, in an inactive conformation confined to the cytoplasmic compartment [Fig. 14 (1)]. The binding of estradiol to the 4 S EBP serves to shift the 4 S EBP from its inhibited complex to an unobstructive 4 S EBP-estradiol complex available for the formation of the 5 S EBP [Fig. 14 (2)]. The final equilibrium is between the 4 S EBP and its complementary monomer (E-?), forming the 5 S EBP dimer [Fig. 14 (3)]. This last equilibrium may be

2. Conformational Forms of the Estrogen Receptor

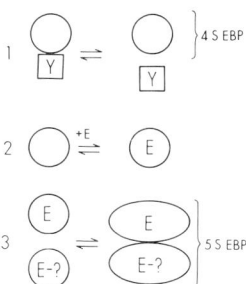

Fig. 14. A hypothetical model of the regulatory interactions of the estrogen receptor *in vivo*. The 4 S EBP in equilibrium with a macromolecule (inhibitor Y) is predominantly in the cytoplasmic compartment (1). Estradiol binding by the 4 S EBP favors the dissociation of the 4 S EBP from the inhibitor Y (2). The 4 S receptor can now dimerize with itself or with a dissimilar monomer to form the 5 S EBP dimer, which translocates into the nucleus (3). Step (2), estradiol binding, serves to shift the equilibrium from an inhibitory oligomeric conformation (1) to an oligomeric conformation (the 5 S EBP) with enhanced biochemical activity.

initiated in the cytoplasm, but could be present in the nuclear compartment as well. Thus, the formation of the 5 S EBP is dependent upon the three equilibrium constants and the concentration of each reactant.

The conversion of the receptor from a dormant to a biochemically active macromolecule, by estradiol, is an essential event in estrogen action. From a variety of experimental evidence, the analysis of the estrogen receptor structure has provided a plausible model for understanding its regulatory mechanism.

ACKNOWLEDGMENT

Investigations described in this report were supported by Research Grant HD 06707 from the National Institute of Child Health and Human Development.

REFERENCES

André, J., and Rochefort, H. (1973). *FEBS Lett.* **32**, 330.
Baulieu, E. E. (1975). *Biochem. Pharmacol.* **24**, 1743.
Baulieu, E. E., Alberga, A., Jung, I., Lebeau, M. C., Mercier-Bodard, C., Milgrom, E., Raynaud, J. P., Raynaud-Jammet, C., Rochefort, H., Truong, H., and Robel, P. (1971). *Recent Prog. Horm. Res.* **27**, 351.
Bresciani, F., Nola, E., Sica, V., and Puca, G. A. (1973). *Fed. Proc., Fed. Am. Soc. Exp. Biol.* **32**, 2126.
Buller, R. E., and O'Malley, B. W. (1976). *Biochem. Pharmacol.* **25**, 1.

Buller, R. E., Toft, D. O., Schrader, W. T., and O'Malley, B. W. (1975). *J. Biol. Chem.* **250**, 801.
Chakrabarti, U., and Kenkare, U. W. (1974). *J. Biol. Chem.* **249**, 5984.
Chamness, G. G., Jennings, A. W., and McGuire, W. L. (1974). *Biochemistry* **13**, 327.
De Sombre, E. R., Mohla, S., and Jensen, E. V. (1972). *Biochem. Biophys. Res. Commun.* **48**, 1601.
Dunne, C. D., and Wood, W. A. (1975). *Curr. Top. Cell. Regul.* **9**, 65.
Edelman, I. S. (1975). *J. Steroid Biochem.* **6**, 147.
Erdos, T. (1968). *Biochem. Biophys. Res. Commun.* **32**, 338.
Erdos, T., and Fries, J. (1974). *Biochem. Biophys. Res. Commun.* **58**, 932.
Frieden, C. (1971). *Annu. Rev. Biochem.* **40**, 653.
Funkhouser, J. D., Abraham, A., Smith, A., and Smith, W. G. (1974). *J. Biol. Chem.* **249**, 5478.
Gerlt, J. A., Rabinowitz, K. W., Dunne, C. P., and Wood, W. A. (1973). *J. Biol. Chem.* **248**, 2800.
Giannopoulos, G. (1975). *J. Biol. Chem.* **250**, 2904.
Giannopoulos, G., and Gorski, J. (1971). *J. Biol. Chem.* **246**, 2524.
Gorell, T. A., De Sombre, E. R., and Jensen, E. V. (1974). *Fed. Proc., Fed. Am. Soc. Exp. Biol.* **33**, 1511.
Gorski, J., and Gannon, F. (1976). *Annu. Rev. Biochem.* **38**, 425.
Gorski, J., Toft, D., Shyamalä, G., Smith, D., and Notides, A. (1968). *Recent Prog. Horm. Res.* **24**, 45.
Higgins, S. J., Rousseau, G. G., Baxter, J. D., and Tomkins, G. M. (1973). *J. Biol. Chem.* **248**, 5866.
Hille, M. B., Barrett, A. J., Dingle, J. T., and Fell, H. B. (1970). *Exp Cell Res.* **61**, 470.
Jensen, E. V., and De Sombre, E. R. (1973). *Science* **182**, 126.
Jensen, E. V., Suzuki, T., Kawashima, T., Stumpf, W. E., Jungblut, P. W., and De Sombre, E. R. (1968). *Proc. Natl. Acad. Sci. U.S.A.* **59**, 632.
Jensen, E. V., Suzuki, T., Numata, M., Smith, S., and De Sombre, E. R. (1969). *Steroids* **13**, 417.
Jensen, E. V., Numata, M., Brecher, P. I., and De Sombre, E. R. (1971). *Biochem. Soc. Symp.* **32**, 133.
Jensen, E. V., Mohla, S., Brecher, P. I., and De Sombre, E. R. (1973). *Adv. Exp. Med. Biol.* **36**, 60.
Jensen, E. V., Mohla, S., Gorell, T. A., and De Sombre, E. R. (1974). *Vitam. Horm. (N.Y.)* **32**, 89.
Klotz, I. M., Darnall, D. W., and Langerman, N. R. (1975). *In* "The Proteins" (H. Neurath and R. L. Hill, eds.), 3rd ed., Vol. 1, pp. 293–411. Academic Press, New York.
Korenman, S. G., and Rao, B. R. (1968). *Proc. Natl. Acad. Sci. U.S.A.* **69**, 3247.
Koshland, D. E., Jr., Némethy, G., and Filmer, D. (1966). *Biochemistry* **5**, 365.
Kuhn, R. W., Schrader, W. T., Smith, R. G., and O'Malley, B. W. (1975). *J. Biol. Chem.* **250**, 4220.
Liao, S. (1975). *Int. Rev. Cytol.* **40**, 87.
Little, M., Szendro, P., Teran, C., Hughes, A., and Jungblut, P. W. (1975). *J. Steroid Biochem.* **6**, 493.
Lohmar, P. H., and Toft, D. O. (1975). *Biochem. Biophys. Res. Commun.* **67**, 8.
Markus, G. (1965). *Proc. Natl. Acad. Sci. U.S.A.* **54**, 253.
Milgrom, E., Atger, M., and Baulieu, E. (1973). *Biochemistry* **12**, 5198.
Mohla, S., De Sombre, E. R., and Jensen, E. V. (1972). *Biochem. Biophys. Res. Commun.* **46**, 661.

Monod, J., Wyman, J., and Changeux, J. P. (1965). *J. Mol. Biol.* **12,** 88.
Mueller, G. C., Vonderhaar, B., Kim, U. H., and Le Mahieu, M. (1972). *Recent Prog. Horm. Res.* **28,** 1.
Nielsen, S., and Notides, A. C. (1975). *Biochim. Biophys. Acta* **381,** 377.
Notides, A. C., and Nielsen, S. (1974). *J. Biol. Chem.* **249,** 1866.
Notides, A. C., and Nielsen, S. (1975). *J. Steroid Biochem.* **6,** 483.
Notides, A. C., Hamilton, D. E., and Rudolph, J. H. (1972). *Biochim. Biophys. Acta* **271,** 214.
Notides, A. C., Hamilton, D. E., and Rudolph, J. H. (1973). *Endocrinology* **93,** 210.
Notides, A. C., Hamilton, D. E., and Auer, H. E. (1975). *J. Biol. Chem.* **250,** 3945.
Notides, A. C., Hamilton, D. E., and Muechler, E. K. (1976). *J. Steroid Biochem.* **7,** 1025.
O'Malley, B. W., Schrader, W. T., and Spelsberg, T. C. (1973). *Adv. Exp. Med. Biol.* **36,** 174.
Phillips, A. T. (1974). *Crit. Rev. Biochem.* **2,** 343.
Puca, G. A., Nola, E., Sica, V., and Bresciani, F. (1971). *Biochemistry* **10,** 3769.
Puca, G. A., Nola, E., Sica, V., and Bresciani, F. (1972). *Biochemistry* **11,** 4157.
Raynaud-Jammet, C., and Baulieu, E. E. (1969). *C. R. Hebd. Seances Acad. Sci., Ser. D* **268,** 3211.
Roark, D. E., and Yphantis, D. A. (1969). *Ann. N.Y. Acad. Sci.* **164,** 245.
Ruh, T. S., Katzenellenbogen, B. S., Katzenellenbogen, J. A., and Gorski, J. (1973). *Endocrinology* **92,** 125.
Samuels, H. H., and Tomkins, G. M. (1970). *J. Mol. Biol.* **52,** 57.
Schrader, W. T., and O'Malley, B. W. (1972). *J. Biol. Chem.* **247,** 51.
Sherman, M. R., Atienza, S. B. P., Shansky, J. R., and Hoffman, L. M. (1974). *J. Biol. Chem.* **249,** 5351.
Sherman, M. R., Tuazon, F. B., Diaz, S. C., and Miller, L. K. (1976). *Biochemistry* **15,** 980.
Shyamala, G., and Gorski, J. (1969). *J. Biol. Chem.* **244,** 1097.
Siegel, L. M., and Monty, K. J. (1966). *Biochim. Biophys. Acta* **112,** 346.
Siiteri, P. K., Schwarz, B. E., Moriyama, I., Ashby, R., Linkie, D., and MacDonald, P. C. (1973). *Adv. Exp. Med. Biol.* **36,** 97.
Simons, S. S., Martinez, H. M., Garcea, R. L., Baxter, J. D., and Tomkins, G. M. (1976). *J. Biol. Chem.* **251,** 334.
Sober, J. A., ed. (1968). "Handbook of Biochemistry." Chem. Rubber Publ. Co., Cleveland, Ohio.
Spelsberg, T. C., Steggles, A. W., Chytil, F., and O'Malley, B. W. (1972). *J. Biol. Chem.* **247,** 1368.
Stancel, G. M., Leung, K. M. T., and Gorski, J. (1973a). *Biochemistry* **12,** 2130.
Stancel, G. M., Leung, K. M. T., and Gorski, J. (1973b). *Biochemistry* **12,** 2137.
Toft, D., and Gorski, J. (1966). *Proc. Natl. Acad. Sci. U.S.A.* **55,** 1574.
Toft, D., Shyamala, G., and Gorski, J. (1967). *Proc. Natl. Acad. Sci. U.S.A.* **57,** 1740.
Van Holde, K. E. (1975). *In* "The Proteins" (H. Neurath and R. L. Hill, eds.), 3rd ed., Vol. 1, pp. 225–291. Academic Press, New York.
Vonderhaar, B. K., Kim, U. H., and Mueller, G. C. (1970). *Biochim. Biophys. Acta* **215,** 125.
Williams, D., and Gorski, J. (1971). *Biochem. Biophys. Res. Commun.* **45,** 258.
Williams, D., and Gorski, J. (1972). *Proc. Natl. Acad. Sci. U.S.A.* **69,** 3464.
Williams, D., and Gorski, J. (1973). *Biochemistry* **12,** 297.
Williams, D., and Gorski, J. (1974). *Biochemistry* **13,** 5537.
Wyss, R. H., Heinrichs, W. L., and Herrmann, W. L. (1968). *J. Clin. Endocrinol. Metab.* **28,** 1227.
Yamamoto, K. R., and Alberts, B. (1972). *Proc. Natl. Acad. Sci. U.S.A.* **69,** 2105.
Zito, R., Antonini, E., and Wyman, J. (1964). *J. Biol. Chem.* **239,** 1804.

3

Nuclear Estrogen Receptor and DNA Synthesis

F. STORMSHAK, J. N. HARRIS, AND J. GORSKI

I.	Introduction	63
II.	Estrogen and the Cell Cycle	64
	A. Duration of the Cell Cycle	64
	B. Biochemical Characteristics of the Prereplicative (G_1) Phase	66
	C. The S Phase: Nuclear Estrogen and DNA Synthesis	67
	D. DNA Polymerase in Estrogen-Stimulated DNA Synthesis	70
III.	Dynamics of DNA Synthesis in Response to Sequential Injections of Estrogen	73
IV.	Antimitotic Effects of Estrogen	78
V.	Conclusions	79
	References	79

I. INTRODUCTION

Cell division is commonly accepted as the terminal event of *in vivo* estrogen action on the target tissue. In fact, knowledge of the ability of estrogens to provoke extensive hyperplasia of target tissues was acquired (Allen *et al.*, 1924, 1937) long before the molecular basis of the mechanism of action of this hormone was elucidated in the mid-1960's. The discovery that the estrogen molecule is bound by a cytoplasmic receptor (Toft and Gorski, 1966) which translocates the hormone to the nucleus (Jensen *et al.*, 1968; Gorski *et al.*, 1968) led to the concept that the nucleus was the primary site of action of this steroid. One might expect discovery of this intracellular translocation phenomenon to be followed by a host of studies whose objectives would be to define the specific estrogen-induced biochemical events which are requisite for DNA synthesis and cell division. A survey of the literature, however, reveals that this has not been the case. Rather, it appears that research efforts during the past decade have focused on characterization of the physical properties of the cytoplasmic and nuclear forms of the receptor protein and the nature and quantitative aspects of various early responses of the cell to estrogen. Since a number of these responses appear to be the consequence of the ability of estrogen to regulate gene expression (Mueller *et al.*, 1972), it is not surprising that considerable more research effort has been devoted to identification of the putative DNA or chromatin acceptor site(s) of this hormone than to the mechanisms regulating DNA synthesis.

In light of our current understanding of the cell cycle, it is perhaps fortuitous that extensive investigations have been conducted to elucidate the early responses of the cell to estrogen. It has been demonstrated that synthesis of DNA is preceded and dependent upon a relatively long period of prereplicative biochemical and cytological changes. This association raises a number of questions regarding the relationship of nuclear estrogen to DNA synthesis. To what extent are the early responses of the estrogen-stimulated cell necessary for DNA synthesis? Is the synthesis of DNA the terminal event of a chain reaction initiated by entry of the hormone into the nucleus, or is the continual presence of nuclear estrogen necessary to ensure synthesis of this macromolecule?

In what follows, an attempt has been made to provide answers to these questions by drawing upon the experimental results of a number of investigators, as well as the authors' own research endeavors in this area. The majority of the experimental results on the relationship of nuclear estrogen to DNA synthesis have been obtained, using as a model the rat and mouse uterus or the chick oviduct. Where relevant, results on the effect of estrogen on the mammary gland will also be included.

II ESTROGEN AND THE CELL CYCLE

A. Duration of the Cell Cycle

The concept of the cell cycle as first introduced by Howard and Pelc (1953) and subsequently expanded by Quastler (1963), consists of the following stages of interphase; G_1, that period during which the cell prepares for DNA synthesis through increased synthesis of RNA and protein; S, the period during which DNA synthesis occurs; G_2, the period following DNA synthesis and during which RNA and protein are synthesized in preparation for M or mitosis. Apparently, cells may pass into a resting stage after mitosis (commonly designated as G_0) or after DNA synthesis (Frankfurt, 1967) from which they may be stimulated to reenter the cell cycle or undergo irreversible changes and gradually proceed towards death. There is some controversy over the existence of a distinct G_0 stage. The argument has been advanced that no biochemical characteristics relevant to the onset of DNA synthesis and cell division have been identified for cells to serve as a basis for such a classification (Baserga, 1968, 1971). Consequently, it has been proposed that the so-called G_0 cell may be an arrested G_1 cell (Baserga, 1971). Regardless of whether the resting cell is in a unique stage of the cycle or merely arrested in G_1, for purposes of this presentation a resting cell will be considered as one which is capable of being provoked by hormonal stimulation to undergo preparations for DNA synthesis.

For a number of years, it was erroneously assumed that the duration of the S phase of the cell cycle was constant from tissue to tissue within the various mammalian species (Cameron and Greulich, 1963; Pilgrim and Maurer, 1965; Thrasher and Greulich, 1965). It is noteworthy that research involving the use of ovarian hormones was instrumental in refuting this dogma. Using a double labeling technique with [^{3}H]thymidine and [^{14}C]thymidine, Bresciani (1964, 1965) found that the duration of the S phase in alveolar cells of the mammary glands of C_3H mice varied from 14.8 to 27.6 hours, with an average of 20.1 hours. Daily administration of 1 μg of estradiol-17β and 1 mg of progesterone to ovariectomized mice for 3–4 days reduced the duration of the S phase in alveolar cells to between 9.5 and 11.9 hours, with an average of 10.7 hours. Similar results were obtained when dosages of hormones were increased by a factor of 10 and treatment extended over a period of 2–3 weeks. Results of these studies suggested that the duration of the S phase could be reduced to a minimum. In addition, Bresciani (1965) found that, under the influence of hormones, the duct cells of the mammary gland had a longer S phase than the alveolar cells, suggesting that the minimum duration of DNA synthesis can be a characteristic of the cell type.

Extensive studies have been conducted on the effects of estrogen on the cell cycle of the uterine epithelium. In ovariectomized mice, the duration of G_1, S, G_2, and M in uterine surface epithelium was found to be 31.5, 8.5, 1, and 1 hour, respectively (Epifanova, 1966). Treatment of ovariectomized mice with two injections of 2.5 μg of estrone at 24-hour intervals caused a threefold increase in the proliferating pool of uterine epithelial cells capable of DNA synthesis. A 1.5-fold reduction in the duration of the cell cycle occurred at the expense of the G_1 and S periods, which were reduced to 18.5 and 5.5 hours, respectively. This observed reduction in the duration of the cell cycle cannot be attributed to dosage or nature of estrogen administered, since Das (1972) reported a similar decrease in the S phase in uterine epithelium of ovariectomized mice following injection with 0.1 μg of estradiol-17β.

The results of these studies leave little doubt that estrogen can reduce the duration of the cell cycle. This means that the presence of estrogen stimulates all the prereplicative preparations and the actual synthesis of DNA in the uterine epithelial cell in approximately one-half the time normally required for these processes. How does estrogen act to promote this reduction in the duration of the G_1 and S periods? It may be hypothesized that estrogen acts to accelerate the rate of synthesis of certain essential substrates and enzymes during these periods of the cell cycle. In the absence of hormone, the population of spontaneously dividing cells is very small, thus precluding their use as a control for identification of the key reaction(s) by which estrogen is able to reduce the duration of these phases of the cell cycle. Nevertheless, the estrogen-provoked biochemical events that occur during the G_1 and S phases may be examined in light of their significance to the synthesis of DNA.

B. Biochemical Characteristics of the Prereplicative (G_1) Phase

As a general rule, among the sequence of biochemical events that characterize the G_1 period, the synthesis of RNA and protein appear to be particularly essential for the subsequent onset of DNA synthesis in a number of cell types (Baserga, 1968). Experimental evidence on the early responses of the target cell to estrogen suggests that this cell is no exception to the rule. The initial studies by Mueller *et al.* (1958), demonstrating that the injection of estrogen stimulated increases in rat uterine RNA and protein, were instrumental in paving the way for a number of subsequent investigations on the mechanism of action of estrogen on the synthesis of these cellular constituents. The results of these latter studies have been reviewed by Hamilton (1968) and, more recently, by O'Malley and Means (1974).

There can be little doubt that the early estrogen-stimulated responses are necessary for the transformation of the resting cell to one which is competent for undergoing DNA synthesis and division. However, it is conceivable that many of the observed initial responses of the cell to estrogen are related more to hypertrophy of the cell than to subsequent DNA synthesis. This is supported by the observations of Gelfant *et al.* (1955) who found that concomitant administration of estrogen and the mitotic inhibitor aminopterin to ovariectomized rats permitted hypertrophy of the uterine epithelial cells in the absence of hyperplasia. This then suggests the possibility that some unique, and as yet unidentified cellular event, occurs during

C. The S Phase: Nuclear Estrogen and DNA Synthesis

It has been demonstrated that the initiation of DNA synthesis requires the synthesis of new RNA and protein. Mueller et al. (1962) found that HeLa cells grown in culture could be synchronized to begin DNA synthesis by the induction and subsequent reversal of a thymidineless state. The addition of thymidine to the culture resulted in an accelerated increase in DNA synthesis. The simultaneous addition to the culture medium of thymidine and actinomycin D (Mueller, 1963) or puromycin (Mueller et al., 1962; Mueller, 1963) blocked DNA synthesis, suggesting that this phenomenon is dependent upon the synthesis of new RNA and protein. Once RNA synthesis had been initiated, the addition of actinomycin D or puromycin failed to completely inhibit the synthesis of this macromolecule but did block cell division (Mueller, 1963). Using a similar technique involving the culture of human oral carcinoma cells, Taylor (1965) found that the ability of actinomycin D or puromycin to block DNA synthesis occurred without altering the synthesis of DNA polymerase or thymidine kinase. Thus, these latter data also are in support of the concept that initiation of DNA synthesis requires the synthesis of a new protein. It can be argued that the intimate relationship between RNA and protein synthesis and the synthesis of DNA may simply be a characteristic of an abnormal cell type. However, investigations on other cell types *in vitro* (Lieberman et al., 1963) and *in vivo* (Estensen and Baserga, 1966) have also indicated that DNA synthesis is dependent upon RNA and protein synthesis.

As determined by the use of [^{3}H]thymidine, Kaye et al. (1972) found that a single injection of estradiol into the immature rat stimulated an increase in uterine DNA synthesis by 18 hours after treatment. Maximal synthesis of DNA occurred by 24 hours and then subsided to control levels by 36 hours after treatment. Although uterine DNA synthesis is maximal at 24 hours after treatment, increases in uterine DNA are not yet detectable at this time (Mueller et al., 1958; Mueller, 1960; Kaye et al., 1972).

Kaye et al. (1972) also reported that the simultaneous injection of 10 μg of actinomycin D with estradiol caused an 8–15% reduction in RNA and a 45% decrease in DNA synthesis as determined at 24 hours after injection. It is likely that the observed actinomycin D-induced reduction in DNA synthesis was a consequence of an overall diminution in the early synthesis of RNA that occurs during the prereplicative phase of the cell cycle and may even be attributed, in part, to subsequent cell death. Thus, for example actinomycin D (Ui and Mueller, 1963), as well as puromycin (Mueller *et al.,* 1961) and cycloheximide (Gorski and Axman, 1964), have been demonstrated to be effective inhibitors of early uterine RNA and protein synthesis. Critical experiments have not been conducted to determine what effect administration of these RNA and protein synthesis inhibitors during the late prereplicative phase of the estrogen-stimulated uterine cell would have on DNA synthesis.

The increases in macromolecular synthesis which occur during the S phase in the estrogen-treated immature rat uterus are accompanied by increases in glucose transport and phosphorylation consistent with the increased energy demand of the cells. Using the labeled glucose analogue, 2-deoxyglucose, Gorski and Raker (1974) found that conversion of 2-deoxyglucose to 2-deoxyglucose 6-phosphate in the uterus of the estrogen treated immature rat was biphasic. *In vitro* conversion of 2-deoxyglucose to 2-deoxyglucose 6-phosphate by uteri was maximal at 2 and 18 hours after a single injection of estradiol. The latter time of increased phosphorylation of this analogue of glucose coincides with the time of increased DNA synthesis.

Gorski and Raker (1974) also reported that a dose of 0.04 μg of estriol is only partially effective in stimulating early responses of the immature rat uterus, whereas a dose of 1 μg of estriol results in a maximal response. Injection of the immature rat with 0.1 μg of estriol has little effect on DNA synthesis as determined 18 hours after treatment, and injection of 1 μg of estriol results in only a partial enhancement of DNA synthesis (Fig. 1A,B; Stormshak *et al.,* 1976). Anderson *et al.* (1975) have also found that single injections of estriol fail to promote uterine cellular proliferation. If administration of 1 μg of estriol is followed 6 hours later with an injection of 1 μg of estradiol-17β, maximal synthesis of DNA occurs at 18 hours, which is comparable in magnitude to that observed when only estradiol is given as the initial treatment. Although 1 μg of estriol is similar to estradiol in stimulating the early (0–6 hours) uterine responses (Gorski and Raker, 1974), it alone is unable to induce DNA synthesis to the fullest extent. Estriol is not retained in the uterine cell as long as estradiol and the equilibrium constant of estriol is only about one-half that of estradiol, suggesting a more rapid rate of dissociation for this estrogen (Gorski and Raker, 1974; Anderson *et al.,* 1975). Consequently, the induction of DNA synthesis by estrogen appears to require the presence of this steroid in the cell for periods in excess of 6 hours after injection.

The enzymes essential for regulation of DNA synthesis and their properties have been recently summarized by Keir and Craig (1973). Generally, information on the activity of these enzymes in relation to

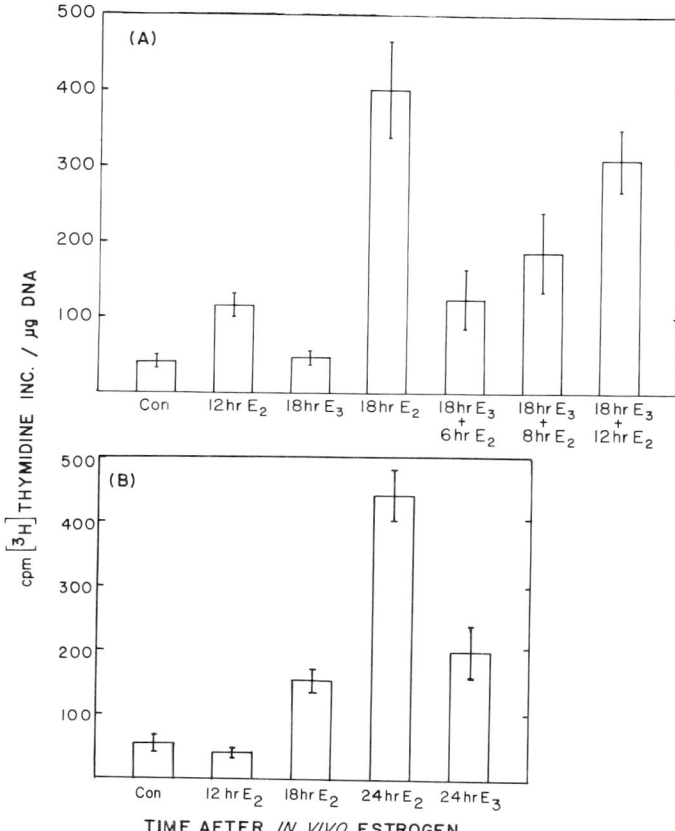

Fig. 1. (A) Changes in uterine DNA synthesis of immature rats following a single injection of 0.1 μg of estriol (E_3) or 1 μg of estradiol-17β (E_2) or 0.1 μg of estriol followed by a single injection of 1 μg of estradiol-17β at 6, 8, or 12 hours prior to sacrifice. Animals were sacrificed at 12 or 18 hours after the initial injection of estriol or estradiol. Incorporation of [^{3}H]thymidine into DNA was determined by incubating the uteri *in vitro* at 37°C for 1 hour. Mean ± SE based on six animals per group. (B) Effect of a single injection of 1 μg of estriol (E_3) or estradiol-17β (E_2) on uterine DNA synthesis at 12, 18, and 24 hours after treatment of immature rats. Mean ± SE based on eight animals per group. (From Stormshak *et al.*, 1976).

estrogen-provoked stimulation of DNA synthesis is, for the most part, lacking. However, Leake *et al.* (1975) have reported that estrogen-stimulated synthesis of DNA in the uterus of the immature rat is accompanied by a parallel increase in thymidine kinase activity. The role of the DNA polymerases in the synthesis of DNA is of particular interest and is discussed below.

D. DNA Polymerase in Estrogen-Stimulated DNA Synthesis

Deoxyribonucleic acid-dependent DNA polymerases (deoxyribonucleosidetriphosphate:DNA deoxynucleotidyltransferase, EC 2.7.7.7) from animal cells have been studied intensively during the last 15 years. Several recent, excellent reviews covering our present knowledge of eukaryotic DNA polymerases are available (Bollum, 1975; Fansler, 1974; Holmes and Johnston, 1975). Only a brief overview of the molecular species described in animal cells and their possible roles in cell proliferation will be presented here. Of the four separate molecular species of DNA polymerases identified in most eukaryotic cells, two are minor activities. Deoxyribonucleic acid polymerase γ (an RNA-directed DNA polymerase activity) and the mitochondrial DNA polymerase together account for a small percentage of the total cellular activity. Deoxyribonucleic acid polymerase α is a high molecular weight enzyme (130,000–450,000) and is the principal activity in rapidly proliferating tissue. Tissue levels of DNA polymerase α fluctuate with the rate of DNA synthesis, and, from this correlation and other characteristics (see references above), it is implicated as having some role in nuclear DNA replication. Deoxyribonucleic acid polymerase β, a low molecular weight enzyme (40,000–50,000), does not fluctuate appreciably in correlation with cellular DNA synthesis and may have some function in DNA repair. By normal aqueous cell fractionation procedures DNA polymerase α is found principally in the soluble cytosol fraction, while DNA polymerase β is located in the nuclear fraction. Recent data suggests this distribution may be artifactual. By using nonaqueous fractionation techniques (Foster and Gurney, 1974) or by using cytochalasin B isolated karyoplasts (Herrick *et al.,* 1976), it has been reported that over 85% of the total DNA polymerase activity was located in the nucleus. Thus, the apparent subcellular distribution using aqueous fractionation procedures may reflect only a relative affinity of DNA polymerase α for the nucleus or its "leakiness" from the nucleus as a function of changes during the cell cycle.

Although DNA polymerases have been studied in several animal and cell tissue culture systems, their function in estrogen-stimulated DNA synthesis has not been extensively examined. Results of early research suggested that estradiol-17α and -17β could directly stimulate partially purified calf thymus DNA polymerase activity, while diethylstilbestrol and other stilbestrol derivatives directly inhibited calf thymus DNA polymerase (Fahmy *et al.,* 1967; Fahmy and Griffiths, 1968). The concentration of steroids used in these studies (40 μM) were over 1300-fold higher than the estrogen concentration necessary to elicit maximal *in vitro* induction of the uterine induced-protein (IP) as reported by Katzenellenbogen and Gorski (1972).

3. Nuclear Estrogen Receptor and DNA Synthesis

Considering the known direct interactions of high concentrations of estrogens with nucleic acids (Ts'o and Lu, 1964), the meaning of this apparent direct estrogen effect is not clear.

In mouse mammary tissue, Banerjee et al. (1971) observed a sixfold increase in the levels of DNA polymerase activity following 48 hours of simultaneous *in vivo* treatment with estradiol-17β and progesterone. This increased DNA polymerase activity was measured in the post-microsomal supernatant fraction and, therefore, was apparently due to DNA polymerase α activity. Interestingly, if the hormones were administered by intraperitoneal injection as opposed to subcutaneously, increased activity was observed as early as 5–7 hours, which is much earlier than increased DNA synthesis is observed in other estrogen-dependent growth systems (Kaye et al., 1972; Oka and Schimke, 1969b).

Fowler et al. (1972) in screening various synthetic estrogenic compounds for the possible induction of Type C RNA virus markers in mouse uterine tissue reported that a DNA polymerase capable of utilizing poly(rA)·oligo(dT) as template primer was stimulated by *in vivo* treatment for 4 days with estradiol-17β. This estrogen-induced polymerase activity was inhibited by antiserum which was also effective in inhibiting mouse leukemia viral RNA-directed DNA polymerase. It was suggested by the authors that the estrogen-stimulated DNA polymerase was an RNA-directed DNA polymerase similar to viral "reverse transcriptase". The ability of DNA polymerases β and γ in several animal tissues to utilize poly(rA)·oligo(dT) as template primer (Bollum, 1975; Fansler, 1974) makes the identification of this estrogen-induced DNA polymerase from the mouse uterus as being a true reverse transcriptase tentative until further characterization.

In a recent report, Schmelck et al. (1975) observed increased DNA polymerase activities in both nuclear and cytoplasmic fractions of estrogen-restimulated chick oviduct. Two- to fivefold increases in both cell fractions were detected 12 hours following estrogen treatment of estrogen-primed chicks. Both cytosol and nuclear DNA polymerases were of high molecular weight as judged by sucrose-density gradient analysis with no change in sedimentation due to hormone treatment. The authors did not state, however, if gradient analysis was performed under high ionic strength conditions, which has been shown to be necessary to resolve aggregation phenomena (Wang et al., 1975; Sedwick et al., 1975). Rohde et al. (1975) examined DNA polymerase activities in the quail oviduct during primary estrogen stimulation and secondary restimulation and found similar increases in activity at both times.

When DNA polymerase activities were examined in the estrogen-stimulated immature rat uterus, increases in both cytoplasmic and nuclear tissue fractions were observed (Harris and Gorski, 1976). The increases in DNA polymerase activities observed followed a time course similar to the kinetics of increased rates of DNA synthesis with no increase observed until 18 hours following a single intraperitoneal injection of estradiol-17β, reaching maximal stimulation between 24 and 30 hours, and then decreasing slowly to near control levels by 72 hours. Cytosol fractions showed the largest stimulation, with from three- to fivefold increases in DNA polymerase activity, while DNA polymerase activity in the high-salt nuclear extract increased twofold. Maximal stimulation was achieved with a dose of 0.1 μg estradiol-17β, while treatment with estradiol-17α or testosterone gave no stimulation. Progesterone (0.1 mg per rat) resulted in a small stimulation of both cytoplasmic and nuclear DNA polymerase activity, but when combined with estradiol-17β, resulted in a small but significant reduction of the full estrogen response (Fig. 2). A similar but more pronounced reduction of the estrogen response by simultaneous progesterone treatment was observed in the restimulated chick oviduct (Schmelck *et al.*, 1975).

In order to determine if RNA synthesis was required for this estradiol-stimulated increase in DNA polymerase activity, rats were injected with a high dose of actinomycin D (440 μg per rat) at various times following estrogen treatment, and the increase in enzyme activity was determined 18 hours later. As shown in Fig. 3, the increases in DNA polymerase activities observed 18 hours after estrogen treatment were not affected by actinomycin D during the last 6 hours of hormone stimulation but were sensitive to the drug for the first 10 hours. A simple interpretation of this

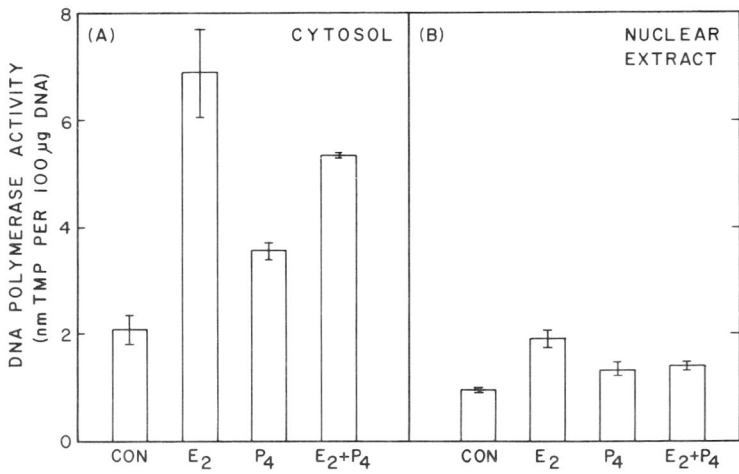

Fig. 2. Cytosol (A) and nuclear extract (B) DNA polymerase activity 24 hours following intraperitoneal injection of 1 μg of estradiol-17β (E_2), 0.1 mg of progesterone (P_4) subcutaneously, or a combination of steroids. Mean ± SE based on four rats per group.

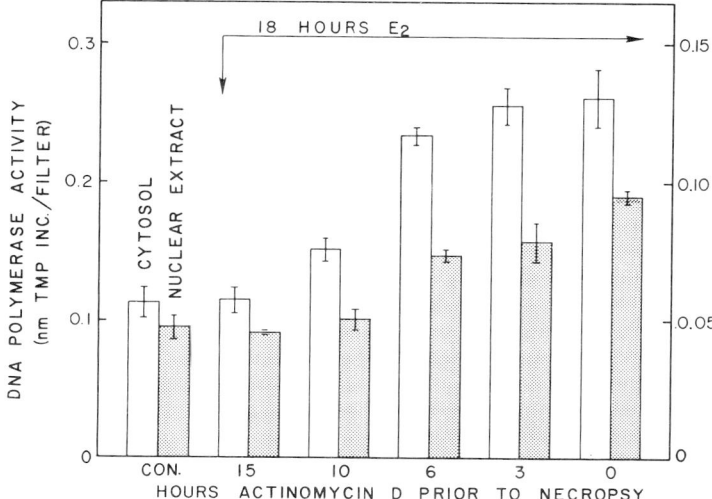

Fig. 3. Inhibition of estradiol-17β (E_2) stimulated DNA polymerase activity by actinomycin D. Control (Con) rats received saline vehicle only. All other groups received 1 μg E_2, and DNA polymerase activity was determined 18 hours later after rats received actinomycin D (440 μg/rat) for the indicated time prior to necropsy. Mean ± SE based on four rats per group.

experiment would be that the mRNA template for *de novo* synthesis of DNA polymerase enzymes occurs primarily during the first 10 hours following hormone treatment. However, the duration of this *in vivo* treatment resulted in drastic systemic effects on the animals (including some mortality by 15 hours of drug treatment). Therefore, conclusions regarding these data must be considered as speculative without more direct evidence.

The cytoplasmic and nuclear DNA polymerase activities from the estrogen-stimulated uterus have been characterized by both sucrose-gradient analysis in the presence of 0.5 M NaCl and by ion exchange chromatography, using DEAE–cellulose. The cytosol contains only high molecular weight DNA polymerase α with a sedimentation coefficient of 7.6 S. The high-salt nuclear extract fraction contains both DNA polymerase α and low molecular weight DNA polymerase β, which has a sedimentation coefficient of 3.6 S (Harris and Gorski, 1976).

III. DYNAMICS OF DNA SYNTHESIS IN RESPONSE TO SEQUENTIAL INJECTIONS OF ESTROGEN

Bullough (1946) was the first to report the response of target cells to repeated injections of estrogen. When mice were given repeated injections of estrone at 12-hour intervals, mitoses of the uterine epithelium were found to increase after one and two injections of hormone and then to decline, until by six injections virtually none were detected. In a later study of a similar nature, Epifanova (1967) studied the rate of mitoses in the uterine epithelium of the mouse during the estrous cycle. Mitoses were found to be considerably greater during proestrus and the early stages of diestrus than during estrus and metestrus. In an attempt to mimic the changes in mitoses observed during estrus and metestrus of the estrous cycle, ovariectomized mice were injected daily with 2.5 μg of estrone for up to 10 days. Mitoses were maximal after two injections of estrone and then declined and remained at the control level for the duration of treatment. If, however, injections of estrone were discontinued after 5 days, there resulted a spontaneous increase in the number of mitoses similar in magnitude to that observed after two injections of estrone. Lee (1972) and Martin et $al.$ (1973) by injecting [^{3}H]thymidine into ovariectomized mice observed a similar pattern of incorporation of this pyrimidine nucleoside into uterine DNA during chronic treatment with estrogen. Likewise, a depressing effect of repeated injections of estradiol on mitoses of the cervical and vaginal epithelium of the neonatal mouse has been reported (Forsberg, 1970). Collectively, the results of these studies suggest that estrogen acts to initially stimulate and subsequently to suppress uterine cell division. The mitotic response of the chick oviduct epithelium to repeated injections of estrogen is, however, in striking contrast to that of the rodent uterus. Daily injection of 1 mg of estradiol-17β into immature chicks results in an increased number of mitoses and a continuous increase in oviductal DNA content, at least for the first 10 days of treatment (Oka and Schimke, 1969b; Socher and O'Malley, 1973). This response of the chick oviduct to repeated injections of estrogen is attributed to the hormone-stimulated differentiation of the surface epithelium into specific cell types, particularly tubular gland cells (Kohler et $al.$, 1969; Oka and Schimke, 1969a). Only when administration of estrogen is discontinued is there a reduction in cell division, but the DNA content of the oviduct never decreases to the level observed for that of the control chicks, suggesting that tubular gland cells persist in the absence of this hormone (Oka and Schimke, 1969b).

The observations of Bullough (1946) and Epifanova (1967) on the mitotic response of the mouse uterine epithelium to repeated injections of estrogen prompted investigations on the biochemical characteristics of the immature rat uterus following sequential injections of estrogen (Stormshak et $al.$, 1976). In these experiments, immature female rats received one injection or two or three sequential injections of estrogen. As determined by in $vitro$ incorporation of [^{3}H]thymidine into uterine DNA, a single intraperitoneal injection of 1 μg of estradiol-17β results in a maximal stimulation of DNA

3. Nuclear Estrogen Receptor and DNA Synthesis

synthesis by 24 hours (Fig. 4) which is comparable to the results of Kaye *et al.* (1972). The synthesis of DNA is reduced with each succeeding injection of estradiol. Thus, by 24 hours after three sequential injections of estradiol, the synthesis of uterine DNA is less than that observed for uteri of control animals. This pattern of DNA synthesis following repeated injections of estradiol is remarkably similar to the pattern of mitoses observed for the uteri of mice subjected to chronic estrogen treatment (Epifanova, 1967).

Since estrogen-stimulated uterine cells at 24 hours after the first injection of hormone are still in the process of preparing for replication, it is not surprising that uterine DNA content at this time is similar to that of control animals (Fig. 4). Only by 24 hours after two sequential injections of estradiol is there a marked increase in uterine DNA content, the quantity of which remains elevated through three sequential injections of hormone. Similar changes in DNA synthesis and uterine DNA content occur following sequential injections of 0.01 or 0.1 μg of estradiol. However, when two sequential injections of 0.01 μg of estradiol are followed by an injection of 1 μg of estradiol, the DNA synthesis as determined 24 hours later was similar in magnitude to that observed at 24 hours after only a single injection of 1 μg of estradiol. These data suggest that treatment of the immature rat with sequential injections of estradiol promotes a dose-dependent state of uterine "refractoriness" in which the target cells become unresponsive to further stimulation by this hormone.

In a subsequent experiment (Fig. 5), it was found that one injection of estriol and two sequential injections of estradiol or two sequential injections of estriol and one injection of estradiol failed to reduce DNA synthesis to the same extent as three sequential injections of estradiol. It appears,

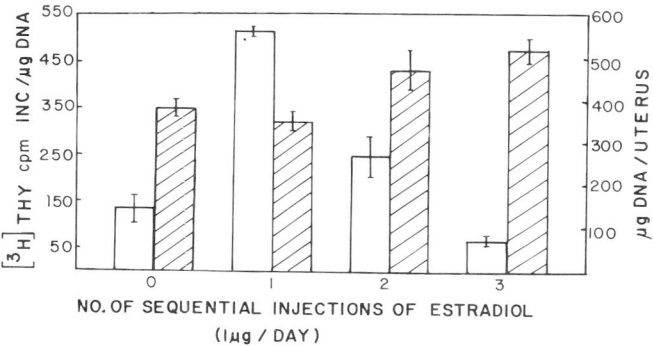

Fig. 4. Changes in uterine DNA synthesis (open bars) and DNA content (hatched bars) 24 hours after one injection or the last of two or three sequential injections of 1 μg of estradiol-17β given at 24-hour intervals. Mean ± SE based on four animals per group. (From Stormshak *et al.*, 1976).

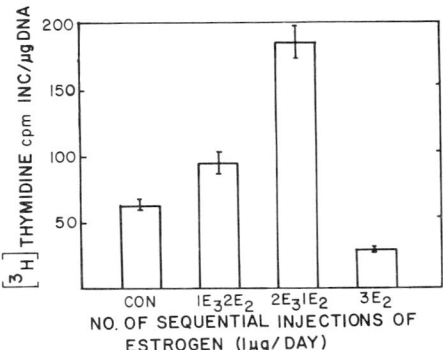

Fig. 5. Effect of sequential injections of 1 μg of estriol (E_3), 1 μg of estradiol-17β (E_2), or three sequential injections of 1 μg of estradiol-17β on uterine DNA synthesis of immature rats. Mean ± SE based on four animals per group. (From Stormshak et al., 1976).

therefore, that the sustained presence of estrogen is necessary to evoke this state of uterine unresponsiveness.

The interesting "refractory" response to chronic estrogen treatment observed with the rates of DNA synthesis in the uterus has also been observed with tissue levels of DNA polymerase activity. Rats were injected once daily for 3 days and the DNA polymerase activity measured after either 1, 2, or 3 days of estrogen stimulation. Nuclear DNA polymerase activity reached a maximum after only a single injection and decreased with further treatment, just as the rate of DNA synthesis decreased, as measured by [³H]thymidine incorporation *in vitro* (J. N. Harris and J. Gorski, unpublished observations). The cytoplasmic DNA polymerase activity did not reach a maximum until after 2 days of treatment, but then it too began to be depressed following 1 more day of treatment. The phenomenon of limited stimulation termed refractoriness in this chapter is of particular interest. In effect, the uterus demonstrates three metabolic states in terms of DNA synthesis and DNA polymerase activity: (a) the nonstimulated resting level, (b) the estrogen-stimulated state of increased activity, and (c) the refractory state after prolonged estrogen stimulation in which levels of DNA synthesis and DNA polymerase activity have returned to the lower resting levels. The refractory phenomenon would appear to be tissue specific. It has been reported that, following 7 days of chronic estrone treatment, pituitaries from male rats displayed a fivefold increase in cytoplasmic DNA polymerase activity and a slightly elevated rate of DNA synthesis in intact nuclei (Mastro and Hymer, 1973). These molecular events are consistent with the biology of these two tissues, as it has been long recognized that chronic estrogen administration can result in pituitary tumors in rats and mice (Furth and Clifton, 1966). This is in contrast to the

3. Nuclear Estrogen Receptor and DNA Synthesis

limited DNA synthetic and DNA polymerase response of uterine tissue, due to multiple doses of estradiol reported here and the lack of an oncogenic response of the rat uterus following chronic estrogen treatment.

It has recently been reported that the antagonistic action of the antiestrogen nafoxidine hydrochloride can be attributed to the failure of this agent to promote the replenishment of the cytoplasmic estrogen receptor (Clark *et al.*, 1974). Apparently, nafoxidine hydrochloride causes the estrogen receptor to become trapped in the nucleus for prolonged periods (Clark *et al.*, 1973). In order to determine whether sequential injections of estrogen altered the amount of cytoplasmic receptor available, uteri of immature rats were removed 24 hours after one or the last of two or three sequential injections of 1 μg of estradiol-17β and the *in vitro* translocation of estrogen–receptor complex into the nucleus determined. Specifically bound nuclear estradiol in uteri of treated animals was, in all cases, greater than or equal to nuclear bound estradiol in uteri of control animals (Fig. 6). Further, as determined by the estrogen-exchange assay of Anderson *et al.* (1972), there was no indication that specifically bound nuclear estradiol measured 24 hours after one, two, or three sequential injections of estradiol was a result of the estradiol–receptor complex being trapped in the nucleus.

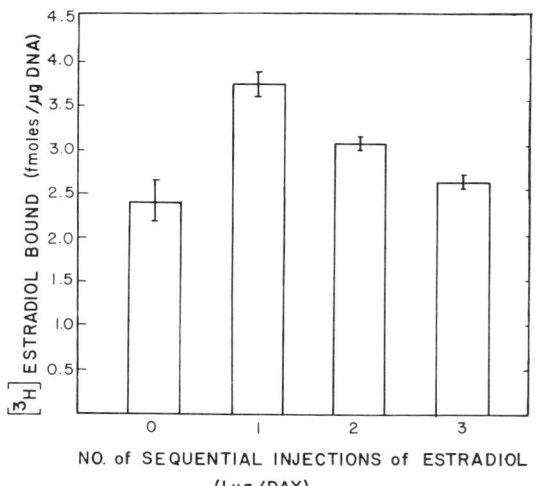

Fig. 6. Nuclear bound estradiol in uteri of immature rats 24 hours after treatment with one, two, or three sequential injections of 1 μg of estradiol-17β. Controls (0) were injected with vehicle only. Uteri were incubated *in vitro* for 1 hour at 37°C in Eagle's HeLa medium containing $1 \times 10^{-8}M$ [³H]estradiol or labeled estradiol and $1 \times 10^{-6}M$ diethylstilbestrol. Specifically bound estradiol was determined by difference. Mean ± SE based on four animals per group.

Thus, it appears that uterine refractoriness once induced is independent of the ability of the hormone to be translocated to the nucleus.

No comparable state of oviductal refractoriness has been reported to occur in the immature chick subjected to chronic estrogen treatment. Yet, in contrast to the failure of repeated injections of estrogen to effect a change in nuclear bound estrogen in the uterus of the rat, a similar treatment regime involving the use of diethylstilbestrol caused a substantial increase in the concentration of nuclear-bound estrogen in the oviduct of the chick during the first 6 days of treatment (Kalimi *et al.*, 1976). This period of treatment is coincident with the greatest growth and cellular differentiation of the oviduct (Oka and Schimke, 1969a,b). After 6 days of treatment, nuclear bound estrogen declined but never reached the concentration found in the oviduct of unstimulated chicks. Since cytoplasmic concentrations of receptor were not determined, it is not known to what extent, if any, the measured nuclear bound estrogen may have represented trapped estrogen–receptor complex in this cell organelle.

IV. ANTIMITOTIC EFFECTS OF ESTROGEN

Bullough (1946) suggested the existence of mitosis inhibitors to explain the reduction in uterine cell division in mice following chronic treatment with estrogen. These substances have come to be referred to as chalones (Bullough, 1973). The estrogen dose-dependent induction of a uterine refractory state may be due to the accumulation of some product which limits the ability of the cell to respond to additional estrogen. The extent or degree of refractoriness would depend on the amount of this product present in the cell. The presence of small amounts of this product, such as after estriol or low doses of estradiol, would render the cell only slightly refractory and capable of responding to additional estrogen.

The sustained presence of estrogen not only suppresses DNA polymerase and DNA synthesis, but also the general metabolic events which precede and are necessary for synthesis of this macromolecule, such as the synthesis of protein and the metabolism of glucose (Stormshak *et al.*, 1976). This is supported, in part, by the recent report of Katzenellenbogen (1975), who found that a very early uterine response to estrogen, the synthesis of a specific protein (IP) is not induced by injection of estrogen if the uterus has been previously exposed to this steroid. In agreement with the conclusions of Epifanova (1967), it appears that chronic estrogen treatment blocks the capacity of the target cell to pass from the resting or presynthetic phase into the S phase of the cell cycle.

V. CONCLUSIONS

Experimental evidence indicates that estrogen acts to reduce the duration of the cell cycle predominantly at the expense of the G_1 and S periods. Although the overall early responses of the target cell to estrogen are requisite for preparing the cell for subsequent replication, they are not solely able to promote the later responses, such as DNA synthesis. Thus, the initial entry of estrogen into the cell does not appear to precipitate a "domino" effect with the first response triggering a chain reaction, ultimately ending with synthesis of DNA and mitoses. Rather, it appears that a sustained presence of estrogen in the nucleus of the previously unstimulated cell is required to elicit maximal DNA synthesis and suggests that this latter process is dependent upon a specific estrogen-regulated event(s) which occurs during the G_1 period. Further research is needed to elucidate the time course and nature of this estrogen-induced event(s) which occurs during the prereplicative period.

In common with other paradoxical actions of estrogen in evoking biologic responses, it appears that this steroid can inhibit, as well as stimulate uterine cell proliferation. Continuous exposure of the uterine cell to estrogen results in a state of refractoriness characterized by failure of additional estrogen to provoke the overall synthesis of protein, DNA polymerase, and, hence, deoxyribonucleic acid. This estrogen-induced uterine refractoriness may be attributed to the emergence of some agent whose function is reminescent of that of a chalone and, thus, serves to regulate mitotic homeostasis. It is apparent, however, that uterine refractoriness, once induced, is not a consequence of impeded translocation of estrogen into the nucleus.

ACKNOWLEDGMENT

Supported in part by the College of Agricultural and Life Sciences, University of Wisconsin, Madison; Ford Foundation Grant 630-0505A; NIH Grant 5-T01-HD00104-10 awarded by the National Institutes of Child Health and Human Development; NIH Grant HD 08192 from the United States Public Health Service and Project No. 160671 from the Graduate School, University of Wisconsin, Madison.

REFERENCES

Allen, E., Francis, B. F., Robertson, L. L., Colgate, C. E., Johnston, C. G., Doisy, E. A., Kountz, W. B., and Gibson. H. V. (1924). *Am. J. Anat.* **34,** 133–181.

Allen, E., Smith, G. M., and Gardner, W. U. (1937). *Am. J. Anat.* **61**, 321–341.
Anderson, J., Clark, J. H., and Peck, E. J., Jr. (1972). *Biochem. J.* **126**, 561–567.
Anderson, J. N., Peck, E. J., Jr., and Clark, J. H. (1975). *Endocrinology* **96**, 160–167.
Banerjee, D. N., Banerjee, M. R., and Wagner, J. (1971). *J. Endocrinol.* **51**, 259–264.
Baserga, R. (1968). *Cell Tissue Kinet.* **1**, 167–191.
Baserga, R. (1971). "The Cell Cycle and Cancer," pp. 191–196. Dekker, New York.
Bollum, F. J. (1975). *Prog. Nucleic Acid Res. Mol. Biol.* **15**, 109–145.
Bresciani, F. (1964). *Science* **146**, 653–655.
Bresciani, F. (1965). *Exp. Cell Res.* **38**, 13–32.
Bullough, W. S. (1946). *Philos. Trans. R. Soc. London, Ser. B* **231**, 453–516.
Bullough, W. S. (1973). *Natl. Cancer Inst., Monogr.* **38**, 5–19.
Cameron, I. L., and Greulich, R. C. (1963). *J. Cell Biol.* **18**, 31–40.
Clark, J. H., Anderson, J. N., and Peck, E. J., Jr. (1973). *Steroids* **22**, 707–718.
Clark, J. H., Peck, E. J., Jr., and Anderson, J. N. (1974). *Nature (London)* **251**, 446–448.
Das, R. M. (1972). *J. Endocrinol.* **55**, 21–30.
Epifanova, O. I. (1966). *Exp. Cell Res.* **42**, 562–577.
Epifanova, O. I. (1967). "Hormones and the Reproduction of Cells." Israel Program Sci. Transl., Jerusalem.
Estensen, R. D., and Baserga, R. (1966). *J. Cell Biol.* **30**, 13–22.
Fahmy, A. R., and Griffiths, K. (1968). *Biochem. J.* **108**, 749–753.
Fahmy, A. R., Griffiths, K., Mahler, R., and Williams, A. R. (1967). *Biochem. J.* **105**, 6c–7c.
Fansler, B. S. (1974). *Int. Rev. Cytol., Suppl.* **4**, 363–415.
Forsberg, J. (1970). *J. Exp. Zool.* **175**, 369–374.
Foster, D. N., and Gurney, T., Jr. (1974). *J. Cell Biol.* **63**, 103a.
Fowler, A. K., Reed, C. D., Todaro, G. J., and Hellman, A. (1972). *Proc. Natl. Acad. Sci. U.S.A.* **69**, 2254–2257.
Frankfurt, O. S. (1967). *Int. J. Cancer* **2**, 304–310.
Furth, J., and Clifton, K. H. (1966). *In* "The Pituitary Gland" (G. W. Harris and B. T. Donovan, eds.), Vol. 2, pp. 460–497. Univ. of California Press, Berkeley.
Gelfant, S., Meyer, R. K., and Ris, H. (1955). *J. Exp. Zool.* **128**, 219–257.
Gorski, J., and Axman, M. C. (1964). *Arch. Biochem. Biophys.* **105**, 517–520.
Gorski, J., and Raker, B. (1974). *Gynecol. Oncol.* **2**, 249–258.
Gorski, J., Toft, D., Shyamalä, G., Smith, D., and Notides, A. (1968). *Recent Prog. Horm. Res.* **24**, 45–80.
Hamilton, T. H. (1968). *Science* **161**, 649–661.
Harris, J. N., and Gorski, J. (1976). *Fed. Proc., Fed. Am. Soc. Exp. Biol.* **35**, 1528.
Herrick, G. B., Spear, B., and Veomett, G. (1976). *ICN-UCLA Winter Conf. Mol. Cell. Biol.* p. 48.
Holmes, A. M., and Johnston, A. R. (1975). *FEBS Lett.* **60**, 233–243.
Howard, A., and Pelc, S. R. (1953). *Heredity, Suppl.* **6**, 261–273.
Jensen, E. V., Suzuki, T., Kawashima, T., Stumpf, W. E., Jungblut, P. W., and DeSombre, E. R. (1968). *Proc. Natl. Acad. Sci. U.S.A.* **59**, 632–638.
Kalimi, M., Tsai, S. Y., Tsai, M. J., Clark, J. H., and O'Malley, B. W. (1976). *J. Biol. Chem.* **251**, 516–523.
Katzenellenbogen, B. S. (1975). *Endocrinology* **96**, 289–297.
Katzenellenbogen, B. S., and Gorski, J. (1972). *J. Biol. Chem.* **247**, 1299–1305.
Kaye, A. M., Sheratzky, D., and Lindner, H. R. (1972). *Biochim. Biophys. Acta* **261**, 475–486.
Keir, H. M., and Craig, R. K. (1973). *Biochem. Soc. Trans.* **1**, 1073–1077.
Kohler, P. O., Grimley, P. M., and O'Malley, B. W. (1969). *J. Cell Biol.* **40**, 8–27.
Leake, R., McNeill, W., and Black, M. (1975). *Biochem. Soc. Trans.* **3**, 1180–1183.

Lee, A. E. (1972). *J. Endocrinol.* **55**, 507–512.
Lieberman, I., Abrams, R., Hunt, N., and Ove, P. (1963). *J. Biol. Chem.* **238**, 3955–3962.
Martin, L., Finn, C. A., and Trinder, G. (1973). *J. Endocrinol.* **56**, 133–143.
Mastro, A., and Hymer, W. C. (1973). *J. Endocrinol.* **59**, 107–119.
Mueller, G. C. (1960). *In* "Biological Activities of Steroids in Relation to Cancer" (G. Pincus and E. P. Vollmer, eds.), pp. 129–145. Academic Press, New York.
Mueller, G. C. (1963). *Exp. Cell Res., Suppl.* **9**, 144–149.
Mueller, G. C., Herranen, A. M., and Jervell, K. F. (1958). *Recent Prog. Horm. Res.* **14**, 95–139.
Mueller, G. C., Gorski, J., and Aizawa, Y. (1961). *Proc. Natl. Acad. Sci. U.S.A.* **47**, 164–169.
Mueller, G. C., Kajiwara, K., Stubblefield, E., and Rueckert, R. R. (1962). *Cancer Res.* **22**, 1084–1090.
Mueller, G. C., Vonderhaar, B., Kim, U. H., and Mahieu, M. L. (1972). *Recent Prog. Horm. Res.* **28**, 1–49.
Oka, T., and Schimke, R. T. (1969a). *J. Cell Biol.* **41**, 816–831.
Oka, T., and Schimke, R. T. (1969b). *J. Cell Biol.* **43**, 123–137.
O'Malley, B. W., and Means, A. R. (1974). *Science* **183**, 610–620.
Pilgrim, C., and Maurer, W. (1965). *Exp. Cell Res.* **37**, 183–199.
Quastler, H. (1963). *In* "Cell Proliferation" (L. F. Lamerton and R. J. M. Fry, eds.), pp. 18–34. Blackwell, Oxford.
Rohde, H. J., Muller, W. E. G., and Zahn, R. K. (1975). *J. Nucleic Acids Res.* **2**, 2101–2109.
Schmelck, P. H., Le Goascogne, C., and Le Beau, M.-C. (1975). *Fed. Eur. Biochem. Soc. Proc.* **31**, Abstr. 1408.
Sedwick, W. D., Wang, T. S. F., and Korn, D. (1975). *J. Biol. Chem.* **250**, 7045–7056.
Socher, S. H., and O'Malley, B. W. (1973). *Dev. Biol.* **30**, 411–417.
Stormshak, F., Leake, R., Wertz, N., and Gorski, J. (1976). *Endocrinology* **99**, 1501–1511.
Taylor, E. W. (1965). *Exp. Cell Res.* **40**, 316–332.
Thrasher, J. D., and Greulich, R. C. (1965). *J. Exp. Zool.* **159**, 39–46.
Toft, D., and Gorski, J. (1966). *Proc. Natl. Acad. Sci. U.S.A.* **55**, 1574–1581.
Ts'o, P. O. P., and Lu, P. (1964). *Proc. Natl. Acad. Sci. U.S.A.* **51**, 17–24.
Ui, H., and Mueller, G. C. (1963). *Proc. Natl. Acad. Sci. U.S.A.* **50**, 256–260.
Wang, T. S. F., Sedwick, W. D., and Korn, D. (1975). *J. Biol. Chem.* **250**, 7040–7044.

4

The Role of Receptors in the Anabolic Action of Androgens

C. WAYNE BARDIN, LESLIE P. BULLOCK,
NATHANIEL C. MILLS,
YEN-CHIU LIN, AND SAMSON T. JACOB

I.	Introduction	83
II.	Metabolism of Androgens by Mouse Kidney	85
III.	Androgen Receptors in Mouse Kidney	87
IV.	Androgen Receptors in Mice with Testicular Feminization (tfm)	90
V.	Effects of Androgen Receptors on RNA Polymerase and Chromatin Template Activation	92
VI.	Role of Androgen Receptors in the Action of Progestins on Mouse Kidney	94
VII.	Effects of Androgens on Kidney Growth	97
VIII.	Summary and Conclusions	100
	References	101

I. INTRODUCTION

The growth-promoting effect of testosterone and its 5α-metabolites on the male reproductive tract is generally referred to as the "androgenic" action of this class of steroids. By contrast, the stimulatory effect of these hormones on body weight and nitrogen balance is termed their "anabolic" action (Kochakian, 1975). These latter effects are due to androgen stimulation of protein synthesis in tissues such as muscle, bone, kidney, and liver which comprise a large portion of body mass. Clinicians were interested in these actions as they were of potential benefit to patients with a variety of diseases. However, since virilization was associated with long-term androgen therapy, an extensive search was conducted for compounds which would promote nitrogen retention with minimal effects on the male reproductive tract. New steroids were synthesized and assayed for their respective androgenic and anabolic activities. This latter effect was quantified by assays with end points as varied as body weight, nitrogen retention, muscle weight, and kidney weight. Each of the assays for anabolic activity has recognized advantages, disadvantages, and limitations which are summarized as follows.

The major extragenital site of androgen action is on skeletal muscle. However, the magnitude of this response varies widely among individual muscles and between species (Kochakian et al., 1956; Kochakian and Tillotson, 1957). Nevertheless, a comparison of several steroids suggested that some may have a preferential effect on muscle when compared to seminal vesicle and prostate (Kochakian and Tillotson, 1957). The rat levator ani has been the most widely used muscle for quantitating anabolic response. However, many investigators feel that it is not representative of other skeletal muscles (Scow, 1952; Nimni and Bavetta, 1961), since it, like the remainder of the male reproductive tract, is dependent upon androgens for differentiation (Hayes, 1965). Furthermore, the apparent separation of androgenic and myotropic activities recorded in animal experiments has not been entirely supported by clinical trials (Kochakian, 1975). In another series of studies, renatropic assay demonstrated that some androgens were more effective on the kidney than the male reproductive tract (Kochakian, 1944, 1946). However, the response of the castrated mouse kidney has not had widespread acceptance as a measure of anabolic activity (Kochakian, 1975). Finally, nitrogen balance studies also demonstrated that some steroids have greater activity than testosterone propionate or methyltestosterone (Kochakian, 1975). The major difficulty with this assay, however, is that relative potency estimates are difficult to obtain. These problems have been discussed in greater detail in several reviews (Overbeek, 1966; Krüskemper, 1968; Segaloff, 1964). Thus, although some dissociation of anabolic and androgenic activities has been demonstrated in several animal bioassays, similar results have not been obtained in man. This is not surprising since dissociation of the androgenic action of a single steroid on two tissues of the reproductive tract such as prostate and seminal vesicle has been observed (Korenchevsky and Dennison, 1935). As a consequence, a complete separation of the action of androgens on extragenital tissue from that on the accessory sex organs does not seem possible at present. A major reason for this is that the basic mechanisms of androgen action on both types of tissue are incompletely understood. In view of these considerations, we thought it pertinent to briefly summarize androgen action on the male reproductive tract as an introduction to a more extensive review of how androgen receptors influence androgen action on mouse kidney, an extragenital tissue which has been used as an index of anabolic activity.

Since the effect of androgens on male accessory sex tissue is covered in several recent reviews (Liao, 1975; Baulieu et al., 1975; Williams-Ashman et al., 1975), it is only briefly discussed in this report. Testosterone is the major androgen in blood, and its action has been studied most extensively in prostate. In this and other reproductive tissues, testosterone is first metabolized by 5α-reductase to dihydrotestosterone (DHT) which, in turn, is bound to a specific intracellular receptor protein. The DHT–receptor complex is transferred to the nucleus where it stimulates a series of metabolic events which, in turn, results in increased RNA synthesis. The increase in RNA results in synthesis of tissue specific proteins and organ growth. Each step in this metabolic cascade is believed essential for the action of testosterone on reproductive tissue. The major question posed in this review is to what extent does the action of testosterone on these organs differ from that on somatic tissues. Accordingly, the mechanism of androgen action on the mouse kidney is examined in detail and when possible compared with that on the male reproductive tract. The recent acquisition of knowledge in this area has been facilitated by studies of two genes in the mouse, *tfm* and *Gur*, which regulate the magnitude of the androgen response on one or several target tissues (Lyon and Hawkes, 1970; Paigen et al., 1975).

II. METABOLISM OF ANDROGENS BY MOUSE KIDNEY

Studies of *in vitro* and *in vivo* androgen metabolism have provided evidence that testosterone rather than one of its metabolites is bound by androgen receptors in kidney. When kidney slices were incubated with testosterone or dihydrotestosterone (10^{-7} M) for 30 minutes, only 3% of the testosterone was metabolized, as compared with 75% of dihydrotestosterone (Bardin et al., 1973). From subsequent studies of cell fractions with optimal substrate and cofactor concentrations, it was concluded that an insignificant amount of testosterone was metabolized to dihydrotestosterone in mouse kidney. These experiments further suggested that when dihydrotestosterone was formed, it was rapidly metabolized to the 5α-androstanediols (Wilson and Gloyna, 1970; Bardin et al., 1973; Mowszowicz and Bardin, 1974). Additional studies indicated that epitestosterone was the major metabolite of testosterone and androstenedione in mouse kidney (Arimasa and Kochakian, 1973).

In vivo experiments confirmed the absence of significant 5α-reductase activity in mouse kidney. Following administration of [³H]testosterone to castrate male mice, testosterone was the predominant steroid in renal cytoplasm and nuclei (Fig. 1). When [³H]androstenedione was administered, testosterone was again the major nuclear steroid and little or no dihydrotestosterone was found. By contrast, after the intravenous administration of [³H]dihydrotestosterone, 5α-androstanediols, and dihydrotestosterone were the predominant cytoplasmic androgens. In these experiments, almost all the nuclear radioactivity was dihydrotestosterone (Bullock and Bardin, 1975) (Fig. 1). A similar pattern was observed when [³H]5α-androstane-3α,17β-diol and its ³H-3β isomer were administered (Fig. 1). These latter studies indicated that the intranuclear androgen in the kidney was directly related to the androgen in the blood. DHT was present in nuclei only when the blood steroid had a 5α-hydrogen. These findings indicated that mouse kidney can concentrate both testosterone and dihydrotestosterone. However, since testosterone is normally the major circulating androgen and is not metabolized by kidney, testosterone is the major effector of androgen action in this organ. This conclusion is based

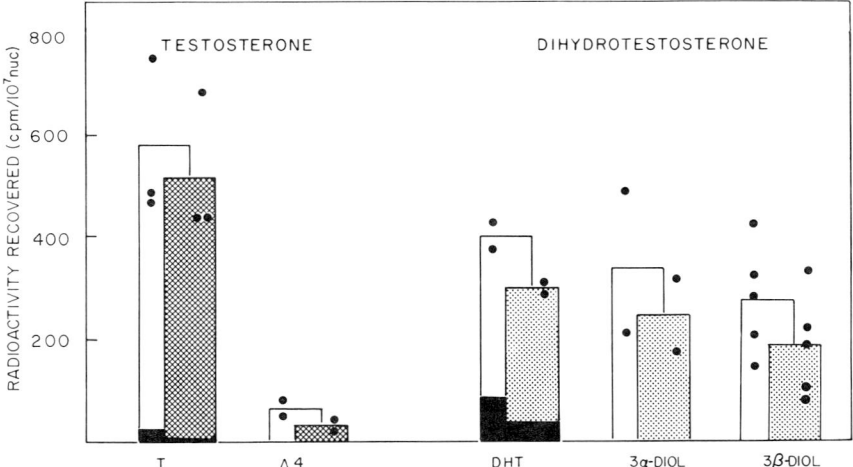

Fig. 1. Nuclear uptake of total radioactivity (open bars) and [³H]androgens (shaded bars) after the intravenous administration of [³H]testosterone (T), [³H]androstenedione (Δ4), [³H]5α-dihydrotestosterone (DHT), [³H]5α-androstane-3α,17β-diol (3α-diol) and [³H]5α-androstane-3β,17β-diol (3β-diol). When either testosterone or androstenedione was administered, testosterone was the predominant androgen isolated from kidney nuclei (left). When one of the 5α-reduced steroids was administered, dihydrotestosterone was the predominant steroid isolated from kidney nuclei (right). The solid portion of the testosterone and dihydrotestosterone bars indicates the nuclear androgen uptake when cyproterone acetate was administered before the [³H]androgen. (From Bardin and Bullock, 1974.)

upon the assumption that specific nuclear binding is required for steroid hormone action and that the nuclear steroids isolated are those that were active at the time the animal was killed.

Subsequent studies by numerous investigators demonstrated little or no 5α-reductase activity in many tissues of mouse and rat, such as brain, pituitary, submaxillary gland, testis, pituitary, and muscle. In these organs, testosterone was usually the dominant steroid found in the nucleus of the cell. This was in contrast to tissues with an active 5α-reductase (such as skin and male reproductive tract) in which DHT was the intranuclear steroid (Bardin et al., 1975b). Although an effective 5α-reductase distinguishes the male reproductive tract from other androgen responsive tissues in adult life, it should be noted that the activity of this enzyme is low in vas deferens and seminal vesicle at the time of differentiation (Siiteri and Wilson, 1974). As a consequence, testosterone is believed to be responsible for the development of these latter tissues, whereas DHT is essential for differentiation of prostate and external genitalia (Imperato-McGinley and Peterson, 1976).

III. ANDROGEN RECEPTORS IN MOUSE KIDNEY

Since the transfer of androgens to the nucleus of the cell is mediated by the cytosol androgen receptor, the *in vivo* studies presented above suggested that testosterone and DHT shared a common intracellular binding site in mouse kidney (Bardin et al., 1973). To confirm this possibility, cytosols were prepared from kidneys of male and female mice and incubated with [^{3}H]testosterone or [^{3}H]dihydrotestosterone. Both ^{3}H-androgens were bound by macromolecules which sedimented in the 8 S portion of sucrose gradients (Fig. 2) and were displaced from their respective binders by unlabeled cyproterone acetate, testosterone, or dihydrotestosterone. These *in vitro* observations were, thus, consistent with the *in vivo* studies. Together, they indicated that testosterone and dihydrotestosterone could bind to the same intracellular binding protein.

Subsequent studies demonstrated that the 8 S androgen binder in kidney cytosol has all the properties usually associated with steroid receptors in general (Table I). It is an asymmetric, acidic molecule with an estimated molecular weight (MW) of 270,000 daltons. Studies with protein-specific reagents suggested that both cysteine and tryptophan residues may be necessary for maintenance of the functional configuration associated with androgen binding. The kidney receptor is heat labile and can promote the association of testosterone with purified DNA. These properties of the

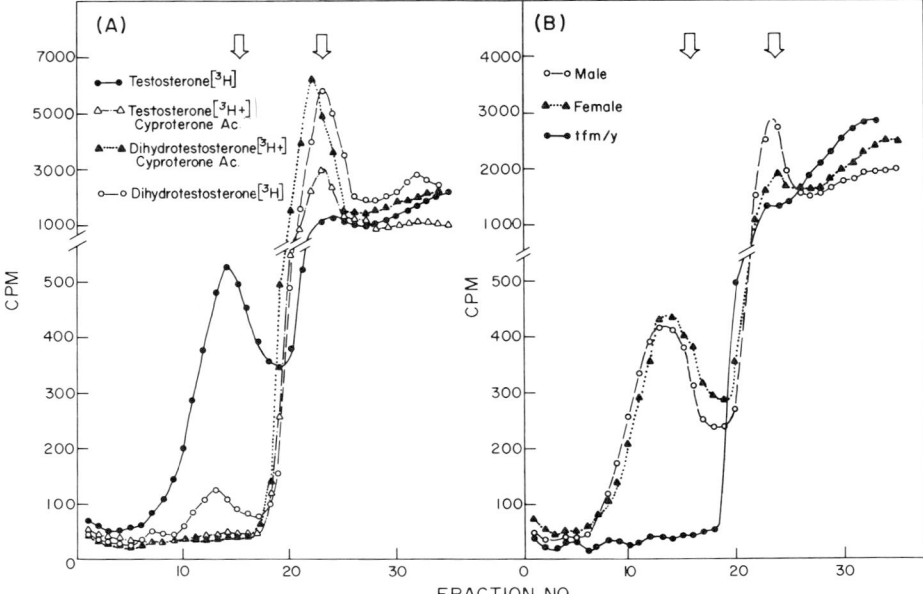

Fig. 2. Sedimentation pattern of androgen receptor from kidney cytosol through 5–20% sucrose gradients. Arrows indicate γ-globulin (7 S) and cortisol-binding globulin (3.5 S). The bottom of the tube is on the left. (A) [^{3}H]Testosterone and [^{3}H]dihydrotestosterone binding to cytosol macromolecules of mouse kidney. Cyproterone acetate completely displaced both [^{3}H]steroids from the cytosol receptor as did cold testosterone and dihydrotestosterone (not shown). (B) [^{3}H]Testosterone binding to receptor from kidney cytosol in male and female mice. No androgen binding could be demonstrated in the tfm/Y mouse. (From Bardin *et al.*, 1973.)

androgen receptor in mouse kidney are remarkably similar to those of male accessory sexual tissue (Bullock *et al.*, 1975b). Since androgen receptors in reproductive and nonreproductive tissues could have similar physical properties but bind different hormones, it was important to compare their steroid specificity.

When the binding of testosterone and dihydrotestosterone to the kidney androgen receptor were compared on sucrose gradient, testosterone appeared to have a higher affinity for this protein than dihydrotestosterone (Fig. 2). Subsequent studies demonstrated, however, that the affinity of this receptor for dihydrotestosterone could not be estimated in crude cytosol preparations due to steroid metabolism by 3-ketosteroid reductase (Bullock and Bardin, 1974). Nonetheless, the binding of testosterone by kidney receptors was strikingly different from that reported for prostate by Fang and Liao (1971). These latter investigators performed an extensive evaluation of the partially purified androgen receptor from rat prostate. In their studies, when sucrose gradients were used to separate bound and free steroid, testosterone demonstrated little, if any, receptor binding. These observations seemed to be in keeping with the results of others (Bardin *et al.*, 1975b), indicating that dihydrotestosterone was the major intranuclear androgen in the prostate. However, recent studies of the male reproductive tract perfused with [^{3}H]testosterone indicated that up to 20% of specifically bound nuclear androgen in prostate and seminal vesicle was testosterone. However, when extracts of these labeled nuclei were examined on sucrose gradients, only dihydrotestosterone was bound to androgen receptor (Baker *et al.*, 1977). The apparent inconsistency of these latter findings with those of Fang and Liao (1971) may be explained, in part, by the recent observations of Verhoeven *et al.* (1975) who showed that testosterone dissociated from prostatic cytoplasmic receptor during the prolonged centrifugation used with sucrose-gradient analysis. When this problem was obviated by use of an ammonium sulfate assay and the bound steroid was in nonequilibrium for a much shorter time, testosterone binding to prostate was demonstrated. Under these conditions the relative binding affinities of the prostate receptor were similar to those of kidney. These latter observations do not explain, however, why testosterone does not dissociate from kidney receptor during fractionation on sucrose gradients.

In conclusion, androgen receptors in the male reproductive tract and in kidney have similar physical properties. These observations, along with genetic studies on androgen-insensitive rodents (mentioned below) suggested that the androgen receptor is the same in all tissues. Additional studies using purified proteins are required to exclude the possibility of organ-specific modifications in the androgen receptor.

TABLE I

Physicochemical Properties of the Cytoplasmic Androgen Receptor from Kidney[a]

Parameter	Receptor (kidney)
Sedimentation coefficient	7.9
Stokes radius (Å)	82
Molecular weight (daltons)	270,000
Frictional ratio (f/f_0)	1.98
Isoelectric point	4.8
Heat stable	No
Binds to DNA	Yes

[a] From Bullock *et al.*, 1975b.

IV. ANDROGEN RECEPTORS IN MICE WITH TESTICULAR FEMINIZATION (tfm)

Lyon and Hawkes (1970) described a mouse with testicular feminization. This disorder, like that of rat (Bardin et al., 1973; Bardin and Bullock, 1974) and man (Naftolin and Judd, 1973) was passed by the female to half her male offspring. The pattern of inheritance along with linkage studies indicated that *tfm* is transmitted as an X-linked recessive gene. Males with this defect (tfm/Y) were characterized by lack of androgen-dependent differentiation resulting from end organ insensitivity to androgens during fetal life. Since affected mice had no prostate or seminal vesicles, studies of androgen action and metabolism were conducted on tissues that are not dependent on androgen for differentiation but are responsive to these steroids. Experiments from our own and other laboratories indicated that kidney (Bardin et al., 1973), submaxillary gland (Lyon et al., 1973; Barthe et al., 1974; Schenkein et al., 1974; Dunn and Wilson, 1975; Bullock et al., 1975a), and pituitary (Itakura and Ohno, 1973; Kan et al., 1974) of adult tfm/Y mice are insensitive to large doses of androgens.

The molecular basis of the tfm defect was first suggested by *in vivo* studies of androgen metabolism in tfm rats (Bullock and Bardin, 1970). In these animals, decreased uptake of [^{3}H]dihydrotestosterone by preputial gland nuclei was demonstrated following administration of [^{3}H]testosterone. Similar experiments with tissues from tfm/Y mice and human fibroblasts indicated that a similar defect could explain many of the conditions characterized by end-organ insensitivity to androgens. These latter observations suggested that some tissues are insensitive to androgens because of their inability to concentrate these steroids at the active site in the cell (Bardin et al., 1973; Amrhein et al., 1976).

One explanation for decreased nuclear androgen uptake in tfm animals was a defective androgen receptor. Subsequent experiments demonstrated that the 8 S androgen receptor present in cytosol of normal animals was undetectable in tfm/Y mice (Bullock and Bardin, 1972). These observations were subsequently confirmed and expanded by numerous investigators, using a variety of techniques and tissues (Attardi and Ohno, 1974; Gehring and Tomkins; 1974; Fox, 1975; Attardi et al., 1976). The relationship of this receptor defect with androgen responsiveness and the *tfm* gene in mouse kidney is summarized in Fig. 3. Unaffected male (+/Y) and female (+/+) mice have normal X chromosomes and a full complement of active androgen receptors. They also are fully (100%) inducible by androgens. The androgen-insensitive pseudohermaphrodite (tfm/Y) carries the tfm defect on the X chromosome in all cells. This animal has no functional androgen

4. Receptors in Anabolic Action of Androgens

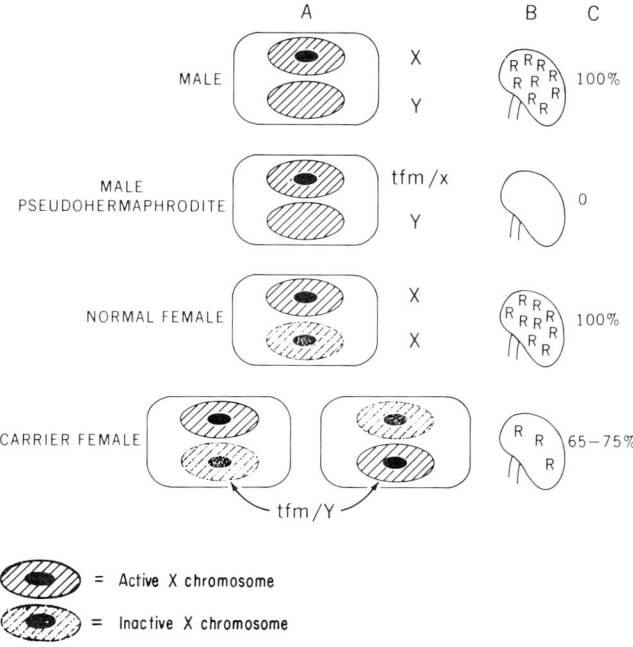

Fig. 3. Correlation of androgen receptor activity, androgen responsiveness and the presence or absence of the *tfm* gene. (A) Genotypes studied. (B) Kidney androgen receptor (R) content; (C) Androgen responsiveness, 100% = maximal response. (From Bardin *et al.*, 1977.)

receptor and is not inducible. By contrast, the heterozygous female (tfm/+) should have two populations of cells as a consequence of random X inactivation. In some cells, the active X chromosome is normal and in others, it carries tfm. As a result, androgen receptor levels in tfm/+ are only 69% of normal, and androgen treatment results in an intermediate response (65–75% of normal) (Bardin *et al.*, 1977). These experiments demonstrate a correlation between androgen receptor activity, androgen responsiveness, and activity of the *tfm* gene. These studies suggest that *tfm* controls either the synthesis or the assembly of the androgen receptor (Bardin *et al.*, 1973). To date, studies on the residual androgen receptor present in tfm/Y cannot distinguish between these two possibilities. Some investigators reported altered receptor affinity (Attardi and Ohno, 1974), and others have shown low levels of normal receptors (Gehring and Tomkins, 1974). Nevertheless, the fact that androgen insensitivity affects all tissues suggests that the initial step of androgen action, formation of an active steroid receptor complex, is the same for the androgenic and anabolic actions of testosterone.

V. EFFECTS OF ANDROGEN RECEPTORS ON RNA POLYMERASE AND CHROMATIN TEMPLATE ACTIVATION

Studies from many laboratories have indicated that steroid hormones regulate target cell function by influencing RNA synthesis, a process which is thought to be regulated by steroid-receptor complex (O'Malley and Means, 1974). Almost all steroid hormones produced very early increases in the formation of DNA-like nuclear RNA, a step that is believed to be essential for the subsequent accumulation of all classes of RNA and for the synthesis of hormone-specific proteins in target organs. Increases in RNA concentrations have been attributed to changes in transcriptional processes, either from enhanced chromatin template activity or from activation of different DNA-directed RNA polymerases.

In order to gain further insight into the role of the steroid receptor in producing the anabolic action of androgens, a series of studies on early transcriptional events in normal and tfm/Y mice were conducted (Jánne et al., 1976). A single subcutaneous injection of testosterone increased RNA polymerase II activity in kidney nuclei by 15 minutes. Activity was maximal at 1 hour and returned to baseline between 2 and 4 hours after hormone administration (Fig. 4). Although RNA polymerase I activity was also increased by 15 minutes, its peak activity occurred at 2 hours, and it slowly declined toward the baseline by 4 hours. Both types of activity increased again (between 4 and 24 hours) without subsequent hormone treatment (Fig. 4). There was no change in nuclear RNA polymerase type I

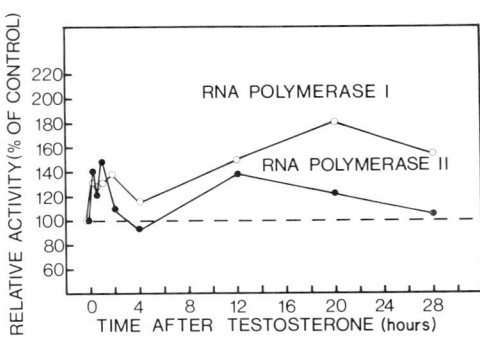

Fig. 4. Effect of testosterone treatment on RNA polymerase activities in mouse kidney nuclei. Young adult female mice (8–10 weeks old in each experimental group) were treated with a single dose of testosterone (1 mg). The changes in RNA polymerase activities (means of two separate experiments) are expressed as percentages of controls (= 100), which were 39 and 369 pmoles UMP incorporated per milligram of DNA for RNA polymerase I and II, respectively. (From Jänne et al., 1976.)

4. Receptors in Anabolic Action of Androgens

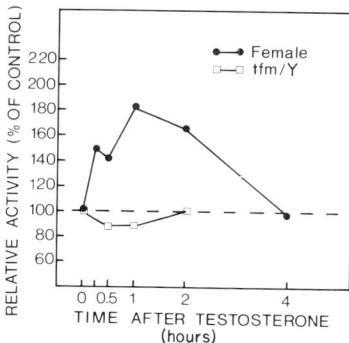

Fig. 5. Action of testosterone on chromatin template capacity in kidney of normal female and androgen-insensitive tfm/Y mice. Testosterone (1 mg) was given to the animals subcutaneously. The measurement of renal chromatin template activity was conducted with RNA polymerase II. The changes in template activity are expressed as percentages of the controls (= 100), which were 7.4 and 11.4 pmoles UMP incorporated per microgram of DNA for normal female and tfm/Y mice. The values given for normal mice are means of two separate experiments, whereas those of tfm/Y animals are means of triplicate assays in one experiment. (From Jänne et al., 1976.)

or II in kidney of tfm/Y mice following exogenous testosterone administration (not shown).

In another series of experiments using normal mice (Jänne et al., 1976), a single subcutaneous injection of testosterone increased template activity of renal chromatin as measured with highly purified renal RNA polymerase II. Template capacity rose progressively for 1 hour and then declined back to baseline by 4 hours. As observed for nuclear RNA polymerase I and II activities, renal chromatin template capacity did not change when tfm/Y mice were treated with testosterone (Fig. 5).

The above results are consistent with the hypothesis that the cytosolic androgen–receptor complex is required for the early transcriptional events elicited by testosterone administration in mouse kidney. The fact that, in normal mice, nuclear testosterone uptake preceded or coincided with early changes in the activities of renal RNA polymerase and chromatin template strengthens the hypothesis that steroid receptor plays an important role in the regulation of gene transcription of the target cell (Jänne et al., 1976). This contention was further supported by recent observations of in vitro activation of kidney chromatin by mouse kidney receptor in the presence of homologous RNA polymerase (Bardin et al., 1975b).

These studies suggested that androgens elicit their initial action in mouse kidney nuclei by preferentially stimulating the fractional activity of RNA polymerase II. Although RNA polymerase I activity began to rise as early as 15 minutes after hormone administration, it peaked at the time when

RNA polymerase II activity was back to control levels. The pattern of RNA polymerase I stimulation resembled that reported by Avdalovic and Kochakian (1969). These latter investigators first measured polymerase activity at 2 hours following hormone treatment, which accounts for their failure to observe an early increase in RNA polymerase activity. It was of interest to note that the secondary increases in renal RNA polymerase activity coincided with the reported time of orotic acid incorporation into RNA and clearly preceded detectable accumulation of RNA and androgen-specific proteins (Frieden and Ku, 1971; Kochakian, 1969).

The results in Fig. 5 indicating very early stimulation of chromatin template activity are similar to those observed for estradiol on uterine chromatin (Glasser et al., 1972). By contrast, Mainwaring et al. (1971) failed to detect a significant early stimulation in rat prostatic chromatin template activity following testosterone treatment although a later increase similar to that observed in the present study occurred. It is not known whether these variations in androgen response between prostate and kidney are due to organ differences or to techniques employed to prepare chromatin and examine its template capacity.

In conclusion, a single dose of testosterone stimulated RNA polymerase and chromatin template activities in renal nuclei. These activations correlated temporally with nuclear steroid accumulation. These changes were qualitatively similar to those produced by other sex steroids on their respective target tissues. At the present time, however, sufficient comparative studies have not been performed to determine whether the androgen-induced early nuclear effects on kidney differ from those on the male reproductive tract.

VI. ROLE OF ANDROGEN RECEPTORS IN THE ACTION OF PROGESTINS ON MOUSE KIDNEY

The ability of progestins to mimic the action of androgens is well recognized. However, demonstration of progestational androgenicity is highly dependent upon the steroid as well as the end point used. When progestins were assayed in the adult rat, progesterone and its C_{21} derivatives had only minimal androgenic effects, whereas progestins structurally related to 19-nortestosterone stimulated the male reproductive tract (Edgren et al., 1967). By contrast, both progesterone and 19-nortestosterone derivatives masculinized the external genitalia (Revesz et al., 1960; Suchowsky and Junkmann, 1961). In addition to their actions on the reproductive tract, a variety of progestins also stimulated androgen action on other tissues such as kidney (Mowszowicz et al., 1974), preputial gland (Bardin et al., 1973), and submaxillary glands (Bullock et al., 1975a).

Although there are many studies indicating that progestins stimulate androgen-responsive tissues, there are few experiments to indicate the mechanism by which this activity is initiated. Observations on the effects of progestins in tfm/Y mice indicated that these animals were also insensitive to the androgenic actions of these steroids. Since tfm animals lack an androgen receptor, it was possible that, in some organs, progestin activation of the cell was mediated by way of the androgen receptor (Mowszowicz et al., 1974; Bullock et al., 1975a). To test this possibility, the binding of progestational steroids to the androgen receptor was studied.

Kidney cytosol was incubated with [^{3}H]testosterone or [^{3}H]medroxyprogesterone acetate (MPA) in the presence or absence of nonradioactive steroids. Samples were sedimented on sucrose gradients, and the results are summarized in Fig. 6. [^{3}H]Testosterone and ^{3}H-MPA-labeled macromolecules sedimented in the 8 S region of the gradient. Nonradioac-

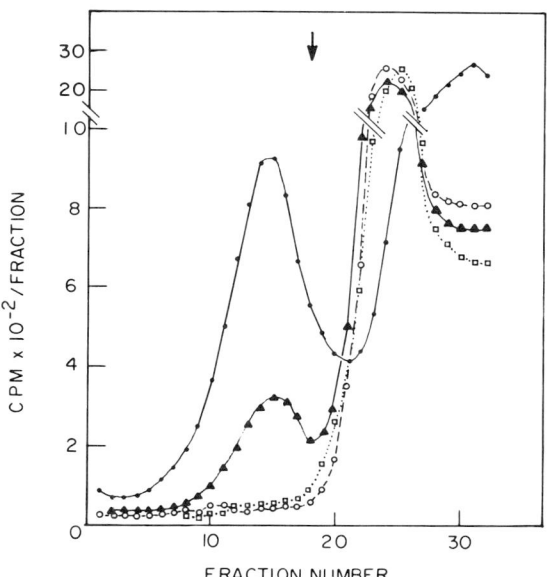

Fig. 6. *In vitro* [^{3}H]testosterone (●———●) and [^{3}H]medroxyprogesterone acetate (▲———▲) (MPA) binding in kidney cytosol. [^{3}H]Steroids were incubated with kidney cytosol from castrated mice and analyzed on sucrose gradients. Cold MPA could displace [^{3}H]testosterone (□·····□) and cold testosterone could displace [^{3}H]MPA (O------O) from their respective binding sites. Neither [^{3}H]testosterone nor [^{3}H]MPA demonstrated specific binding in the cytoplasm of tfm/Y mice (not shown). Arrow indicate γ-globulin. (From Bardin et al., 1975a.)

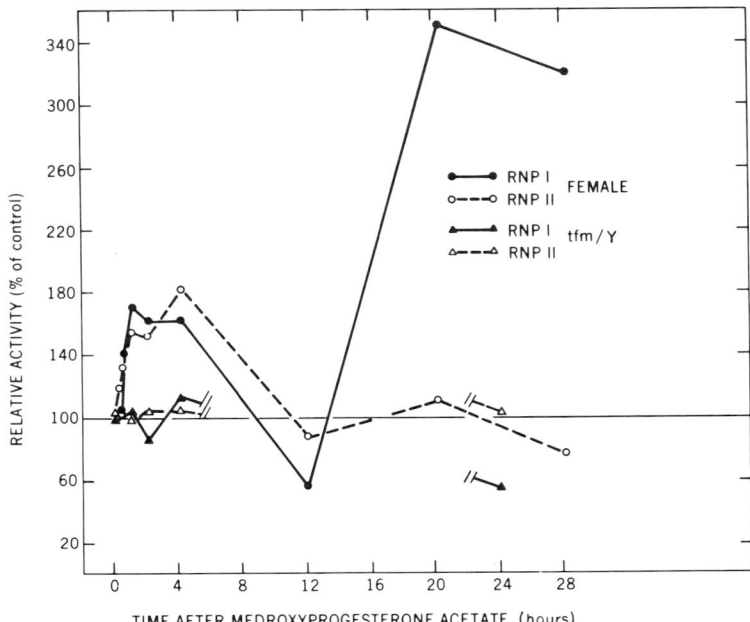

Fig. 7. Effect of medroxyprogesterone acetate treatment on RNA polymerase activities in kidney nuclei from normal female and tfm/Y mice. Animals were treated with a single dose of medroxyprogesterone acetate (10 mg). The changes in RNA polymerase activities (means of two experiments) are expressed as percentages of controls (= 100).

tive testosterone and MPA competed with both ^{3}H ligands for their binding sites. Additional *in vivo* studies demonstrated that MPA and testosterone could inhibit the uptake of [^{3}H]testosterone and ^{3}H-MPA, respectively, by kidney nuclei. Furthermore, neither [^{3}H]testosterone or ^{3}H-MPA were concentrated by kidney cytosol or nuclei from tfm/y mice. These experiments demonstrated that MPA binds to the androgen receptor in kidney (Bardin *et al.*, 1975a). Although all progestins studied to date bind to kidney androgen receptor, it is significant that not all are androgenic. Some are antiandrogenic and some have little, if any, biologic action on kidney.

Since the above studies suggested that the long-term effects of MPA on mouse kidney were mediated by the androgen receptor, it was of interest to determine the early effects of this progestin in normal and tfm/Y animals. The RNA polymerase I and II activities in whole nuclei following the administration of MPA are shown in Fig. 7. The pattern of response is similar to that of testosterone.

VII. EFFECTS OF ANDROGENS ON KIDNEY GROWTH

The stimulatory effect of androgens on the growth of the mouse kidney has been known for over 35 years (Kochakian, 1975). Morphological studies indicated that the cells of Bowman's capsule and the proximal convoluted tubule of male mice were more cuboidal than those of female mice (Crabtree, 1941; Dunn, 1949) and that this sexual dimorphism was dependent upon endogenous or exogenous androgens (Muller and von Deimling, 1971). Analysis of the mouse kidney before and after androgen treatment indicated that renal enlargement was secondary to cellular hypertrophy, rather than hyperplasia, since there was an increase in total protein and RNA but no change in DNA content (Kochakian, 1975). In this regard, the kidney differs from the male reproductive tract where androgens produce cellular hyperplasia as well as hypertrophy.

The androgen-induced hypertrophy of the mouse kidney is associated with the increase in a number of specific kidney proteins, some of which are summarized in Table II. In some instances, histochemical studies demonstrated that the increased activity of these proteins was primarily in the proximal convoluted tubule (Brandt *et al.,* 1975). Of the many androgen-responsive renal proteins, β-glucuronidase is perhaps the best studied. Testosterone increased the rate of β-glucuronidase synthesis, which resulted in a 20- to 50-fold increase in specific activity (Swank *et al.,* 1973). Concomitant with the increase in tissue enzyme, there is a marked increase

TABLE II

Androgen Responsiveness of Mouse Kidney Can Be Demonstrated As Increases in the Activities or Levels of the Following End Points during Testosterone Treatment

End point	Reference
Glutamic-pyruvic transaminase	Schwarzlose and Heim, 1973
Glutamatic-oxaloacetate transaminase	Schwarzlose and Heim, 1973
Glutamate dehydrogenase	Schwarzlose and Heim, 1973
Free amino acids	Kochakian, 1974
D-Amino acid oxidase	Frieden *et al.,* 1964
β-Glucuronidase	Plaut and Fishman, 1963; Frieden *et al.,* 1964; Frieden and Fishel, 1968
Arginase	Kochakian *et al.,* 1948; Frieden and Fishel, 1968
Digalactosylceramide	Gray, 1971
Esterases	Staeudinger *et al.,* 1974; Shaw and Koen, 1963; Ruddle, 1966
Alcohol dehydrogenase	Ohno *et al.,* 1970
3-Keto-reductase	Mowszowicz and Bardin, 1974

in β-glucuronidase excretion into the urine (Fig. 8). Even though β-glucuronidase is one of the major excretory renal proteins in the mouse, it makes only a minor contribution to total urinary proteins (Fig. 9). The many urinary proteins in the mouse are probably synthesized in liver (Bao-Linh et al., 1964) and, in this regard, are analogous to the androgen-responsive α_{2u}-globulin in rat urine (Roy, 1973). The fact that a large portion of β-glucuronidase activity is excreted emphasizes that tissue activity is determined by the rate of enzyme loss (excretion plus proteolysis) as well as by rate of enzyme synthesis.

Paigen and his associates (1975) recently reviewed a number of genes which determine β-glucuronidase activity in kidney. Of these, the effects of Gur were particularly important for defining the mechanism by which androgens regulate the activity of this protein. A survey of inbred strains of mice revealed two classes with respect to stimulation of β-glucuronidase activity in kidney (Swank et al., 1973). One group, typified by strain A/J (Gur^a), had a short lag period and a rapid rise of β-glucuronidase activity reaching a high maximum activity. The other group, typified by C57BL/6J (Gur^b), induced with a longer lag period and a slower rise to a lower maximum enzyme activity (Fig. 10). Genetic studies using a set of a recombinant-inbred lines derived from a cross between high- and low-inducing strains suggested that a single genetic locus (Gur) appeared to determine

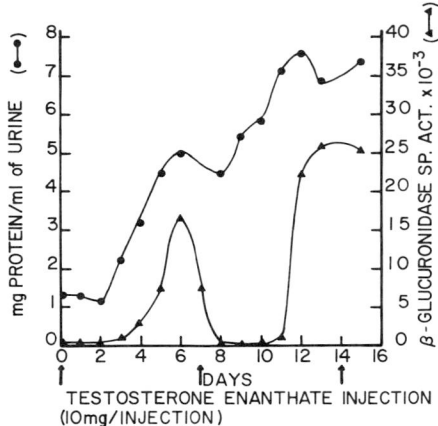

Fig. 8. Mouse urinary proteins and β-glucuronidase secretion. Mouse urine was collected in metabolic cages for continuous 24-hour periods. An aliquot from each period was dialyzed against 20 mM sodium phosphate buffer, pH 7.8, for 36 hours at 4°C. β-Glucuronidase activity was assayed using 1 mM p-nitrophenyl-β-D-glucuronide as a substrate. Specific activity is expressed as nmoles of p-nitrophenol release per hour at 56°C per milligram of urinary protein. Day 0 represents activity in a pooled urine collection over a period of approximately 2 weeks from untreated A/J female mice 6–10 weeks of age.

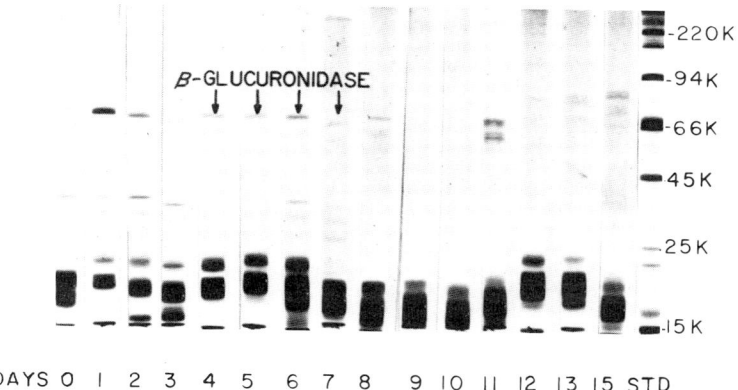

Fig. 9. SDS polyacrylamide gels with proteins of mouse urine after testosterone at 0, 7, and 14 days. Urinary proteins (25 μg) from the dialyzed samples assayed in Fig. 8 were applied to 5-mm diameter SDS polyacrylamide gels. The standard MW proteins used were: myosin, 220,000; phosphorylase A, 94,000; bovine serum albumin, 66,000; ovalbumin, 45,000; chymotrypsinogen A, 25,000. The major urinary proteins have MW's between 15,000 and 25,000, while β-glucuronidase subunit has an MW of 70,000.

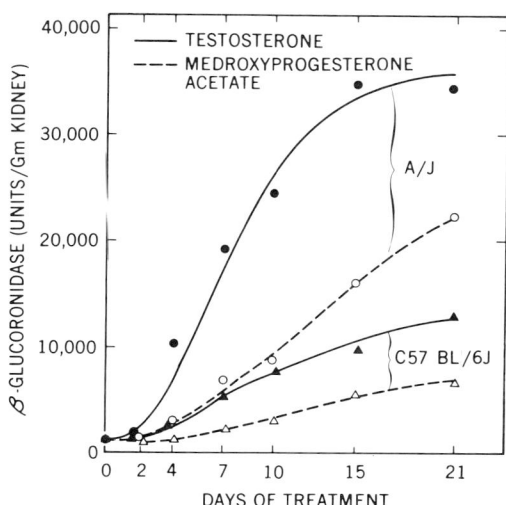

Fig. 10. The effect of testosterone and medroxyprogesterone acetate on β-glucuronidase activity in mouse kidney. Females of each strain received daily injections of testosterone (2 mg/day) or medroxyprogesterone acetate (5 mg/day). The responses of 5 animals were assayed separately at each point and the means are shown. A/J mice have the Gur^a allele and C57BL/6J animals carry the Gur^b allele.

both the duration of the lag and the subsequent rate of enzyme activity increase. The final plateau appeared to be determined by that locus in combination with one or more additional sites (Swank and Bailey, 1973). Pulse-labeling experiments using immunoprecipitation indicated that Gur regulates the rate of β-glucuronidase synthesis in the proximal convoluted tubule, but not any of the other androgen responsive proteins in the kidney or liver (Paigen et al., 1975). When the F_1 hybrid of A/J × C57BL/6J was treated with testosterone, the rate of enzyme synthesis was intermediate between that of the two parent strains. This experiment demonstrated that the alleles of Gur (Gur^a, Gur^b) showed additive inheritance (Paigen et al., 1975). In addition, Gur was closely linked to the glucuronidase structural gene (Gus) on chromosome 5, and its activity was not mediated through a diffusible product. Gur was, therefore, thought to be the cis-acting regulatory element, which presumably controls the rate of androgen-induced RNA synthesis from the nearby glucuronidase structural gene. As noted by Paigen and his colleagues (1975), this is the first known mammalian regulatory element that controls the response of an enzyme through its physiological signal.

In view of the regulatory role of the Gur locus on the androgen induction of β-glucuronidase, it was pertinent to determine whether another class of β-glucuronidase inducers would be recognized by the two Gur alleles. A/J and C57BL/6J mice (with Gur^a and Gur^b, respectively) were treated with MPA for varying periods of time. As was the case with testosterone, MPA produced a greater stimulation of β-glucuronidase activity in A/J animals (Fig. 10). It is significant that in either strain of animals MPA was as potent as testosterone.

VIII. SUMMARY AND CONCLUSIONS

The mouse kidney has been used by some investigators to assay the anabolic action of steroids, although others do not believe that it is representative of other nonreproductive tissues. The kidney differs primarily from reproductive tract in that it lacks the ability to divide in response to androgens and has an insignificant 5α-reductase. It is of interest, however, that when kidney cells are placed in culture, they divide in the presence of serum and acquire a 5α-reductase (Mowszowicz and Bardin, 1977).

In spite of the above differences, there are many features of androgen action on kidney which are similar to other androgen-responsive tissues. First, they have a common androgen receptor mechanism which is believed to initiate hormone action. The early activation of RNA polymerase and chromatin template in kidney appear to be similar to that of accessory sex tissues. Finally, weak inducers, such as MPA, stimulate the kidney in a fashion analogous to other androgen-responsive tissues.

ACKNOWLEDGMENT

This study was supported in part by NIH Grant HD-05276 and NIH Contract No. NO1-HD-2-2730.

REFERENCES

Amrhein, J. A., Meyer, W. J., III, Jones, H. W., Jr., and Migeon, C. J. (1976). *Proc. Natl. Acad. Sci. U.S.A.* **73**, 891–894.
Arimasa, N., and Kochakian, C. D. (1973). *Endocrinology* **92**, 72–82.
Attardi, B., and Ohno, S. (1974). *Cell* **2**, 205–212.
Attardi, B., Geller, L. N., and Ohno, S. (1976). *Endocrinology* **98**, 864–874.
Avdalovic, N., and Kochakian, C. D. (1969). *Biochim. Biophys. Acta* **182**, 382–393.
Baker, H. W. G., Bailey, D. J., Feil, P. D., Jefferson, L. S., Santen, R. J., and Bardin, C. W. (1977). *Endocrinology* **100**, 709–721.
Bao-Linh, D., Hermann, G., and Grabar, P. (1964). *Bull. Soc. Chim. Biol.* **46**, 255–269.
Bardin, C. W., and Bullock, L. P. (1974). *J. Invest. Dermatol.* **63**, 75–84.
Bardin, C. W., Bullock, L. P., Sherins, R. J., Mowszowicz, I., and Blackburn, W. R. (1973). *Recent Prog. Horm. Res.* **29**, 65–109.
Bardin, C. W., Bullock, L. P., Jänne, O., and Jacob, S. T. (1975a). *J. Steroid Biochem.* **6**, 515–520.
Bardin, C. W., Jänne, O., Bullock, L. P., and Jacob, S. T. (1975b). *In* "Hormonal Regulation of Spermatogenesis" (F. S. French *et al.*, eds.), pp. 237–255. Plenum, New York.
Bardin, C. W., Bullock, L. P., Gupta, C., and Brown, T. (1977). *Proc. Int. Congr. Endocrinol., 5th, 1976* **1**, 481–485.
Barthe, P. L., Bullock, L. P., Mowszowicz, I., Bardin, C. W., and Orth, D. N. (1974). *Endocrinology* **95**, 1019–1025.
Baulieu, E. E., Le Goascogne C., Groyer, A., Feyel-Cabanes, T., and Robel, P. (1975). *Vitam. Horm. (N.Y.)* **33**, 1–38.
Brandt, E. J., Elliott, R. W., and Swank, R. T. (1975). *J. Cell Biol.* **67**, 774–788.
Bullock, L., and Bardin, C. W. (1970). *J. Clin. Endocrinol. Metab.* **31**, 113–115.
Bullock, L. P., and Bardin, C. W. (1972). *J. Clin. Endocrinol. Metab.* **35**, 935–937.
Bullock, L. P., and Bardin, C. W. (1974). *Endocrinology* **94**, 746–756.
Bullock, L. P., and Bardin, C. W. (1975). *Steroids* **25**, 107–119.
Bullock, L. P., Barthe, P. L., Mowszowicz, I., Orth, D. N., and Bardin, C. W. (1975a). *Endocrinology* **97**, 189–195.
Bullock, L. P., Mainwaring, W. I. P., and Bardin, C. W. (1975b). *Endocr. Res. Commun.* **2**, 25–45.
Crabtree, C. (1941). *Anat. Rec.* **79**, 395, 413.
Dunn, J. F., and Wilson, J. D. (1975). *Endocrinology* **96**, 1571–1578.
Dunn, T. B. (1949). *J. Natl. Cancer Inst.* **9**, 285–301.
Edgren, R. A., Jones, R. C., and Petersen, D. L. (1967). *Fertil. Steril.* **18**, 238–256.
Fang, S., and Liao, S. (1971). *J. Biol. Chem.* **246**, 16–24.

Fox, T. O. (1975). *Proc. Natl. Acad. Sci. U.S.A.* **72**, 4303–4307.
Frieden, E. H., and Fishel, S. S. (1968). *Biochem. Biophys. Res. Commun.* **31**, 515–521.
Frieden, E. H., and Ku, C.-C. (1971). *Proc. Soc. Exp. Biol. Med.* **137**, 1110–1114.
Frieden, E. H., Harper, A. A., Chin, F., and Fishman, W. H. (1964). *Steroids* **4**, 777–786.
Gehring, U., and Tomkins, G. M. (1974). *Cell* **3**, 59–64.
Glasser, S. R., Chytil, F., and Spelsberg, T. C. (1972). *Biochem. J.* **130**, 947–957.
Gray, G. M. (1971). *Biochim. Biophys. Acta* **239**, 494–500.
Hayes, K. J. (1965). *Acta Endocrinol. (Copenhagen)* **48**, 337–347.
Imperato-McGinley, J., and Peterson, R. E. (1976). *Am. J. Med.* **61**, 251–272.
Itakura, H., and Ohno, S. (1973). *Clin. Genet.* **4**, 91–97.
Jänne, O., Bullock, L. P., Bardin, C. W., and Jacob, S. T. (1976). *Biochim. Biophys. Acta* **418**, 330–343.
Kan, J., Mackinnon, P. C. B., Ohno, S., and Younglai, E. V. (1974). *J. Physiol. (London)* **242**, 103P.
Kochakian, C. D. (1944). *Am. J. Physiol.* **142**, 315–325.
Kochakian, C. D. (1946). *Vitam. Horm. (N.Y.)* **4**, 255–310.
Kochakian, C. D. (1969). *Gen. Comp. Endocrinol.* **13**, 146–150.
Kochakian, C. D. (1974). *Ala. J. Med. Sci.* **11**, 333–339.
Kochakian, C. D. (1975). *Pharmacol. & Ther., Part B* **1**, 149–177.
Kochakian, C. D., and Tillotson, C. (1957). *Endocrinology* **60**, 607–618.
Kochakian, C. D., Garber, E. E., and Bartlett, M. N. (1948). *Am. J. Physiol.* **155**, 265–271.
Kochakian, C. D., Tillotson, C., and Endahl, G. L. (1956). *Endocrinology* **58**, 226–231.
Korenchevsky, V., and Dennison, M. (1935). *Biochem. J.* **29**, 2122–2130.
Krüskemper, H. L. (1968). "Anabolic Steroids." Academic Press, New York.
Liao, S. (1975). *Int. Rev. Cytol.* **41**, 87–171.
Lyon, M. F., and Hawkes, S. G. (1970). *Nature (London)* **227**, 1217–1219.
Lyon, M. F., Hendry, I., and Short, R. V. (1973). *J. Endocrinol.* **58**, 357–362.
Mainwaring, W. I. P., Mangan, F. R., and Peterken, B. M. (1971). *Biochem. J.* **123**, 619–628.
Mowszowicz, I., and Bardin, C. W. (1974). *Steroids* **23**, 793–807.
Mowszowicz, I., and Bardin, C. W. (1977). *Mol. Cell. Endocrinol.* **8**, 15–26.
Mowszowicz, I., Bieber, D. E., Chung, K. W., Bullock, L. P., and Bardin, C. W. (1974). *Endocrinology* **95**, 1589–1599.
Müller, H.-C., and von Deimling, O. (1971). *Histochemie* **28**, 145–159.
Naftolin, F., and Judd, H. L. (1973). In "Obstetrics and Gynecology Annual" (R. W. Wynn, ed.), pp. 25–53. Appleton, New York.
Nimni, M. E., and Bavetta, L. A. (1961). *Proc. Soc. Exp. Biol. Med.* **106**, 738–740.
Ohno, S., Stenius, C., Christian, L., Harris, C., and Ivey, C. (1970). *Biochem. Genet.* **4**, 565–577.
O'Malley, B. W., and Means, A. R. (1974). *Science* **183**, 610–620.
Overbeek, G. A. (1966). "Anabolic Steroids." Springer-Verlag, Berlin and New York.
Paigen, K., Swank, R. T., Tomino, S., and Ganschow, R. E. (1975). *J. Cell. Physiol.* **85**, 379–392.
Plaut, A. G., and Fishman, W. H. (1963). *J. Cell Biol.* **16**, 253–258.
Revesz, C., Chappel, C. I., and Gaudry, R. (1960). *Endocrinology* **66**, 140–144.
Roy, A. K. (1973). *J. Endocrinol.* **56**, 295–301.
Ruddle, F. H. (1966). *J. Histochem. Cytochem.* **14**, 25–32.
Schenkein, I., Levy, M., Bueker, E. D., and Wilson, J. D. (1974). *Endocrinology* **94**, 840–844.
Schwarzlose, W., and Heim, F. (1973). *Life Sci.* **12**, 107–115.
Scow, R. O. (1952). *Endocrinology* **51**, 42–51.
Segaloff, A. (1964). *Adv. Chem. Ser.* **45**, 204–220.

Shaw, C. R., and Koen, A. L. (1963). *Science* **140**, 70–71.
Siiteri, P. K., and Wilson, J. D. (1974). *J. Clin. Endocrinol. Metab.* **38**, 113–125.
Staeudinger, M., Wienker, T., and von Deimling, O. V. (1974). *Histochemistry* **39**, 361–370.
Suchowsky, G. K., and Junkmann, K. (1961). *Endocrinology* **68**, 341–349.
Swank, R. T., and Bailey, D. W. (1973). *Science* **181**, 1249–1252.
Swank, R. T., Paigen, K., and Ganschow, R. E. (1973). *J. Mol. Biol.* **81**, 225–243.
Verhoeven, G., Heyns, W., and DeMoor, P. (1975). *Steroids* **26**, 149–167.
Williams-Ashman, H. G., Tadolini, B., Wilson, J., and Corti, A. (1975). *Vitam. Horm. (N.Y.)* **33**, 39–60.
Wilson, J. D., and Gloyna, R. E. (1970). *Recent Prog. Horm. Res.* **26**, 309–336.

5

Androgen Receptors and Biologic Responses: A Survey

W. I. P. MAINWARING

I.	Introduction	105
II.	General Model for the Mechanism of Action of Androgens	106
III.	Desirable Trends in Future Research	111
	A. Purification of Receptor Complexes	111
	B. Wider Use of Genetic Mutants	113
	C. Exploitation of New Experimental Systems	114
	D. The Use of More Sophisticated Methods	116
IV.	Summary	117
	References	117

I. INTRODUCTION

About 10 years ago, studies on the mechanism of action of androgens were entrusted in the hands of a small but valiant band of pioneers. Since then, there has been a tremendous resurgence of interest in this area of contemporary endocrinology and the ranks of investigators have increased almost exponentially. As a result of this increased work force, impressive advances have been made in our understanding of androgen action in molecular terms. Some insight into the rate of progress may be gained by comparing reviews of this subject, notably those by Ofner (1968), Liao and Fang (1969), Williams-Ashman and Reddi (1971), King and Mainwaring (1974), Liao (1975), and Mainwaring (1975a,b). From understandably hesitant beginnings, the general application of sophisticated methods has enabled many aspects of the interactions of androgens and mammalian cells to be elucidated. It would be fallacious, however, to assume that we understand fully the manifestation of androgenic responses. The principal objectives of this survey are to present a personal appraisal of current research and to attempt to predict important trends in the future.

II. GENERAL MODEL FOR THE MECHANISM OF ACTION OF ANDROGENS

For over a decade, the rat ventral prostate has almost invariably been the system of choice for investigations on the mechanism of action of androgens. Based on the current literature, a working model for the inception of androgenic responses in this male accessory sexual gland may be proposed (Fig. 1).

The interaction and retention of androgens with their "target" cells is not a haphazard process but is mediated, rather, by an integrated series of molecular events.

The major androgen, testosterone, is transported in the plasma in the form of stable complexes with plasma proteins. For details of the distribution of testosterone in the peripheral circulation, the reference work by Westphal (1971) is strongly recommended.

Testosterone enters all cells to a certain extent by processes that remain to be unequivocally defined but almost certainly include simple diffusion. Largely from the work of Giorgi and her associates, it remains a distinct possibility that androgen target cells may possess a carrier mechanism on the plasma membrane that promotes the facilitated entry of testosterone and closely related steroids. A lucid evaluation of the present status of this work may be found in the recent article by Giorgi (1976).

Exclusively within androgen target cells, testosterone is extensively metabolized, the principal products being 5α-dihydrotestosterone (17β-hydroxy-5α-androstan-3-one) and a spectrum of 5α-androstanediols. The original observation on the formation of 5α-dihydrotestosterone must be credited to Farnsworth and Brown (1963), but the full implication of their work was evident only later, largely through the innovative contributions of Bruchovsky and Wilson (1968) and Anderson and Liao (1968).

The 5α-dihydrotestosterone is a powerful androgen, and it is selectively bound with a high affinity (K_d approximately 1×10^{-9} M) to a cytoplasmic receptor protein, forming an androgen–receptor protein complex.

By subtle alterations in the tertiary or quaternary structure of the receptor complex, an activated form results that has a stronger ability to interact with a limited number of binding sites within nuclear chromatin. The latter

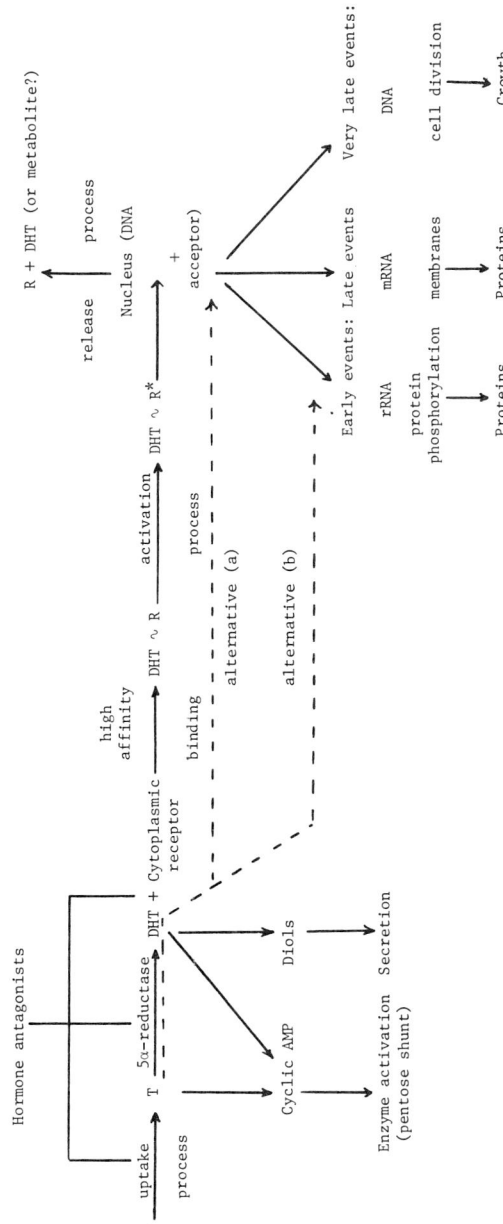

Fig. 1. A simplified mechanism of action of androgens. It is suggested that the nuclear binding of androgens is particularly important, particularly with respect to the activation of processes that require DNA as template. Alternative (a) suggests that certain nuclear events may be stimulated without any involvement of the receptor system; alternative (b) suggests that certain processes are stimulated without the activation of nuclear events or the involvement of the receptor system in any way. Abbreviations: P, steroid-binding proteins in plasma; T, testosterone; DHT, 5α-dihydrotestosterone; R, receptor protein; R*, activated configuration of the receptor; diols, various 5α-androstanediols.

are generally termed the acceptor sites, and their characterization is presently of widespread interest.

The activated complex is translocated into the nucleus and is retained at this intracellular locus for a significant but finite time.

The arrival of the receptor complex stimulates many processes which essentially require DNA as template, the principal being genetic transcription and DNA replication itself. These steroid-mediated events proceed in an ordered temporal sequence and may be classified as initial, early and late responses. Examples of each category of response are given in Fig. 1.

The androgen–receptor protein complex is finally degraded or displaced from the nucleus by mechanisms that are far from clear. Nozu and Tamaoki (1975) suggest that further metabolism of 5α-dihydrotestosterone, while an integral part of the receptor complex, may feature in the release process. This concept needs to be validated, and it also runs counter to the suggestion of Casteñada and Liao (1975) that receptor-bound steroids are enveloped deep within the complex and, hence, inaccessible to catabolic enzymes. An alternative mechanism, that of receptor cycling, has been proposed by Liao *et al.* (1973a,b). In their concept, the receptor complex associates with newly synthesized ribonucleoprotein particles and is ultimately transported from the nucleus to the cytoplasm. While not rigorously proved, this concept is consistent with the observation that an acceleration of ribosomal RNA synthesis is an initial or rapid androgenic response (Mainwaring *et al.*, 1971).

As yet, androgen–receptor protein complexes have resisted all attempts at their extensive purification. Until this is accomplished, the role of receptor complexes in the regulation of metabolic processes remains somewhat imprecise. Nevertheless, many lines of circumstantial evidence support the authenticity of the model presented in Fig. 1 and suggest that it is applicable, at least in principle, to androgen target cells other than rat ventral prostate.

To date, receptorlike proteins have been found in most, if not all, cells that are sensitive to androgenic stimulation or control. As an illustration, high-affinity binding components for androgens have been identified in cells as diverse as rat brain (Thieulant *et al.*, 1975; Kato, 1975), hamster costovertebral glands (Adachi and Kano, 1972), rat skin (Eppenberger and Hsia, 1972), human prostate (Mainwaring and Milroy, 1973; Rosen *et al.*, 1975), rat uterus (Giannopoulos, 1973), fibroblasts derived from human perineal skin (Keenan *et al.*, 1975), cockerel comb and wattles (Dubé *et al.*, 1975), human mammary carcinomas (Poortman *et al.*, 1975), and mouse kidney (Bullock *et al.*, 1971; Bullock and Bardin, 1975a).

The Tfm mouse carries a stable, inherited defect in that the male genitalia fail to develop, despite the presence of the X chromosome and admittedly restricted concentrations of circulating androgens. Certain androgen target organs persist in this mutant, such as the kidney and preputial gland, but, unlike the wild type, androgen receptors are absent (Bullock et al., 1975; Attardi and Ohno, 1974). A general absence of androgen receptors provides a plausible explanation of this syndrome, because the administration of even massive doses of testosterone fails to promote the appearance of male somatic characteristics or other androgen-mediated phenomena.

There are two sublines of Shionogi tumors, an androgen-dependent S115 line and an androgen-independent S42 line (Minesita and Yamaguchi, 1965). While there is neither karyotypic nor morphological evidence to suggest that these sublines have an identical origin, differences in the uptake (Matsumoto et al., 1972) and binding (Mainwaring and Mangan, 1973) of androgens are probably responsible for their contrasted responses to hormonal stimulation.

Perhaps the most impressive evidence supporting the receptor concept comes from studies on antiandrogens. Such androgen antagonists fall into two categories, with either steroidlike or nonsteroidal chemical structures. Taking cyproterone acetate and flutamide as typical representatives of each category, both compounds negate the uptake (Sakiz et al., 1976) or binding (Liao and Fang, 1969; Mainwaring et al., 1974a) of androgens and similarly suppress the manifestation of most androgenic responses (Geller et al., 1969; Mainwaring et al., 1971, 1974a,b,c; Mainwaring and Wilce, 1973; Mangan et al., 1973).

By contrast, other lines of evidence expose the limitations of the model system presented in Fig. 1. In many respects, this is not surprising, as androgens and their metabolites influence such a bewildering array of cell types that a unifying mechanism of action is hardly to be expected.

The model places heavy emphasis on an enhancement of genetic transcription after hormonal stimulation. In rat prostate (Ichii et al., 1974) and other systems (Irving et al., 1976), androgens and related steroids directly influence protein synthesis by translational mechanisms in the cytoplasmic compartment.

Hormones often act synergistically on mammalian cells and, in the case of many male accessory glands, it has long been recognized that prolactin can potentiate the effects of testosterone (Grayhack and Lebovitz, 1967). Hormonal synergism is not adequately explained by the model, but prolactin may stimulate the uptake of testosterone (Resnick et al., 1974). From the work of Rolland and Hammond (1975) and others, techniques have been developed for identifying the specific binding sites for prolactin.

It now appears that testosterone increases the number of prolactin receptor sites in rat prostate (Kledzik et al., 1976), thus providing some indication of the complexity of hormonal synergism.

Contrary to our working model, there are two instances where target cells accumulate androgens directly in the nucleus in the seeming absence of cytoplasmic receptor protein, namely bone marrow (Minguell and Valladares, 1974) and vagina (Shao et al., 1975).

A unique feature of androgenic responses is their acute tissue specificity. For example, certain basic proteins are characteristic of the secretion of the seminal vesicle (Mányai et al., 1965) and alcohol dehydrogenase may be induced by androgens only in mouse kidney (Ohno et al., 1970). Such stringent specificity is not compatible with a simplistic model and from the recent work of Mainwaring et al. (1976), tissue specificity cannot be attributed to receptor mechanisms alone. There are clearly other regulatory elements in mammalian chromatin which control such unique functions and their nature and properties remain totally unknown.

It cannot be overemphasized that a model based on the selective binding of 5α-dihydrotestosterone is not applicable to all androgen target cells because of the critical importance of steroid metabolism in the mechanism of action of androgens and related steroids. It is now clear that the putative "active" steroid can vary enormously, being 5α-dihydrotestosterone in most male accessory sexual glands (Mainwaring and Mangan, 1973) but not dog prostate, where it is clearly 5α-androstane-$3\alpha,17\alpha$-diol (Evans and Pierrepoint, 1975), testosterone itself in muscle (Powers and Florini, 1975) and rat uterus (Giannopoulos, 1973), androstenedione in liver (Gustafsson et al., 1975), Δ^5-androstenediol ($3\beta,17\beta$-dihydroxyandrost-5-ene) in vagina (Shao et al., 1975), and 5β-reduced steroids such as etiocholanolone (3α-hydroxy-5β-androstan-3-one) in fetal chick blastoderm (Iriving et al., 1976).

Hormonal responses essentially fall into two categories: switch or amplification processes. Switch processes involve qualitative changes, whereas amplification processes involve quantitative changes where the hormone simply accelerates events which proceed at much slower rates in the absence of the hormonal stimulus. Most androgenic responses proceed by amplification, but an example of a switch mechanism is the development of the masculine phenotype. All aspects of this complex phenomenon, including the differentiation of the male urogenital tract, are instigated by the fetal secretion of testosterone (Jost, 1953, 1959). The simplistic model cannot satisfactorily explain how androgens promote switch as against amplification processes.

Despite these reservations, the present model of androgen action is a considerable achievement, and it will undoubtedly provide the essential framework for future research on androgen-sensitive cells in general.

III. DESIRABLE TRENDS IN FUTURE RESEARCH

A. Purification of Receptor Complexes

If the role played by androgen–receptor complexes in the regulation of biochemical processes is to be elucidated precisely, then the receptor complexes must first be extensively purified. Creditable attempts by Davies and Griffiths (1974, 1975) and Mainwaring and Jones (1975) to investigate the influence of receptor complexes on the transcription of chromatin were somewhat marred by the use of impure preparations. Conventional methods of protein fractionation have not been particularly successful in the purification of androgen–receptor complexes, the best achievement being the 5000-fold purification reported by Mainwaring and Irving (1973); the final purity of the complex, however, was estimated at best to be only 5–10%. Despite this seeming disclaimer of conventional methods, Schrader et al. (1974) have demonstrated that the sequential application of ion-exchange procedures can achieve extensive purification of the progesterone receptor complexes from chick oviduct and their methodology could be usefully applied to androgen–receptor preparations.

Recent studies from many laboratories raise justifiable hopes that the extensive purification of androgen–receptor complexes may now be possible.

First, there have been considerable improvements in the assay of androgen receptors (Boesel and Shain, 1974; Grover and O'Dell, 1975; Casteñada and Liao, 1975). In addition, Bonne and Raynaud (1975) have made an invaluable contribution by demonstrating that [^{3}H]methyltrienolone (the synthetic androgen, R1881 or 17β-hydroxy-17α-methylestra-4,9,11-trien-3-one) is an ideal radioactive ligand for androgen–receptor proteins but not the plasma protein, sex steroid-binding β-globulin (SBG), which often contaminates receptor preparations and especially those from human sources (Mainwaring and Milroy, 1973; Steins et al., 1974; Rosen et al., 1975). The importance of [^{3}H]methyltrienolone is highlighted by the fact that benign hyperplastic nodules of human prostate possibly represent the most plentiful source of androgen-sensitive tissues for the purification of androgen–receptor complexes on a large scale.

Second, many research teams have successfully exploited the extreme specificity of affinity chromatography for the purification of steroid hormone–receptor protein complexes to a state approaching homogeneity (Sica et al., 1973; Kuhn et al., 1975; Smith et al., 1975), and this sophisticated procedure should be applied to androgen receptors as a matter of priority. To date, affinity matrices containing immobilized androgens have not been developed specifically for receptor proteins, but several have been advocated for the purification of SBG (Burstein, 1969; Mickelson and

Pétra, 1975; Rosner and Smith, 1975), and there is no *a priori* reason why these should not be applied for androgen–receptor complexes. In particular, the matrix developed by Rosner and Smith (1975) has much to recommend its wider use, for unlike other alternatives (Burstein, 1969; Mickelson and Pétra, 1975), it contains 5α-dihydrotestosterone covalently linked via a hemisuccinate bridge at the C-3 position, thus leaving the important C-17β-hydroxyl group accessible for the binding of the androgen–receptor protein. Studies by Liao *et al.* (1973a) and Skinner *et al.* (1975) have shown that the 17β-hydroxyl group is probably the most important structural determinant in steroid ligands for their recognition by the high-affinity binding sites within the androgen receptor molecule. In addition, Rosner and Smith (1975) demonstrated that 4,4′-azodianiline is a superior spacer moiety to bovine serum albumin, poly(L-lysine-DL-alanine) or 3,3′-diaminodipropylamine (Mickelson and Pétra, 1975), enabling proteins adsorbed on the matrix to be efficiently eluted under very mild conditions. Affinity chromatography would yield receptor–protein complexes contaminated with SBG or other androgen-binding proteins.

There seem to be three potential methods for selectively isolating the androgen–receptor complexes from eluates of affinity matrices: (a) physicochemical methods, such as isoelectric focusing (Coffer *et al.*, 1977) or agar gel electrophoresis (Wagner and Jungblut, 1976) where differences in pI or charge may be usefully exploited; (b) passage through columns containing immobilized prostate nuclear proteins, including putative acceptor molecules, since these do not recognize SBG or low-affinity, androgen-binding proteins (Mainwaring *et al.*, 1976); (c) passage through columns containing immobilized antibodies raised against androgenic steroids, since these would impede only the elution of androgen-containing complexes with SBG or other proteins (Casteñada and Liao, 1975), leaving the androgen–receptor complexes in the "flow-through" fraction. By a combination of these approaches, androgen–receptor complexes may soon be available in a highly purified form.

While receptor proteins themselves have been rather neglected, it has become rather fashionable to examine in detail the binding of androgens to nonreceptor, androgen-binding proteins, including uteroglobin (Beato, 1976), human erythrocytes and hemoglobins (Ige and Adadevoh, 1975), and nonspecific binding proteins of rat prostate (Heyns *et al.*, 1976). It is difficult to envisage how these studies can further knowledge considerably on the mechanism of steroid hormone action. This criticism cannot be justifiably leveled at studies on SBG–androgen interactions because the homogeneous protein is now available in quantity, and sequence analysis, combined with affinity labeling of the single steroid-binding site, may provide the first real clues to the nature of high-affinity binding in this important plasma protein. Such studies would be an invaluable guide to future work on receptor–androgen interactions.

B. Wider Use of Genetic Mutants

The importance of mutants to the development of molecular biology and biochemistry over the last two decades is incalculable. Largely through advances in cell biology and, in particular, to improvements in cloning techniques, it has proved possible to isolate mammalian cell types with grossly different responses to steroid hormones. These have provided unique systems for unraveling the molecular basis for hormone action. As an example, the spectrum of glucocorticoid-sensitive and -insensitive lymphoma lines pioneered, among others, by Horibata and Harris (1970), have been studied from the standpoint of comparative binding mechanisms. The exemplary study by Yamamoto *et al.* (1974) revealed several categories of mutants with distinctive deletions in either the glucocorticoid receptor proteins, the nuclear translocation process or other discrete stages of the overall mechanism responsible for glucocorticoid-mediated responses. It is imperative that these genetic approaches be adopted in a wider context in the future.

With respect to androgen action, the Tfm mouse (Lyon and Hawkes, 1970) and the pseudohermaphrodite rat (Stanley and Gumbreck, 1964) are stable mutants suitable for detailed investigation. Both mutants provide experimental models for the testicular feminization syndrome. They have a male genotype and female phenotype, and the failure to develop external male genitalia, plus other aspects of masculine differentiation, cannot be rectified even by the administration of massive doses of androgens. The mutants present the classical symptoms of androgen insensitivity, and this is best explained by the virtual absence of androgen–receptor proteins (Attardi and Ohno, 1974; Bullock *et al.*, 1975). To emphasize the specificity of this genetic aberration, the full complement of estrogen receptor proteins persists in all the expected target sites of the Tfm mouse (Bullock and Bardin, 1975b). It is also important to stress that these experimental models have provided a plausible explanation in molecular terms for testicular feminization in man (Keenan *et al.* 1975; Wilson, 1975). Bardin (1977) has reported very recently that all manifestations of androgen action are not completely suppressed in the Tfm mouse. Many microsomal enzymes in mouse liver are subject to androgenic modulation, but some persist and respond to androgens even in the Tfm mutation. This study provides a novel insight into the subtleties of androgen action in a given cell type and presents a unique opportunity for contrasting the molecular mechanisms for androgenic responses, notably receptor-dependent and -independent processes.

Paigen and his collaborators have also demonstrated the impact of genetic mutants in a very elegant manner, using β-glucuronidase of mouse kidney as a tissue-specific marker for androgenic induction. The culmination of this work was the publication of a sophisticated model for the regulation of enzyme synthesis in mammalian cells (Paigen et al., 1975), and, in the present author's view, it represents the most exciting contribution to our understanding of androgen action for many years. Drawing heavily on recombinant and inbred strains of mice (Swank and Bailey, 1973), each bearing stable mutations in the genetic loci responsible for regulating the activity of β-glucuronidase, Paigen et al. (1975) proposed four categories of regulatory elements as (a) structural, (b) processing, (c) regulatory, and (d) temporal genes. Together, these regulate the synthesis, intracellular distribution, sensitivity to hormones, developmental modulation, and secretion of kidney β-glucuronidase. Aside from conceptual importance, two aspects of this brilliant work warrant particular comment. First, the regulatory Gur locus, where the kidney androgen–receptor complex is bound, is the first genetic site under stringent hormonal control to be identified unequivocally in any eukaryotic cell. Second, the study indicates that it is not always necessary to monitor the synthesis, processing, and translation of a specific species of messenger RNA in order to elucidate mechanisms of hormonal control, provided that alternative approaches can be used instead. In the work of Paigen et al. (1975), genetic analysis combined with detailed studies on the molecular architecture of β-glucuronidase provided all the necessary information.

As reviewed by Mainwaring (1975b) and Yamamoto and Alberts (1975), binding mechanisms alone cannot provide a convincing explanation for the tissue specificity of hormonal responses. The study by Mainwaring et al. (1976) suggests that the chromatin of hormone-sensitive cells is somehow imparted with a unique, tissue-specific character during the process of cellular differentiation. The nature of the regulatory elements remains unknown, but studies of mutants may provide vital clues. What investigators need are cell lines containing normal or functional receptor mechanisms, but with imparied or defective responses to steroid hormones. Gehring (1977) has indicated the existence of such mutants, and the report by Bardin (1977) also offers hope in this direction.

C. Exploitation of New Experimental Systems

The rat ventral prostate has occupied the center of the stage for so long that its limitations have tended to be overlooked. Indeed, future progress may well depend more on the development of new experimental systems than to any other single factor. To take full advantage of contemporary advances in molecular biology, the ideal system for studies on androgen action should satisfy the following criteria. (a) The androgen target cell should contain a macromolecular marker, preferably a protein, whose synthesis is totally regulated by androgens. (b) The marker should constitute a major proportion of the synthetic output of the target cell. This consideration dashed our earlier hopes that prostate aldolase would be a suitable marker (Mainwaring et al., 1974c). (c) The marker should have a known function and its structure should be well characterized.

Recent studies by Higgins et al. (1976) indicate that certain basic proteins in rat seminal vesicle may fulfill these requirements. (a) Two basic proteins are selectively induced by androgens in seminal vesicle; they cannot be detected in any other tissue of the male rat. (b) These proteins are probably necessary for the formation of the vaginal plug after copulation and may be related to the "clotting proteins" described by other investigators (Mányai, 1964; Notides and Williams-Ashman, 1967). (c) The two proteins have almost identical physicochemical properties, yet may be resolved and purified by preparative polyacrylamide electrophoresis in the presence of sodium dodecyl sulfate into SVBP/F (faster migration; MW 17000) and SVBP/S (slower migration; MW 18,500). Both have a pI of 9.7 and contain carbohydrate moieties. (d) Together, these two glycoproteins constitute 25-30% of the total protein synthesized in the seminal vesicle. These favorable properties should enable the regulation of their synthesis to be determined, with the long-term objective of simulating these regulatory processes in reconstituted, cell-free systems.

With a few notable exceptions, androgen target cells cannot be satisfactorily maintained in any quantity as separated cells *in vitro*. Human fibroblasts derived from perineal skin are an exception, but even these have certain limitations which preclude their widespread adoption for general studies on the mechanism of action of androgens. Despite the unquestionable presence of androgen receptors (Keenan et al., 1975) and steroid-metabolizing enzyme systems (Wilson, 1975) in cultured fibroblasts, there is no convincing evidence to date that supplementation of the culture medium with physiological concentrations of androgens stimulates classical androgenic responses, such as cellular proliferation. Tissue explants of male accessory sexual glands can be maintained, but these often lose their characteristic responsiveness to androgens *in vitro*, particularly in terms of an acceleration of RNA synthesis (Alfheim and Fjell, 1973). However, the activation of cultures of rat epididymal cells by androgens *in vitro* (Blaquier et al., 1975) may point to a more favorable trend for the future. Tumor cells often adapt well to conditions of cell culture, but there have been few reports of the successful maintenance of tumors from androgen target cells. Aside from variability in the induction of rat prostate tumors by chemical carcinogens (Dunning et al., 1946) or oncogenic viruses (Fraley and Ecker, 1971), the resulting tumors can only be maintained satisfactorily in immunosuppressed animals. Attempts to culture cells from human prostatic tumors have met with only limited success. Many research groups have maintained viable cultures, but except for the report by McRae et al. (1973), the tumor cells are either refractory to androgens (McMahon et al., 1974; Harbitz et al., 1974) or have lost all the classical markers for androgens, especially the hormone-inducible acid phosphatase (Schroeder and Mackensen, 1974). The spontaneous tumors of the rat prostate described by Pollard and Luckert (1975) seem the best available at the present time, and it would be a very significant step forward if stable yet hormone-responsive cell lines could be derived from these primary, transplantable tumors.

It is widely accepted that androgenic responses originate from the activation of transcriptional processes. However, Ichii et al. (1974) have rightly emphasized the importance of translational control mechanisms, and these seem singularly applicable to the enhancement of fetal hemoglobin synthesis by androgen-related steroids (Irving et al., 1976). These cultures of chick blastoderm are also distinctive in that the erythropoietic response to 5β-reduced steroids may be elicited under conditions in vitro.

As an overview, then, it would appear that rat prostate will not invariably be the experimental system of choice in the future. Systems will be selected for their suitability for certain aspects of androgen action only, for no system can be considered ideal in all respects. The development of stable cell lines of androgen target cells remains a high priority, especially in experimental cancer research, because they offer the potential advantages of stability, reproducibility, and ease of handling.

D. The Use of More Sophisticated Methods

The principal objective in many laboratories is to reproduce faithfully many aspects of the mechanism of action of androgens in reconstituted systems, in vitro, particularly from the standpoint of the activation of genetic transcription (Davies and Griffiths, 1974, 1975; Mainwaring and Jones, 1975). The precise role of nonhistone proteins in the regulation of transcription is also the center of considerable interest (Nyberg and Wang, 1976; Webster et al., 1976).

It is worthwhile, however, to consider how these experiments can be improved and, thus, provide a more significant insight into the activation of chromatin by androgen–receptor complexes. The use of highly purified preparations of androgen–receptor complexes has been mentioned earlier but cannot be overemphasized. In view of the recent studies by Spelsberg (1976) and Pikler et al. (1976), it is now evident that optimum conditions for the transfer of receptor complexes into chromatin *in vitro* must be determined very carefully; otherwise the results are open to serious criticism. In addition, Simons et al. (1976) have indicated the artifacts that may so easily be created in these reconstituted systems. Yamamoto and Alberts (1975) have also drawn attention to the fact that present methods for assessing receptor complex–acceptor interactions are imprecise and may give a serious overestimate of the number of molecules of receptor complex that are really necessary to evoke the hormonal activation of chromatin. For this and other reasons, more precise methods must be used for analyzing the RNA synthesized on the chromatin template *in vitro*. Nucleic acid hybridization offers perhaps the only hope in this context and was wisely incorporated into the recent study of prostate chromatin by Nyberg and Wang (1976). The real importance of this powerful technique is evident from the elegant studies on chromatin transcription performed by Wilson *et al.* (1975) and Schwartz *et al.* (1975).

IV. SUMMARY

Considerable progress has been made in elucidating the mechanism of action of androgens. However, if this impetus is to be maintained, investigations will have to be carried out in a more sophisticated manner than practiced hitherto. Some of the more desirable trends for the future have been briefly discussed and in the interests of constructive self-criticism, the author intends to improve his own approach to this complex yet fascinating problem.

ACKNOWLEDGMENT

The author wishes to thank Mrs. Margaret Barker for her patient and painstaking assistance in the preparation of the manuscript.

REFERENCES

Adachi, K., and Kano, M. (1972). *Steroids* **19**, 567.
Alfheim, I., and Fjell, B. (1973). *Acta Endocrinol. (Copenhagen).* **73**, 189.
Anderson, K. M., and Liao, S. (1968). *Nature (London)* **219**, 277.

Attardi, B., and Ohno, S. (1970). *Cell* **2**, 205.
Bardin, C. W. (1977). *Proc. Int. Congr. Endocrinol. 5th 1976* (in press).
Beato, M. (1976). *J. Steroid Biochem.* **7**, 327.
Blaquier, J., Breger, D., Cameo, M. S., and Calandra, R. (1975). *J. Steroid Biochem.* **6**, 573.
Boesel, R. W., and Shain, S. A. (1974). *Biochem. Biophys. Res. Commun.* **61**, 1004.
Bonne, C., and Raynaud, J.-P. (1975). *Steroids* **26**, 227.
Bruchovsky, N., and Wilson, J. D. (1968). *J. Biol. Chem.* **243**, 2012.
Bullock, L. P., and Bardin, C. W. (1975a). *Steroids* **20**, 107.
Bullock, L. P., and Bardin, C. W. (1975b). *Endocrinology* **97**, 1106.
Bullock, L. P., Bardin, C. W., and Ohno, S. (1971). *Biochem. Biophys. Res. Commun.* **44**, 1537.
Bullock, L. P., Mainwaring, W. I. P., and Bardin, C. W. (1975). *Endocr. Res. Commun.* **2**, 25.
Burstein, S. H. (1969). *Steroids* **14**, 263.
Casteñada, E., and Liao, S. (1975). *J. Biol. Chem.* **250**, 883.
Coffer, A. I., Milton, P. J. D., Pryse-Davis, J., and King, R. J. B. (1977). *Mol. Cell. Endocr.* **6**, 231.
Davies, P., and Griffiths, K. (1974). *Biochem. J.* **136**, 611.
Davies, P., and Griffiths, K. (1975). *Mol. Cell. Endocrinol.* **3**, 143.
Dubé, J. Y., Tremblay, R. R., Lesage, R., and Vierret, G. (1975). *Mol. Cell. Endocrinol.* **2**, 213.
Dunning, W. F., Curtis, M. R., and Segaloff, A. (1946). *Cancer Res.* **6**, 256.
Eppenberger, U., and Hsia, S. L. (1972). *J. Biol. Chem.* **247**, 5463.
Evans, C. R., and Pierrepoint, C. G. (1975). *J. Endocrinol.* **64**, 539.
Farnsworth, W. E., and Brown, J. R. (1963). *Natl. Cancer Inst., Monogr.* **12**, 323.
Fraley, E. E., and Ecker, S. (1971). *J. Urol.* **106**, 95.
Gehring, U. (1977). *Proc. Int. Congr. Endocrinol., 5th, 1976* (in press).
Geller, J., van Damme, O., Garabieta, G., Loh, A., Rettura, J., and Seifter, E. (1969). *Endocrinology* **84**, 1330.
Gianopoulos, G. (1973). *J. Biol. Chem.* **248**, 1004.
Giorgi, E. P. (1976). *J. Endocrinol.* **68**, 109.
Grayhack, J. T., and Lebovitz, J. M. (1967). *Invest. Urol.* **5**, 87.
Grover, P. K., and O'Dell, W. D. (1975). *J. Steroid Biochem.* **6**, 1373.
Gustafsson, J-Å., Pousette, Å., Stenberg, Å., and Wrange, Ö. (1975). *Biochemistry* **14**, 3942.
Harbitz, T. B., Falkanger, B., and Sanger, S. (1974). *Acta Pathol. Microbiol. Scand., Sect. A., Suppl.* **248**, 89.
Heyns, W., Verhoeven, G., and de Moor, P. (1976). *J. Steroid Biochem.* **7**, 987.
Higgins, S. J., Burchell, J. M., and Mainwaring, W. I. P. (1976). *Biochem. J.* (in press).
Horibata, K., and Harris, A. W. (1970). *Exp. Cell Res.* **60**, 61.
Ichii, S., Izawa, M., and Murakami, N. (1974). *Endocrinol. Jpn.* **21**, 267.
Ige, R. O., and Adadevoh, B. K. (1975). *J. Steroid Biochem.* **6**, 1253.
Irving, R. A., Mainwaring, W. I. P., and Spooner, P. M. (1976). *Biochem. J.* **154**, 83.
Jost, A. (1953). *Recent Prog. Horm. Res.* **8**, 379.
Jost, A. (1959). *Harvey Lect.* **55**, 201.
Kato, J. (1975). *J. Steroid Biochem.* **6**, 979.
Keenan, B. S., Meyer, W. T., Hadjian, A. J., and Migeon, C. T. (1975). *Steroids* **25**, 535.
King, R. J. B., and Mainwaring, W. I. P. (1974). "Steroid-Cell Interactions." Butterworth, London.
Kledzik, G. S., Marshall, S., Campbell, G. A., Gelato, M., and Meites, J. (1976). *Endocrinology* **98**, 373.

Kuhn, R. W., Schrader, W. T., Smith, R. G., and O'Malley, B. W. (1975). *J. Biol. Chem.* **250**, 4220.
Liao, S. (1975). *Int. Rev. Cytol.* **41**, 87.
Liao, S., and Fang, S. (1969). *Vitam. Horm. (N.Y.)* **27**, 17.
Liao, S., Liang, T., Fang, S., Casteñada, E., and Shao, T.-C. (1973a). *J. Biol. Chem.* **248**, 6514.
Liao, S., Liang, T., Shao, T.-C., and Tymoczko, J. L. (1973b). *Ann. Exp. Biol. Med.* **36**, 232.
Liao, S., Liang, T., and Tymoczko, J. L. (1973c). *Nature (London), New Biol.* **241**, 211.
Lyon, M. F., and Hawkes, S. G. (1970). *Nature (London)* **227**, 1217.
McMahon, M. J., Butler, A. V. J., and Thomas, G. H. (1974). *Acta Endocrinol. (Copenhagen)* **77**, 784.
McRae, C. V., Ghanadian, R., Fotherby, K., and Chisholm, G. D. (1973). *Br. J. Urol.* **45**, 156.
Mainwaring, W. I. P. (1975a). *J. Reprod. Fertil.* **44**, 377.
Mainwaring, W. I. P. (1975b). *Vitam. Horm. (N.Y.)* **33**, 223.
Mainwaring, W. I. P., and Irving, R. A. (1973). *Biochem. J.* **134**, 113.
Mainwaring, W. I. P., and Jones, D. A. (1975). *J. Steroid Biochem.* **6**, 475.
Mainwaring, W. I. P., and Mangan, F. R. (1973). *J. Endocrinol.* **59**, 121.
Mainwaring, W. I. P., and Milroy, E. J. G. (1973). *J. Endocrinol.* **57**, 371.
Mainwaring, W. I. P., and Wilce, P. A. (1973). *Biochem. J.* **134**, 795.
Mainwaring, W. I. P., Mangan, F. R., and Peterken, B. M. (1971). *Biochem. J.* **123**, 619.
Mainwaring, W. I. P., Mangan, F. R., Feherty, P. A., and Friefeld, M. (1974a). *Mol. Cell. Endocrinol.* **1**, 113.
Mainwaring, W. I. P., Wilce, P. A., and Smith, A. E. (1974b). *Biochem. J.* **137**, 513.
Mainwaring, W. I. P., Mangan, F. R., Irving, R. A., and Jones, D. A. (1974c). *Biochem. J.* **144**, 413.
Mainwaring, W. I. P., Symes. E. K., and Higgins, S. J. (1976). *Biochem. J.* **156**, 129.
Mangan, F. R., Pegg, A. E., and Mainwaring, W. I. P. (1973). *Biochem. J.* **134**, 129.
Mányai, S. (1964). *Acta Physiol. Acad. Sci. Hung.* **24**, 419.
Mányai, S., Beney, L., and Czuppon, A. (1965). *Acta Physiol. Acad. Sci. Hung.* **28**, 108.
Matsumoto, K., Kotoh, K., Kasai, H., Minesita, T., and Yamaguchi, K. (1972). *Steroids* **20**, 311.
Mickelson, K. E., and Pétra, P. H. (1975). *Biochemistry* **14**, 957.
Minesita, T., and Yamaguchi, K. (1965). *Cancer Res.* **25**, 1168.
Minguell, J., and Valladares, L. (1974). *J. Steroid Biochem.* **5**, 649.
Notides, A., and Williams-Ashman, H. G. (1967). *Proc. Natl. Acad. Sci. U.S.A.* **58**, 1991.
Nozu, K., and Tamaoki, B.-I. (1975). *J. Steroid Biochem.* **6**, 1319.
Nyberg, L. M., and Wang, T. Y. (1976). *J. Steroid Biochem.* **7**, 267.
Ofner, P. (1968). *Vitam. Horm. (N.Y.)* **26**, 237.
Ohno, S., Stenius, S., Christian, L., Harris, C., and Ivey. C. (1970). *Biochem. Genet.* **4**, 565.
Paigen, R., Swank, R. T., Tomino, S., and Ganschow, R. E. (1975). *J. Cell. Physiol.* **85**, 379.
Pikler, G. M., Webster, R. A., and Spelsberg, T. C. (1975). *Biochem. J.* **156**, 399.
Pollard, M., and Luckert, P. H. (1975). *J. Natl. Cancer Inst.* **54**, 643.
Poortman, J., Prenen, J. A. C., Schwartz, F., and Thijssen, J. H. H. (1975). *J. Clin. Endocrinol. Metab.* **40**, 373.
Powers, M. L., and Florini, J. R. (1975). *Endocrinology* **97**, 1043.
Resnick, M. I., Walvoord, D. J., and Grayhack, J. T. (1974). *Surg. Forum* **25**, 70.
Rolland, R., and Hammond, J. M. (1975). *Endocrinol. Res. Commun.* **2**, 281.
Rosen, V., Jung, I., Baulieu, E.-E., and Robel, P. (1975). *J. Clin. Endocrinol. Metab.* **41**, 761.
Rosner, W., and Smith, R. N. (1975). *Biochemistry* **14**, 4813.

Sakiz, E., Azadian-Boulanger, G., Bonne, C., Perronet, J., and Raynaud, J.-P. (1976). "Androgens and Antiandrogens" (in press).
Schrader, W. T., Buller, R. E., Kuhn, R. W., and O'Malley, B. W. (1974). *J. Steroid Biochem.* **5**, 989.
Schroeder, F. M., and Mackensen, S. J. (1974). *Invest. Urol.* **12**, 176.
Schwartz, R. J., Tsai, M-J., Tsai, S. Y., and O'Malley, B. W. (1975). *J. Biol. Chem.* **250**, 5175.
Shao, T.-C., Casteñada, E., Rosenfield, R. L., and Liao, S. (1975). *J. Biol. Chem.* **250**, 3095.
Sica, V., Parikh, I., Nola, E., Puca, G. A., and Cuatrecasas, P. (1973). *J. Biol. Chem.* **248**, 6543.
Simons, S. S., Martinez, H. M., Garcea, R. L., Baxter, J. D., and Tomkins, G. M. (1976). *J. Biol. Chem.* **251**, 334.
Skinner, R. W. S., Pozderac, R. V., Counsell, R. E., and Weinhold, P. M. (1975). *Steroids* **25**, 185.
Smith, R. G., Iramain, C. A., Buttram, V. C., and O'Malley, B. W. (1975). *Nature (London), New Biol.* **253**, 271.
Spelsberg, T. C. (1976). *Biochem. J.* **156**, 391.
Stanley, A. J., and Gumbreck, L. G. (1964). *Proc. Am. Endocr. Soc.* **31**, 40.
Steins, P., Kreig, M., Hollmann, H. J., and Voigt, K.-D. (1974). *Acta Endocrinol. (Copenhagen)* **75**, 773.
Swank, R. T., and Bailey, D. W. (1973). *Science* **181**, 1249.
Thieulant, M. L., Mercier, L., Samparez, S., and Juoan, P. (1975). *J. Steroid Biochem.* **6**, 1257.
Wagner, R. K., and Jungblut, P. W. (1976). *Mol. Cell. Endocrinol.* **4**, 13.
Webster, R. A., Pikler, G. M., and Spelsberg, T. C. (1976). *Biochem. J.* **156**, 409.
Westphal, U. (1971). "Steroid-Protein Interactions." Springer-Verlag, Berlin.
Williams-Ashman, H. G., and Reddi, A. H. (1971). *Annu. Rev. Physiol.* **33**, 31.
Wilson, G. N., Steggles, A. W., Kantor, J. A., Niehuis, A. W., and Anderson, W. F. (1975). *J. Biol. Chem.* **250**, 8604.
Wilson, J. D. (1975). *J. Biol. Chem.* **250**, 3498.
Yamamoto, K. R., and Alberts, B. M. (1975). *Cell* **4**, 301.
Yamamoto, K. R., Stampfer, M. R., and Tomkins, G. M. (1974). *Proc. Natl. Acad. Sci. U.S.A.* **71**, 3901.

6

Androgen Receptor Interactions in Target Cells: Biochemical Evaluation

JOHN L. TYMOCZKO, TEHMING LIANG,
AND SHUTSUNG LIAO

I.	Evidence for Existence of Androgen Receptors	122
II.	Identification and Characterization of Androgen Receptors	123
	A. Cellular Localization	123
	B. Sedimentation Properties	126
	C. Characterization by Antisteroid Antibody	126
	D. Characterization by Other Methods	129
III.	Specificities in Androgen–Receptor Interactions	130
	A. Target Tissue Specificity	130
	B. Steroid Specificity	132
IV.	Cell Nucleus and Chromatin Binding of Androgen Receptor	136
	A. Steroid and Receptor Interdependence	136
	B. Receptor Transformation	137
	C. Acceptor Concepts	138
	D. Characterization of Acceptor Molecules	139
	E. Histones and Nuclear Acceptor Activity	143
	F. Release of Receptor From Chromatin	144
V.	Interaction of Androgen Receptors with Other Cellular Components	144
	A. Divalent Metal Cations and Mononucleotides	144
	B. Polynucleotides and Ribonucleoproteins	146
VI.	Concluding Remarks	148
	A. Action of Antiandrogens	148
	B. RNA Synthesis	149
	C. Ribonucleoprotein Function	150
	D. Protein Synthesis	151
	References	153

I. EVIDENCE FOR EXISTENCE OF ANDROGEN RECEPTORS

Studies in the 1950's (Barry et al., 1952; Greer, 1959) indicated that the sexual accessory glands were capable of retaining radioisotope-labeled androgen in higher amounts than muscle, adrenals, or salivary glands. The pattern of uptake did not follow that of blood, indicating a selective retention of androgen by the target tissues. The specific radioactive metabolites retained were not identified in these investigations, however. In studies by Pearlman and Pearlman (1961), in which tritiated androstenedione was infused into adult rats, the pattern of metabolites in the ventral prostate resembled that of plasma, but the concentrations of the metabolites identified as testosterone, 3α-hydroxy-5α-androstan-17-one, 3α-hydroxy-5β-androstan-17-one, 5α-androstane-3,17-dione, and injected androstenedione were significantly higher in the accessory glands than in blood or muscle. Harding and Samuels (1962) found that the concentration of chloroform-soluble radioactivity in rat ventral prostate was twice that in blood, even though the total radioactivity in the ventral prostate was only slightly higher than that of blood following injection of [^{14}C]testosterone in the animals. Androstenedione was the major chloroform-soluble isotope in the ventral prostate. Both Pearlman's and Samuel's groups found that blood or liver contained a large quantity of conjugated metabolites which are essentially absent in the ventral prostate, suggesting that this tissue has a selective process for the uptake of free metabolites, but not of conjugated androgens.

The demonstration of the selective accumulation of radioactive androgens by androgen-responsive tissues became easier with the availability, from commercial sources, of testosterone having a high specific radioactivity. In rats, radioactive androgens are retained by the ventral and dorsal prostate, seminal vesicles, and coagulating gland, against concentration gradients, from blood at 1–3 hours after the injection of [^{3}H]testosterone (Tveter and Attramadal, 1968; Bruchovsky and Wilson, 1968; Anderson and Liao, 1968; Belham et al., 1969; Fang et al., 1969; Liao and Fang, 1969). Radioactivity in samples taken from the blood, spleen, lung, thymus, and diaphragm is rapidly cleared within the first hours after androgen injection, but significant amounts of radioactive androgens can be found in the prostate and seminal vesicles 6–10 hours later. These findings were confirmed by autoradiographic studies (Tveter and Attramadal, 1969; Sar et al., 1970). Within a few minutes after injection of [^{3}H]testosterone into rats, radioactivity could be detected in the sex accessory glands and the seminal vesicles, although very little radioactive material was found in the glandular lumina, connective tissue, or stromal tissues.

The key finding that led to the discovery of a specific androgen receptor was made by Bruchovsky and Wilson (1968), and independently by

Anderson and Liao (1968) who reported that prostate cell nuclei can retain 5α-dihydrotestosterone (DHT). The latter group initiated its research after failure to (a) mimic the rapid *in vivo* stimulatory effect of androgen on nuclear RNA synthesis (Liao *et al.,* 1965) by the addition of testosterone to the isolated prostate cell nuclei, and (b) demonstrate a specific receptor protein for testosterone. It was suspected, therefore, that a metabolite of the testicular androgen, rather than testosterone itself, is the cellular androgen functioning in prostate cell nuclei, possibly by binding to a specific receptor protein.

In rats injected with [^{3}H]testosterone, the cell nuclei of the ventral prostate could, *in vivo,* retain DHT and, to a lesser extent, testosterone, at the time when the prostatic cytoplasm contained large quantities of other radioactive steroids. The nuclear retention of DHT was tissue specific and was not clearly observable in the liver and in other tissues that are less responsive to androgens. The phenomenon can be reproduced *in vitro* by incubation of minced rat ventral prostate with a radioactive androgen (Anderson and Liao, 1968). The possibility that the nuclear retention is due to cytoplasmic contamination or nonspecific adsorption of [^{3}H]DHT was eliminated by removal of the nuclear membranes by use of a nonionic detergent and by the demonstration that there is no exchange between the nuclear steroid labeled *in vivo* and the 100-fold excess of unlabeled androgens added to the homogenization medium (Fang *et al.,* 1969). The autoradiographic studies mentioned above also showed that the nuclear concentration of radioactive materials can occur in the muscle cells of the seminal vesicles, coagulation gland, and epididymis. Under the light microscope, the radioactive steroid appeared to be dispersed to all areas of the nuclear chromatin and were not concentrated in the nucleolar regions or nuclear membranes.

DHT is a more potent androgen than testosterone in a number of androgen bioassay systems, including prostate growth (cf. Liao and Fang, 1969), and these androgens can significantly affect nuclear RNA synthesis very rapidly (Liao *et al.,* 1965; Mainwaring *et al.,* 1971). Therefore, the above findings strongly indicate that the prostate has a specific mechanism for concentrating DHT in the cell nuclei, and that such a mechanism may be related to the early molecular process involved in androgen action.

II. IDENTIFICATION AND CHARACTERIZATION OF ANDROGEN RECEPTORS

A. Cellular Localization

Soon after it had been discovered that DHT can be retained selectively by prostate nuclei, several groups of investigators were able to demonstrate specific binding of DHT by proteins from this target tissue (Fang *et al.*, 1969; Fang and Liao, 1969; Liao and Fang, 1969; Mainwaring, 1969a,b; Unhjem *et al.*, 1969; Baulieu and Jung, 1970). Our studies have suggested that the cytosol fraction of ventral prostate contains at least two proteins that bind DHT preferentially over other natural steroid hormones (Fang and Liao, 1971). One of them (β-protein) binds DHT specifically and very tightly (K_a, 10^{11} M^{-1}). At low concentrations of DHT, the androgen binds exclusively to this high-affinity, low-capacity protein and forms a complex that we have called complex II. This protein binds testosterone, but with much lower affinity (Liao *et al.*, 1973b; Castañeda and Liao, 1975). If DHT is present in excess of the high-affinity binding sites, the androgen may bind to another low-affinity (K_a, 10^7 M^{-1}), high-capacity protein (α-protein) and form a complex that we have named complex I (Liao and Fang, 1970; Fang and Liao, 1971). The low-affinity protein also binds estradiol, but not cortisol. These two types of complexes (or proteins) can be separated easily by ammonium sulfate fractionation or by Sephadex gel chromatography. The most significant difference between the two DHT-binding proteins (Table I) is that only complex II can be retained by the prostate nuclear chromatin. Some of the high-affinity androgen-binding proteins that are fractionated together with complex II are also incapable of becoming the precursor for the nuclear complex. It is not clear whether these proteins are altered forms of complex II or whether they represent another class of biologically important androgen-binding proteins.

The cytoplasmic microsomal fraction of the prostate also contains a specific high-affinity and low-capacity DHT-binding protein that can be solubilized by 0.4 M KCl (Liao and Fang, 1970; Liao *et al.*, 1971). The microsomal protein is very similar to the cytosol β-protein in its steroid specificity, heat sensitivity, sedimentation properties, and capacity to be translocated eventually into prostate cell nuclei.

The prostate cell nuclei of castrated rats contain very few proteins that can bind steroid hormones (including DHT) specifically and tightly (Fang *et al.*, 1969). DHT-protein complex can be detected in the cell nuclei, however, shortly after testosterone or DHT is injected into the castrated animals. Several properties of the nuclear complex are very similar to those of the complex transformed from the cytoplasmic complex II (see Section IV). Other *in vivo* and *in vitro* cell-free studies have also shown that the nuclear complex originates in the cytoplasm and that it is transferred into the nucleus only after it interacts with and binds DHT (Liao and Fang, 1970; Fang and Liao, 1971). It is now generally agreed that the β-protein retainable by prostate cell nucleus is an intracellular androgen receptor.

Attempts at purification of an androgen receptor have not been very successful, due mainly to the difficulty of obtaining large quantities of the

TABLE I

DHT-Binding Protein Isolation from Cellular Fractions of Rat Ventral Prostate[a]

Cellular localization	Binding protein	DHT–receptor complex[b]	Properties
Cytoplasm			
Soluble (cytosol)	α-Protein	Complex I, 3.5 S	Binds DHT, testosterone, and estradiol, but not cortisol; K_a for DHT: $10^7\ M^{-1}$, stable at 40°C, cannot bind to nuclei or RNP; precipitated by ammonium sulfate at 55–70% saturation
	β-Protein	Complex II, 3.8 S	Binds DHT and some potent synthetic androgens, but not androstanediols, estradiol, or cortisol; K_a for DHT, $10^{11}\ M^{-1}$, unstable at 40°C, can be converted to nuclear form; precipitated by ammonium sulfate at 0–35% saturation
	β-Protein	Complex II-TR 3.0 S	Transformed from complex II; many properties similar to those of complex II; can bind to nuclei and RNP
	β'-Protein	Complex II' 3.0 S	Properties similar to those of complex II, but cannot bind to nuclei or RNP
Membrane-bound (microsomal)	β-Protein	Complex II-TR 3.0 S	Can be solubilized by 0.4 M KCl; properties similar to those of cytosol complex II-TR; can bind to nuclei and RNP
Nucleus			
Intact	β-Protein	Complex II-TR	Properties similar to those of cytosol complex II-TR; can bind to nuclei and RNP; can be dissociated from chromatin by 0.4 M KCl; probably associated with acceptor proteins that can be extracted by 0.4–2 M KCl
Disrupted	β-Protein	Complex II-TR (aggregated)	Some of the complexes bind factitiously to histones and denatured DNA, and cannot be dissociated from the chromatin by 0.4 M KCl

[a] From Liao et al., 1975.
[b] Sedimentation coefficients were measured in media containing 0.4 M KCl.

target tissue, the instability of the receptor, and loss of androgen from the receptor protein during purification. Using DNA–cellulose chromatography and isoelectric focusing, Mainwaring and Irving (1973) showed that the cytosol receptor of rat ventral prostate can be purified about 3500-fold as measured by recovery of protein, or 350-fold on the basis of specific radioactivity. The purification factor required for obtaining pure receptor is about 10^5-fold. The cytosol androgen receptors isolated from the seminal vesicles, testis, epididymis, kidney, uterus, ovaries, brain, and other organs (Attramadal et al., 1976) appear to have similar physicochemical properties, such as sedimentation patterns thermolability, electrophoretic mobility, isoelectric point (pI, 5.8), and capability to be translocated into cell nuclei and bound to chromatin after a temperature-dependent activation.

B. Sedimentation Properties

The prostate cytosol DHT–receptor complex (complex II), carefully prepared at low temperatures, can form complexes that sediment as 7–12 S and 3–5 S units. The larger complexes can be transformed to the smaller forms by incubation at 20°–30°C or by adjustment of the salt concentrations to 0.4 M KCl (Baulieu et al., 1971). The sedimentation properties of the DHT–receptor complex can vary with changes in the pH of the medium (Liao et al., 1975). At 0.1 M KCl and a pH below 7.5, both the 8 S and 3.5 S complexes gradually aggregate to larger forms. If the pH of the medium is raised from 7 to 9, the quantity of aggregated materials decreases, and the 8 S and 3 to 4 S forms emerge (Fig. 1). At pH 9.5, only a 7 S form is clearly visible. Aggregation as well as the formation of the 8 S form obviously involve other cellular materials, since the gradient- and hydroxylapatite-purified complexes do not aggregate and sediment at about 3 S (Liao and Liang, 1974).

In 0.4 M KCl, prostate cytosol complex II (3.8 ± 0.3 S) sediments somewhat faster than the nuclear complex (2.9 ± 0.3 S). Since this difference can be observed even in 2 M urea (Liao et al., 1975), it may be due to an intrinsic property of the complexes, rather than to association of other macromolecules. At urea concentrations higher than 3 M, DHT is gradually released from the receptor.

In crude extract, various steroid–receptor complexes can sediment at the 8 S region in a medium having a low ionic strength; this provides a convenient method for the detection of the cellular receptor. The 8 S form is rather unstable, however, and its formation is dependent on the pH and other conditions. Therefore, the level of the 8 S form does not represent the total receptor content in the tissue sample.

C. Characterization by Antisteroid Antibody

Under certain conditions, antibodies against DHT and testosterone are effective in removing steroid bound to nonreceptor proteins of blood (including human blood) and prostate, but are not capable of removing

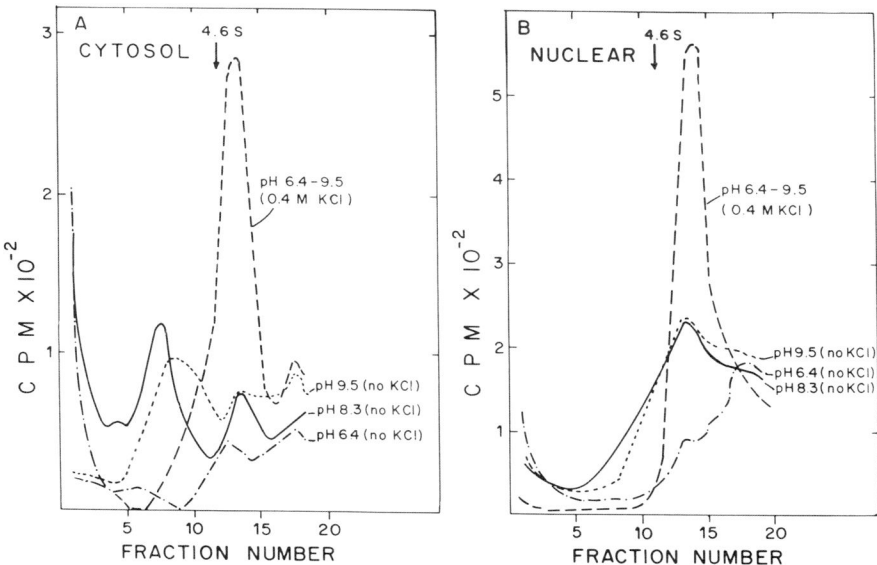

Fig. 1. Effect of pH on the sedimentation pattern of cytosol complex II (A) and nuclear (B) [^{3}H]DHT–receptor complex of rat ventral prostate. The glycerol gradient (10–22%) solution contained 1.5 mM EDTA, 20 mM Tris–HCl buffer at the pH shown, with or without 0.4 M KCl. Fractions were collected and numbered from the bottom of the tube. Bovine serum albumin (4.6 S) sedimented at the position shown by the arrow; (----), pH 6.4–9.5, 0.4 M KCl; (· · · ·) pH 9.5, no KCl; (———) pH 8.3, no KCl; (— · —) pH 6.4, no KCl (Liao et al., 1975).

DHT bound to the high-affinity receptor. Testosterone that may be bound to the same receptor is readily removed by the anti-steroid antibody (Fig. 2), possibly because of its low affinity or high rate of dissociation from the androgen receptor (Castañeda and Liao, 1975).

Utilizing this property, we have devised a simple assay method for the qualitative and quantitative characterization of the steroid–receptor complexes. The sample solution containing ^{3}H-labeled steroid–receptor complexes is mixed with anti-steroid antibody that has the capacity to bind essentially all of the ^{3}H-labeled steroid present. The mixture is made to 0.4 M with respect to KCl and analyzed by gradient centrifugation. Under the conditions of the assay, the ^{3}H-labeled steroid molecules, in the free form or released from nonreceptor proteins, are bound by the antibody and sediment at 8 S, whereas the receptor-bound ^{3}H-steroid remains at the 3–4 S region and can be measured. The assay method can be simplified considerably if the antibody is coupled to a solid phase such as Sepharose. The assay mixture can then simply be centrifuged in a clinical centrifuge for

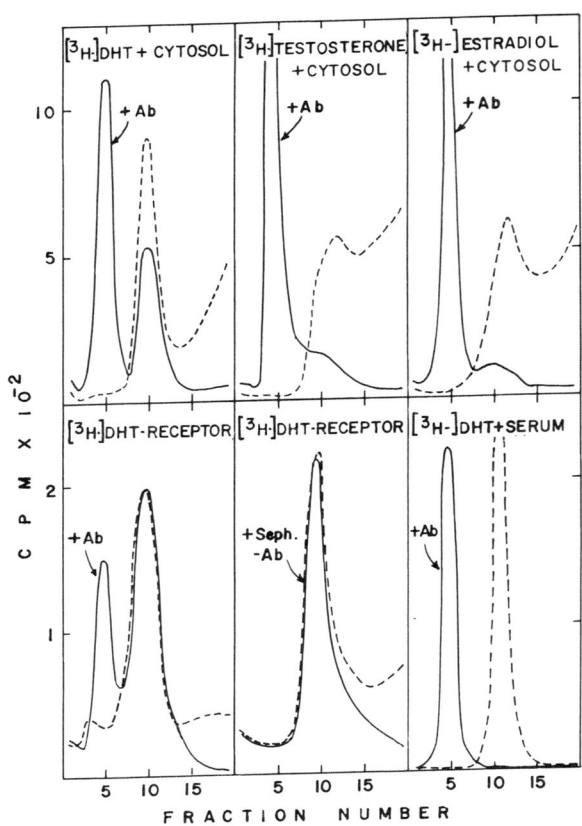

Fig. 2. Effect of an antisteroid antibody (Ab) on the sedimentation pattern (in 10–30% sucrose) of [³H]DHT, [³H]testosterone, or [³H]estradiol bound to the cytosol proteins or receptors of rat ventral prostate, or to the human serum proteins. The graphs in the upper row were obtained from experiments in which 0.4 ml of prostate cytosol containing 12,000 cpm of a [³H]steroid was incubated alone (---) or in the presence of an appropriate antibody (20 µg of protein). For the graphs shown in the lower row, [³H]DHT–receptor complex (complex II), 4000 cpm/0.28 mg of protein, was incubated alone or in the presence of antiDHT antibody, free (left figure) or bound to an insoluble Sephadex gel (middle figure). When [³H]DHT was mixed with human (adult female) serum, a 4–5 S steroid–protein peak appeared, but this was eliminated completely by the addition of the antiDHT antibody that forms a 7–8 S peak with [³H]DHT. Testosterone could bind to the receptor, but only weakly. Estradiol might bind to a specific estrogen receptor in the prostate cytosol. Free steroids that stayed at the upper portion of the centrifuge tube could be eliminated completely by forming a 7–8 S complex with the antibody. If an insolubilized Sephadex gel-bound antibody was used, this complex could be removed by prior centrifugation. In each figure, the 7–8 S complex and the 3–4 S complex sediment, respectively, in the vicinity of fraction numbers 5 and 10 (Castañeda and Liao, 1975).

6. Androgen Receptor Interactions in Target Cells

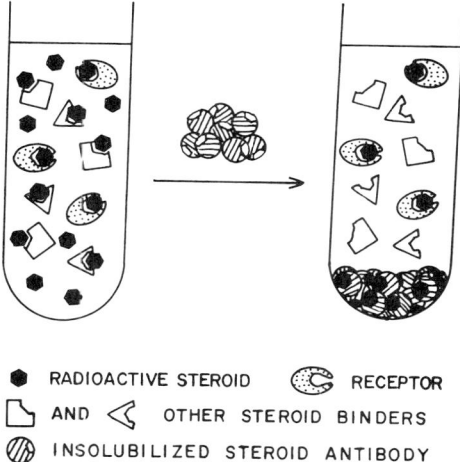

● RADIOACTIVE STEROID   ◉ RECEPTOR
◻ AND ◁ OTHER STEROID BINDERS
◉ INSOLUBILIZED STEROID ANTIBODY

Fig. 3. Diagram illustrating a method for the characterization of [³H]steroid–receptor complex by use of a steroid antibody attached to a solid phase. The radioactive steroid, either free or bound to nonreceptor proteins, can be removed from the solution (left tube) by precipitation with the insolubilized steroid antibody (right tube). The [³H]steroid that binds tightly to the hydrophobic pocket of the receptor is not affected and, therefore, can be estimated from the soluble fraction directly (Castañeda and Liao, 1974).

sedimentation of the steroid molecules that were not attached to the receptor originally, but are now bound to the insolubilized antibody (Fig. 3). The receptor content can, therefore, be determined directly from the radioactivity of the supernatant (Castañeda and Liao, 1974, 1975).

By using this method, we have been able to show that the cell nuclei and cytoplasm of normal, hyperplastic, and cancerous human prostate contain DHT–receptor complexes that sediment at about 3 S in media with 0.4 M KCl.

D. Characterization by Other Methods

Many other techniques have been employed for the qualitative and quantitative analysis of androgen–receptor complex. As described above, ammonium sulfate at 35–40% saturation can effectively precipitate the high-affinity receptor (Fang and Liao, 1971; Mainwaring and Peterken, 1971; Verhoeven *et al.*, 1975). Dextran-coated charcoal has been used for removal of unbound or nonspecifically bound [³H]steroid, but this method has been rather unsatisfactory in the quantitative determination of the receptor in the rat prostate (Blondeau *et al.*, 1975). The method has been improved considerably by Shain et al. (1975). Sephadex gel exclusion column chromatography (Attramadal et al., 1975; Bruchovsky and Craven, 1975) and thin-layer gel filtration (Töpert et al., 1974) have also been employed for measurements of the protein-bound androgens. Other methods useful for characterization of the receptors are DNA–cellulose column retention (Mainwaring and Irving, 1973); electrofocusing (Katsumata and Goldman, 1974); polyacrylamide gel electrophoresis (Ritzén et al., 1974); and agar gel electrophoresis (Krieg et al., 1974a).

The above techniques for the measurement of various physical constants and receptor contents must be used with great care. Receptor alteration, aggregation, and inactivation, steroid dissociation from receptor sites, and nonspecific adsorption of [^{3}H]steroids by chromatographic materials, tubes, etc., often cause serious errors. The lack of a reliable biochemical assay for the determination of the native form and function of the receptors also make it difficult to evaluate the importance of many properties exhibited by the androgen–receptor complex.

III. SPECIFICITIES IN ANDROGEN–RECEPTOR INTERACTIONS

A. Target Tissue Specificity

Most androgen-sensitive tissues appear to have receptor proteins that can bind both DHT and testosterone. Therefore, the relative metabolic activities of these two androgens and their relative affinities toward the cellular receptors may be the important factors determining which of the two androgens can play key roles in androgenic responses.

As reviewed by Attramadal et al. (1975, 1976), DHT plays a major role in the ventral prostate (Liao et al., 1973b), seminal vesicles (Liao et al., 1971; Tveter and Unhjem, 1969), and epididymis (Blaquier and Calandra, 1973; Hansson and Djøseland, 1972; Tindall et al., 1972), since it not only is formed readily from testosterone and binds to prostate receptor more firmly than testosterone, but also is metabolized to hydroxylated compounds (diols) at a slower rate. In other tissues, such as the kidney (Bardin et al., 1975; Gehring et al., 1971; Gustafsson and Pousette, 1975; Ritzén et al., 1972),uterus (Giannopoulos, 1973; Jungblut et al., 1971), ovary (Louvet et al., 1975), submaxillary gland (Dunn et al., 1973; Gustafsson and Pousette, 1975), and possibly certain areas of brain (Fox, 1975; Jouan et al., 1973; Kato, 1975; Loras et al., 1974; Naess et al., 1975), the formation of DHT from testosterone takes place at moderate rates, whereas its metabolism to diols occurs rapidly. In these tissues, both androgens may be effective because the receptor binds both DHT and testosterone well. Since DHT is formed slowly or not at all in the adult testis (Galena *et al.,* 1974; Hansson *et al.,* 1974), levator ani muscle (Jung and Baulieu, 1972; Krieg *et al.,* 1974b), and thigh muscle (Gustafsson and Pousette, 1975), testosterone binding by the receptor may be important regardless of differences in the affinity of the receptor for these androgens.

It has been reported that receptor proteins for DHT or testosterone are present in other target tissues, such as the sebaceous and preputial glands (Bullock and Bardin, 1970; Eppenberger and Hsia, 1972; Gustafsson and Pousette, 1975; Takayasu and Adachi, 1975), coagulating gland (Gustafsson and Pousette, 1975), hair follicles (Fazekas and Sandor, 1973), spermatozoa (Wester and Foote, 1972), bone marrow (Valladares and Mingnell, 1975), chick magnum (Palmiter *et al.,* 1973), cock's comb and other head appendages (Dubé and Tremblay, 1974), the pineal gland (Cardinali *et al.,* 1975), and androgen-sensitive tumors (Bruchovsky *et al.,* 1975; Mainwaring and Mangan, 1973; Norris *et al.,* 1974). In liver, a tissue normally considered to be androgen-insensitive, androgens can enhance nuclear RNA synthesis (Tata, 1966), the production of hepatic α_2-globulin, and DHT-binding activity (Roy *et al.,* 1974). Estradiol antagonized the latter effects of androgens.

The biologic response to DHT and testosterone may be discriminatory in some of the target tissues. In some species, for example, anovulatory sterility (Whalen and Luttge, 1971a) and sexual behavior (Beyer *et al.,* 1973; Whalen and Luttge, 1971b) are affected by testosterone, but not by DHT. Testosterone is also much more effective than DHT in stimulating glandular secretion. In the rat uterus, it increases the height of the luminal epithelium (Gonzales-Diddi *et al.,* 1972); in bull seminal vesicles, it enhances the secretory output of fructose and citric acid (Mann *et al.,* 1971). These differential effects may be due to differences in the metabolic or binding activities of the two androgens; alternatively, the receptor may interact with the two (or with other) androgens and form dissimilar complexes that can induce different biologic responses.

The biologic action of certain androgenic compounds, for example, androsta(e)ne derivatives other than DHT or testosterone, may involve different types of receptors. In the vagina, the production of mucus by the superficial cells is stimulated by 3α-hydroxy- and 3-ketoandrostanes, whereas the deeper layer are affected by the 3β-hydroxyl steroids. Only $3\beta,17\beta$-dihydroxyandrost-5-ene (Δ^5-diol) behaves like estrogens and causes keratinization of the uterine epithelium (Huggins *et al.,* 1954). Receptor proteins for some of these hydroxylated androsta(e)nes have been isolated from cell nuclei of the vagina and uterus (Shao *et al.,* 1975). In human myometrial and mammary cancer tissues, the Δ^5-diol has been shown to interfere with receptor binding of estradiol and DHT (Poortman et al., 1975). Other examples are receptorlike proteins which bind 5β-DHT in bone marrow cells (Valladares and Mingnell, 1975) and liver (Lane et al., 1975), and androstenedione-binding proteins in liver (Gustafsson et al., 1975).

B. Steroid Specificity

1. Gross Structure

Earlier investigators predicted how androgens might interact with hypothetical receptors by comparing chemical structure and end-point activity (see a review by Liao and Fang, 1969). This semiempirical approach was complicated by adsorption, transport, and metabolic processes that involve different types of protein binding, but it was suggested that receptors may bind androgens from the α-face, β-face, and peripheral sides of the steroid, and that the steric and not the electronic characteristics of the steroid are the most important factor in eliciting the biologic response (Vida, 1969; Wolff and Zanati, 1970).

These predictions are well in line with our experimental findings (Liao et al., 1973b) on the study of the structural requirements for steroid binding to the isolated androgen receptor of rat ventral prostate. As the results summarized in Table II show, there is an excellent correlation between the androgenicity and receptor-binding affinity of many steroids tested. In regard to receptor binding, the bulkiness and flatness of the steroid molecule, especially at the ring A area, appear to play a more important role than the detailed electronic structure of the steroid nucleus. The steroids having an A/B cis structure, including the inactive (in prostate) 5β-isomer of DHT, are not bound by the prostate receptor. Other relatively flat steroids with rings A/B in the trans form also differ in their receptor-binding affinity according to the structural differences at the ring A/B area.

For example, competition and anti-steroid antibody assays indicate that testosterone binds less firmly to the receptor (possibly due to a higher dissociation rate) than DHT. The presence or absence of unsaturation at ring A per se does not appear to be crucial to binding, since 7α,17α-dimethyl-19-nortestosterone (DMNT) and 2-oxa-17α-methyl-17β-hydroxyestra-4,9,11-trien-3-one can bind to the androgen receptor more tightly than DHT. By having conjugated double bonds extending from rings A and B to C, the 2-oxatriene and the related estratrienes are indeed very flat molecules. The importance of the gross geometric structure in androgen binding by receptors may also explain why A-nor-17β-acetoxyestra-4,9,11-trien-3-one, with five carbons in ring A, is a very potent androgen, whereas

TABLE II
Relative Androgenic Activities and Relative Competition Indexes of Various Androgens[a]

Steroid	Relative androgenicity (RA)	Relative competition index for receptor binding (RCI)
Group A		
Testosterone (T)	0.4	0.2[b]
$7\alpha, 17\alpha\text{-}(CH_3)_2\text{-}T$	0.6	0.2
$7\beta, 17\alpha\text{-}(CH_3)_2\text{-}T$	0.1	0.1
DHT	1.0	1.0
$7\alpha, 17\alpha\text{-}(CH_3)_2\text{-}DHT$	1.5	0.6
$7\beta, 17\alpha\text{-}(CH_3)_2\text{-}DHT$	0.0	0.1
19-Nortestosterone (NorT)	0.2	0.9
$7\alpha, 17\alpha\text{-}(CH_3)_2\text{-}NorT$ (DMNT)	5.7	3.5
19-Nor-DHT (Nor-DHT)	0.1	0.5
$7\alpha, 17\alpha\text{-}(CH_3)_2\text{-}Nor\text{-}DHT$	0.3	1.0
Group B		
2-Oxa-17β-hydroxyestra-4,9-dien-3-one	3.2	1.4
2-Oxa-17β-hydroxyestra-4,9,11-trien-3-one	8–12	3.2
2-Oxa-17α-methyl-17β-hydroxyestra-4,9,11-trien-3-one	80–120	3.8
17α-Methyl-17β-hydroxyestra-4,9,11-trien-3-one	24	2.3
3α,17β-Dihydroxy-5α-androstane	0.2	0.0
5α-Androstane-3,17-dione	0.2	0.0
5α-Androstane	—	0.0
5α-Androstan-3-one	—	0.0
17β-Hydroxy-5α-androstane	—	0.0
3α-Hydroxy-5α-androstan-17-one	0.2	0.0

[a] The relative activities of the androgens shown in Group A were calculated from our own results, with DHT taken as 1.0. Test steroids were injected subcutaneously into castrated rats daily for 7 days, and the wet weights of the ventral prostates were compared. The prostate weights for the control group were 11.2 ± 0.5 mg. The daily dose of DHT needed to maintain the weight of the ventral prostate in the steroid-injected rats at twice that of the control castrates was 0.8 ± 0.1 μg per rat (body weight, 50 g). The relative activities of the androgens shown in Group B were calculated from the results of other workers, some of whom used the value 1.0 for 17α-methyltestosterone in their reports. To facilitate comparison with other data, we recalculated the figures, using DHT as 1.0. The relative activity for 17α-methyltestosterone was assumed to be 0.4.

The relative competition indexes were measured by methods based on the capability of various steroids of competing with [^{3}H]DHT for binding to β-protein in a cell-free system.

[b] RCI for testosterone in six experiments which we performed recently are in the range of 0.2 ± 0.1. The difference in the affinity constants for DHT and testosterone may be due primarily to the rate of dissociation, rather than to the rate of association (cf. Fig. 2). (From Liao et al., 1973b.)

A-homotestosterone and A-homo-DHT, with seven carbons in ring A, are virtually inactive. An additional carbon in rings B or D does not distort the gross geometry of androstanes very much. Thus, B-homo-DHT and D-homo-DHT (see references cited in the article by Liao et al., 1973b) are potent androgens and probably can bind to the prostate receptor protein. The lack of binding of nonandrogenic natural steroids to the prostatic androgen receptor is easily understood. For example, ring A of 17β-estradiol bends appreciably toward the β-side of the steroid, and the bulky 17-substitution on ring D (glucocorticoids, mineral corticoids, and progestins) can hinder receptor binding.

2. *M Site*

The binding affinity of DMNT to the prostate androgen–receptor is several times greater than that of DHT. The androgen action of DMNT, therefore, may not require reduction of the Δ^4-bond. Using ^{3}H-labeled DMNT, we have found that this very potent androgen is not reduced by prostate 5α-reductase. The chemically reduced form, 7α,17α-dimethyl-19-nor-DHT, is considerably less active in receptor binding and less potent as an androgen than the unsaturated form (Liao et al., 1973b).

We have proposed that the receptor protein has a specific (M) site for binding the 7α-methyl group (Fig. 4), and that this is responsible for the increase in the binding affinity and the androgenicity of DMNT. The substitution of the 7α-methyl group to DHT or to 17α-methyl-19-nor-DHT does not significantly enhance this binding affinity or the androgenicity, perhaps because the 7α-methyl group in these molecules is oriented differently and may not fit perfectly on the M site of the receptor. We have suggested that the terminal methyl group on diethylstilbestrol, a potent synthetic estrogen, may also behave like the 7α-methyl group on the 19-nortestosterone in enhancing the ability of the synthetic estrogen to bind to the estrogen receptor and increasing its estrogenicity (Liao, 1974). If this is a correct view, the M site binding must play only an accessory role and must, therefore, not be absolutely necessary for functioning of sex steroids, since the natural steroids do not have the methyl group. If the 7-methyl substitution is made on the 7β position, both the receptor-binding affinity and the androgenicity are reduced by more than 90%. Apparently, the 7β-methyl group cannot be accommodated into the receptor-binding cavity (Liao et al., 1973b).

3. *Metabolic Conversion*

Some androgens, such as 17β-hydroxy-5α-androstane and 17α-methyl-17-β-hydroxy-5α-androstane (cf. Liao and Fang, 1969), do not have an oxygen at the C-3 position. Since these steroids do not bind tightly to the prostate receptor (Table II), their androgenic action may depend on their

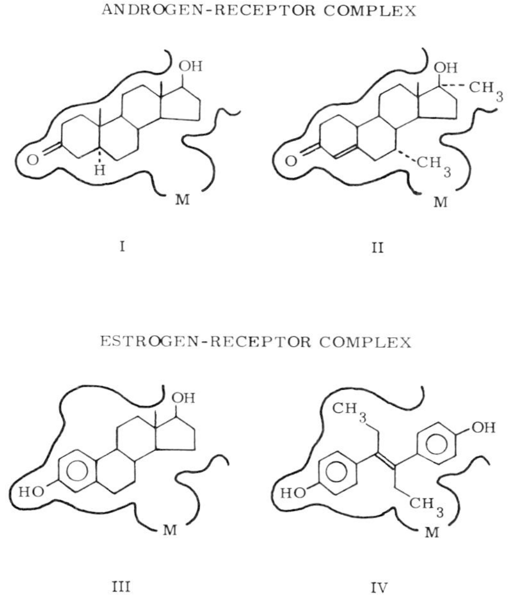

6. Androgen Receptor Interactions in Target Cells

Fig. 4. Schematic representation of the interaction of sex steroids with their receptor protein. (See text for explanation.) Steroid structures shown are for DHT (I), $7\alpha,17\alpha$-dimethyl-19-nortestosterone (II), 17β-estradiol (III), and diethylstilbestrol (IV) (Liao, 1974).

oxygenation in animals (Wolff and Kasuya, 1972). The action of androstanediols and of some other androgens that do not bind tightly to the prostate receptors may depend on their metabolizing to DHT (Bruchovsky, 1971), although they may bind to another receptor and may function differently in certain tissues, such as vagina and uterus (Shao *et al.*, 1975).

With the exception of a possible involvement of a 17α-hydroxylated androgen in the dog prostate (Evans and Pierrepoint, 1975), a 17β-hydroxy group appears to be essential for the androgenicity and high-affinity binding to the androgen receptor. Steroids without this group, such as androstanedione, 5α-androstan-3-one, and the 17α-isomer of testosterone and DHT, do not bind to the androgen receptor of the rat ventral prostate (Table II). If the role of the 17β-hydroxyl group is strictly for maintaining high-affinity binding to the receptor and not for eliciting a biologic function, however, some of these compounds may, at high concentrations, function without metabolic conversion to the 17β-hydroxylated androgens. There are indications that estrone (having no 17β-hydroxy group) at high concentrations can bind to the estrogen receptor, be retained by cell nuclei, and presumably function like 17β-estradiol in the rat uterus (Ruh *et al.*, 1973).

4. Steroid Enveloping

We have suggested that the potent androgens are bound by the prostate receptor from several sides, as if the androgens were being "enveloped" in the hydrophobic cavity. The localization of steroid-binding sites well inside the receptor proteins may be responsible for the very slow rates of association or dissociation of steroids from the receptor proteins at low temperatures, the very high affinity constants (K_a, 10^{11} M^{-1}), the acceleration of the rates of exchange of unbound steroids with bound steroids by freezing and thawing, and the fact that the receptor-bound androgens are rather stable in ethanol (30%) or detergents (2% Triton X100 or deoxycholate).

The concept of steroid enveloping supports the suggestion that the receptor protein, and not the specific functional group on the steroids, participates in the key event leading to steroid hormone action (Fang et al., 1969; Liao and Fang, 1969; Liao et al., 1973b). This view may be applicable to other steroid hormones as well and may provide an explanation for the overlap in the actions of some steroids. In the case of glucocorticoids, Bell and Munck (1973) have also concluded that the thymus receptor binds an active steroid from both the α and β sides. They suggested that certain functional groups (11-OH, 9-F) on the steroid may interact with receptor sites after the steroids has entered the receptor-binding cavity.

The steroid-metabolizing enzymes or blood steroid-binding proteins generally recognize only a portion of the steroid molecule. As described in Section II,C, this differential property has been used for quantitative and qualitative analysis of the steroid–receptor complexes in tissue samples.

IV. CELL NUCLEUS AND CHROMATIN BINDING OF ANDROGEN RECEPTOR

A. Steroid and Receptor Interdependence

Essentially all DHT that is tightly bound to isolated prostate cell nuclei *in vivo* is in a protein-bound form that can be solubilized by 0.4–0.6 M KCl and sedimented as a 3 S form. The cell nuclei in the ventral prostate of castrated rats, however, contain very little salt-extractable receptor for androgens. This, together with the fact that these cell nuclei are not capable of retaining DHT specifically in a protein-bound form unless a cytoplasm protein fraction is supplemented, indicated that the nuclear DHT–receptor complex originates in the cytoplasm (Fang et al., 1969; Liao and Fang, 1969). The time course for the appearance of the androgen–receptor complexes in the cytosol fraction and nuclei of the prostate, after a single injection of ^{3}H-labeled testosterone into castrated rats, also indicates that, *in* vivo, ³H-DHT is first bound to the receptor protein in the cytoplasm and then translocated to the nuclear sites (Fang et al., 1969). This conclusion is supported by the observation that β-protein can be retained more readily by isolated prostate cell nuclei if the receptor protein is first allowed to bind DHT (Fang and Liao, 1971).

The nuclear retention of the DHT–protein complex, therefore, appears to depend on both the β-protein and the hormone. One can conjecture that the β-protein must associate with DHT to remove the protein from a specific subcellular site and to translocate it to another, such as cytoplasmic membranes or nuclei. During such a translocation, a steroid hormone may stabilize the protein or supply an essential structural requirement (including conformational changes or subunit rearrangements) so that the binding protein can transfer and bind to a specific target site (Fang and Liao, 1971; Liao et al., 1975).

The retention of hormone by purified prostate nuclei is hormone specific. When various hormones were mixed with whole prostate cytosol or β-protein, and, subsequently, were incubated with prostate nuclei, only ³H-DHT was retained by the nuclei. Radioactive testosterone, 17β-estradiol, progesterone, and cortisol were ineffective (Liao and Fang, 1970). Specificity is also displayed by the nuclei. Very few [³H]DHT–receptor complexes can be retained by liver nuclei *in vitro*. Cell nuclei isolated from the thymus, brain, and diaphragm of rats were even less effective than liver nuclei in the receptor retention (Liao and Fang, 1970; Fang and Liao, 1971). Similar tissue specificity has also been seen when the receptor-binding capacities of chromatin preparations from various tissues were compared (Steggles et al., 1971; Mainwaring and Peterken, 1971; Tymoczko and Liao, 1971).

B. Receptor Transformation

Studies by autoradiography (Sar et al., 1970) and by reconstruction of cellular fractions (Fang and Liao, 1971) have shown that receptor retention by cell nuclei is temperature dependent; more retention occurs at 20°–40°C than at °C. The temperature effect is primarily on the cytosol DHT–receptor complex, which apparently has to be transformed to fit the nuclear binding sites (Table III). Mainwaring and Irving (1973) have also shown that brief heating of the 8 S cytosol ³H-DHT–receptor complex before its incubation with chromatin markedly accelerated the rate, but not the overall extent of the transfer of the complex into prostate chromatin. The temperature-dependent alteration of the androgen–receptor complex appeared to involve a pronounced decrease in the sedimentation coefficient from 8 S to 4.2 S, and the isoelectric point changed from 5.8 to 6.5. We have also shown that the freshly prepared prostate cytosol receptor (3.8 S in

TABLE III
Retention of DHT-Receptor by Cell Nuclei of Rat Ventral Prostate[a]

Incubation Temperature (°C)	[³H]DHT	Radioactivity (dpm/100 μg DNA) associated with receptor protein in nuclei during incubation of		
		Minced tissue	Homogenate	Receptor[b]
0	−[c]	55	33	24
0	+	528	1295	633
10	+	1339	1674	1467
20	+	2142	2323	1946
30	+	1876	1700	1588
40	+	534	353	427

[a] Male Sprague-Dawley rats (weighing 300–450 g) were castrated 18 hours before they were killed. Minced prostates or prostate homogenates were incubated with [³H]DHT for 20 minutes at the temperatures shown. Nuclei were isolated, and the [³H]DHT-receptor complex was extracted and analyzed by gradient centrifugation. The radioactivity associated with the 3 S protein fractions was measured. (From Liao and Liang, 1974).

[b] Only the receptor preparation was incubated at the temperature shown. After incubation, prostate nuclei were added and the mixture was incubated at 0°C for 30 minutes. See Fang and Liao (1971) for experimental conditions.

[c] [³H]DHT was omitted from the incubation mixture, but was added after nuclear extract had been obtained.

0.4 M KCl) can be changed to the nuclear form (3 S in 0.4 M KCl) under conditions favoring nuclear retention (Liao, 1975; cf. Fig. 8). It is not clear whether the temperature-dependent "receptor transformation" involves a change in receptor conformation (Jensen et al., 1974), a proteolytic action (Bresciani et al., 1973), or a bimolecular reaction (Yamamoto and Alberts, 1974; Notides et al., 1975).

C. Acceptor Concepts

The precise way in which steroid–receptor complex is retained by the target cell nuclei *in vivo* is not clear. The indication that there may be specific acceptor molecules to interact with and retain steroid receptors was first observed in our study of the phenomena in the rat ventral prostate (Liao and Fang, 1969, 1970), and in the chick oviduct in O'Malley's laboratory (see their article in this volume).

In the prostate study, the acceptor molecule was believed to be more abundant in the cell nuclei of the androgen-sensitive tissues than in less responsive tissues such as the liver. Since the nuclear–receptor binding activity, as assayed in the cell-free system, could be saturated with the DHT–receptor complex, and since this activity was inactivated by heating at temperatures higher than 40°C (Fig. 5) the acceptor molecule was considered to be a specific heat-labile protein. It was suggested that the acceptor can participate actively in specifying the nuclear sites where the androgen–receptor complex is to bind and exert its cellular action (Liao and Fang, 1970; Fang and Liao, 1971; Liao et al., 1971). In contrast, other workers (Mainwaring and Peterken, 1971; King and Gordon, 1972) have proposed that DNA is the acceptor and that certain proteins may act passively by restricting the receptor-binding sites available on DNA.

The clarification of these two apparently contradictory views depends on further experimental evidence; there is considerable debate, however, as to whether, in general, the cell nuclei of the target tissues of steroid hormones have a limited number of specific sites for receptor binding.

D. Characterization of Acceptor Molecules

1. By Reconstruction from DNA and Solubilized Nuclear Proteins

Solubilization and isolation of nuclear proteins that may have acceptor activity were first achieved in the androgen–prostate system by Tymoczko and Liao (1971), and in the progesterone–oviduct system by Spelsberg et al. (1971).

In the work by Tymoczko and Liao (1971), fractionated prostate nuclear

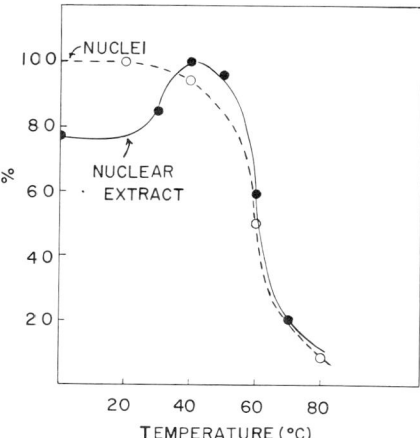

Fig. 5. Heat stability of the nuclear acceptor activity of prostate nuclei and the proteins extracted from the nuclei by 0.4 M KCl. [^{3}H]DHT–receptor complex of the rat ventral prostate was mixed with the nuclei or with a nuclear protein fraction that had been incubated for 10 minutes at various temperatures. The capacity of the nuclear preparations to retain the receptor complex was compared (data from Fang and Liao, 1971; Tymoczko and Liao, 1971).

proteins were mixed with DNA to form a nucleoprotein aggregate. The reconstructed chromatin was then tested for its capacity to bind the prostate [^{3}H]DHT–receptor complex (acceptor activity). Such an assay must rely on the binding of [^{3}H]DHT, rather than on the function of the receptor protein or of the acceptor material. The appropriateness of the assay method, however, can be evaluated by the study of various properties which characterize the retention of the DHT–receptor complex by the intact cell nuclei. Some properties which we have employed for this purpose are β-protein dependence, tissue specificity, heat lability, the ability to solubilize, by 0.4 M KCl, the retained [^{3}H]DHT–receptor complex, and identification of the complex as a 3 S component in gradient centrifugation (Tymoczko and Liao, 1971).

When purified prostate cell nuclei from castrated rats are extracted with a 0.4 M KCl solution, a protein fraction containing a large quantity of nonhistone protein as well as some histone (mainly lysine-rich H-1 histone) is obtained. When this nuclear protein fraction is incubated with [^{3}H]DHT–receptor protein, in the presence of either endogenous or exogenous DNA or other polynucleotides, a nucleoprotein aggregate is formed. This material can be collected by centrifugation and washed with 0.2 M KCl to remove unbound or nonspecifically bound DHT–receptor complex. Alternatively, the nucleoprotein aggregates can be collected on Millipore filters in a vacuum. The DHT–receptor complex can be extracted from the nucleoprotein aggregates by treatment with 0.4 M KCl. As shown in Fig. 6, the salt extract of the prostate cell nuclei demonstrated a very high acceptor activity, which was not observed for the equivalent nuclear extract of rat liver (Tymoczko and Liao, 1971). Normally, addition of the ventral prostate extract resulted in a 5- to 10-fold increase in acceptor activity over the control values. The lack of acceptor activity exhibited by the liver nuclear extract is in keeping with the lack of nuclear retention of DHT–protein complex by liver nuclei in the cell-free system (Fang et al., 1969; Fang and Liao, 1971).

The crude 0.4 M KCl extract of prostate nuclei, which contains nonhistone proteins and H-1 histone, is rich in acceptor molecules, although more acceptor protein(s) can be extracted from the residue by 2 M KCl or 2 M NaCl (Tymoczko, 1973). The acceptor proteins are heat-labile at temperatures above 50°C. Their heat denaturation curve is identical to that for the DHT–receptor binding activity of the intact prostate cell nuclei (Fig. 5). The heat-labile factor is not dialyzable; it can be fractionated by ammonium sulfate and ethanol or precipitated from the solution at pH 4.5.

The salt concentration (0.4 M KCl) employed for the extraction of receptor or acceptor molecules is ideal because, under these conditions, there is

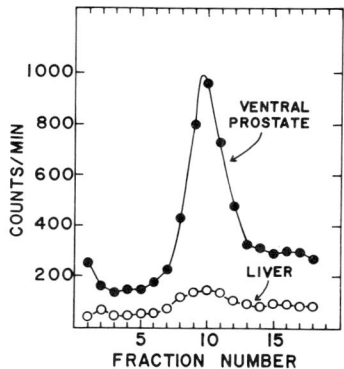

Fig. 6. Retention of [³H]DHT–receptor complex by nuclear extracts of rat liver and ventral prostate. Gradient-purified nuclei of liver and ventral prostate prepared from 18-hour castrates were extracted with a 0.4 M KCl solution. The nuclear acceptor activity of the extract was determined by the centrifugation assay. Since relatively large amounts of nuclear extract (1.28 mg protein, 0.19 mg DNA) were used in each tube, no additional DNA was necessary. The [³H]DHT–receptor preparation added to each tube contained 48,000 counts/minutes/12.4 mg protein. The [³H]DHT–receptor retained by the nucleoprotein aggregates was extracted by 0.4 M KCl, and an aliquot (0.2 ml) was analyzed by gradient centrifugation on a 5–20% sucrose gradient containing 0.4 M KCl in 20 mM Tris–HCl, pH 7.5, and 1.5 mM EDTA, in an SW 56 rotor at 297,000 g and 2°C for 18 hours. Tubes were fractionated and numbered from the bottom (Tymoczko and Liao, 1971).

very little release of DNA from the nuclei. In the aforementioned study, the nuclear extract generally contained about 5% (by weight) nucleic acids and 95% proteins. Addition of an adequate amount of calf thymus DNA enhanced the acceptor activity severalfold. This stimulation was abolished if DNA was denatured by heating. Excess DNA showed a striking inhibitory effect. One possible explanation is that excess DNA, especially single-stranded DNA, binds the nuclear acceptor molecules of the DHT–receptor complex nonspecifically and does not allow the formation of the specific DHT–receptor–acceptor–DNA complex that can be dissociated in 0.4 M KCl and, therefore, assayed (Tymoczko and Liao, 1971). With the Millipore filter assay and gradient centrifugation, DNA without the nuclear extract retains considerable amounts of [³H]DHT–receptor complex. The retained complex could not be extracted with 0.4 M KCl, however, and, therefore, did not exhibit acceptor activity as defined by our assay procedure.

Ventral prostate DNA showed activity equivalent to that of calf thymus DNA, and DNA's from other sources (including bacteria) were also active. The significance of the differences in activity among the different DNA's could not be determined, since various DNA preparations may differ in physical status (extent of shearing and denaturation), rather than in chemical specificity (nucleotide sequences).

2. By Sequential Deproteinization of Chromatin

Recently, Klyzsejko-Stefanowicz and co-workers (1976) studied the chromatin acceptor molecules by sequentially removing urea-soluble chromosomal nonhistone proteins, histones, and DNA-associated nonhistone proteins from the chromatin of the rat ventral prostate and testis. The prostate ^{3}H-DHT–receptor complex was found to bind much better to the partially deproteinized chromatin, which still contains the DNA-binding nonhistone proteins, than to purified DNA. The receptor-binding activity of rat DNA was enhanced significantly by the addition of the DNA-associated nonhistone protein of the prostate or testis, but not the liver. The tissue specificity is in agreement with the results of the study described in the preceding sections.

The need for the nuclear protein in receptor binding, in the study, may be difficult to explain, since pure DNA (or chromatin from which all three classes of proteins were removed) was capable of binding as much androgen–receptor complex as the native chromatin that was not subjected to deproteinization. The binding assay done with the Millipore retention technique may be complicated by nonspecific histone and DNA binding of the radioactive androgen–receptor complex. As we noted above, most of the nuclear androgen–receptor complex retained *in vivo* can be solubilized by 0.4 M KCl, whereas the radioactive complex bound nonspecifically to histone and DNA *in vitro* (in the assay with broken nuclei or chromatin preparations) are difficult to wash away from the aggregate and may, thus, complicate the outcome of the experiments. For this reason, it is advisable to measure the complex that is soluble in 0.4 M KCl (see above section).

3. By Affinity Chromatography with Sepharose-Bound Nuclear Proteins

Puca *et al.* (1974) used covalent linkage of nuclear components to Sepharose to study their interaction with the cytosol estrogen–receptor complex of the uterus. They suggested that the nuclear acceptor molecule or molecules may be basic proteins. Mainwaring *et al.* (1976), who also used this technique, found that certain nonhistone basic proteins in the prostate nuclei, when bound to Sepharose, can retain the prostate cytosol ^{3}H-DHT–receptor complex. Androgens present in free form or bound to the sex steroid-binding globulin were not retained. The acceptor activity was higher in the nuclear preparations from the prostate than in those from the liver, spleen, or other tissues which are relatively insensitive to androgens. When various radioactive steroids were incubated with the prostate cytosol as the source of the steroid–receptor complexes, ^{3}H-DHT was about five times more active than labeled testosterone. Dexamethasone, progesterone, and androsterone were essentially inactive.

These results are in good agreement with those of our earlier studies on purified nuclei or solubilized acceptor preparations.

E. Histones and Nuclear Acceptor Activity

The 0.4 M KCl nuclear extract which we have used as the source of acceptor molecules contains some histones (cf. Johns, 1971). Since the equivalent fraction prepared from liver nuclei was nearly devoid of acceptor activity (Fig. 6), histones extractable by 0.4 M KCl from mammalian cell nuclei may not be the acceptor molecules. The steroid receptor complex and its nuclear acceptor protein, however, may interact with H-1 histone and affect its cellular function.

Although basic proteins such as histones and protamines can bind steroid–receptor complexes, this binding activity is rather stable with respect to heating (Tymoczko, 1973). Besides the heat stability, these basic proteins also differ from the acceptor molecules described above in their sensitivity to trypsin treatment. With the prostate nuclear acceptor preparation, limited digestion enhanced the acceptor activity, but further treatment resulted in complete loss of activity. In contrast, more than 70% of the receptor binding activity by histones was rather stable to a prolonged period of trypsin digestion. The response of the acceptor activity of the nuclear extract to addition of exogenous DNA also differs substantially from that shown by calf thymus histones. As described in Section IV,D,1, the acceptor activity of the prostate extract could be stimulated severalfold by the addition of DNA, but excess DNA resulted in the reduction of this activity close to the background level shown by DNA alone. Such a dramatic response was not observed when calf thymus histones were used.

In earlier studies, the acceptors in nuclei of the prostate (Tymoczko and Liao, 1971) and chick oviduct (Steggles *et al.,* 1971) were found in the acidic nuclear protein fractions; in the studies with affinity chromatography by Puca *et al.* (1974) and Mainwaring *et al.* (1976), however, the acceptor molecules appear to be in the nonhistone basic protein fractions. One of the unique properties of the acceptor molecules may be that they contain both acidic and basic ends, which can interact with either the basic or the acidic molecules. Such a dual interaction may play a role in an orderly alteration of chromatin structures, or in allowing key proteins (such as steroid receptor) to interact specifically with DNA and histones to bring about new genomic programs.

F. Release of Receptor from Chromatin

Whether there is a specific mechanism which regulates the interaction of the activated steroid–receptor complex and the nuclear chromatin is not clear. In fact, very little consideration has been given to the process of receptor release from the acceptor site for recycling (Liao *et al.*, 1973a, 1975). The possibility that there is a macromolecular factor that serves such a regulatory purpose was first indicated by the isolation of a protein fraction, from the prostate cytosol, capable of inhibiting the nuclear chromatin retention of the cytosol DHT–receptor complex in a cell-free system (Fang and Liao, 1971). Subsequently, other investigators suggested the presence of similar inhibitors in the cytosols of rat uterus (Chamness *et al.*, 1974), chick oviduct (Buller *et al.*, 1975), rat liver (Milgrom and Atger, 1975), and rat hepatoma cells (Simons *et al.*, 1976). Since bovine serum albumin was also inhibitory in many of these systems, the inhibition has not been regarded as a highly specific phenomenon.

We recently purified the prostate inhibitor more than 100-fold and identified it as a protein. This partially purified inhibitor was active at 50 to 100 μg/ml, whereas bovine serum albumin was totally inactive at 1 to 5 mg/ml of the incubation mixture. The inhibition is reversible; removal of the inhibitor from the incubation medium completely restores the capability of the DHT–receptor complex and the nuclear chromatin to interact and bind to each other. The protein factor can also release the DHT–receptor complex from the chromatin by a temperature-dependent process.

One of the most likely mechanisms for the inhibitory action is that the protein factor is capable of modifying the chromatin from a receptor-binding status to one not favorable for such binding. It is conceivable that the steroid–receptor complex is also a chromatin modifier that can maintain the genomic structure needed for the hormone induction of cellular functions.

V. INTERACTION OF ANDROGEN RECEPTORS WITH OTHER CELLULAR COMPONENTS

A. Divalent Metal Cations and Mononucleotides

Since the steroid receptor may interact with certain divalent cations and nucleotides (such as in RNA synthesis), we have studied this interaction by gradient centrifugation (Fig. 7). For this purpose, the androgen–receptor complex was incubated with the metal ion at 0° or 20°C prior to centrifugation in a gradient medium containing 0.4 M KCl, but no divalent cation. In such a study, we found that $CoCl_2$ facilitated aggregation of the complex and reduced the 3–4 S peak markedly, whereas $MnCl_2$, $MgCl_2$, and $CaCl_2$ had no significant effect at concentrations of 1–5 mM. The most dramatic effect, however, was observed when the DHT–receptor complex was incubated with 1–3 mM $ZnCl_2$ at 0°C for 20 minutes. This resulted in a shift of the sedimentation coefficient from 3.8 S to 4.5 S without a change in the total [^{3}H]DHT bound to the receptor. Incubation under identical conditions, except for an increase in temperature of 20°C, resulted in a broad radioactivity peak (5 S ± 2 S) accompanied by a release of much of the bound androgen. These results imply that the interaction of Zn^{2+} with the receptor protein may change the configuration of the receptor protein, thereby decreasing the steroid binding affinity and possibly altering the way in which the receptor can interact with other cellular molecules (Liao et al., 1975; Liao, 1976).

In the absence of nucleotide, the incubation of the freshly prepared prostate cytosol DHT–receptor complex at 20°C can cause a shift in the sedimentation coefficient of the complex from 3.8 S to 3.0 S (Section

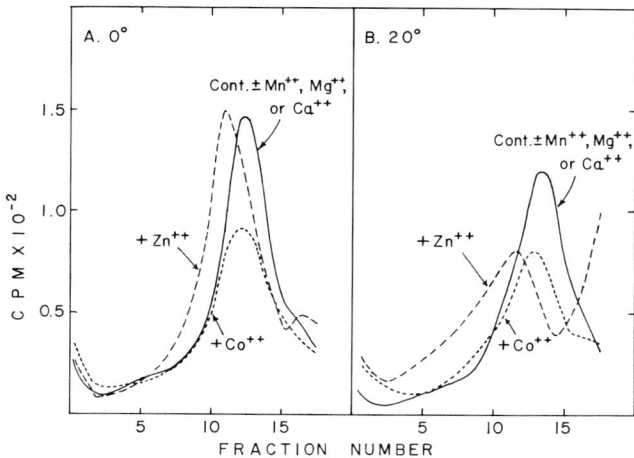

Fig. 7. Interaction of metal ions with [^{3}H]DHT-receptor complex of rat ventral prostate. The cytosol complex II was incubated with 3 mM of $ZnCl_2$, $CoCl_2$, $MgCl_2$, or $CaCl_2$ for 20 minutes at 0°C (A) or 20°C (B) before it was layered on the top of a glycerol gradient (10 to 22%) solution and analyzed by gradient centrifugation. Centrifugation was performed at 54,000 rpm for 18 hours. The solid lines represent results with the samples containing no metal ion, or in the presence of $MnCl_2$, $MgCl_2$, or $CaCl_2$ which had no visible effect on the sedimentation patterns; (---), Zn^{2+}; (····), Co^{2+}. The gradient medium had pH of 7.5. The sedimentation was from right to left (Liao et al., 1975).

IV,B). If GTP or ATP is present, a small shift in the coefficient can be observed even when the sample is maintained at 0°C (Fig. 8). Additional incubation at 20°C does not change the sedimentation property further. Both CTP and UTP also demonstrate some effect, but this is not clear as with ATP and GTP. The effectiveness of ADP, AMP, and cyclic AMP is much smaller. Addition of ATP and GTP to the heat-transformed complex does not result in very significant change in the sedimentation pattern. The effect is clearly not due to the phosphate moiety alone, as inorganic mono- or pyrophosphate at these concentrations is not effective. It may be that ATP and GTP can also specifically induce a biologically important conformational change of the DHT–receptor complex (Liao *et al.*, 1975).

B. Polynucleotides and Ribonucleoproteins

The prostate DHT–receptor complex is also capable of binding to certain polynucleotides. If nucleic acids with known sedimentation coefficients are mixed with a cytosol preparation containing [³H]DHT–receptor complex, new radioactivity peaks appear, the size of which depends on the type, size, and amount of nucleic acid employed (Tymoczko, 1973). With polymers having sedimentation coefficients of about 4 ± 1 S, poly(A) and poly(G)

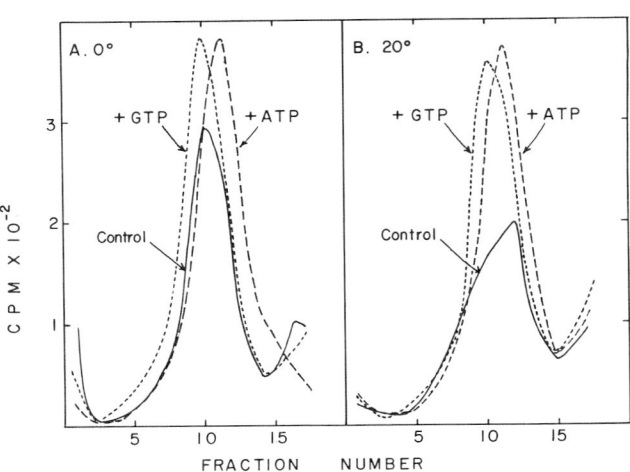

Fig. 8. Interaction of nucleoside triphosphates with [³H]DHT–receptor complex of rat ventral prostate. The cytosol complex II was incubated with 4 mM of GTP or ATP for 20 minutes at 0°C (A) or 20°C (B) before it was layered on the top of a glycerol gradient (10–20%) solution and analyzed by gradient centrifugation. The control tube (———) contained no nucleotide; (– – –), + ATP; (·····), + GTP. The sedimentation was from right to left (Liao *et al.*, 1975).

gave distinct radioactivity peaks which were heavier than 25 S; poly(U) gave a radioactive shoulder that was only slightly heavier than the nucleic acid itself; and the effect of poly(C), liver tRNA, and *Escherichia coli* tRNA was barely apparent. Incubation of 5 S poly(A) with the DHT–receptor complex resulted in radioactivity peaks between 50 and 70 S. The formation of the peaks heavier than the nucleic acids themselves may involve fortuitous binding of nonreceptor proteins in the receptor preparation.

Rat ventral prostate 16 S and 28 S ribosomal RNA, as well as DNA from the ventral prostate, calf thymus, salmon sperm, *Escherichia coli*, and *Bacillus subtilis* bind to the DHT–receptor complex, forming radioactivity peaks which are detectable by gradient centrifugation. On the basis of radioactivity per unit quantity of DNA, no specificity for DNA was found.

In our acceptor assay (Section IV,D,1), the stimulation of the acceptor activity by DNA can be mimicked by liver ribosomal RNA, poly(G), or poly(A); or by poly(U) and poly(C), however, these polymers are much less effective (Tymoczko and Liao, 1971). Whether the action of nucleic acid is dependent largely on the purine nucleotide components remains to be determined. Under our assay conditions, various regions of these active synthetic polymers may form multiple helical structures; therefore, it is possible that the acceptor activity depends on certain secondary or tertiary structures of the polynucleotides. On the other hand, DNA and the polynucleotides may each have their distinct binding sites on the ternary complex of nuclear acceptor molecules and on the steroid–receptor complexes.

These studies have prompted us also to consider the possibility that certain ribonucleoprotein (RNP) particles in the nuclei and cytoplasm may interact with the steroid–receptor complex in biologically meaninfgul ways (Liao *et al.*, 1973a). We, therefore, isolated nuclear RNP particles according to the method developed by Hu and Wang (1971) and incubated them with DHT–receptor complex at 0°C for 30 minutes. The mixture was then subjected to gradient centrifugation. The sedimentation pattern showed the formation of a new radioactive peak in the 60–80 S region of the gradient. The formation of this new complex was accompanied by a concomitant loss of the unbound ^{3}H-DHT–receptor complex. The 80 S radioactivity peak was not formed in the presence of 0.4 M KCl, and a KCl concentration of 0.15 M or higher resulted in the dissociation of the 80 S complex. The efficiency of the association between the DHT–receptor complex and the RNP was dependent on the pH of the incubating medium and the gradient solution, the optimum being in the vicinity of pH 8.1. Treatment of the RNP with RNase prevented the formation of the 60–80 S radioactivity peak, presumably by destroying the RNA component of the RNP. Destruction of the RNP particles was probably also responsible for the loss of receptor binding capacity after the RNP had been heated at 70°C for 20 minutes. Treatment of the RNP with DNase had no effect.

The receptor binding sites on the RNP particles could be saturated with excess DHT receptor, indicating that a limited number of binding sites exist. The apparent association constant calculated from such experiments is of the order of 10^{10} M^{-1}. Under saturating conditions with respect to the DHT receptor, less than 5% of the isolated RNP particles can bind to the steroid–receptor complex. It is possible that only those RNP with heat-labile acceptor factors can associate with the DHT–receptor complex.

Experiments with excess RNP demonstrate that only about 30–50% of the total DHT–receptor complex is capable of binding to the RNP particles (cf. Table I). This might indicate that only certain forms of the steroid–receptor complex are capable of interacting with the RNP particles. Receptor specificity is also demonstrated by the inefficient binding found for [^{3}H]progesterone and [^{3}H]17β-estradiol complexes of the calf uterus to the nuclear RNP particles of rat ventral prostate. Free DHT and heated DHT–receptor complex failed to produce the 80 S RNP particle when they were incubated with the nuclear RNP particle.

The cytoplasmic polysome or 80 S monosome forms of ribosomes do not bind the DHT–receptor complex at all, although the 40 S and 60 S subunit particles prepared from them can bind the complex readily. Radioactive steroids alone do not associate with any of these ribosomal particles. Preliminary experiments suggested that naked receptor, unattached to an androgen, does not bind to the particles.

VI. CONCLUDING REMARKS

A. Action of Antiandrogens

Steroid binding by cellular receptors is of biologic importance since many steroid hormone antagonists can interfere with the formation of steroid–receptor complexes in the target cells. For antiandrogens, this interference was first shown by the use of cyproterone and its 17α-acetate (Fang and Liao, 1969; Liao and Fang, 1969). Other antagonists, such as SK and F 7690 (17α-methyl-B-nortestosterone; Tveter and Aakvagg, 1969), R-2956 (17β-hydroxy-2α,2β,17α-trimethylestra-4,9,11-trien-3-one; Baulieu and Jung, 1970), BOMT (6α-bromo-17β-hydroxy-17α-methyl-4-oxa-5α-androstan-3-one; Mangan and Mainwaring, 1972), and flutamide behave in a similar way. Flutamide (Peets *et al.*, 1974; Liao *et al.*, 1974; Mainwaring *et al.*, 1974a) appears to be metabolized outside the prostate to a more potent hydroxylated form (Neri, 1976) that can suppress the receptor binding of androgens.

The cellular action of certain antiandrogens may be more complex, however. For example, cyproterone and its acetate may affect the androgen transport and clearance mechanism, possibly at the cell membranes (Giorgi 1976). Theoretically, certain antagonist–receptor complexes may also compete with the androgen–receptor complexes for the nuclear acceptor sites and, thus, prevent the normal function of the ternary complex. Although estrogens can inhibit androgen binding to prostate receptors (Fang et al., 1969), there are specific estradiol-binding proteins in the prostate which are distinguishable from the specific DHT–receptor proteins (Jungblut et al., 1971; Armstrong and Bashirelahi, 1974; Van Beurden-Lamers et al., 1974). The estrogen–receptor complex may function independently from the androgen–receptor complex and cause inhibition. In the liver of adult rats, the antagonistic action of estradiol on the androgen induction of α_2-globulin is thought to be due to binding of estrogen to the androgen receptor at a distinct site, inducing an allosteric effect and preventing androgen binding at a distant site of the receptor protein (Roy et al., 1974).

B. RNA Synthesis

Since androgens can rapidly effect RNA synthesis in the cell nuclei of target tissues (Liao et al., 1965; Liao and Fang, 1969), the selective retention of the cytoplasmic androgen–protein complex by prostate cell nuclei appears to be very important in androgen action. This view is corroborated by the observation that these rapid effects can be antagonized by antiandrogens that also inhibit receptor binding of androgens (Anderson et al., 1972; Mainwaring et al., 1974b). Persuasive support comes from Davies and Griffiths (1974), who reported that certain prostate cytosol preparations containing the DHT–receptor complex can enhance the RNA-synthesizing activity of the prostate nuclear chromatin in cell-free systems. (As described in other articles of this book, this type of study has been performed with other steroid–receptor complexes).

However, the way in which the androgen–receptor complex acts in prostate cell nuclei remains a mystery. It is not clear, for example, whether the receptor (or androgen) is directly involved in the activation of specific genes or whether it acts at a distant site. Our study suggests that the receptor protein is not retained by the nuclear acceptor sites if the androgen is not present. As has been described for various hormones (Jensen et al., 1974), binding of an androgen to a receptor protein may result in a change of the structure of the receptor protein so that it conforms with the nuclear acceptor site (Liao, 1975). Our suggestion that DHT is enveloped by the receptor protein (Section III,B,4) supports the concept that the function of the steroid hormone is to fulfill the structural requirement of the steroid–receptor complex, and that the hormone itself may not be directly involved in the biochemical reaction.

It can be conjectured that either the receptor proteins or the nuclear acidic proteins may be part of the regulatory or catalytic proteins of the RNA–polymerase complex (positive control). Earlier suggestions that steroid hormones act by binding to an inactivating repressor molecule would suggest that the steroid receptors themselves are the repressors. If so, it would be difficult to understand the significance of the binding of the steroid–repressor complex to the nuclear chromatin, or the presence of large amounts of the repressor in the cytoplasm. It is more likely that, if derepression is involved, it is the steroid–receptor complex, rather than the steroid alone, which interacts with nuclear repressors and prevents their functioning (negative control). Alternatively, the steroid–receptor complex may interact with acceptor molecules and alter the chromatin structures in such a way that a new genomic program can be initiated (Section IV,E).

C. Ribonucleoprotein Function

The finding that certain nuclear RNP particles bind steroid–receptor complex in a specific manner raises the new possibility that some of the hormone actions may be related to the functions performed by these particles, e.g., the regulation of the synthesis and processing of RNA because the particles serve as ribosomal precursors (Burdon, 1971; Kumar and Warner, 1972), mRNA carriers (i.e., informosomes, informofers, etc.) (Spirin, 1969; Samarina *et al.,* 1968), and gene regulators (Paul, 1971; Britten and Davidson, 1969). The elimination of any of these possibilities is difficult at this time. Many properties of these particles in animal cells in general are not well understood, and the DHT-receptor-binding particles are only a small portion of the total particles in the preparations being analyzed. In addition, the isolated RNP particles may be altered forms of the intact particles.

In a hypothetical model, the steroid–receptor complex may enter the nucleus and associate with the nuclear acceptor proteins (regulatory or catalytic proteins) on the chromatin. The formation of this "trigger complex" may permit initiation of transcription at previously restricted portions of the genome. The trigger complex, or a portion of the complex that involves the receptor, may then participate in the processing or packaging of the RNA. The RNA product may form an RNP particle which can still retain the androgen–receptor complex. The RNP particle is then processed and transported to the cytoplasm where it may become involved in protein synthesis. Thus, the nuclear chromatin or RNP binding of the DHT–receptor complex is considered to be a dynamic phenomenon. Both the steroid and the receptor protein may be reutilized; thus, a receptor cycle (Liao et al., 1973a) can be envisaged. This suggestion implies that, if the target cells have large quantities of RNP particles which simply lack the steroid hormone for further processing or utilization, the effect of replenishing of the steroid hormone on protein synthesis may not depend entirely on the RNA synthesis itself. This may explain some of the anomalous findings that certain steroid hormone effects are not sensitive to actinomycin D inhibition of gene transcription (Smith and Ecker, 1971; Schuetz, 1974; see also references cited in Liang, Castañeda, and Liao, 1977).

D. Protein Synthesis

Although there is no compelling reason for the belief that androgens act in the cell cytoplasm, such a possibility cannot be excluded completely (see review by Liao, 1976). There are, in fact, many reports describing androgen effects that are insensitive to actinomycin D or are not likely to be critically dependent on new RNA synthesis. Among them are the effects of androgens on chick comb growth (Talwar et al., 1965), arginase synthesis and incorporation of amino acids into bulk proteins of the mouse kidney (Frieden and Fishel, 1968), early increase in prostatic NADH (Ritter, 1966), cation transport by prostate cell membranes (Farnsworth, 1968), protein kinase activity (Ahmed and Wilson, 1975), and lysosome–nucleus interaction (Szego, 1972; cf. Sepsenwol and Hechter, 1976). Many of these findings have not been confirmed, however, and need more extensive investigation.

The high protein-synthesizing activity in the prostate cell stimulated by androgens can be attributed to an increase in the mRNA content (Liao and Williams-Ashman, 1962; Liao, 1965, 1968) and to protein synthesis initiation and elongation factors (Ichii et al., 1974). We have shown (Fig. 9) that the [^{35}S]Met-tRNA$_f$ (initiator tRNA) binding activity of the initiation factor, eIF-2, in the prostate cytosol is reduced rapidly within hours after castration, and that this effect is reversed within 10–30 minutes by an intravenous injection of DHT into the castrated rats (Liang and Liao, 1975). Castañeda (see Liao et al., 1975) has found that actinomycin D and cycloheximide injected into experimental animals in quantities that inhibit 75% and 95% of RNA synthesis and protein synthesis, respectively, in the

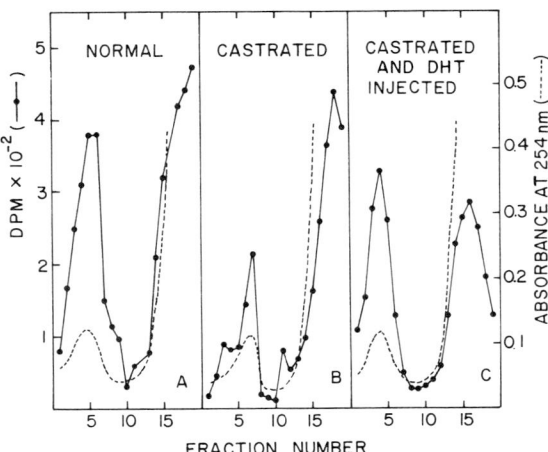

Fig. 9. Effect of androgen *in vivo* on the prostate cytosol initiation factor eIF-2 activity. Adult Carworth CFE male rats (300 g body weight) were used. Two groups of rats were castrated; 16 hours later, one group was injected intravenously with 20 µg of 5α-dihydrotestosterone (in 0.1 ml saline containing 10% ethanol) and another with the vehicle solution alone, 10 minutes before they were killed. The cytosol preparations were obtained from the normal control (A), castrated (B), and castrated and androgen-treated (C) rats by the method described previously (Liang and Liao, 1975). The preparations were assayed for their capacity to promote [^{35}S]met-tRNA$_f$ binding to the 40 S prostate ribosomal particles from the normal rats. The assay medium (0.3 ml) contained 300 µg cytosol proteins, 0.6 A_{260} unit of 40 S ribosomal particles, 404,00 cpm [^{35}S]met-tRNA$_f$ (0.9 pmole) in 5.9 µg liver tRNA, 2 mM GTP, 5 mM MgCl$_2$, 25 mM KCl, 3 mM dithiothreitol. 10 µg poly(A:U:G), and 20 mM Tris–HCl, pH 7.5. The mixture was incubated at 30°C for 30 minutes and fixed with 5 µl of 25% glutaraldehyde (adjusted by 1 N NaOH to pH 6). Two-tenths milliliter of the fixed sample was layered on the top of a linear 5–20% sucrose gradient medium containing 5 mM MgCl$_2$, 25 mM KCl, and 20 mM Tris–HCl, pH 7.5, and centrifuged at 54,000 rpm for 100 min in a Beckman swinging bucket rotor No. 56. Fractions (0.2 ml each) were analyzed for absorbancy at 254 nm and for the radioactivity that could be retained on Millipore HA filters. The fractions were numbered from the bottom of the centrifuged samples. The 40 S ribosomal particles sedimented near fraction No. 5.

prostate, were not able to eliminate the androgen-dependent increase in eIF-2 activity. However, cyproterone acetate, which can inhibit the receptor binding of DHT, can eliminate the androgen effect *in vivo*. An involvement of DHT–receptor complex in this very rapid effect is, therefore, conceivable. It may be worthwhile to pursue further the possibility that certain steroid hormones control factors that have dual roles in the transcription and translation processes and can assure a well-coordinated and efficient regulation of gene expression in the steroid target cells.

ACKNOWLEDGMENT

Research carried out in this laboratory was supported by NIH Grants AM-09461 and HD-07110 and by Grant BC-151 from the American Cancer Society, Inc.

REFERENCES

Ahmed, K., and Wilson, M. J. (1975). *J. Biol. Chem.* **250**, 2370.
Anderson, K. M., and Liao, S. (1968). *Nature (London)* **219**, 277.
Anderson, K. M., Cohn, H., and Samuels, S. (1972). *FEBS Lett.* **27**, 149.
Armstrong, E. G., and Bashirelahi, N. (1974). *Biochem. Biophys. Res. Commun.* **61**, 578.
Attramadal, A., Tveter, K. J., Weddington, S. C., Djøseland, O., Naess, O., Hansson, V., and Torgersen, O. (1975). *Vitam. Horm. (N.Y.)* **33**, 247.
Attramadal, A., Weddington, S. C., Naess, O., Djøseland, O., and Hansson, V. (1976). In "Prostate Disease" (H. Marberger, H. Haschek, H. K. A. Schirmer, J. A. C. Colston, and E. Witkin, eds.), p. 189. Alan Liss, New York.
Bardin, W., Bullock, L. P., and Mowszowicz, I. (1975). In "Methods in Enzymology" (B. W. O'Malley and J. G. Hardman, eds.), Vol. 39, Part D, p. 454. Academic Press, New York.
Barry, M., Eidinoff, M. C. L., Dobriner, K., and Gallagher, T. F. (1952). *Endocrinology* **50**, 587.
Baulieu, E.-E., and Jung, I. (1970). *Biochem. Biophys. Res. Commun.* **38**, 599.
Baulieu, E.-E., Jung, I., Blondeau, J. P., and Robel, P. (1971). *Adv. Biosci.* **7**, 180.
Belham, J. E., Neal, G. E., and Williams, D. C. (1969). *Biochim. Biophys. Acta* **187**, 159.
Bell, P. A., and Munck, A. (1973). *Biochem. J.* **136**, 97.
Beyer, C., Larsson, K., Perez-Palacios, G., and Morali, G. (1973). *Horm. Behav.* **4**, 99.
Blaquier, J. A., and Calandra, R. S. (1973). *Endocrinology* **93**, 51.
Blondeau, J. P., Corpechot, C., LeGoascogne, C., Baulieu, E. E., and Robel, P. (1975). *Vitam. Horm. (N.Y.)* **33**, 319.
Bresciani, F., Nola, E., Sica, V., and Puca, G. A. (1973). *Fed. Proc., Fed. Am. Soc. Exp. Biol.* **32**, 2126.
Britten, R. H., and Davidson, E. H. (1969). *Science* **165**, 349.
Bruchovsky, N. (1971). *Endocrinology* **89**, 1212.
Bruchovsky, N., and Craven, S. (1975). *Biochem. Biophys. Res. Commun.* **4**, 837.
Bruchovsky, N., and Wilson, J. D. (1968). *J. Biol. Chem.* **243**, 2012.
Bruchovsky, N., Sutherland, D. J. A., Meakin, J. W., and Minesita, T. (1975). *Biochim. Biophys. Acta* **381**, 61.
Buller, R. E., Schrader, W. T., and O'Malley, B. W. (1975). *J. Biol. Chem.* **250**, 809.
Bullock, L., and Bardin, C. W. (1970). *J. Clin. Endocrinol. Metab.* **31**, 113.
Burdon, R. H. (1971). *Prog. Nucleic Acid. Res. Mol. Biol.* **11**, 33.
Cardinali, D. P., Nagle, C. A., and Rosner, J. M. (1975). *Life Sci.* **16**, 93.
Castañeda, E., and Liao, S. (1974). *Endocr. Res. Commun.* **1**, 271.
Castañeda, E., and Liao, S. (1975). *J. Biol. Chem.* **250**, 883.
Chamness, G. G., Jennings, A. W., and McGuire, W. L. (1974). *Biochemistry* **13**, 327.
Davies, P., and Griffiths, K. (1974). *Biochem. J.* **140**, 565.
Dubé, J. Y., and Tremblay, R. R. (1974). *Endocrinology* **95**, 1105.
Dunn, J. F., Goldstein, J. L., and Wilson, J. D. (1973). *J. Biol. Chem.* **348**, 7819.

Eppenberger, U., and Hsia, S. L. (1972). *J. Biol. Chem.* **247**, 5463.
Evans, C. R., and Pierrepoint, C. G. (1975). *J. Endocrinol.* **64**, 539.
Fang, S., and Liao, S. (1969). *Mol. Pharmacol.* **5**, 428.
Fang, S., and Liao, S. (1971). *J. Biol. Chem.* **246**, 16.
Fang, S., Anderson, K. M., and Liao, S. (1969). *J. Biol. Chem.* **244**, 6584.
Fansworth, W. F. (1968). *Biochim. Biophys. Acta* **150**, 446.
Fazekas, A. G., and Sandor, T. (1973). *Endocrinol., Proc. Int. Symp., 4th, 1972* Excerpta Med. Found. Int. Congr. Ser. No. 203, Abstract, p. 80.
Fox, T. O. (1975). *Proc. Natl. Acad. Sci. U.S.A.* **72**, 4303.
Frieden, E. H., and Fishel, S. S. (1968). *Biochem. Biophys. Res. Commun.* **31**, 515.
Galena, H. J., Pillai, A. K., and Terner, C. (1974). *J. Endocrinol.* **63**, 223.
Gehring, U., Tomkins, G. M., and Ohno, S. (1971). *Nature (London), New Biol.* **232**, 106.
Giannopoulos, G. (1973). *J. Biol. Chem.* **248**, 1004.
Giorgi, E. P. (1976). *J. Endocrinol.* **68**, 109.
Gonzalez-Diddi, M., Komisaruk, B., and Beyer, C. (1972). *Endocrinology* **91**, 1130.
Greer, D. S. (1959). *Endocrinology* **64**, 898.
Gustafsson, J.-A., and Pousette, A. (1975). *Biochemistry* **14**, 3094.
Gustafsson, J.-A., Pousette, A., Stenberg, A., and Wrange, O. (1975). *Biochemistry* **14**, 3942.
Hansson, V., and Djøseland, O. (1972). *Acta Endocrinol. (Copenhagen)* **71**, 614.
Hansson, V., Trygstad, O., French, F. S., McLean, W. S., Smith, A. A., Tindall, D. J., Weddington, S. C., Petrusz, P., Nayfeh, S. N., and Ritzén, E. M. (1974). *Nature (London)* **250**, 387.
Harding, B. W., and Samuels, L. T. (1962). *Endocrinology* **70**, 109.
Hu, A. L., and Wang, T. Y. (1971). *Arch. Biochem. Biophys.* **144**, 549.
Huggins, C., Jensen, E. V., and Cleveland, A. S. (1954). *J. Exp. Med.* **100**, 225.
Ichii, S., Izawa, M., and Murakimi, N. (1974). *Endocrinol. Jpn.* **21**, 267.
Jensen, E. V., Mohla, S., Gorrel, T. A., and De Sombre, E. R. (1974). *Vitam. Horm. (N.Y.)* **32**, 89.
Johns, E. W. (1971). *In* "Histones and Nucleohistones" (D. M. P. Phillips, ed.), p. 2. Plenum, New York.
Jouan, P., Samperez, S., and Thieulant, M. L. (1973). *J. Steroid Biochem.* **4**, 65.
Jung, I., and Baulieu, E. E. (1972). *Nature (London), New Biol.* **237**, 24.
Jungblut, P. W., Hughes, S. F., Gorlich, L., Gowers, U., and Wagner, R. K. (1971). *Hoppe-Seyler's Z. Physiol. Chem.* **352**, 1603.
Kato, J. (1975). *J. Steroid Biochem.* **6**, 979.
Katsumata, M., and Goldman, A. S. (1974). *Biochim. Biophys. Acta* **359**, 112.
King, R. B., and Gordon, J. (1972). *Nature (London), New Biol.* **240**, 185.
Klyzsejko-Stefanowicz, L., Chiu, J. F., Tsai, Y. H., and Hnilica, L. S. (1976). *Proc. Natl. Acad. Sci. U.S.A.* **73**, 1954.
Krieg, M., Steins, P., Szalay, R., and Voigt, K. D. (1974a). *J. Steroid Biochem.* **5**, 87.
Krieg, M., Szalay, R., and Voight, K. D. (1974b). *J. Steroid Biochem.* **5**, 453.
Kumar, A., and Warner, J. R. (1972). *J. Mol. Biol.* **63**, 233.
Lane, S. E., Gidari, A. S., and Levere, R. D. (1975). *J. Biol. Chem.* **250**, 8209.
Liang, T., and Liao, S. (1975). *Proc. Natl. Acad. Sci. U.S.A.* **72**, 706.
Liang, T., Castañeda, E., and Liao, S. (1977). *J. Biol. Chem.* **252**, 5692.
Liao, S. (1965). *J. Biol. Chem.* **240**, 1236.
Liao, S. (1968). *Am. Zool.* **8**, 233.
Liao, S. (1974). *In* "Biochemistry of Hormones" (H. V. Rickenberg, ed.), p. 154. Medical and Technical Publ. Co., Oxford.
Liao, S. (1975). *Int. Rev. Cytol.* **41**, 87.

Liao, S. (1977). *Biochem. Actions Horm.* **4**, 351.
Liao, S., and Fang, S. (1969). *Vitam. Horm. (N.Y.)* **27**, 17.
Liao, S., and Fang, S. (1970). *In* "Some Aspects of Aetiology and Biochemistry of Prostate Cancer" (K. Griffiths and C. G. Pierrepoint, eds.), p. 105. Alpha Omega Alpha Publ., Cardiff, Wales.
Liao, S., and Liang, T. (1974). *In* "Hormones and Cancer" (K. W. McKerns, ed.), p. 229. Academic Press, New York.
Liao, S., and Williams-Ashman, H. G. (1962). *Proc. Natl. Acad. Sci. U.S.A.* **48**, 1956.
Liao, S., Leinninger, K. R., Sagher, D., and Barton, R. W. (1965). *Endocrinology* **77**, 763.
Liao, S., Tymoczko, J. L., Liang, T., Anderson, K. M., and Fang, S. (1971). *Adv. Biosci.* **7**, 155.
Liao, S., Liang, T., and Tymoczko, J. L. (1973a). *Nature (London), New Biol.* **241**, 211.
Liao, S., Liang, T., Fang, S., Castañeda, E., and Shao, T.-C. (1973b). *J. Biol. Chem.* **248**, 6154.
Liao, S., Howell, D. K., and Chang, T. M. (1974). *Endocrinology* **94**, 1205.
Liao, S., Tymoczko, J. L., Castañeda, E., and Liang, T. (1975). *Vitam. Horm. (N.Y.)* **33**, 297.
Loras, B., Genot, A., Monbon, M., Beucher, F., Reboucl, J. P., and Bertrand, J. (1974). *J. Steroid Biochem.* **5**, 425.
Louvet, J. P., Harman, S. M., Schreiber, J. R., and Ross, G. T. (1975). *Endocrinology* **97**, 368.
Mainwaring, W. I. P. (1969a). *J. Endocrinol.* **44**, 323.
Mainwaring, W. I. P. (1969b). *J. Endocrinol.* **45**, 531.
Mainwaring, W. I. P., and Irving, R. (1973). *Biochem. J.* **134**, 113.
Mainwaring, W. I. P., and Mangan, F. R. (1973). *J. Endocrinol.* **54**, 121.
Mainwaring, W. I. P., and Peterken, B. M. (1971). *Biochem. J.* **125**, 285.
Mainwaring, W. I. P., Mangan, F. R., and Peterken, B. M. (1971). *Biochem. J.* **123**, 619.
Mainwaring, W. I. P., Mangan, F. R., Feherty, P. A., and Freifeld, M. (1974a). *Mol. Cell. Endocrinol.* **1**, 113.
Mainwaring, W. I. P., Mangan, F. R., Irving, R. A., and Jones, D. A. (1974b). *Biochem. J.* **144**, 413.
Mainwaring, W. I. P., Symes, E. K., and Higgins, S. J. (1976). *Biochem. J.* **156**, 129.
Mangan, F. R., and Mainwaring, W. I. P. (1972). *Steroids* **20**, 331.
Mann, T., Rowson, L. E. A., Baronos, S., and Karagiannidis, A. (1971). *J. Endocrinol.* **51**, 707.
Milgrom, E., and Atger, M. (1975). *J. Steroid Biochem.* **6**, 487.
Naess, O., Hansson, V., Djoseland, O., and Attramadal, A. (1975). *Endocrinology* **97**, 1355.
Neri, R. (1976). *Advan. Sex Hormone Res.* **2**, 233.
Norris, J. S., Gorski, J., and Kohler, P. O. (1974). *Nature (London)* **248**, 422.
Notides, A. C., Hamilton, D. E., and Aver, H. E. (1975). *J. Biol. Chem.* **250**, 3945.
O'Malley, B. W., and Means, A. R., eds. (1973). "Receptors for Reproductive Hormones." Plenum, New York.
Palmiter, R. D., Catlin, G. H., and Cox, R. F. (1973). *Cell Differ.* **2**, 163.
Paul, J. (1971). *Curr. Top. Dev. Biol.* **5**, 317.
Pearlman, W. H., and Pearlman, M. R. (1961). *J. Biol. Chem.* **236**, 1321.
Peets, E. A., Henson, M. F., and Neri, R. (1974). *Endocrinology* **94**, 532.
Poortman, J., Prenen, J. A. C., Schwarz, F., and Thijssen, J. H. H. (1975). *J. Clin. Endocrinol. Metab.* **40**, 373.
Puca, G. A., Sica, V., and Nola, E. (1974). *Proc. Natl. Acad. Sci. U.S.A.* **71**, 979.
Ritter, C. (1966). *Mol. Pharmacol.* **2**, 125.
Ritzén, E. M., Nayfeh, S. N., French, F. S., and Aronin, P. A. (1972). *Endocrinology* **91**, 116.

Ritzén, E. M., French, F. S., Weddington, S. C., and Nayfish, S. N. (1974). *J. Biol. Chem.* **249,** 6597.
Roy, A. K., Milin, B. S., and McMinn, D. M. (1974). *Biochim. Biophys. Acta* **354,** 213.
Ruh, T. S., Katzenellenbogen, B. S., Katzenellenbogen, J. A., and Gorski, J. (1973). *Endocrinology* **92,** 125.
Samarina, O. P., Lukanidin, E. M., Molnar, J., and Georgiev, G. P. (1968). *J. Mol. Biol.* **33,** 251.
Sar, M., Liao, S., and Stumpf, W. E. (1970). *Endocrinology* **86,** 1008.
Schuetz, A. W. (1974). *Biol. Reprod.* **10,** 150.
Sepsenwol, W., and Hechter, O. (1976). *Mol. Cell. Endocrinol.* **4,** 115.
Shain, S. A., Boesel, K. W., and Axelrod, L. R. (1975). *Arch. Biochem. Biophys.* **167,** 247.
Shao, T.-C., Castañeda, E., Rosenfield, R. L., and Liao, S. (1975). *J. Biol. Chem.* **250,** 3095.
Simons, S. S., Martinez, H. M., Garcea, R. L., Baxter, J. D., and Tomkins, G. M. (1976). *J. Biol. Chem.* **251,** 334.
Smith, L. D., and Ecker, R. E. (1971). *Dev. Biol.* **25,** 232.
Spelsberg, T. C., Steggles, A. W., and O'Malley, B. W. (1971). *J. Biol. Chem.* **246,** 4188.
Spirin, A. S. (1969). *Eur. J. Biochem.* **10,** 20.
Steggles, A. W., Spelsberg, T. C., Glasser, S. R., and O'Malley, B. W. (1971). *Proc. Natl. Acad. Sci. U.S.A.* **68,** 1479.
Szego, C. M. (1972). *Gynecol. Invest.* **3,** 63.
Takayasu, S., and Adachi, K. (1975). *Endocrinology* **96,** 525.
Talwar, G. P., Modi, S., and Rao, K. N. (1965). *Science* **150,** 1315.
Tata, J. R. (1966). *Prog. Nucleic Acid. Res. Mol. Biol.* **5,** 191.
Tindall, D. J., French, F. S., and Neyfeh, S. N. (1972). *Biochem. Biophys. Res. Commun.* **49,** 1391.
Töpert, M., Zabel, I., and Ziegler, M. (1974). *Anal. Biochem.* **62,** 514.
Tveter, K. J., and Aakvaag, A. (1969). *Endocrinology* **85,** 683.
Tveter, K. J., and Attramadal, A. (1968). *Acta Endocrinol. (Copenhagen)* **59,** 218.
Tveter, K. J., and Attramadal, A. (1969). *Endocrinology* **85,** 350.
Tveter, K. J., and Unhjem, O. (1969). *Endocrinology* **84,** 963.
Tymoczko, J. L. (1973). Ph.D. Dissertation, University of Chicago, Chicago, Illinois.
Tymoczko, J. L., and Liao, S. (1971). *Biochim. Biophys. Acta* **252,** 607.
Unhjem, O., Tveter, K. J., and Aakvagg, A. (1969). *Acta Endocrinol. (Copenhagen)* **62,** 153.
Valladares, L., and Mingnell, J. (1975). *Steroids* **25,** 13.
Van Beurden-Lamers, W. M. O., Brinkman, A. O., Mulder, E., and Van der Molen, H. J. (1974). *Biochem. J.* **140,** 492.
Verhoeven, G., Heyns, W., and De Moor, P. (1975). *Vitam. Horm. (N.Y.)* **33,** 265.
Vida, J. A. (1969). "Androgens and Anabolic Agents." Academic Press, New York.
Wester, R. C., and Foote, R. H. (1972). *Proc. Soc. Exp. Biol. Med.* **141,** 26.
Whalen, R. E., and Luttge, W. G. (1971a). *Horm. Behav.* **2,** 117.
Whalen, R. E., and Luttge, W. G. (1971b). *Endocrinology* **89,** 1320.
Wolff, M. E., and Kasuya, Y. (1972). *J. Med. Chem.* **15,** 87.
Wolff, M. E., and Zanati, G. (1970). *Experientia* **26,** 1115.
Yamamoto, K. R., and Alberts, B. (1974). *J. Biol. Chem.* **249,** 7076.

7

Biology of Progesterone Receptors

WENDELL W. LEAVITT, TONG J. CHEN,
YUNG S. DO, BETSY D. CARLTON,
AND THOMAS C. ALLEN

I.	Introduction	157
II.	Progesterone Action in the Hamster	159
III.	Progesterone Uptake *in Vivo*	160
IV.	Methods for Studying Cytosol Progesterone Receptor	161
	A. Buffers	162
	B. Dextran-Coated Charcoal	162
	C. Cytosol and Serum Preparation	163
	D. Sucrose–Glycerol Gradient Centrifugation	163
	E. Scatchard Assay	164
	F. Competition Assay	168
V.	Progesterone Receptor Distribution in Different Tissues	169
	A. Endometrium and Myometrium	169
	B. Deciduoma	169
	C. Vagina	171
	D. Pituitary and Hypothalamus	171
	E. Mammary Gland	173
VI.	Regulation of Progesterone Receptor Levels	173
	A. Estrous Cycle	173
	B. Pregnancy	175
	C. Estrogen Action	176
	D. Progesterone Action	179
VII.	Progesterone Receptor Synthesis *in Vitro*	184
	References	186

I. INTRODUCTION

The classic experiments of Fraenkel (1903) and Allen and Corner (1930) demonstrated the requirement of corpus luteum hormone ("progestin") for pregnancy maintenance in the rabbit. Following these pioneering studies, progestins were detected in the ovaries of many animal species. Since progesterone is an important precursor utilized in the synthesis of several steroid hormones, its presence in the endocrine tissues of most vertebrate and some invertebrate species is not surprising. Progestin synthesis has been demonstrated in virtually all types of vertebrate steroidogenic tissues, e.g., ovaries, testes, adrenals, and placenta, and progesterone is produced by enzymatic conversion (3β-hydroxysteroid dehydrogenase-Δ^{4-5} isomerase system) from the precursor, pregnenolone (Fig. 1). Although the classic function ascribed to progesterone is pregnancy maintenance in mammals, progestins are now known to elicit many other biologic responses that are not necessarily related to the pregnancy state. Recent studies indicate that progesterone participates in the regulation of ovulation at neural and/or ovarian loci in amphibians, birds, and mammals. A dramatic central neural effect of progesterone is evidenced by its ability to induce sexual receptivity in the female of several mammalian species (Kow et al., 1974), and behavioral responses to progesterone have been observed in birds (Goldman and Zarrow, 1973).

Although progesterone is known to play a fundamental role in the regulation of female reproductive processes, the mechanism of progesterone action is poorly understood. Comprehensive studies with the chick oviduct system by O'Malley and co-workers have demonstrated the importance of specific progesterone receptors in the binding and transport (translocation) of receptor–hormone complex into active intranuclear sites (O'Malley and Means, 1974). Specific progesterone-binding components have been demonstrated in the mammalian uterus, but the intracellular function of these putative receptor molecules in the mechanism of progesterone action has not been elucidated.

Considerable evidence found elsewhere in this book is available to support the receptor hypothesis of steroid hormone action. According to this concept, the binding of steroid hormone by a specific cytoplasmic receptor protein initiates the intracellular translocation of hormone–receptor complex to responsive binding sites in the target cell nucleus (Baulieu et al., 1975). In the case of estrogen, hormone binding and translocation of the receptor–estradiol complex to acceptor sites in the nuclear chromatin occurs without significant metabolism of the estradiol molecule (Jensen and De Sombre, 1973). In contrast, androgens are actively metabolized within the target cell. For example, testosterone is rapidly converted by a 5α-reductase enzyme to the potent metabolite, 5α-dihydrotestosterone (DHT), which, in turn, interacts preferentially with an androgen receptor, i.e., the receptor has a higher binding affinity for DHT than for testosterone (Baulieu et al., 1975). The mechanism of progestin action remains to be

7. Biology of Progesterone Receptors

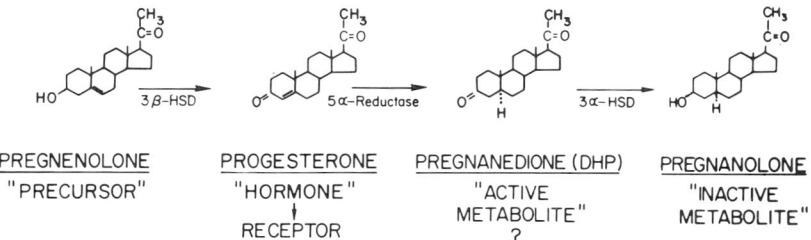

Fig. 1. Progesterone synthesis and metabolism. See text for details. HSD (3α and 3β) is hydroxysteroid dehydrogenase.

clarified. Following uptake by the target tissue, progesterone undergoes an extensive reductive metabolism, and a variety of metabolites are produced including 5α-pregnanedione (dihydroprogesterone, DHP) and 5α-pregnanolone (Fig. 1). Thus, in order to account for the mechanism of progestin action, several possibilities have to be considered. First, progestin action may be triggered by progesterone interaction with a receptor system specific for progesterone. Second, a progesterone metabolite, such as DHP, might be the active intracellular mediator of progestin action (Fig. 1). Third, the mechanism of progestin action might vary in different target cells so that certain cells respond to progesterone, while others are regulated by progesterone metabolite(s). In this chapter, pertinent new information will be reviewed on the regulation and function of progestin receptors in several target tissues, including the myometrium, endometrium, deciduoma, vagina, anterior pituitary gland, and hypothalamus.

II. PROGESTERONE ACTION IN THE HAMSTER

Although several laboratory species have been employed previously for the study of progesterone action, we and others have found the golden hamster to be an excellent model system. The female hamster exhibits an extremely regular 4-day estrous cycle, and ovarian functions during the cycle can be predicted with considerable accuracy (Bosley and Leavitt, 1972a; Fitzgerald and Zucker, 1976). Female sexual behavior, implantation, and pregnancy maintenance are clearly dependent on ovarian progesterone action in the hamster (Goldman and Zarrow, 1973; Harper *et al.,* 1969; Leavitt and Blaha, 1970). Furthermore, the predominant progestin present in the circulation is progesterone, as opposed to the significant levels of 20α-hydroxyprogesterone (20α-hydroxy-4-pregnen-3-one) which are found in the serum of the rat and rabbit (Leavitt *et al.,* 1973).

Several progesterone-dependent events are observable during the hamster estrous cycle. On cycle day 4, the ovulatory surge of gonadotropin is initiated by a neurogenic stimulus occurring between 1300 and 1400 hours in animals exposed to a regular photoperiod (lights on 0500–1900 hours) (Bosley and Leavitt, 1972a). The ovulatory surge of gonadotropin (primarily LH) stimulates ovarian interstitial and follicular elements to synthesize and secrete progesterone (Leavitt *et al.*, 1971). The gonadotropin surge triggers the ovulatory process in the Graafian follicles, and ovulation occurs predictably at 0100–0200 hours early on cycle day 1. The possibility exists for a direct action of preovulatory progesterone in the ovulatory process at the follicular level (Rondell, 1974). However, it is definitely established that preovulatory progesterone secretion stimulates (a) the release of uterine luminal fluid, and (b) the onset of sexual receptivity in the female as evidenced by the lordosis response which can be elicited by the male or by other procedures (Bosley and Leavitt, 1972a). Additionally, there is evidence suggesting that the feedback of preovulatory progesterone at the level of hypophysiotropic hypothalamic centers and/or the pituitary gland facilitates gonadotropin release during this interval of the cycle (Bosley and Leavitt, 1972b). These observations serve to emphasize the importance of preovulatory progesterone secretion in the regulation of the uterine, neuroendocrine, and behavioral responses that occur during the ovulatory phase of the hamster estrous cycle. The next major question to be considered is how progestin action is mediated in the different target tissues.

III. PROGESTERONE UPTAKE *IN VIVO*

Many factors affect the target organ response to any hormone; these include the biosynthesis, secretion, transport, uptake, and metabolism of the hormone. Furthermore, these factors have been found to vary considerably between species. In the case of progesterone, the metabolic clearance rate (MCR) ranges between 40 and 180 liters/day/kg in the different animals examined, and the major sites of clearance include liver, brain, and uterus (Herrmann *et al.*, 1973; Little *et al.*, 1975). By using the pulse technique, in which high specific activity [^{3}H]progesterone is injected into the animal, several workers have attempted to measure specific progestin uptake and retention by various organs according to their total radioactivity content. However, the extensive reductive metabolism of [^{3}H]progesterone by target and nontarget tissues has to be considered before this technique can be employed for this purpose, and specific [^{3}H]progesterone retention by target and nontarget tissues has been measured in just a few cases (Falk and Bardin, 1970; Leavitt and Blaha, 1972). In these latter studies, results were obtained supporting the existence of an estrogen-sensitive, progesterone-binding system in the uterus and vagina of the hamster and guinea pig.

Autoradiography has been applied to the study of [^{3}H]progesterone localization in various tissues of the guinea pig and rat (Stumpf and Sar, 1973; Sar and Stumpf, 1973, 1974; Warembourg, 1974). Although an intranuclear concentration of [^{3}H]"progestin" (either progesterone or metabolites) was found in target cells of oviduct, uterus, vagina, and perhaps brain, the chemical nature of the radioactive steroid associated with the nucleus has not been established. It is pertinent that estrogen priming of the animal enhanced the ability of target cells to localize [^{3}H]progestin in the nucleus (Sar and Stumpf, 1973, 1974), and these observations, coupled with those from previous autoradiographic studies of [^{3}H]estradiol localization (Stumpf, 1968, 1969), indicate that both estrogen and progestin are concentrated by the same cell types. Thus, it would appear that most estrogen target cells possess the ability to selectively bind progestin (W. E. Stumpf, personal communication), and estrogen action increases the progestin-binding capacity of the target cell.

IV. METHODS FOR STUDYING CYTOSOL PROGESTERONE RECEPTOR

Specific progesterone-binding components have been characterized in the uterine cytosol fraction of several mammalian species. The cytosol progesterone receptor in guinea pig uterus is a thermolabile protein which sediments at 6.7 S with a 4–5 S shoulder upon sucrose density gradient centrifugation (Milgrom *et al.*, 1970; Corvol *et al.*, 1972). In the presence of 0.3 M KCl, a lighter form is observed with a 4 S sedimentation coefficient. Binding of [^{3}H]progesterone is inhibited by the sulfhydryl blocking agent, *para*-hydroxymercuribenzoate, and it has a K_D in the order of 10^{-9} M. This [^{3}H]progesterone-binding component exhibits hormonal specificity in that competition is observed with unlabeled progesterone, but not with cortisol, estradiol, or testosterone.

Studies of rat uterine cytosol by Milgrom and Baulieu (1970) indicated the presence of a limited-capacity progesterone-binding component with sedimentation (4 S) and binding properties similar to those of corticosteroid-binding globulin (CBG). More recent evidence has indicated that rat uterine cytosol contains, in addition to the 4 S CBG-like protein, a specific progesterone-binding component with physicochemical properties that are different from those of CBG (Feil *et al.*, 1972). When 10% glycerol was incorporated into the buffer systems used to prepare cytosol, a specific binding component with a 6–7 S sedimentation coefficient was resolved in uterine cytosol from the estrogen-primed rat and mouse. Apparently, the progesterone receptor of rat and mouse uterus is extremely labile, and it can be easily modified or destroyed during preparation of cytosol. Thus, special precautions must be taken to preserve the cytosol progesterone receptor through the use of (a) buffer media containing glycerol (or other protein stabilizing agents) and (b) cold temperature (0–4°C). The same is true for the uterine progesterone receptors of other species as well. From the literature, there appear to be some variations in the kinetics of progesterone binding to the receptor protein in different species (Rao and Wiest, 1974). However, the physicochemical properties of progesterone receptors from different species appear to be quite similar.

In general, three techniques are adequate to determine whether a progesterone-binding protein has the physicochemical properties expected of a hormone receptor, i.e., high binding affinity, limited binding capacity, hormonal binding specificity, and target tissue specificity. The procedures are (a) sucrose–glycerol density gradient centrifugation (for sedimentation and general binding properties); (b) equilibrium binding assay (for binding affinity, K_A, and binding capacity); and (c) competitive binding assay (for steroid binding specificity). Recently, Clark et al. (1976) presented a comprehensive review of procedures used for the characterization and quantification of estrogen receptors, and additional information is contained in other sections of this book. Inasmuch as we have evaluated and modified several assay procedures in experiments done with the progesterone receptor of hamster, rat, mouse, and human, the following reagents and procedures are offered as the ones which have produced the most reliable and reproducible results in our experience.

A. Buffers

Buffer A contains 50 mM Tris–HCl (Schwarz/Mann, ultrapure) 1 mM EDTA, 12 mM monothioglycerol (Sigma), pH 7.5. Glycerol (Fisher reagent) is added to buffer A at either 10% (v/v) or 30% (v/v) concentration. Buffer B is 10 mM Tris–HCl, 1 mM EDTA, 12 mM monothioglycerol, pH 7.5. Buffer C contains 10 mM Tris–HCl, 1 mM EDTA, 20% glycerol (v/v), pH 7.5. Buffer D consists of 10 mM Tris–HCl, 1 mM EDTA, and 0.05% (w/v) dextran-70 (Pharmacia), pH 7.5. Saline (150 mM NaCl) is buffered with 10 mM Tris–HCl, pH 7.4.

B. Dextran-Coated Charcoal

Charcoal (Norit A, activated) is suspended (0.5%, w/v) in buffer D. The suspension is mixed and allowed to incubate in the cold (4°C) for 20–24

7. Biology of Progesterone Receptors

hours. The charcoal solution is used after it has been shown to be capable of removing more than 95% of [^{3}H]progesterone from buffer solution.

C. Cytosol and Serum Preparation

Trunk blood is collected at autopsy, chilled on ice, allowed to clot, and serum is obtained after centrifugation of the blood sample at 1000 g for 10 minutes at 4°C. Tissues are excised and chilled rapidly on saline-soaked filter paper at 4°C. Tissues are weighed, minced, rinsed with cold saline, and homogenized in 4 volumes of buffer A (v/w) at 2°C with a Polytron Pt-10 (Brinkman Instruments) using three 5-second bursts at rheostat setting 5. Cytosol is prepared by centrifugation of the homogenate in polyallomer tubes (Beckman) at 170,000 g for 1 hour at 2°C.

D. Sucrose–Glycerol Gradient Centrifugation

Linear sucrose gradients (5–20% sucrose in buffer B + 10% glycerol) are prepared in 5-ml polyallomer tubes using a Beckman gradient former. Cytosol (diluted 1:4, w/v, with buffer A + 10% glycerol) is incubated with a 250-fold excess (5.3 × 10^{-6} M) of unlabeled cortisol for 15 minutes at 4°C to saturate CBG-like components. Then [^{3}H]progesterone (2.1 × 10^{-8} M) is incubated with the cytosol for 1 hour, and the labeled cytosol is layered on the top of sucrose–glycerol gradients (0.2 ml/gradient). The gradients are centrifuged in a Spinco SW 50.1 rotor at 202,000 g for 18–20 hours at 2°C using a preparative ultracentrifuge. Gradients are fractionated from the bottom, and 15-drop fractions (20-21 fractions/gradient) are collected in the cold using an ISCO fractionator. To each fraction is added 0.5 ml buffer A + 30% glycerol (v/v), and free or loosely bound [^{3}H]progesterone is eliminated by treatment with 0.5 ml of dextran–charcoal solution in the cold (Fig. 2). The dextran–charcoal is removed by centrifugation in the cold for 3 minutes at 1000 g, and the supernatant containing bound [^{3}H]steroid is added to scintillation cocktail. The bound radioactivity is counted in a liquid scintillation spectrometer at 35% efficiency for ^{3}H. Sedimentation coefficients of the [^{3}H]progesterone-binding substances are estimated by the method of Martin and Ames (1961) using appropriate standards such as bovine serum albumin (BSA).

To evaluate tissue specificity, serum and cytosol from target and nontarget tissues are analyzed for specific progesterone-binding components. Density gradient centrifugation studies have revealed two distinct types of progesterone-binding substances. The progesterone binder (component 1) in cytosol from hamster vagina and uterus has a 6–7 sedimentation coefficient in low ionic strength medium, and it is thermolabile

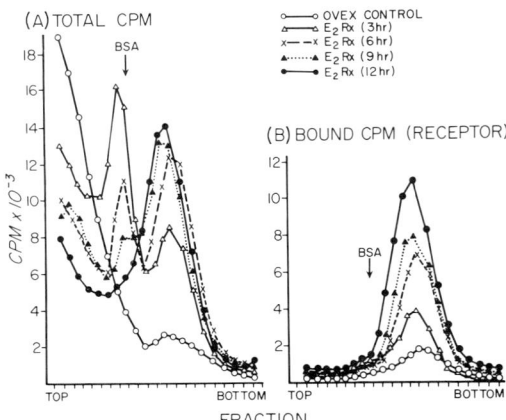

Fig. 2. Sucrose-glycerol gradient centrifugation of [^{3}H]progesterone-binding components in hamster uterine cytosol. Ovariectomized (OVEX) hamsters were treated with estradiol-17β (15 μg/animal, E_zRx) at time 0. Uterine cytosol was incubated with an excess of unlabeled cortisol prior to labeling with [^{3}H]progesterone. Two progesterone-binding components are apparent when the distribution of total radioactivity is plotted (panel A). However, when the gradient fractions were treated with dextran-charcoal solution to remove free or loosely bound hormone, a single binding component (receptor) with a 6-7 S sedimentation coefficient was resolved (panel B). Bovine serum albumin (BSA) was the standard (4.6 S).

and insensitive to cortisol competition. Another progesterone binder (component 2) is found in serum and cytosol derived from nontarget tissues. The properties of component 2 are similar to those of CBG, i.e., 4-5 S sedimentation coefficient, heat stable (37°C for 90 minutes), and sensitive to cortisol competition. Thus, receptor (component 1) is found to be restricted to the target tissues, while component 2 is not.

Although the progesterone receptor sediments at 6-7 S in sucrose-glycerol gradients prepared with low ionic strength medium, a smaller form (4-5 S) is observed following exposure to high salt conditions (0.3 M KCl). Presumably, the faster sedimenting form (6-7 S) of the receptor is a dimer of two smaller subunits (Schrader et al., 1975), and the subunits can be dissociated in a high salt environment. However, it should be noted that exposure of the mammalian progesterone receptor to 0.3 M KCl also causes a rapid degradation of the receptor molecules unless glycerol is used in the buffer media.

E. Scatchard Assay

Serum and cytosol fractions are diluted to a final concentration ranging between 1:10 and 1:20 (w/v) using buffer A + 30% glycerol. Aliquots

(0.3 ml) of the diluted serum or cytosol are incubated for 16-18 hours with varying amounts of [^{3}H]progesterone (final concentration range = 0.8 nM– 12 nM) in the presence (competed) or absence (noncompeted) of unlabeled progesterone (final concentration = 4×10^{-6} M). The binding data from noncompeted tubes (total binding) minus that from the competed tubes (nonspecific binding) provide the measure of specific binding.

Following incubation at 2°C, the samples are treated in the cold with 0.5 ml of dextran–charcoal solution for 30–45 seconds. Then the samples are centrifuged for 3 minutes at 800 g. The supernatant fractions containing the bound ^{3}H-steroid are decanted into counting vials, and the radioactivity is measured by liquid scintillation counting procedures. Specific binding data are analyzed according to Scatchard (1949). The relationship between the bound to free ratio (B/F) and the concentration (nanomolar) of specifically bound hormone is subjected to linear regression analysis, providing a correlation coefficient (linearity), slope (equilibrium association constant, K_A), and the concentration of specific binding sites (pmole/ml incubation mixture) from the intercept on the abscissa.

Scatchard plot analysis of [^{3}H]progesterone binding data has been used by many investigators to measure the progesterone-binding capacity of cytosol. According to Milgrom et al. (1972a), this technique is valid even in the presence of endogenous progesterone, provided that the time of incubation is long enough to permit exchange between endogenous unlabeled hormone and exogenous [^{3}H]progesterone. Leavitt et al. (1974) showed with hamster uterine progesterone receptor that (a) an equilibrium between exogenous [^{3}H]progesterone and endogenous unlabeled progesterone for receptor sites was reached within 16–18 hours of incubation at 2°C; (b) the receptor remained stable in glycerol-containing medium for the 16–18 hour incubation period; and (c) [^{3}H]progesterone would exchange with unlabeled bound hormone in uterine cytosol. Thus, Milgrom et al. (1972a) and Leavitt et al. (1974) could estimate the total (occupied plus unoccupied) receptor sites in uterine cytosol using these assay conditions. However, the validity of the Scatchard assay for the measurement of total receptor in other tissues was not known. Therefore, the Scatchard assay system has been tested with respect to the influence of unlabeled progesterone addition on the estimation of vaginal receptor levels. Vaginal and uterine cytosol (diluted 1:16, w/v, with buffer A + 10% glycerol) from proestrous hamsters was incubated for 90 minutes in the presence (final concentrations = 5nM and 15nM) and absence of unlabeled progesterone. Then aliquots of the progesterone-pretreated cytosols were assayed for receptor in the usual manner. Increasing the concentration of unlabeled progesterone reduced the slope of the Scatchard plot relationship for the cytosol fractions of both tissues (Fig. 3). However, there was no significant effect on the extrapolated

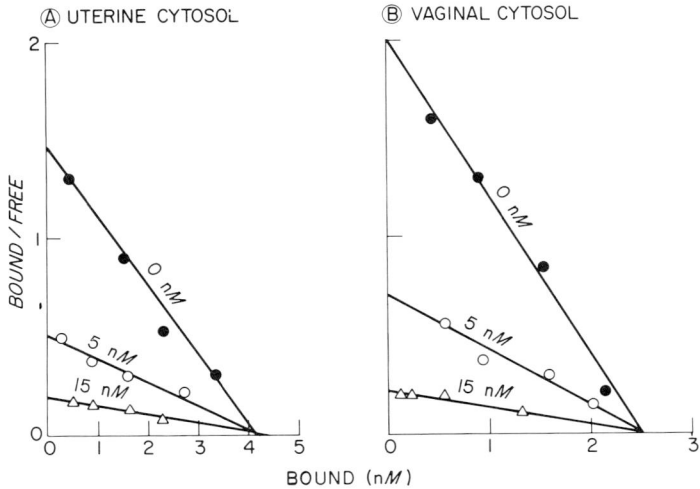

Fig. 3. Scatchard assay of specific [^{3}H]progesterone binding data from uterine (A) and vaginal (B) cytosols derived from the proestrous hamster. Cytosols were preincubated for 90 minutes with a final concentration of 0 nM (●———●), 5 nM (○———○), or 15 nM (△———△) unlabeled progesterone. The specific binding of [^{3}H]progesterone was determined by the dextran–charcoal technique. The number of binding sites relative to tissue weight is indicated by the intercept on the abscissa. Unlabeled progesterone decreased the slope of the Scatchard relationship, but did not change the intercept on the abscissa. Therefore, the assay is capable of measuring total receptor (occupied plus unoccupied).

value of receptor concentration (X intercept). Therefore, the accumulation of physiological (nanomolar) levels of endogenous progesterone in the cytosol fraction of vagina or uterus would produce a similar result. Such an effect would be evident from a change (decrease) in the slope of the Scatchard plot of specific [^{3}H]progesterone-binding data.

Cytosol derived from uterus and vagina contains a high-affinity ($K_A = 1 \times 10^9\ M^{-1}$), limited-capacity progesterone binder (component 1), whereas cytosol from liver and kidney has a binding macromolecule (component 2) with a lower affinity ($K_A = 3 \times 10^7\ M^{-1}$) for progesterone. Cytosol fractions from heart, duodenum, and spleen have no detectable amounts of either of the progesterone binding components using this method (Allen and Leavitt, 1975). In some cases, particularly with the pregnant or pseudopregnant animal, component 2 levels are high enough in the cytosol fraction so as to interfere with component 1 (receptor) measurement. For example, in the pseudopregnant, decidualized hamster, the Scatchard plot of total specific [^{3}H]progesterone-binding data from deciduomal and myometrial cytosol exhibits a curvilinear relationship (Fig. 4). Since the CBG-like protein (component 2) can influence the estimation of receptor capacity using total specific binding data, a method was developed and validated for the separate measurement of each binding component in cytosol (Do et al., 1976). The methodology is based on the observed differences in the physicochemical properties of components 1 and 2. Progesterone receptor has a low affinity and the CBG-like protein a high affinity for cortisol (Table I). Thus, receptor capacity can be measured in cytosol after component 2 is saturated by preincubation with an excess amount of nonradioactive cortisol for 1 hour at 4°C (Fig. 4). Since the receptor is thermolabile and component 2 is heat stable, component 2 can be determined after the receptor is inactivated by incubating the cytosol at 37°C for 60–90 minutes (Fig. 4).

When the amount of target tissue is limited, e.g., in the fetal or neonatal animal, a modification of the Scatchard assay can be used (Carlton and Leavitt, 1977). In this assay, the concentration of [^{3}H]progesterone (0.4 nM) is held constant, and the cytosol concentration is varied. Cytosol is diluted serially with buffer A + 30% glycerol as follows: 1/12, 1/24, 1/48, 1/96 (w/v). In one series of tubes, [^{3}H]progesterone is used to measure total binding. Another set of tubes contains [^{3}H]progesterone plus a 250-fold M excess of unlabeled progesterone for the determination of nonspecific binding. After incubation in the cold for 18 hours, samples are treated with dextran–charcoal solution, and bound hormone is measured as before. The

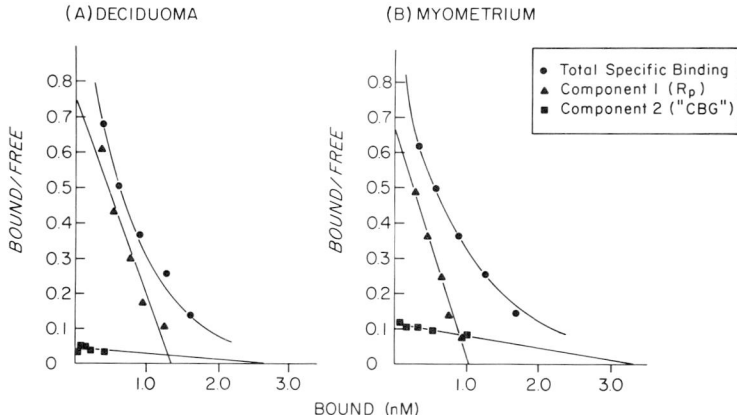

Fig. 4. Scatchard assay of progesterone-binding components in deciduomal (A) and myometrial (B) cytosol from the decidualized, pseudopregnant hamster. Total specific binding data exhibit a curvilinear relationship (●———●). Component 1 (receptor, Rp) was measured in cytosol after treatment with excess unlabeled cortisol (▲———▲). Component 2 (CBG-like protein) was determined using cytosol that was incubated at 37°C for 90 minutes to destroy receptor (■———■).

difference between total and nonspecific binding is the measure of specific [^{3}H]progesterone binding. The estimation of progesterone receptor levels with this method (dilution assay) can be validated by correlation with results obtained using the Scatchard assay (Carlton and Leavitt, 1977).

F. Competition Assay

The hormonal binding specificity of the progesterone binding components in cytosol is evaluated by competitive binding assay (Leavitt et al., 1974). Cortisol-competed cytosol can be used to determine the hormonal binding specificity of receptor, and cytosol that has been preincubated at 37°C for 90 minutes can be used to evaluate the binding specificity of CBG-like proteins. Cytosol fractions are diluted at about 1/12 (w/v) with buffer C. A 0.3-ml aliquot of diluted serum or cytosol is incubated with 0.1 ml of [^{3}H]progesterone in buffer C (final concentration = 5×10^{-9} M), and different concentrations (4×10^{-10} M to 4×10^{-6} M) of unlabeled steroid competitor are added in 0.1 ml of buffer C. After incubation for 16–18 hours at 4°C, bound and free [^{3}H]progesterone are separated by the dextran–charcoal absorption method. The relative binding affinity (RBA) of each steroid is determined at the 50% competition level. The RBA of progesterone is arbitrarily set at 100. The binding specificity of progesterone receptor (component 1) as compared to CBG-like protein (component 2) is shown in Table I.

TABLE I

Relative Binding Affinity of Progesterone-Binding Components in Deciduoma, Myometrium, and Serum of the Pseudopregnant, Decidualized Hamster

	Component 1[a]		Component 2[b]		
	Deciduoma	Myometrium	Deciduoma	Myometrium	Serum
Progesterone	100[c]	100	100	100	100
Deoxycorticosterone	20	20	160	160	130
5α-Pregnanedione (DHP)	40	40	11	23	16
Testosterone	3	3	200	200	200
Estradiol-17β	< 1	< 1	< 1	< 1	< 1
Cortisol	< 1	< 1	500	500	300

[a] Progesterone receptor; cytosol preincubated with an excess amount of unlabeled cortisol before assay.

[b] CBG-like substance; cytosol preincubated at 37°C for 90 minutes before assay.

[c] The relative binding affinity (RBA) of each steroid was determined as described in the text.

V. PROGESTERONE RECEPTOR DISTRIBUTION IN DIFFERENT TISSUES

A. Endometrium and Myometrium

Some variations have been observed in the progesterone receptors of different species (Smith *et al.*, 1974; Kontula *et al.*, 1975), but it is still not certain whether progesterone receptors vary in the different target cell types within the same animal. Distinct progesterone-binding components have been described in endometrium and myometrium (Davies and Ryan, 1973; Rao and Wiest, 1974), suggesting that these compartments might contain receptors with dissimilar properties. When this possibility was examined, comparing endometrium and myometrium in the hamster, guinea pig, and sheep (Grossman and Leavitt, 1974; Luu Thi *et al.*, 1975; Kontula, 1975), the physicochemical properties of endometrial and myometrial receptors in these species appeared to be identical, e.g., the hamster receptors had the same sedimentation coefficient (6–7 S), binding affinity ($K_A = 1 \times 10^9$ M^{-1}) and ligand specificity (progesterone > deoxycorticosterone > DHP > testosterone > estradiol > cortisol) (Grossman and Leavitt, 1974). Although the binding and sedimentation properties of the myometrial and endometrial receptors seem to be the same on the basis of the limited data now available, important undetermined differences may exist either in the chemical composition, e.g., amino acid sequence, or physical structure of the receptors in the different target cell types. Additional biochemical studies with purified receptors are needed to resolve this point (Kuhn *et al.*, 1975; Smith *et al.*, 1975).

B. Deciduoma

During deciduomal development, ovarian steroid hormones act to stimulate the hyperplasia, hypertrophy, and differentiation of the endometrial stromal cells and the resultant deciduomal cells (Psychoyos, 1973; Finn and Martin, 1974). Biochemical analysis of the rat uterus has documented an increase in DNA, RNA, and protein content during decidualization (Glasser and Clark, 1975; Yochim, 1975). Evidence from studies performed with the rat (Glasser and Clark, 1975) and hamster (Harper, 1970) demonstrated that deciduomal growth and maintenance is primarily dependent upon progesterone action, and the deciduomal response has served as a classic endpoint of progesterone action in the uterus (Astwood, 1939; Miyake *et al.*, 1963).

Information is lacking on the nature of the progesterone receptor system in the deciduoma. Efforts to delineate the role of progesterone in rat deciduomal formation through measurement of endogenous uterine progesterone levels have provided indirect evidence for the possible existence of a progestin-binding system in decidualized uterine tissue (Rao and Wiest, 1974). A progesterone-binding macromolecule with properties similar to CBG has been described in the uterine cytosol from the decidualized rat and rabbit (Reel *et al.,* 1971), but it remains to be determined whether this substance is a specific progesterone receptor. Two progesterone-binding components have been identified in the cytosol fraction of hamster deciduomal tissue (Leavitt and Reuss, 1975; Do *et al.,* 1976). Density gradient centrifugation studies performed with deciduomal and myometrial cytosol revealed that component 1 had a 6–7 S sedimentation coefficient, was heat labile (37°C, 90 minutes), and insensitive to cortisol competition. Component 2 had a 4–5 S sedimentation coefficient, was heat stable, and sensitive to cortisol competition. Serum contained a progesterone binder with properties similar to component 2. Competitive binding studies demonstrated that component 1 possessed hormonal binding specificity (progesterone > DHP > deoxycorticosterone > testosterone > estradiol > cortisol), and the binding specificity of component 2 was similar to that of serum CBG (Table I). Neither one of these components bound [^{3}H]dexamethasone, but a [^{3}H]dexamethasone binder with a 7–8 S sedimentation coefficient was identified as a presumptive glucocorticoid receptor. Thus, the physicochemical properties of component 1 were consistent with those expected of a progesterone receptor, and those of component 2 were similar to serum CBG (Do *et al.,* 1976). Component 1 was measured using cytosol preincubated with an excess of unlabeled cortisol, while component 2 was determined after preincubation of cytosol at 37°C for 90 minutes. Component 1 had a high binding affinity for progesterone ($K_A = 1 \times 10^9$ M^{-1}) with a concentration of 38.6 ± 8.4 pmole/g deciduomal tissue and 29.1 ± 6.5 pmole/g myometrial tissue. Component 2 exhibited a lower binding affinity for progesterone ($K_A = 3 \times 10^7$ M^{-1}). Treatment of the pseudopregnant, decidualized hamster with progesterone for 2 hours prior to sacrifice caused a significant depletion of component 1 from the cytosol fraction in both uterine compartments, but no response of component 2 was observed. Similar treatment with cortisol for 2 hours had no effect on component 1, but component 2 levels decreased significantly. Estrogen treatment initiated 24 hours before autopsy increased component 1 levels. These results demonstrate the existence of an estrogen-inducible progesterone receptor (component 1) in the cytosol fraction of deciduomal tissue in the pseudopregnant hamster (Do *et al.,* 1976). The source and functional significance of component 2 remains to be determined. However, these and other results (Do and Leavitt, unpublished) support the idea that component 2 is CBG distributed primarily in the extracellular space (Fig.

7. Biology of Progesterone Receptors

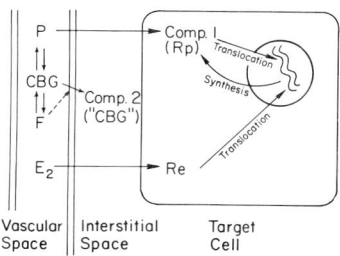

Fig. 5. Proposed distribution of progesterone-binding components in the decidualized hamster uterus. Serum corticosteroid-binding globulin (CBG) binds cortisol (F) and progesterone (P), and component 2 is proposed to be CBG which is extravasated into the interstitial space. Cortisol (F) decreases vascular permeability and, thus, prevents CBG entry into the interstitial space. Component 1 is progesterone receptor (Rp), and the interaction of progesterone (P) with Rp causes the translocation of hormone–receptor complex to active intranuclear sites. Estrogen (E_2) interaction with estrogen receptor (Re) induces translocation of $E_2 \cdot Re$ complex to the nucleus, and this triggers the events which stimulate Rp synthesis.

5). The extravasation of CBG may be regulated by factors such as estrogen and corticosteroid, which are known to affect capillary permeability (Bell, 1974; Szego, 1974).

C. Vagina

In the few studies done on the identification and characterization of specific progesterone-binding components in the vagina, a specific progesterone binder, similar to the uterine progesterone receptor, was identified in vaginal cytosol from the guinea pig and hamster (Atger *et al.*, 1974; Allen and Leavitt, 1975; Leavitt *et al.*, 1977). The vaginal receptor has a high binding affinity for progesterone (Fig. 3), a 6–7 S sedimentation coefficient in low ionic strength medium, and it exhibits hormonal binding specificity. The concentration of progesterone receptor is lower in the vagina than in the uterus, and estrogen action increases the receptor capacity of both organs (Atger *et al.*, 1974; Leavitt *et al.*, 1977). Thus, although uterus and vagina develop from different embryonic sources (Müllerian ducts and sinus epithelium, respectively), the progesterone receptor molecules present in these organs are remarkably similar. This would support the hypothesis that different target cell types contain identical receptor molecules.

D. Pituitary and Hypothalamus

The mechanism of progesterone action in the brain and anterior pituitary gland remains to be clarified. Although previous studies did not detect a cytosol progesterone receptor in these target tissues (Atger *et al.,* 1974; Reel and Shih, 1975), we have been able to identify a putative progesterone receptor in hamster pituitary and hypothalamus (Leavitt *et al.,* 1977). When the cytosol fraction of anterior pituitary tissue from ovariectomized hamsters was subjected to sucrose–glycerol gradient centrifugation, a specific progesterone-binding component with a 6–7 S sedimentation coefficient was resolved (Fig. 6). However, a 6–7 S receptor was not detected in hypothalamic cytosol from the ovariectomized animal by this method (Fig. 6). In the estrogen-primed hamster, pituitary cytosol contained a greater quantity of receptor, and a similar substance was observed in hypothalamic cytosol (Fig. 6). Labeling of pituitary cytosol with equimolar amounts of [^{3}H]progesterone or [^{3}H]DHP established that the pituitary receptor had a higher binding affinity for progesterone than for DHP. These results establish the existence of an estrogen-inducible progesterone binder in the pituitary and hypothalamus, and this putative receptor has sedimentation and binding properties similar to those determined previously for hamster uterine and vaginal receptor (Leavitt *et al.,* 1974; Allen and Leavitt, 1975).

Preliminary density gradient studies with rat pituitary cytosol have verified the existence of a specific progesterone receptor with a 6–7 S sedimentation coefficient (Evans *et al.,* 1977). However, the rat pituitary recep-

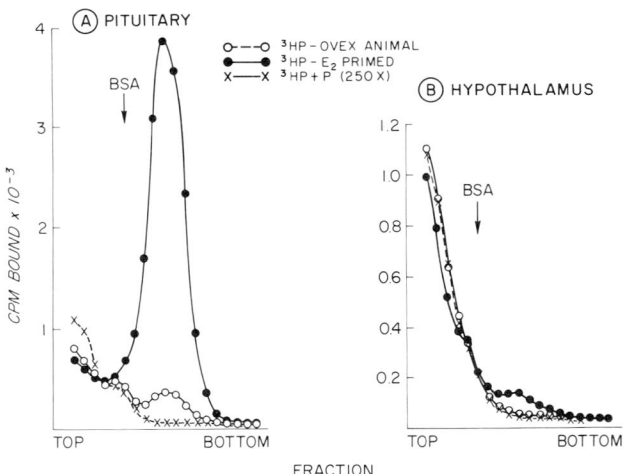

Fig. 6. Sucrose–glycerol gradient centrifugation of pituitary (A) and hypothalamic (B) cytosol. Cytosol was labeled with [^{3}H]progesterone (^{3}HP) or ^{3}HP plus a 250-fold excess of unlabeled progesterone (P) (X----X). A progesterone receptor with a 6–7 S sedimentation coefficient was evident in the pituitary, but not the hypothalamus, of the ovariectomized (OVEX) hamster. Estrogen (E$_2$) priming caused receptor to increase in both pituitary and hypothalamic cytosols (●———●).

tor is more easily demonstrated with [^{3}H]R5020 ([6,7-^{3}H]17,21-dimethyl-19-norpregna-4,9-diene-3,20-dione) than with [^{3}H]progesterone, and this is consistent with previous results with [^{3}H]R5020 as applied to the uterine progesterone receptor of the rat and mouse (Philibert and Raynaud, 1973). Since the rat adrenal is a significant source of progesterone, particularly in the stressed state (Feder and Ruf, 1969; Resko, 1969), caution should be exercised in the handling of rats prior to autopsy because both uterine and pituitary progesterone receptor levels in cytosol can be reduced significantly in response to stress-induced adrenal progesterone release (Evans *et al.*, 1977).

E. Mammary Gland

Small amounts of progesterone receptor may exist in normal breast tissue (Atger *et al.*, 1974). However, the evidence to date is equivocal at best, and additional studies are required to resolve this point. Specific progesterone receptors have been detected in mammary tumor tissue from the mouse and human (Horwitz and McGuire, 1975; Sluyser *et al.*, 1976), and the presence of progesterone receptor in breast tumors is of value in identifying those patients who will show objective remissions of breast tumors in response to endocrine therapy (Horwitz *et al.*, 1975a). Interesting studies with a human breast cancer cell line (MCF-7) have demonstrated the existence of progesterone receptor as well as estrogen, androgen, and glucocorticoid receptors in these cells (Horwitz *et al.*, 1975b). This is the first demonstration of four different steroid-hormone receptors in the same cell type, and the MCF-7 cell line may be useful as a model system for studies of receptor regulation and steroid interactions with different receptor systems.

VI. REGULATION OF PROGESTERONE RECEPTOR LEVELS

A. Estrous Cycle

Studies performed with the guinea pig, rat, and mouse demonstrated that there were significant fluctuations in the concentration of progesterone receptor in uterine cytosol during the female reproductive cycle (Feil *et al.*, 1972; Milgrom *et al.*, 1972b). During the hamster estrous cycle, we established that the variations in uterine progesterone receptor levels were correlated with the pattern of estrogen and progesterone secretion (Leavitt *et al.*, 1974). The cellular concentration of receptor increased during diestrus (day 3) to a maximum at proestrus on day 4 coincident with a ris-

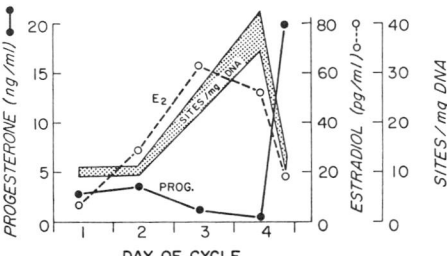

Fig. 7. Cellular concentration of progesterone receptor sites during the hamster estrous cycle. Receptor sites were measured in uterine cytosol by Scatchard assay. Serum estradiol (E_2) was determined by radioimmunoassay and serum progesterone (PROG.) by competitive protein-binding assay. Modified from Leavitt et al. (1974).

ing serum estradiol level (Fig. 7). The uterine receptor concentration decreased slowly following ovariectomy at proestrus, and the level was rapidly restored by estrogen treatment suggesting that the increased number of receptor sites during the cycle was caused by estrogen action. The formation of progesterone receptor with a 6–7 S sedimentation coefficient occurred during the follicular phase of the cycle and also following estrogen treatment of the ovariectomized hamster (Leavitt et al., 1974). These results supported the hypothesis that estrogen action during the cycle promoted formation of progesterone receptor.

The cellular concentration of uterine progesterone receptor dropped markedly between proestrus (AM) and estrus (PM) on day 4 of the hamster cycle during the time of preovulatory progesterone secretion (Fig. 7). The abrupt depletion of receptor from the cytosol fraction at estrus could be attributed to ovarian progesterone action because (a) it was prevented by ovariectomy at proestrus, and (b) progesterone treatment given early on day 4 caused a rapid premature depletion of receptor from the cytosol fraction (Leavitt et al., 1974). Thus, it was possible to demonstrate with the cyclic hamster that the variations of progesterone receptor levels observed in uterine cytosol are a result of the cyclic pattern of estrogen and progestin secretion.

Acute ovariectomy experiments were carried out to determine the role of ovarian and adrenal function in the regulation of uterine receptor levels during the hamster cycle. Ovariectomy performed on either cycle day 1, 2, or 3 reduced receptor levels in all cases on the morning of day 4, and the decrement in receptor titer was greater with increasing time of ovariectomy. This experiment established that the ovaries and not the adrenals were responsible for stimulating the uterine progesterone-binding capacity during the hamster cycle. However, it was not clear when, during the cycle, the ovaries exerted this effect on the receptor system. This information was provided by a second experiment in which hamsters were ovariectomized on cycle day 1 and autopsied on either day 2, 3, or 4. By comparing the uterine receptor titer in ovariectomized animals and sham controls on each successive day of the cycle, it was determined that ovarian stimulation of the uterine receptor capacity occurred between cycle days 2 and 4, and this corresponded to the time of increased estradiol secretion (Fig. 7). Thus, the quantity of uterine progesterone receptor increased during the follicular phase of the female cycle in response to increased ovarian estrogen secretion, while the depletion of cytosol receptor during the ovulatory phase of the cycle can be ascribed to progesterone uptake and action in the target cell.

If the uterine receptor functions in a manner similar to that of other steroid hormone receptors, then it would be expected that progesterone binding to the cytosol receptor would cause translocation of receptor–hormone complex to active intracellular sites.

B. Pregnancy

Studies with the rat and rabbit have established that pregnancy maintenance is correlated with the uterine progesterone level (Csapo and Wiest, 1969; Challis *et al.*, 1974). Experiments with the pregnant rat have established that progesterone levels above 20 μg/g uterine tissue are commensurate with pregnancy maintenance, and levels below 13 μg progesterone/g tissue are associated with increased myometrial activity and delivery (Csapo and Wiest, 1969). Although many factors are known to be involved in the regulation of gestation and parturition, the experimental evidence from the rat and rabbit serves to document the fact that a relationship exists between the uterine progesterone concentration and the continuation of gestation.

Progesterone-binding components have been measured in myometrial cytosol during pregnancy in the rat and rabbit (Davies and Ryan, 1973; Davies *et al.*, 1974). In the pregnant rat, myometrial progesterone-binding sites increased from days 3 to 9, and then the concentration of binding sites decreased to a low value on day 15, and low levels were observed until term (day 22). In the pregnant rabbit, the concentration of progesterone-binding sites in myometrial cytosol was stable from days 3 to 15, decreased somewhat on days 15–24, and then increased on days 27–30 before term (day 31). In both species during the first two-thirds of pregnancy, the myometrial cytosol had a progesterone-binding site concentration that exceeded the plasma progesterone concentration (Davies and Ryan, 1973; Davies *et al.*, 1974). This may account for the ability of the myometrium to maintain a higher concentration of progesterone than is present in the plasma. During the last third of pregnancy, the titer of progesterone binder in myometrial cytosol fell below plasma progesterone levels, and the tissue progesterone concentration remained similar to that of plasma.

Specific progesterone-binding components have been studied in the pregnant hamster (Leavitt and Reuss, 1975). Myometrium, endometrium, and implantation sites were demonstrated to contain a specific progesterone-binding component which had properties consistent with those of the uterine receptor previously characterized (Leavitt et al., 1974). Placental tissue, fetuses, and serum did not contain detectable levels of receptor. In myometrial cytosol, the receptor level decreased gradually from days 2 to 10 and remained low until term (day 16). A significant amount of CBG-like binder (component 2) was detected near term (days 13-15) in myometrial cytosol, and this was thought to reflect the high serum CBG titers which were present during late pregnancy (see Fig. 5).

Additional studies are necessary to distinguish between myometrial progesterone receptor and CBG-like protein before the actual relationship between cytosol receptor and serum progesterone levels can be established. Also, it will be important to measure nuclear progesterone receptor levels to determine whether they vary during gestation. At the present time, there is no information available on nuclear receptor levels during pregnancy, and the development of methods for measuring nuclear progesterone receptor will permit studies on this point.

C. Estrogen Action

It is now well established that estrogen priming of the immature or ovariectomized animal augments progesterone receptor titers in the target cell, and estrogen induction of progesterone receptor formation would seem to provide a basis for the priming effect of estrogen in the preparation of target tissues for subsequent progestational response (Leavitt et al., 1977). The temporal pattern of uterine progesterone receptor production during estrogen stimulation has been determined (Toft and O'Malley, 1972; Milgrom et al., 1973; Leavitt et al., 1974; Freifeld et al., 1974), and estrogen action causes a rapid production of receptor which is evident within 3-6 hours (Fig. 2). After several days of estrogen treatment, the progesterone-receptor capacity of uterine cytosol is increased severalfold on a tissue weight, DNA, or cytosol protein basis (Fig. 8). Thus, the estrogen-mediated augmentation of the uterine receptor capacity can be attributed in part to an increased cellular concentration of receptor. In addition, estrogen stimulates target cell proliferation, and the uterine progesterone receptor response appears to result from addition of intracellular receptors plus new cells containing receptor.

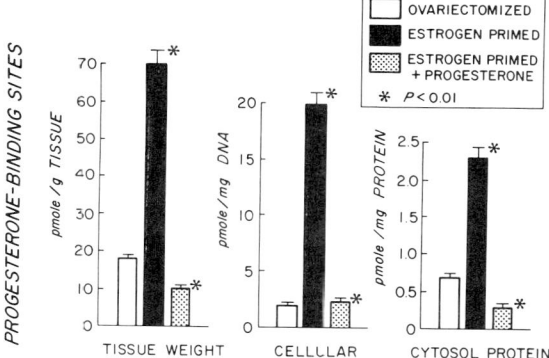

Fig. 8. The concentration of progesterone-binding sites (receptor) in uterine cytosol from ovariectomized hamsters as influenced by priming with estradiol-17β (15 μg/day) for 3 days or by progesterone treatment (2 mg) of the estrogen-primed hamster for 2 hours. Each bar represents the mean ± SEM for four determinations. Significant differences ($P < 0.01$) were observed between the ovariectomized and estrogen-primed groups, and the estrogen-primed and estrogen-primed plus progesterone-treated groups.

The responsiveness of uterus and vagina have been evaluated in terms of estradiol-induced progesterone receptor formation (Leavitt et al., 1977). Ovariectomized hamsters were primed with different doses of estradiol (0.1, 1, 10, or 100 μg per animal per day) or oil vehicle (control) for 3 days. In the control preparation, measurable amounts of receptor were present in uterine and vaginal cytosol. The control receptor level is referred to as estrogen independent because it is maintained in the absence of ovarian estrogen (Leavitt et al., 1974). The concentration of estrogen-independent receptor in uterus (32 pmole/g tissue) was four times greater than the vaginal level (8 pmole/g tissue).

A significant increase in receptor concentration was obtained with 0.1 μg estradiol/day in both uterus and vagina, and maximal stimulation of estrogen-dependent receptor was achieved with the 1 μg dose in both organs. However, the magnitude of the uterine response was four-fold greater than the vaginal response. These results suggested that the amplitude of the estrogen-induced progesterone receptor response was related to the estrogen-independent receptor level. Additional support for this idea was provided by the dose-response relationship observed for uterine and vaginal progesterone receptor content. In the control, uterine receptor content was higher than vaginal receptor content, and estrogen treatment was more effective in raising the uterine receptor level. However, the uterine receptor content relative to that of the vagina remained constant. When estrogen-induced receptor levels were expressed relative to control values (estrogen-independent receptor content), no difference was observed between the relative responses of uterus and vagina. These results indicate that uterus and vagina are equally sensitive to estrogen action, but the uterus has a great capacity to produce progesterone receptor in response to a given dose of estrogen. On the basis of this evidence, the following hypothesis was proposed. Estrogen-independent progesterone receptor (RpI) resides in estrogen target cells, and the RpI concentration is a function of the relative concentration of estrogen target cells. Each target cell has approximately the same sensitivity to estrogen action, and a similar number of estrogen-dependent receptor (RpD) molecules are produced per cell in response to estrogen action. According to this hypothesis, the amount of RpD formation would depend primarily on the number of estrogen target cells present in each target tissue. The relative concentration of estrogen target cells in uterus and vagina, as estimated by the estrogen receptor concentration in tissue obtained from ovariectomized animals, verified that uterus had a higher concentration of estrogen target cells (Leavitt et al., 1977).

The previous results suggested an involvement of the estrogen receptor system in the induction of progesterone receptor, but additional evidence was needed to establish this concept. Such evidence was provided by showing that a correlation existed between receptor binding and biologic activity. Different estrogens and "antiestrogens" (weak agonists) were tested for the ability to promote formation of uterine progesterone receptor in the ovariectomized hamster, and the relative binding affinity of each compound for uterine estrogen receptor was measured by a competitive binding assay (Leavitt et al., 1977).

Hamster uterine estrogen receptor had the highest affinity (RBA) for estradiol (100) followed by diethylstilbestrol (DES) (50), estrone (24), estriol (10), CI-628 (2), *cis*-clomiphene (1), nafoxidine (0.2), TACE (0.1), *trans*-clomiphene (0.08), and MER-25 (0.01). All compounds, except MER-25, stimulated progesterone receptor production and uterine weight gain. Comparison of the relative uterotropic and progesterone receptor responses for steroidal estrogens revealed that the relative progesterone receptor response was greater than relative uterotropic response in all cases. Similar findings were obtained with the antiestrogens. Thus, the progesterone receptor response is a more sensitive end point of estrogen action than is the uterine weight response. With the antiestrogens, it was possible to show that a progesterone receptor response could be obtained with doses below the amount needed to significantly increase uterine weight. *trans*-Clomiphene produced full uterotrophic and progesterone receptor responses. In contrast, *cis*-clomiphene, nafoxidine, and CI-628 produced incomplete uterine weight responses, and the progesterone receptor response was correspondingly less than that produced by the steroidal estrogens.

Correlation of binding and biologic activity data demonstrated that there was good agreement between the binding affinity for estrogen receptor and biologic activity (uterotropic and progesterone receptor responses) particularly in the case of estradiol, DES, estrone, cisclomiphene, and nafoxidine (Fig. 9). With estriol and CI-628, the binding affinity for estrogen receptor exceeded biologic activity, and binding activity was lower than biologic activity with transclomiphene and TACE. These discrepancies may be accounted for by various factors, such as drug metabolism, half-life in the circulation, and nuclear estrogen receptor retention, and additional studies are required to explain the deviations observed.

These results (a) established that a variety of estrogenic compounds can stimulate progesterone receptor production, and (b) provided evidence for the participation of the estrogen receptor system in the induction of progesterone receptor. Several antiestrogens were found to stimulate uterine progesterone receptor formation, indicating that these compounds are weak estrogens which possess the ability to increase the target cell responsiveness to progestin action. As is shown in Fig. 10, estrogen receptor replenishment and progesterone receptor synthesis are different end points of the estrogenic response. The antiestrogens are weak or incomplete agonists (estrogens) which act by the estrogen receptor system to increase progesterone receptor formation. Since these agents do not stimulate estrogen receptor replenishment to the same extent as do more potent estrogens, such as estradiol (Clark *et al.*, 1973, 1974), it is proposed that antiestrogens preferentially increase progesterone receptor titers in the target cell. This would render the target cell more responsive to progestin action. Progesterone has been shown to inhibit estrogen receptor replenishment (Hseuh *et al.*, 1976). Therefore, exposure of the antiestrogen-primed target cell to progestin derived from either ovarian or adrenal sources would be expected to reduce estrogen receptor levels and blunt the target cell response to estrogen action. These results suggest that regulation of progesterone receptor levels could be an important part of antiestrogen action in the target cell, and this hypothesis should be tested in future experiments done with these agents.

D. Progesterone Action

The participation of uterine progesterone receptor in the mechanism of progestin action is suggested by the rapid depletion response that is observed following progesterone administration *in vivo* (Milgrom *et al.*,

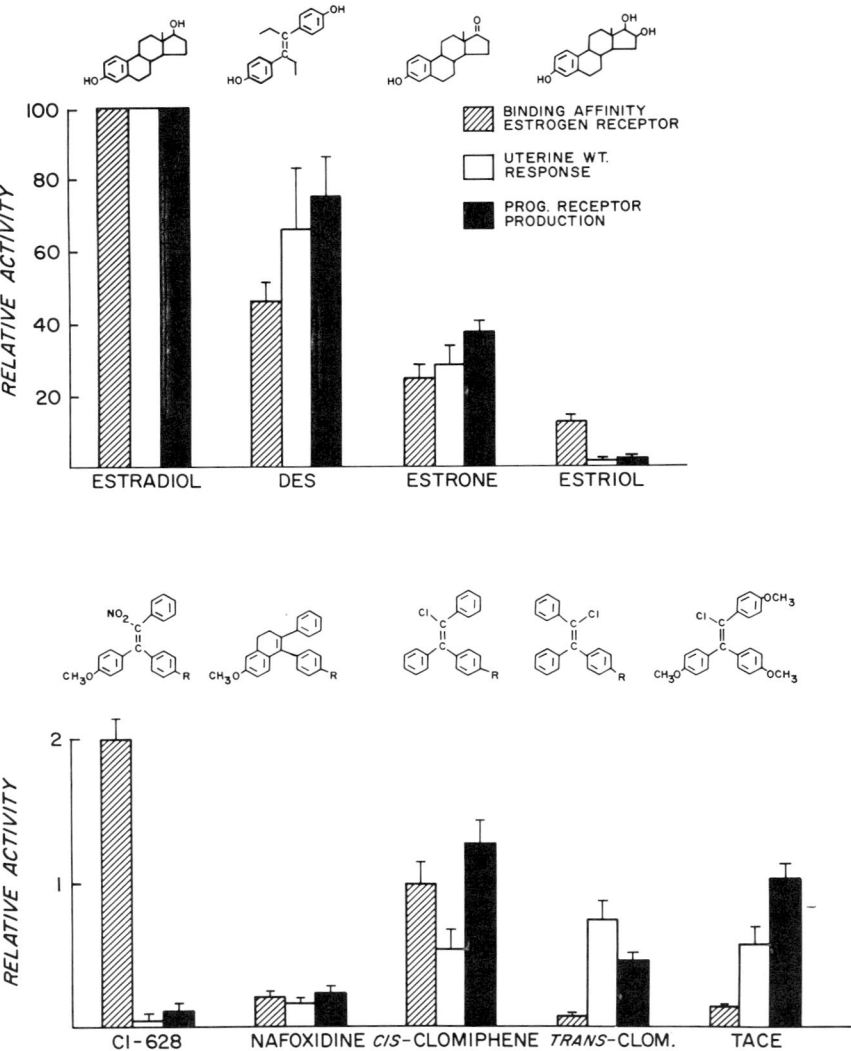

Fig. 9. Correlation between binding affinity for estrogen receptor and biologic activity. The binding and biologic activities are expressed on a molar basis relative to the activity of estradiol which was arbitrarily set at 100. The relative binding affinity of hamster uterine estrogen receptor (hatched bar) was determined by competitive binding assay. Relative uterotropic activity (open bar) was calculated from the amount of compound needed to elicit a half-maximal response. The relative progesterone receptor induction activity (solid bar) was calculated from the amount of compound required to produce a fourfold increase in receptor content. Each bar represents the mean ± SEM of four or more determinations.

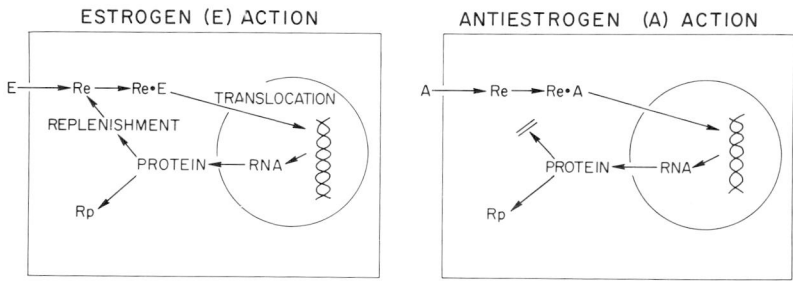

Re = ESTROGEN RECEPTOR
Rp = PROGESTERONE RECEPTOR

Fig. 10. Proposed mechanism of estrogen and antiestrogen action. Estrogen (E) acts via the estrogen receptor (Re) system to stimulate progesterone receptor (Rp) synthesis and Re replenishment. Antiestrogen (A) appears to work through the Re system to stimulate Rp synthesis, but A does not cause Re replenishment to the same extent as with E.

1973; Leavitt et al., 1974; Freifeld et al., 1974). Shortly after progesterone treatment, there is a marked reduction in the concentration of cytosol progesterone receptor (Fig. 8). Progesterone-induced depletion of receptor sites from the cytosol fraction supports the potential involvement of these macromolecules in the translocation of hormone–receptor complex to active intranuclear sites (Milgrom et al., 1973; Feil and Bardin, 1975).

It is well known that progesterone is actively metabolized by uterine tissue to a variety of metabolites, and the possibility exists that a progesterone metabolite, e.g., dihydroprogesterone (DHP), might be the intracellular mediator of hormone action (Fig. 1). Several lines of evidence argue against this possibility. DHP possesses little progestational activity in the rat uterus (Sanyal and Villee, 1973; Stromberg and Wiest, 1976), and a similar lack of uterotropic activity has been observed in the hamster following direct intrauterine application of DHP (Blaha, 1974). If DHP were the true intracellular mediator of progestin action, uterine tissue would be expected to exhibit two fundamental properties: (a) uterine cytosol would contain a specific receptor molecule for DHP; and (b) following progesterone uptake, DHP should accumulate as a result of progesterone metabolism and DHP binding. Hamster uterine cytosol was examined for the presence of specific binding macromolecules for DHP, and none were found (Leavitt and Grossman, 1974). Furthermore, the inactive metabolite, 3α-hydroxy-5α-pregnan-20-one (5α-pregnanolone, Fig. 1), was produced in greater quantity than DHP following progesterone uptake by uterine tissue, and evidence was obtained indicating that the accumulation of DHP in uterine tissue was related to the amount of nonspecifically bound progesterone which was available for metabolism (Leavitt and Grossman,

1974). Thus, the available evidence supports the concept that specific progesterone receptors exist in the cytoplasm of uterine target cells and that progesterone, rather than a progesterone metabolite, mediates the uterine progestational response by interacting with this specific receptor system.

The results of studies with the hamster model system support the following mechanism of progesterone action in the uterine target cell (Fig. 11). When progesterone enters the target cell, it binds either to the specific high-affinity receptor system or to a nonspecific low-affinity system. Nonspecific binding favors the metabolism of progesterone to inactive polar metabolites. DHP appears to function primarily as an intermediate in the conversion of progesterone to these inactive products. The hamster progesterone receptor has a higher binding affinity for progesterone than for DHP (Leavitt *et al.*, 1974), and this favors progesterone binding to the receptor. Since the receptor has a low binding affinity for DHP, it is possible that DHP could interact with the receptor if the concentration of DHP relative to progesterone were high enough. However, DHP accumulation is unlikely because it is rapidly converted to pregnanolone. Therefore, interaction of progesterone with the cytosol receptor appears to initiate the translocation step, i.e., the depletion of hormone–receptor complex from the cytosol fraction. The binding of receptor–hormone complex with specific acceptor sites in the nucleus is proposed to be the event which triggers nuclear reactions leading to the progestational response.

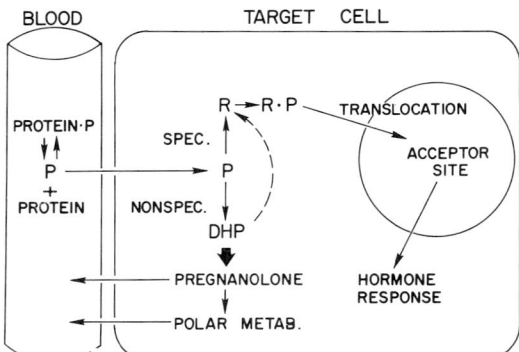

Fig. 11. Proposed mechanism of progestin action in uterus. Progesterone (P) enters the target cell and binds either to a specific receptor system or to a nonspecific binding system. Nonspecific binding favors progesterone metabolism to 5α-dihydroprogesterone (DHP), pregnanolone (3α-hydroxy-5α-pregnan-20-one), and polar metabolites. Specific binding by the progesterone receptor (R) causes formation of hormone–receptor complex (R·P) and translocation of the complex to nuclear acceptor sites. Binding of the hormone–receptor complex by nuclear acceptor sites is proposed to trigger reactions leading to the hormone response.

7. Biology of Progesterone Receptors

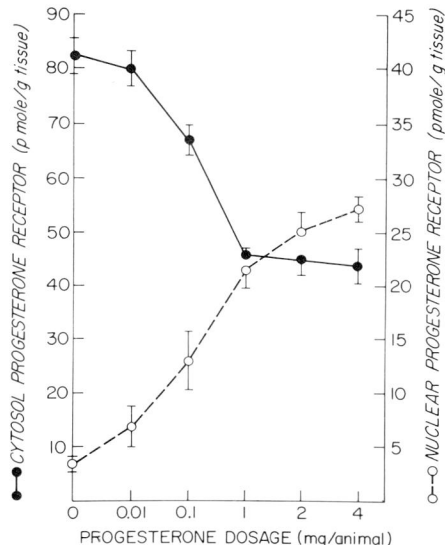

Fig. 12. Nuclear progesterone receptor response to progesterone treatment *in vivo*. Ovariectomized estrogen-primed hamsters were treated with different doses of progesterone for 2 hours, and the uterine cytosol and uterine nuclear fractions were assayed for receptor content. Cytosol receptor was measured by the Scatchard assay, and nuclear receptor was determined by the method of Chen and Leavitt (1977).

Studies on the nuclear progesterone receptor are lacking primarily because appropriate methodology for the measurement of nuclear receptor has not been developed (Faber *et al.*, 1976). Preliminary results suggest that nuclear progesterone receptor can be measured by a [³H]progesterone exchange assay (Hseuh *et al.*, 1974). However, this procedure is carried out at 15°C with intact nuclei, and, at this temperature, [³H]progesterone metabolism by the nuclear 5α-reductase enzyme is a serious problem (Morgan and Wilson, 1970). We have developed an exchange assay for nuclear progesterone receptor in which [³H]progesterone exchange is accomplished using nuclear receptor that is extracted with 0.5 *M* KCl in 50 m*M* Tris buffer + 30% glycerol (Chen and Leavitt, 1977). Exchange is carried out at low temperature, and the nuclear receptor level is estimated by Scatchard plot analysis of specific [³H]progesterone-binding data. Dose-response results obtained using the estrogen-primed ovariectomized hamster demonstrate that the dose of progesterone (about 100 μg/animal) which causes a significant intranuclear receptor translocation (Fig. 12) is the same as that required for progestational response in the hamster (Bosley and Leavitt, 1972a; Reuter *et al.*, 1970). These observations on the function of progesterone receptors in the mammalian uterus are consistent with the more elaborate model forwarded by O'Malley and colleagues for the chick oviduct system (Schrader et al., 1977).

VII. PROGESTERONE RECEPTOR SYNTHESIS IN VITRO

Experiments performed *in vivo* suggested that estrogen action increased progesterone receptor formation via RNA and protein synthesis (Milgrom et al., 1973; Reel and Shih, 1975). In order to study progesterone receptor synthesis under *in vitro* conditions, a hamster uterine strip system was developed (Chen and Leavitt, 1975; Leavitt et al., 1977). The rationale for the experimental design was as follows. Uterine tissue was exposed to estradiol during preincubation for 1 hour at 25°C to permit formation of estradiol–receptor complex and translocation of the complex to nuclear acceptor sites (Kessel and Leavitt, 1977). After this, hormone was removed from the medium during subsequent incubation at 37°C.

In a time-course study, done with control and estradiol-treated uterine strips, it was established that progesterone receptor production could be measured with the *in vitro* system. Although a substantial amount of progesterone receptor was lost during preparation and preincubation of the strips, receptor levels increased significantly in control strips during incubation for up to 24 hours. Furthermore, progesterone receptor production by estradiol-treated strips was significantly enhanced, as compared to the production by control strips. The responsiveness of the *in vitro* system to estrogen action was evaluated in a dose-response study, and a significant progesterone receptor response was obtained with 3×10^{-11} M estradiol, and a maximum response occurred after treatment with 3×10^{-8} M estradiol. If the estrogen-induced progesterone receptor response was mediated by estrogen receptor, it was reasoned that (a) the amount of estrogen needed to produce a progesterone receptor response should approximate the amount of estrogen receptor available for binding, and (b) the progesterone receptor response should be specific for estrogen. Uterine strips before incubation contained 7.1 ± 0.3 pmole estrogen receptor/g tissue or about 0.8 pmole receptor/flask. A half-maximal progesterone receptor response was achieved with somewhat less than 3×10^{-10} M estradiol (1.2 pmole estradiol/flask). Thus, there was reasonable agreement between the dose of estradiol needed for a progesterone receptor response and the amount of estrogen receptor available for binding. The specificity of the response was evaluated using different hormonal steroids (3×10^{-8} M) during preincubation at 25°C. Subsequent incubation of paired strips at 37°C in hormone-free Medium 199 revealed that receptor synthesis was increased only by estradiol, as compared to treatment with testosterone, 5α-dihydrotestosterone, or cortisol.

The progesterone receptor synthesized by both control and estrogen-treated strips had a 6-7 S sedimentation coefficient in low ionic strength medium. In addition, the size of the receptor peak increased with time of incubation in both groups, and this was consistent with the results obtained by Scatchard assay of the receptor binding capacity.

The protein synthesis inhibitor, cycloheximide, was used to study the involvement of protein synthesis in progesterone receptor production. When uterine strips were exposed to cycloheximide (10 μg/ml) at time 0, receptor synthesis was blocked in control strips, as well as estrogen-treated strips. This indicated that receptor production was dependent on protein synthesis in both the control and estrogen-stimulated preparations. When estrogen-treated strips were exposed to cycloheximide at 6 hours of incubation, receptor synthesis was inhibited from 6 to 12 hours. Thus, estrogen-induced progesterone receptor production appears to be dependent on continued protein synthesis throughout the time course of the response. Similar studies performed using actinomycin D determined that receptor synthesis was dependent on RNA. As was the case with cycloheximide, application of actinomycin D (10 μg/ml) at time 0 blocked subsequent receptor production in both control and estrogen-treated strips. Thus, progesterone receptor synthesis in both preparations appeared to be dependent on nuclear RNA synthesis. However, when estrogen-treated strips were exposed to actinomycin D at 6 hours, receptor synthesis was not inhibited when measured at 12 hours. This was interpreted to indicate that enough estrogen-dependent RNA was produced during the first 6 hours of estrogen action to sustain receptor synthesis in the absence of new RNA synthesis from 6 to 12 hours of incubation.

The results of these *in vitro* studies are consistent with the following model of progesterone receptor synthesis. The estrogen target cell is capable of synthesizing progesterone receptor in the absence of estrogen support, and this basal level of receptor synthesis is dependent on continued RNA and protein synthesis. The augmentation of progesterone receptor synthesis by estrogen action involves stimulation of RNA and protein synthesis, and this response appears to be regulated by the estrogen receptor system. Presumably, the uterine strip system can serve as a model for the study of estrogen-induced progesterone receptor synthesis. In addition, the *in vitro* approach may be of value in the clinical evaluation of hormone-dependent tumors. The finding of progesterone receptor in breast cancer tissue is useful in the identification of patients who will show objective remissions to endocrine therapy (Horwitz *et al.*, 1975a). This suggests that an incubation system could be used for the identification of endocrine-dependent tumor tissues on the basis of a progesterone receptor response to an estrogen challenge given *in vitro*.

ACKNOWLEDGMENT

The studies reported here were supported by Population Council Grant M74.113; USPHS Grant HD 06982, and NSF Grant PCM 75-16135.

Special thanks are due Ms. Karen Albaugh for typing the manuscript.

REFERENCES

Allen, T. C., and Leavitt, W. W. (1975). *Fed. Proc., Fed. Am. Soc. Exp. Biol.* **34**, 279.
Allen, W. M., and Corner, G. W. (1930). *Proc. Soc. Exp. Biol. Med.* **27**, 403–405.
Astwood, E. B. (1939). *J. Endocrinol.* **1**, 49–55.
Atger, M., Baulieu, E.-E., and Milgrom, E. (1974). *Endocrinology* **94**, 161–167.
Baulieu, E.-E., Atger, M., Best-Belpomme, M., Corvol, P., Courvalin, J.-C., Mester, J., Milgrom, E., Robel, P., Rochefort, H., and De Catalogne, D. (1975). *Vitam. Horm. (N.Y.)* **33**, 649–736.
Bell, C. (1974). *Med. Biol.* **52**, 219–228.
Blaha, G. C. (1974). *Anat. Rec.* **178**, 311.
Bosley, C. G., and Leavitt, W. W. (1972a). *Am. J. Physiol.* **222**, 129–133.
Bosley, C. G., and Leavitt, W. W. (1972b). *Fed. Proc., Fed. Am. Soc. Exp. Biol.* **31**, 257.
Carlton, B. D., and Leavitt, W. W. (1977). *Fed. Proc., Fed. Am. Soc. Exp. Biol.* **36**, 344.
Challis, J. R. G., Davies, I. J., and Ryan, K. J. (1974). *Endocrinology* **95**, 160–164.
Chen, T. J., and Leavitt, W. W. (1975). *Physiologist* **18**, 166.
Chen, T. J., and Leavitt, W. W. (1977). *Program. 59th Annu. Meet. Endocr. Soc.* p. 89.
Clark, J. H., Anderson, J. N., and Peck, E. J., Jr. (1973). *Steroids* **22**, 707–718.
Clark, J. H., Peck, E. J., Jr., and Anderson, J. N. (1974). *Nature (London)* **251**, 446–448.
Clark, J. H., Peck, E. J., Jr., Schrader, W. T., and O'Malley, B. W. (1976). *Methods Cancer Res.* **12**, 367–417.
Corvol, P., Falk, R., Freifeld, M., and Bardin, C. W. (1972). *Endocrinology* **90**, 1464–1469.
Csapo, A. I., and Wiest, W. G. (1969). *Endocrinology* **85**, 735–746.
Davies, I. J., and Ryan, K. J. (1973). *Endocrinology* **92**, 394–401.
Davies, I. J., Challis, J. R. G., and Ryan, K. J. (1974). *Endocrinology* **95**, 165–173.
Do, Y. S., Baldwin, D. M., and Leavitt, W. W. (1976). *Program 9th Meet. Soc. Study Reprod.* p. 61.
Evans, R. W., Sholiton, L. J., and Leavitt, W. W., (1977). *Program 10th Meet. Soc. Study Reprod.* (in press).
Faber, L. E., Saffran, J., Chen, T. J., and Leavitt, W. W. (1976). *In* "Steroid Hormone Action and Cancer" (K. M. J. Menon and J. R. Reel, eds.), pp. 68–84. Plenum, New York.
Falk, R. J., and Bardin, C. W. (1970). *Endocrinology* **86**, 1059–1063.
Feder, H. H., and Ruf, K. B. (1969). *Endocrinology* **84**, 171–174.
Feil, P. D., and Bardin, C. W. (1975). *Endocrinology* **97**, 1398–1407.
Feil, P. D., Glasser, S. R., Toft, D. O., and O'Malley, B. W. (1972). *Endocrinology* **91**, 738–746.
Finn, C. A., and Martin, L. (1974). *J. Reprod. Fertil.* **39**, 195–206.

7. Biology of Progesterone Receptors

Fitzgerald, K. M., and Zucker, I. (1976). *Proc. Natl. Acad. Sci. U.S.A.* **73**, 2923–2927.
Fraenkel, K. (1903). *Arch. Gynäkol.* **68**, 438–545.
Freifeld, M. L., Feil, P. D., and Bardin, C. W. (1974). *Steroids* **23**, 93–103.
Glasser, S. R., and Clark, J. H. (1975). *In* "The Developmental Biology of Reproduction" (C. L. Markert and J. Papaconstantinou, eds.), pp. 311–345. Academic Press, New York.
Goldman, B. D., and Zarrow, M. X. (1973). *Handb. Physiol., Sect. 7: Endocrinol.* **2**, 547–572.
Grossman, C. J., and Leavitt, W. W. (1974). *Fed. Proc., Fed. Am. Soc. Exp. Biol.* **33**, 268.
Harper, M. J. K. (1970). *Anat. Rec.* **167**, 225–230.
Harper, M. J. K., Dowd, D., and Elliot, A. S. W. (1969). *Biol. Reprod.* **1**, 253–257.
Herrmann, W. L., Heinrichs, W. L., and Tabei, T. (1973). *Am. J. Obstet. Gynecol.* **117**, 679–688.
Horwitz, K. B., and McGuire, W. L. (1975). *Steroids* **25**, 496–505.
Horwitz, K. B., McGuire, W. L., Pearson, O. H., and Segaloff, A. (1975a). *Science* **189**, 726–727.
Horwitz, K. B., Costlow, M. E., and McGuire, W. L. (1975b). *Steroids* **26**, 785–795.
Hseuh, A. J. W., Peck, E. J., Jr., and Clark, J. H. (1974). *Steroids* **24**, 599–611.
Hseuh, A. J. W., Peck, E. J., Jr., and Clark, J. H. (1976). *Endocrinology* **98**, 438–444.
Jensen, E. V., and De Sombre, E. R. (1973). *Science* **182**, 126–134.
Kessel, B., and Leavitt, W. W. (1977). *Fed. Proc., Fed. Am. Soc. Exp. Biol.* **36**, 344.
Kontula, K. (1975). *Acta Endocrinol. (Copenhagen)* **78**, 593–603.
Kontula, K., Jänne, O., Vihko, R., deJager, E., deVisser, J., and Zeelen, F. (1975). *Acta Endocrinol. (Copenhagen)* **78**, 574–592.
Kow, L.-M., Malsbury, C. W., and Pfaff, D. W. (1974). *In* "Reproductive Behavior" (W. Montagna and W. A. Sadler, eds.), pp. 179–210. Plenum, New York.
Kuhn, R. W., Schrader, W. T., Smith, R. G., and O'Malley, B. W. (1975). *J. Biol. Chem.* **250**, 4220–4228.
Leavitt, W. W., and Blaha, G. C. (1970). *Biol. Reprod.* **3**, 353–361.
Leavitt, W. W., and Blaha, G. C. (1972). *Steroids* **19**, 263–274.
Leavitt, W. W., and Grossman, C. J. (1974). *Proc. Natl. Acad. Sci. U.S.A.* **71**, 4341–4345.
Leavitt, W. W., and Reuss, B. J. (1975). *Program 57th Annu. Meet. Endocr. Soc.* p. 273.
Leavitt, W. W., Bosley, C. G., and Blaha, G. C. (1971). *Nature (London)* 234, 283–284.
Leavitt, W. W., Basom, C. R., Bagwell, J. N., and Blaha, G. C. (1973). *Am. J. Anat.* **136**, 235–249.
Leavitt, W. W., Toft, D. O., Strott, C. A., and O'Malley, B. W. (1974). *Endocrinology* **94**, 1041–1053.
Leavitt, W. W., Chen, T. J., Allen, T. C., and Johnston, J. O. (1977). *Ann. N.Y. Acad. Sci.* **286**, 210–225.
Little, B., Billiar, R. B., Rahman, S. S., Johnson, W. A., Takaoka, Y., and White, R. J. (1975). *Am. J. Obstet. Gynecol.* **123**, 527–534.
Luu Thi, M. T., Baulieu, E.-E., and Milgrom, E. (1975). *J. Endocrinol.* **66**, 349–356.
Martin, R. G., and Ames, B. N. (1961). *J. Biol. Chem.* **236**, 1372–1379.
Milgrom, E., and Baulieu, E.-E. (1970). *Endocrinology* **87**, 276–287.
Milgrom, E., Atger, M., and Baulieu, E.-E. (1970). *Steroids* **16**, 741–754.
Milgrom, E., Perrot, M., Atger, M., and Baulieu, E.-E. (1972a). *Endocrinology* **90**, 1064–1070.
Milgrom, E., Atger, M., Perrot, M., and Baulieu, E.-E. (1972b). *Endocrinology* **90**, 1071–1078.
Milgrom, E., Luu Thi, M. T., Atger, M., and Baulieu, E.-E. (1973). *J. Biol. Chem.* **248**, 6366–6374.
Miyake, T., Kakushi, H., and Hara, K. (1963). *Steroids* **2**, 749–763.
Morgan, M. D., and Wilson, J. D. (1970). *J. Biol. Chem.* **245**, 3781–3789.

O'Malley, B. W., and Means, A. R. (1974). *Science* **183**, 610–620.
Philibert, D., and Raynaud, J.-P. (1973). *Steroids* **22**, 89–98.
Psychoyos, A. (1973). *Vitam. Horm. (N.Y.)* **31**, 201–256.
Rao, B. R., and Wiest, W. G. (1974). *Gynecol. Oncol.* **2**, 239–248.
Reel, J. R., and Shih, Y. (1975). *Acta Endocrinol. (Copenhagen)* **80**, 344–354.
Reel, J. R., VanDewark, S. D., Shih, Y., and Callantine, M. R. (1971). *Steroids* **18**, 441–461.
Resko, J. A. (1969). *Science* **64**, 70–71.
Reuter, L. A., Ciaccio, L. A., and Lisk, R. D. (1970). *Endocrinology* **86**, 1286–1297.
Rondell, P. (1974). *Biol. Reprod.* **10**, 199–215.
Sanyal, M. K., and Villee, C. A. (1973). *Endocrinology* **92**, 83–93.
Sar, M., and Stumpf, W. E. (1973). *Science* **183**, 1266–1268.
Sar, M., and Stumpf, W. E. (1974). *Endocrinology* **94**, 1116–1125.
Scatchard, G. (1949). *Ann. N.Y. Acad. Sci.* **51**, 660–672.
Schrader, W. T., Heuer, S. S., and O'Malley, B. W. (1975). *Biol. Reprod.* **12**, 134–142.
Schrader, W. T., Kuhn, R. W., Buller, R. E., Schwartz, R. T., and O'Malley, B. W. (1977). *In* "Receptors in Pharmacology" (J. R. Smythies, ed.), pp. 67–95, Dekker, New York.
Sluyser, M., Evers, S. G., and DeGoeij, C. C. J. (1976). *Nature (London)* **263**, 386–389.
Smith, H. E., Smith, R. G., Toft, D. O., Neergaard, J. R., Burrows, E. P., and O'Malley, B. W. (1974). *J. Biol. Chem.* **249**, 5924–5932.
Smith, R. G., Iramain, C. A., Buttram, V. C., Jr., and O'Malley, B. W. (1975). *Nature (London)* **253**, 271–272.
Stromberg, B. V., and Wiest, W. G. (1976). *J. Steroid Biochem.* **7**, 51–53.
Stumpf, W. E. (1968). *Endocrinology* **83**, 777–782.
Stumpf, W. E. (1969). *Endocrinology* **85**, 31–37.
Stumpf, W. E., and Sar, M. (1973). *J. Steroid Biochem.* **4**, 477–481.
Szego, C. M. (1974). *Recent Prog. Horm. Res.* **30**, 171–233.
Toft, D. O., and O'Malley, B. W. (1972). *Endocrinology* **90**, 1041–1045.
Warembourg, M. (1974). *Endocrinology* **94**, 665–670.
Yochim, J. M. (1975). *Biol. Reprod.* **12**, 106–133.

8

Molecular Structure and Analysis of Progesterone Receptors

WILLIAM T. SCHRADER AND BERT W. O'MALLEY

I.	Introduction	189
	A. General Features of the Chick Oviduct System	189
II.	The Progesterone Receptor Protein	193
	A. Progesterone Receptor Subunit Structure	193
	B. Purification and Properties of Receptor Proteins	200
III.	Effects of Progesterone *in Vivo* on Chromatin Gene Transcription	207
	A. Assay of Chromatin RNA Initiation Sites	207
	B. Assay of Ovalbumin mRNA Induction by Hybridization	210
IV.	Effect of Purified Progesterone–Receptor Complexes *in Vitro* on Chromatin Gene Transcription	210
	A. Assay of Chromatin RNA Initiation Sites	211
	B. Tissue Specificity	214
	C. Stimulation *in Vitro* of Ovalbumin mRNA Synthesis from Oviduct Chromatin	215
	D. Differential Activity of Receptor Subunits on Chromatin Transcription *in Vitro*	216
V.	A Proposed Model for Steroid Hormone Regulation of Gene Transcription	218
	References	222

I. INTRODUCTION

A. General Features of the Chick Oviduct System

1. Effect of Steroids on Gene Transcription

The chick oviduct provides an excellent model system for studying the hormonal control of cellular differentiation and gene expression (O'Malley *et al.*, 1969). Chronic administration of estrogen over a period of 10–14 days results in growth and differentiation of the chick oviduct. Previous studies from this laboratory have shown that estrogen-mediated growth and differentiation of the chick oviduct involve significant alterations in gene transcription. Competitive hybridization experiments have demonstrated qualitative changes in RNA synthesized from the repetitive sequences of nuclear DNA during estrogen-mediated differentiation (O'Malley and McGuire, 1968). More recent studies have also demonstrated increased transcription of unique sequence DNA during oviduct growth (Liarakos *et al.*, 1973). Concomitant with steroid-mediated oviduct differentiation, increased levels of nuclear RNA, RNA polymerase activity (O'Malley *et al.*, 1969; Cox *et al.*, 1973), chromatin template capacity, and changes in chromatin nonhistone proteins (Spelsberg *et al.*, 1972) were also found in the oviduct. Preceding the well-documented specific changes in protein synthesis (Rosenfeld *et al.*, 1972; Means *et al.*, 1972; Comstock, *et al.*, 1972), previous studies have demonstrated an unequivocal net accumulation of specific, biologically active messenger RNA, coding for ovalbumin (Chan *et al.*, 1973; Rhoads *et al.*, 1971; Harris *et al.*, 1975).

When estrogen treatment of the chicks is discontinued, a reduction in the overall level of RNA and protein synthesis occurs, and the cells' ability to synthesize specific proteins, such as ovalbumin, decreases (Chan *et al.*, 1973; Palmiter, 1973). After 12 days of hormone withdrawal, the rate of ovalbumin biosynthesis is less than 1% of that observed in hormonally stimulated chicks (Harris *et al.*, 1975). If either estrogen or progesterone is readministered (secondary stimulation), there is a rapid increase in the production of ovalbumin mRNA, and the induction of other egg white proteins begins again (Palmiter, 1973). Therefore, the chick oviduct provides a system to study a specific endocrine response in which overall gene expression can be dramatically altered while a specific marker for measuring changes in the transcription rate of a single gene is also available. Figure 1 is a schematic representation of the principal hormonal events in the oviduct as described above.

These transcription events are regulated by the appearance in the nucleus of steroid bound to receptor proteins of cytoplasmic origin. Correlation of growth or genetic activity with nuclear receptor levels has provided the strongest evidence for a cause-and-effect relationship (Anderson *et al.*, 1973; S. Y. Tsai *et al.*, 1975). The temporal sequence of events, together with studies on the nature of the nuclear acceptor sites (Spelsberg *et al.*, 1971; O'Malley and Means, 1974; Buller and O'Malley, 1976), seem to fit the following overall scheme. (a) Steroids enter the cell and bind to specific cytoplasmic receptor proteins; (b) the steroid–receptor complex is translocated into the nuclear compartment; (c) receptor–hormone complex binds

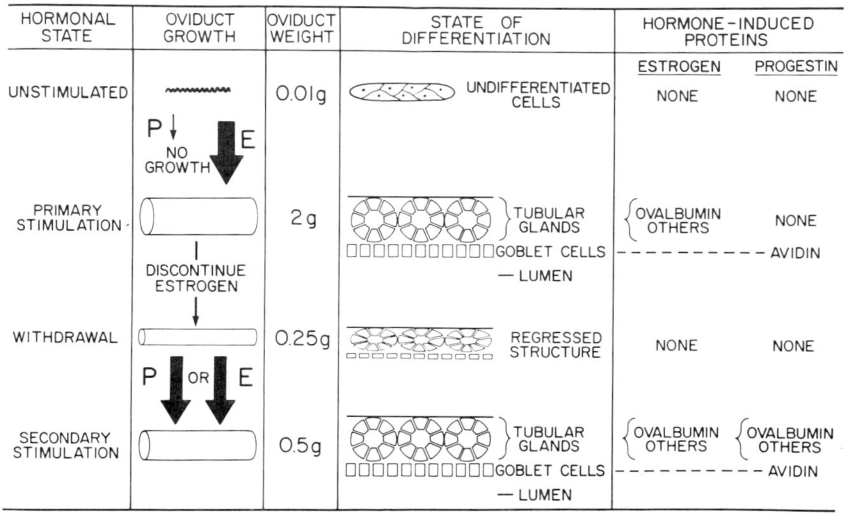

HORMONAL STATE	OVIDUCT GROWTH	OVIDUCT WEIGHT	STATE OF DIFFERENTIATION	HORMONE-INDUCED PROTEINS	
				ESTROGEN	PROGESTIN
UNSTIMULATED	~~~~~~ P↓ ⬇E NO GROWTH	0.01g	UNDIFFERENTIATED CELLS	NONE	NONE
PRIMARY STIMULATION	⬜ | DISCONTINUE ESTROGEN ↓	2g	TUBULAR GLANDS / GOBLET CELLS — LUMEN	OVALBUMIN OTHERS --------- AVIDIN	NONE
WITHDRAWAL	⬜ P⬇ OR ⬇E	0.25g	REGRESSED STRUCTURE	NONE	NONE
SECONDARY STIMULATION	⬜	0.5g	TUBULAR GLANDS / GOBLET CELLS — LUMEN	OVALBUMIN OTHERS --------- AVIDIN	OVALBUMIN OTHERS

Fig. 1. Schematic diagram of the hormonal events in the immature chick oviduct. Degree of growth and cell types produced are shown as a function of the hormonal regimen described in the text. Cell-specific marker proteins produced under influence of these hormones are indicated on the right. Of particular interest is the induction of ovalbumin by progesterone during secondary stimulation.

to acceptor sites on nuclear chromatin; and finally, activation of the transcriptional process occurs, followed by the appearance of specific new RNA species.

2. Progesterone Receptor Protein Characteristics

To elucidate further the mechanism of steroid hormone action, it is necessary to examine the process by which biochemical information held by the steroid receptor complex is transferred or decoded by the transcriptional apparatus. Our efforts have been along two lines: (a) to characterize receptor proteins as completely as possible, and (b) to develop a cell-free transcription system for studying effects of purified receptor–hormone complexes on gene expression *in vitro*.

Steroid hormone receptor proteins have been the subject of intensive study for over 10 years. These studies have shown that receptor proteins are structurally complex, undergoing changes in aggregation, conformation, and binding activities before and during their interaction with nuclear acceptor sites (O'Malley and Means, 1974; Jensen and De Sombre, 1974). The importance of these properties is apparent from the extensive similarities among all steroid receptor proteins studied, regardless of source or steroid-binding specificity.

Work in this laboratory has centered on the purification and characterization of progesterone receptors in chick oviduct. This steroid receptor was chosen for study because it is present in oviducts of immature chicks in concentrations about 10-fold higher than that observed for other receptors. Second, the oviducts grow to nearly 2 g in size under estrogen administration, but in the absence of progesterone. Thus, the progesterone receptors in the tissue are not complexed to their steroid, and are accessible for labeling with radioactive progesterone *in vitro*.

Since the initial detection of this receptor (O'Malley *et al.*, 1969; Sherman *et al.*, 1970) considerable physical and chemical characterization of the protein has been undertaken. Chick oviduct progesterone receptor contains two 4 S components, designated A and B, which can be resolved by chromatography on a variety of ion-exchange resins (Schrader and O'Malley, 1972; Clark *et al.*, 1976). These two components which are present in approximately equal amounts in crude oviduct cytoplasmic extracts (Schrader *et al.*, 1972) are interconvertible. They have similar hormone binding sites, with respect to equilibrium and kinetic binding constants, as well as hormone stereospecificity (Schrader and O'Malley, 1972).

Although both receptor forms are taken up by oviduct nuclei *in vitro* Schrader *et al.*, 1972; O'Malley *et al.*, 1971), they have distinct specificities for binding to nuclear components. The receptor A component binds only to DNA, while the B component binds only to chromatin (Schrader *et al.*, 1972). Furthermore, the B component binding to chromatin is target tissue specific (Schrader *et al.*, 1972; O'Malley *et al.*, 1972; Jaffe *et al.*, 1975).

3. Proposed Model for Effect of Receptors on Transcription

These properties of the progesterone receptor led us to propose (Schrader and O'Malley, 1972; O'Malley and Schrader, 1972; Schrader *et al.*, 1972) that both chromatin and DNA-binding forms might be necessary for receptor function *in vivo*. In our hypothetical model, the chromatin-binding B protein would function to specify regions in the chromatin adjacent to a hormonally regulated gene. This "specifier" activity would then direct the "effector" A protein to its site of action, where it would bind to the DNA and, thus, modify transcription by RNA polymerase (O'Malley *et al.*, 1973).

This model would suggest that aggregated forms of the receptor containing both A and B subunits might be important in receptor function. The concept of coupled A and B receptor subunits was strengthened by our observation (Schrader *et al.*, 1972) that both A and B could be extracted from nuclei in nearly equal amounts. The simplest explanation for this relationship was that A and B were coupled together as a dimer. Some of the experiments described below were designed to examine the subunit structure of the progesterone receptor, and the relationship this quaternary structure has to the functional activities of the A and B receptor forms.

Thus, we have studied these proteins in order to gain information on the relationship between their structure and function. Secondly, we have developed purification techniques for isolation independently of subunits A and B as well as the intact AB dimers. These techniques are described below.

Finally, according to the model mentioned above, the ultimate test of receptor activity is its effect on gene transcription. To develop such an assay, initial efforts in our laboratory have been to characterize the interaction of purified RNA polymerase with intact chromatin. The process of initiation of RNA synthesis has received special attention, since the step appears to be regulated by steroids (M. J. Tsai *et al.,* 1975; Schwartz *et al.,* 1975). The *in vitro* chromatin transcription assay has now been used to test the biologic function of purified receptor–hormone complexes and subunits (Schwartz *et al.,* 1976; Buller *et al.,* 1976b) under cell-free conditions. In this article, we will discuss also our recent evidence on the progesterone-dependent transcription of oviduct chromatin.

II. THE PROGESTERONE RECEPTOR PROTEIN

A. Progesterone Receptor Subunit Structure

1. Subunit Interconversion to Aggregates

A common characteristic of steroid hormone receptors is their tendency to undergo salt-dependent aggregation (Jensen and De Sombre, 1974). Chick oviduct progesterone receptor exhibits this characteristic behavior, as shown by sucrose-gradient ultracentrifugation analysis (Sherman *et al.,* 1970; Schrader *et al.,* 1975a). In gradients containing 0.3 M KCl, progesterone receptor sediments as a single sharp peak at approximately 4 S. In the absence of salt, however, receptor components are observed which sediment at approximately 6 and 8 S. We, therefore, examined these aggregated receptor forms to determine their relationship to the 4 S A and B components.

Results in Fig. 2 show that the 8 S aggregate is unstable to dialysis and dilution. This form is apparently converted to 4 S components, while the 6 S form is relatively unaffected. This concentration dependence of receptor aggregation has been observed for other steroid hormone receptors (Stancel

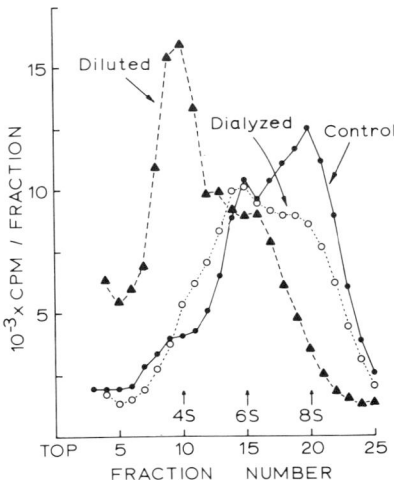

Fig. 2. Effect of dilution and dialysis on the sedimentation properties of the chick oviduct progesterone receptor proteins. Gradients (5–20% sucrose) in 10 mM Tris buffer, pH 7.4, were run in a Beckman SW-50.1 rotor at 45,000 rpm for 16 hours. Labeled control cytosol sedimented as shown (●———●) as a pair of peaks at 6 S and 8 S with a 4 S shoulder (arrows). Companion samples were diluted 10-fold (▲---------▲) or dialyzed against Tris buffer (O·····O) for 4 hours before centrifugation. The diluted sample radioactivity has been multiplied by 10 to allow direct comparison with the other two.

et al., 1973), and may be due to artifactual aggregation of receptor with other cytoplasmic proteins. The relative stability of the 6 S form, and the fact that its molecular weight was approximately equal to the sum of the A and B components, led us to study this aggregate further.

The results of Fig. 2 demonstrated that 8 S aggregates dissociated to 4 S subunits, rather than to the 6 S form. To confirm this, the kinetics of conversion were studied using the sucrose-gradient technique. The results of Fig. 3 were obtained by dialyzing labeled cytosol for various times and then measuring sucrose-gradient peak heights for the 4 S, 6 S, and 8 S forms. The semilogarithmic plots in Fig. 3 show dissociation half-lives for the 6 S and 8 S forms of 17 and 7 hours, respectively. Linearity of the 6 S plot is further evidence that 8 S aggregates do not convert to the 6 S form; a longer half-life would have been seen at early times if this event could occur. The 4 S plot is curved, indicating its appearance is not a first-order process. This behavior is to be expected, since both the 8 S and 6 S forms dissociate and contribute 4 S monomers at different rates.

A major analytical tool for the study of aggregated receptor forms was provided by our discovery (Schrader *et al.,* 1975a) that these proteins pass unretarded through phosphocellulose columns under conditions where 4 S A and B components are quantitatively adsorbed. We used this technique in combination with sucrose-gradient analysis to isolate and study 6 S and 8 S receptor aggregates.

We isolated 6 S hormone–receptor complex from the unadsorbed fraction after phosphocellulose chromatography of cytosol and treated it with high salt or brief warming at room temperature. These treatments resulted in substantial conversion to receptor forms which adsorbed to phosphocellulose. Subsequent elution of this resin with a KCl gradient resolved two equal peaks of radioactivity at 0.22 and 0.26 M KCl (Schrader et al., 1975a; Clark et al., 1976). These peaks were identified as B and A components, respectively, by rechromatography on phosphocellulose and co-elution with the 4 S receptor forms isolated by DEAE–cellulose chromatography. These results suggest that the 6 S receptor form is a dimer containing equal amounts of A and B subunits.

The presence of progesterone had a dramatic effect on the stability of the 6 S receptor dimer. Unlabeled cytosol was warmed as described above, then cooled to 0°C and labeled for 1 hour with [³H]progesterone before application to a phosphocellulose column. As shown by the dotted line in Fig. 4, the 6 S receptor had not dissociated to A and B subunits and, hence, did not bind to the column. The labeled column drop-through fraction was collected, rewarmed, and rechromatographed. As shown by the solid line in Fig. 4, the expected production of equal amounts of A and B subunits occurred.

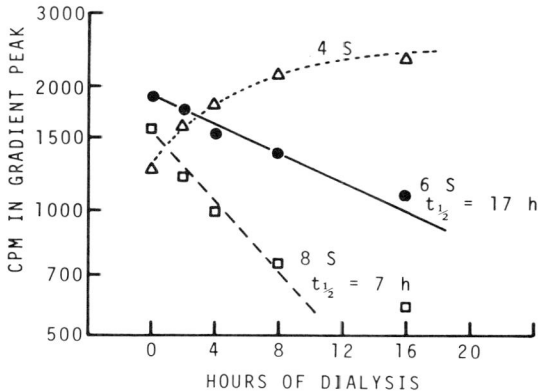

Fig. 3. Effect of prolonged dialysis on receptor subunit structure and aggregation. Labeled cytosol receptors were dialyzed for the indicated times at 0°C and then analyzed by sucrose gradient ultracentrifugation as described in Fig. 2. The radioactivity in the 4 S (△·····△), 6 S (●———●), and 8 S (□--------□) peaks fractions (tubes 10, 15, and 20, respectively) was plotted on a semilogarithmic scale to determine half-lives for the complexes.

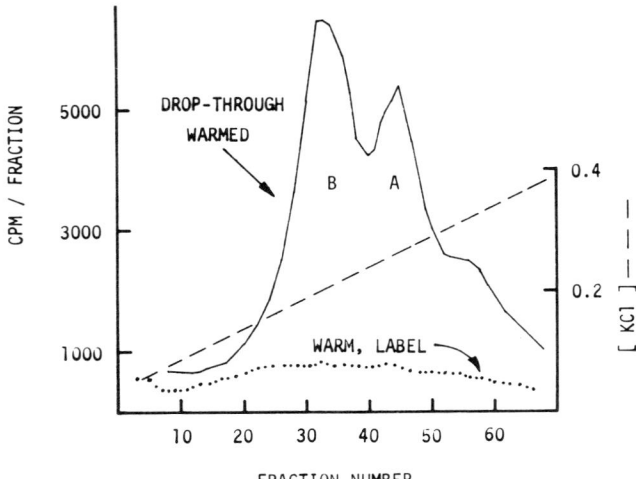

Fig. 4. Phosphocellulose chromatography of receptor subunits obtained by warming 6 S receptor–hormone complexes of cytosol. Oviduct cytosol without hormone was warmed (25°C, 30 minutes), then cooled to 0°C, labeled with [^{3}H]progesterone, and chromatographed on the small phosphocellulose column. Receptor 6 S forms were still present, and passed through column unretarded. Very little radioactivity adsorbed (·······). Subsequent warming of the labeled complexes in the drop-through fraction promoted dissociation to monomers; rechromatography on phosphocellulose (———) showed B and A receptor subunits. From Schrader et al., 1977b.

We also tested the stability of this 6 S species to dissociation by KCl, using sucrose-gradient ultracentrifugation. Oviduct cytosol, with or without bound [^{3}H]progesterone, was run on gradients containing various amounts of KCl. As shown in Fig. 5, aporeceptor did not associate at up to 0.25 M KCl. However, the labeled complex was metastable at physiological concentrations of KCl, and completely dissociated by 0.2 M KCl. These results show that hormone binding results in destabilization of the subunit interactions in the 6 S progesterone receptor dimer. Thus, hormone binding could regulate the subunit structure of the receptor as well as its nuclear localization.

2. *Functional Activities of the Dimer and Subunits*

Since the 6 S receptor contains both DNA- and chromatin-binding subunits, we examined whether these activities were expressed in the intact dimer. Results in Table I show that the 6 S dimer binds to chromatin. Binding was essentially complete within 15 minutes at 0°C; no further binding was observed after 60 minutes. This suggests that the dimer binds directly to chromatin, since very little dissociation into subunits would be expected in this time interval.

We also examined receptor binding to DNA-cellulose, as shown in Fig. 6. Binding of the A subunit to DNA was nearly complete, while no significant binding of the B subunit was observed, in agreement with our earlier results (Schrader *et al.*, 1972). The 6 S dimer also did not bind to DNA. Thus, the DNA-binding activity of the A subunit is not expressed in the intact dimer, perhaps due to blocking or conformational alteration of the DNA-binding site through subunit–subunit interactions.

These properties of the 6 S receptor dimer are consistent with our proposed model of receptor action, which suggests that both DNA- and chromatin-binding activities are required for receptor function. This may also be a general property of all steroid hormone receptors; two receptor forms on DEAE-cellulose chromatography have been observed for other steroid receptors (Norris and Kohler, 1976).

3. *Hormone-Binding Kinetics*

The receptor subunits each bind [^{3}H]progesterone. One test of their identification as functional receptors was to test both A and B for hormone-binding specificity and kinetics. When these studies were done (Schrader and O'Malley, 1972), both A and B bound progesterone better than any

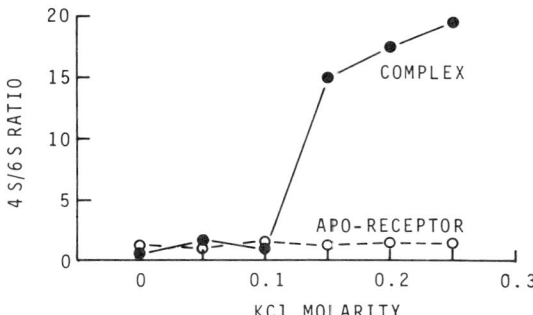

Fig. 5. Effect of bound hormone on stability of intact 6 S receptors to dissociation by KCl. Oviduct cytosol was prepared and either labeled with [^{3}H]progesterone (●———●) or kept uncomplexed (○--------○). Samples were applied to sucrose gradients containing the indicated KCl molarities and centrifuged as described in Fig. 2. The gradients containing labeled complexes were fractionated and counted for ^{3}H. The aporeceptors were fractionated in the cold. Excess [^{3}H]progesterone (20,000 cpm/tube) was added, and the tubes kept at 0°C for 2 hours. Then [^{3}H]progesterone–receptor complexes were collected by adsorption to DEAE-cellulose filters (Whatman DE-81), washed, and the filters counted for ^{3}H. The receptor concentrations in the 4 S (fraction 10) and 6 S (fraction 15) regions were calculated, and the 4 S/6 S ratio plotted as an index of subunit/intact complex ratio. From Schrader *et al.*, 1977b.

TABLE I

Binding of Intact 6 S Receptor to Oviduct Chromatin[a]

Microliters 6 S receptor added[b]	Incubation time[c] (min)	Receptor bound (cpm)	
		Control	+ Chromatin[d]
100	15	3100	15,100
	60	2600	10,300
250	15	6300	24,500
	60	7400	29,500

[a] From Schrader et al., 1977b.

[b] Labeled cytosol 6 S receptors (400,000 cpm/ml) prepared in 0.1 M KCl by phosphocellulose exclusion.

[c] Receptors incubated at 0°C in final volume of 1.0 ml, and tubes processed according to Schrader et al. (1975b).

[d] Oviduct chromatin (500 µg DNA) added to experimental tubes to start binding reaction.

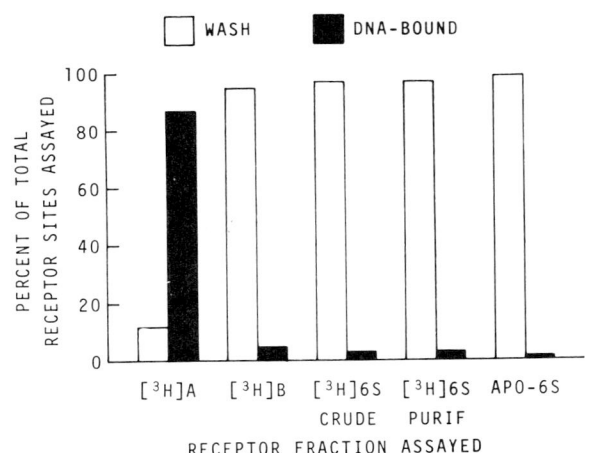

Fig. 6. DNA–cellulose column chromatography of receptor subunits and intact 6 S complexes. Purified A subunit, B subunit, and 6 S intact receptor were prepared as described in the text and applied to 1 ml DNA–cellulose columns. Unbound receptors were washed through with dilute Tris buffer (open bars) and then adsorbed radioactive receptors were eluted stepwise with 0.4 M KCl (solid bars). In addition, a crude labeled 6 S receptor preparation was made by applying diluted cytosol to a 5-ml phosphocellulose column and collecting the drop-through fraction. The receptors in this fraction were then either complexed with labeled progesterone (^{3}H–6 S crude) or left unlabeled (Apo–6 S). These two fractions were then assayed for DNA–cellulose adsorption also. Only receptor A protein adsorbed significantly to DNA–cellulose, identical to the behavior of crude A subunits studied earlier (Schrader, 1975; Schrader et al., 1975b). From Coty et al., 1977.

other ligand. All of the progesterone analogues tested (Smith et al., 1974) bound in reasonable correlation to their *in vivo* biologic potency. Thus, both A and B in cytosol appeared to be authentic progesterone receptor molecules.

The rate kinetics for association and dissociation at 0°C showed evidence of only a single class of hormone-binding sites, whether the study was done on isolated subunits (Schrader and O'Malley, 1972) or on cytosol (Hansen et al., 1976). Furthermore, an Arrhenius plot of the dissociation rate constant data showed no evidence for a change in binding energy over the temperature range at which subunit-subunit dissociation to monomers occurs (Hansen et al., 1976). Therefore, there appears to be little or no cooperation between the hormone sites on the A and B subunits.

There was a distinct discrepancy in the hormone-binding data, however, as shown in Table II. If the pathway of binding obeyed the simple equation

$$RS \rightleftharpoons R + S$$

then the ratio of rate constants should equal the equilibrium constant. As shown in Table II, this is not the case. Furthermore, the deviation between the two determinations increases dramatically with temperature. Thus, the hormone-binding mechanism is more complex than originally thought. When the dissociation of hormone was studied by both dialysis and displacement (addition of excess nonradioactive progesterone), the half-life of complexes was not the same under both experimental methods (Schrader et al., 1974). Thus, dissociation of hormone is not simple by itself. We conclude that the binding reaction probably involves some sort of "helper" site on the molecules whose occupancy may control access to the strong binding site.

TABLE II
Progesterone–Receptor Binding Kinetics[a]

Temperature	Rate constants			Equilibrium constant	
	Association $10^{-7} \times k_a$ ($M^{-1} s^{-1}$)	Dissociation $10^4 \times k_d$ (s^{-1})	Half-life from k_d (min)	from rates $10^9 \times k_d/k_a$ (M)	from Scatchard plot $10^9 \times K_d$ (M)
0	0.077	0.21	540	0.027	5.09
15	7.9	1.4	82	0.0018	5.59
24	405	4.9	24	0.00012	9.0
31	—	17	6.6	—	—
42	—	385	3.0	—	—

[a] From Hansen et al., 1976.

B. Purification and Properties of Receptor Proteins

We have developed techniques for purification of the progesterone receptor A and B subunits and the intact 6 S dimer by three independent methods (Kuhn et al., 1975; Schrader et al., 1977a; Coty et al., 1977). Details of methods for preparation of crude extracts and use of various chromatographic techniques have been covered in detail in earlier reviews and will not be discussed here (Schrader, 1975; Clark et al., 1976).

The receptor A subunit was purified to homogeneity, using a technique we have termed "differential chromatography" (Coty et al., 1977). This procedure takes advantage of the fact that the intact 6 S dimer does not bind to phosphocellulose or DNA-cellulose, while after dissociation the A subunit does. Since few proteins undergo such a dramatic alteration in binding behavior, this has proven to be an extremely powerful purification technique.

1. Purification of Receptor Subunit A

The purification procedure for the A protein consists of the following sequence of steps. First, a crude oviduct soluble cytoplasmic extract containing receptor aggregates is chromatographed on phosphocellulose and DNA-cellulose to remove proteins capable of binding to these resins. The receptor is then labeled by incubation with [^{3}H]progesterone and dissociated into A and B subunits by precipitation with ammonium sulfate at 30% saturation. The A and B subunits are separated by chromatography on DEAE-cellulose, and the A subunit is then subjected to the second phase of differential chromatography: rechromatography on DNA-cellulose and phosphocellulose. The A protein obtained by this procedure is purified approximately 20,000-fold to apparent homogeneity.

Analysis of the purified A subunit by SDS gel electrophoresis shows a single protein band with an apparent molecular weight (MW) of 79,000 g/mole as shown in Fig. 7. This polypeptide MW is in agreement with the native protein MW of 72,000 determined by the Svedberg equation from the sedimentation coefficient and Stokes radius (Coty et al., 1977; Sherman et al., 1976). Thus, the receptor A subunit appears to be a single polypeptide chain. The purity of the A protein was verified in a second denaturing gel electrophoresis system in the presence of acid and urea.

The A protein purified by differential chromatography retained the characteristics observed in crude and partially purified preparations. Values obtained for Stokes radius, sedimentation coefficient, rate of hormone dissociation, and hormone-binding specificity were in excellent agreement with previously reported values (Coty et al., 1977). Finally, the homogenous protein retains its ability to bind to DNA-cellulose.

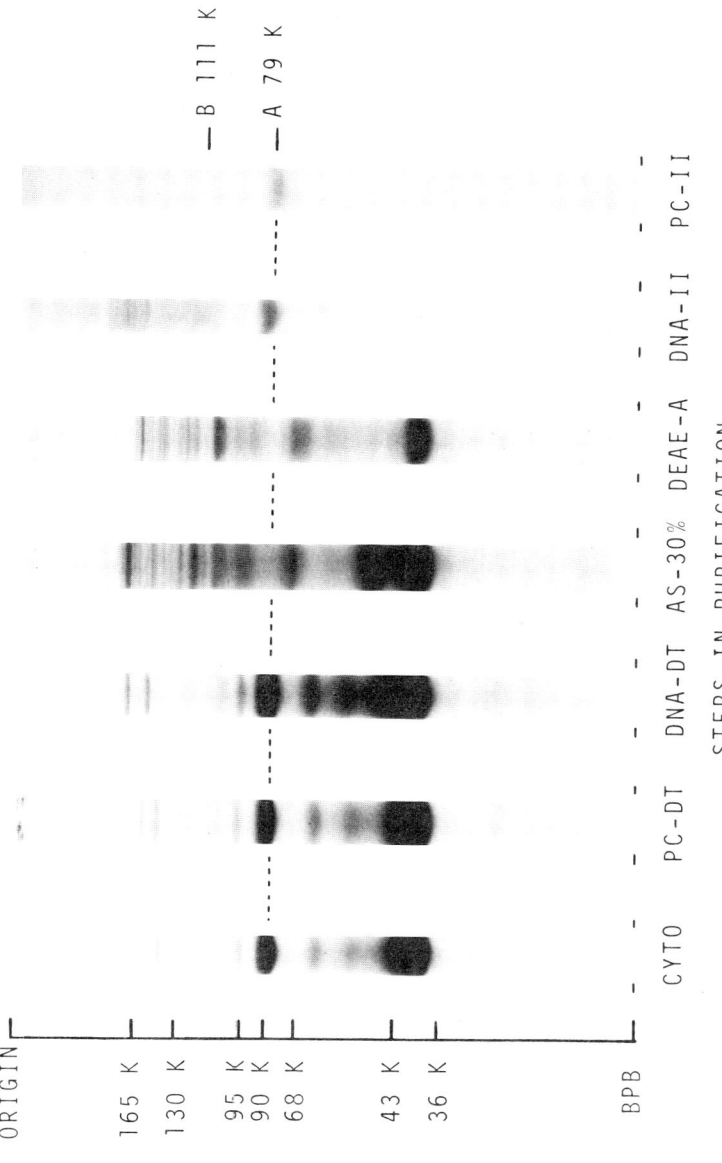

Fig. 7. SDS-polyacrylamide gel electrophoresis of steps in receptor subunit A purification. Aliquots of each step were denatured in 1% sodium dodecyl sulfate containing 100 mM 2-mercaptoethanol and run on 6% acrylamide gels containing 1% SDS. Gels were Cyto, crude cytosol; PC-DT, phosphocellulose drop-through; DNA-DT, DNA-cellulose drop-through; AS-30%, 30% saturation ammonium sulfate precipitate; DEAE-A, receptor A protein fraction eluting between 0.1 and 0.15 M KCl from DEAE; DNA-II, receptor A protein fraction eluting at 0.18 M KCl from DNA–cellulose; PC-II, receptor A protein fraction eluting at 0.26 M KCl from phosphocellulose. Molecular weight standards and migration of purified B protein are shown. From Coty et al., 1977.

2. Purification of Receptor Subunit B

We have obtained the progesterone receptor B subunit from laying hen oviduct by a series of conventional protein purification procedures (Schrader *et al.*, 1977a). Cytosol containing crude [^{3}H]progesterone-labeled receptor is precipitated with ammonium sulfate to 40% saturation. This material is then subjected to chromatography on DEAE–cellulose, phosphocellulose, hydroxylapatite, and agarose A-1.5 M columns.

The purity of this preparation was assessed by gel electrophoresis, as shown in Fig. 8. The B protein preparation exhibits a single stained band after electrophoresis in both a nondenaturing gel system and in the presence of SDS. In the native state, the bound [^{3}H]progesterone migrated with the same R_f as the protein band.

The MW determined by SDS gel electrophoresis is 117,000 g/mole. As in the case of the A subunit, the B protein appears to consist of a single polypeptide chain. The receptor B protein was also denatured with 6.0 M guanidine hydrochloride and analyzed by gel filtration. The MW by this method was in agreement with the value obtained from gel filtration and sucrose gradient ultracentrifugation (Kuhn *et al.*, 1977). After denaturation with guanidine hydrochloride and gel filtration, the B protein again migrated in SDS gels as a single polypeptide chain of MW 117,000 g/mole.

The purified receptor B subunit was also tested for functional activity. The B subunit labeled with [^{3}H]progesterone bound to both nuclei and chromatin with the same affinity exhibited by the crude and partially purified preparations, and did not bind to DNA (Kuhn *et al.*, 1977). In addition, the hormone-binding characteristics of the purified [^{3}H]progesterone-labeled B subunit were unchanged from those of the starting material (Schrader *et al.*, 1977a).

The receptor B subunit can be prepared from laying hen oviduct in sufficient quantities for physical and chemical analysis of the protein (Kuhn *et al.*, 1977). When we examined the B protein by electron microscopy, it appeared to have an elongated shape, with a long axis of 114 Å. A protein of these dimensions would have an MW of 106,000 g/mole which is in excellent agreement with values obtained by other methods. The asymmetric shape is also consistent with the hydrodynamic behavior of the B protein (Sherman *et al.*, 1970; Schrader and O'Malley, 1972).

The UV spectrum of the purified receptor B subunit shown in Fig. 9 exhibited a feature not characteristic of most proteins. The absorbance reached a peak at 280 nm, but did not significantly decline in the region between 280 and 250 nm. When the protein was denatured in guanidine hydrochloride and dialyzed, the absorbance at 250 nm decreased, indicating the loss of UV-absorbing ligand, progesterone. When we added an equimolar

8. Molecular Structure and Analysis of Progesterone Receptors

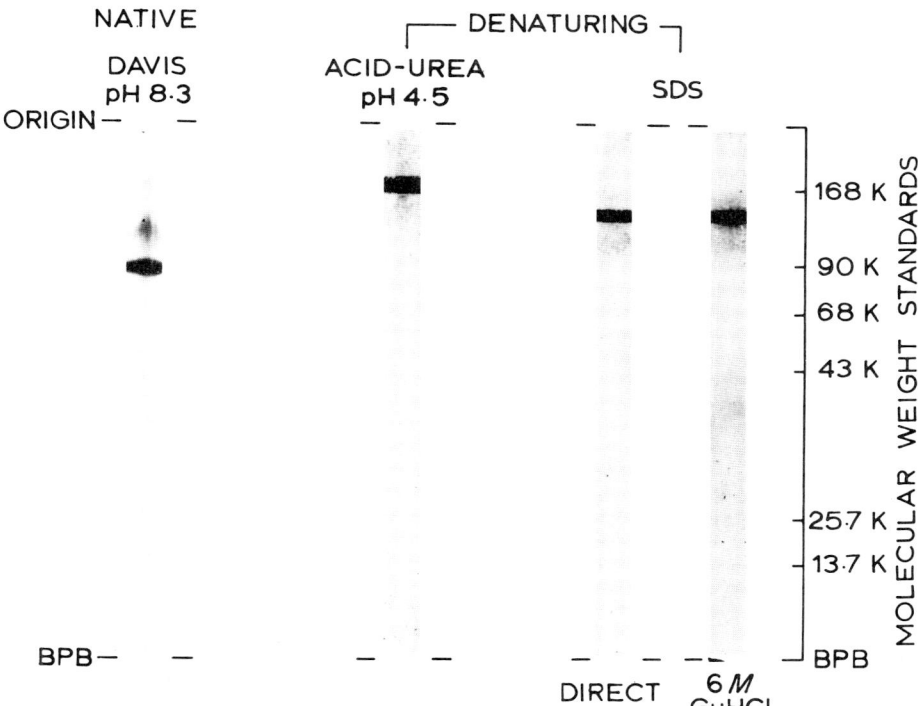

Fig. 8. Polyacrylamide gel electrophoresis of purified receptor B subunit from laying hen oviducts. Labeled receptor–hormone complexes were analyzed by three different gel systems. Left-hand gel: electrophoresis of the native labeled receptor B subunits on a 6.5% acrylamide gel at pH 8.3. One gel was stained for protein; a companion gel was sliced and counted for ^{3}H. The bar shows migration of the peak ^{3}H fraction and its comigration with the major protein band. Second gel from left: electrophoresis at pH 4.5 in 8.6 M urea on 6.6% acrylamide gel. Protein stained with amido black and destained electrophoretically. Third gel from left: SDS–polyacrylamide gel electrophoresis on 8.75% acrylamide in 1% SDS. Protein stained with Coomassie blue and destained by diffusion. Migration of molecular weight standards shown on right: 20 K marker shows lack of stainable band of "mero-receptor," produced if protease is present (Sherman *et al.*, 1974). Right-hand gel: SDS electrophoresis under same conditions of a receptor B sample after it was first chromatographed by gel filtration under highly denaturing conditions in 6 M guanidine hydrochloride and 100 mM 2-mercaptoethanol. Sample from the A-1.5 M column was detected by uv absorbance at 235 nm, pooled, dialyzed in 1% SDS, and electrophoresed. Again no subunits or fragments were seen. From Schrader *et al.*, 1976; Kuhn *et al.*, 1977.

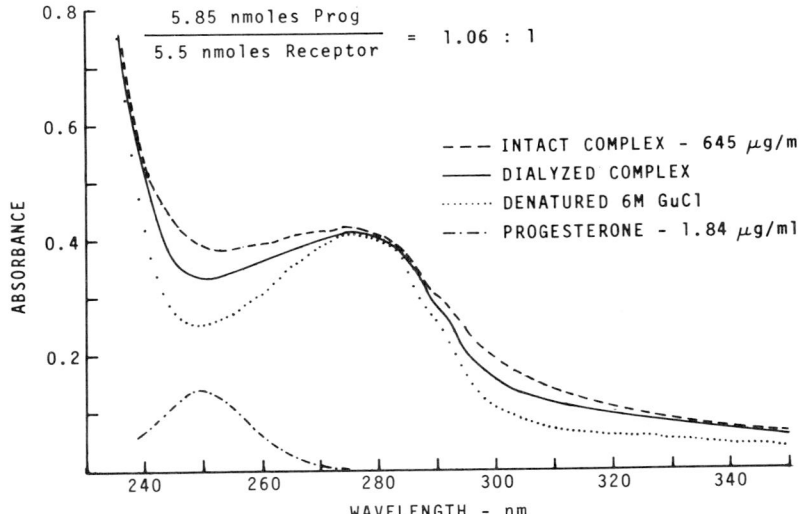

Fig. 9. UV spectra of pure receptor B subunits from laying hen oviducts (645 µg/ml): (---------), intact B receptor-hormone complexes immediately after isolation; (———) same preparation after dialysis first against 6 M guanidine HCl for 48 hours followed by dialysis into buffer; (-·--·--) spectrum of free progesterone (1.84 µg/ml) determined in the presence of guanidine-denatured receptor. From Kuhn *et al.*, 1977.

amount of progesterone to the denatured, dialyzed receptor protein, the original ratio of absorbance at 280 and 250 nm was restored. From the absorbance of receptor and progesterone, we calculated the stoichiometry of progesterone binding to be one molecule of progesterone bound per molecule of receptor B protein. If there is a similar stoichiometry of binding to the A subunit, then there are two progesterone binding sites in the intact 6 S dimer.

3. *Purification of Receptor A-B Dimers*

The purification procedures described above for receptor subunits are not appropriate for the intact 6 S dimer, due to the high salt concentrations necessary for elution of receptor from ion-exchange columns. We, therefore, employed the technique of steroid affinity chromatography (Kuhn *et al.*, 1975; Sica *et al.*, 1973). The resin used contains deoxycorticosterone hemisuccinate linked to Sepharose through a denatured bovine serum albumin (BSA) backbone. This BSA linkage allows multiple attachment points for the hormone to the support, resulting in a more stable resin, and performs a spacer function, allowing the hormone to be attached distant from the Sepharose beads.

The intact 6 S dimer was precipitated from oviduct cytosol with ammonium sulfate at 50% saturation. This removed enzymatic activities which cause release of deoxycorticosterone from the affinity resin. The receptor was redissolved in buffer A and incubated with the resin overnight at 0°C. The resin was then washed to remove unbound protein, and eluted with an excess of [^{3}H]progesterone (20 μM) as previously described (Kuhn et al., 1975). The affinity eluate was then purified by DEAE–Sephadex chromatography to yield receptor in homogeneous form. As shown in Fig. 10, two bands of equal intensity can be seen on SDS–polyacrylamide gels which comigrate with the A and B proteins prepared by the procedures described above.

One major problem encountered with this procedure has been low yield of receptor from the affinity resin. We have recently determined that this is due to extremely efficient coupling of steroid to the affinity resin. The yield of receptor obtained by Kuhn et al. (1975) from the affinity resin was approximately 70%. However, when resins containing as much as 20-fold more bound hormone were used, the yield was reduced to about 4%. The most effective way to overcome this problem is to limit coupling of steroid

Fig. 10. SDS–polyacrylamide gel electrophoresis of receptors obtained by affinity chromatography and DEAE–Sephadex ion exchange. Gel was 8.75% acrylamide containing 1% SDS, stained with Coomassie Blue. From Kuhn et al., 1975.

TABLE III
Molecular Properties of Receptor Forms[a]

Parameter	Method	A	B	Dimer
Sedimentation coefficient (s)	Sucrose gradient	3.6	4.2	6
Stokes radius R_s (Å)	Gel filtration	46	63	80
Frictional ratio (f/f_0)	s and R_s	1.74	1.9	—
Axial ratio (prolate ellipsoid)	s and R_s	14	18	—
Partial specific volume (cm³/g)	Buoyancy in NaBr	0.73	0.73	0.73
Diffusion coefficient $10^7 \times D$ (cm²/sec)	f/f_0	3.89	3.38	—
Molecular weight	s and R_s	71,000	114,000	205,000
	SDS gels	79,000	117,000	194,000
	EM	—	106,000	—
Particle dimensions (Å)	EM	—	114 × 29	—
Isoelectric point (pI)	Isoelectric focus	4.5	4.0	—
N-terminal amino acid	Dansyl chloride	Lysine	Lysine	2 Lys
Number of progesterone sites	UV spectroscopy	1	1	2
Percent α-helical content	Circular dichroism	—	12%	—
Nuclear-binding specificity	Receptor titration	DNA	Chromatin	Chromatin
K_d for nuclear interaction (M)	Receptor titration	—	1.5×10^{-9}	2×10^{-9}
Half-maximal effect on transcription (M)	Rifampicin challenge	50×10^{-9}	None	5×10^{-9}

[a] Values in this table were obtained from the following sources: Coty et al., 1977; Schrader et al., 1972, 1975a, 1976; Schrader and O'Malley, 1972; Kuhn et al., 1977; Sherman et al., 1970; Buller et al., 1975a,b, 1976b; Jaffe et al., 1975.

to the resin by lowering the concentration of the carbodiimide. In this way, the concentration of bound steroid can be kept low enough for reasonable recovery during elution.

The purity and concentration of intact 6 S dimer obtained by this procedure is adequate for use in the *in vitro* assay for chromatin transcription described below (Schwartz *et al.*, 1976). However since there is always dissociation of intact 6 S receptor into subunits, a final purification step was employed. The eluted receptors were passed through a small (0.4 ml) phosphocellulose column immediately before use. Monomers adsorbed to the resin, whereas intact 6 S dimers passed through the column unretarded.

The receptor subunits and intact dimer purified in this way have retained the characteristics of the cruder preparations. These are summarized in Table III.

III. EFFECTS OF PROGESTERONE *IN VIVO* ON CHROMATIN GENE TRANSCRIPTION

A. Assay of Chromatin RNA Initiation Sites

The capacity of oviduct chromatin to serve as a template for *Escherichia coli* RNA polymerase has previously been shown to increase following estrogen administration to the immature chick (Cox *et al.*, 1973; Spelsberg *et al.*, 1973). While chromatin template activity measurements may generally reflect the amount of DNA sequences made available to RNA polymerase, the components of such a reaction are so complex that these experiments shed little light on the biochemical mechanisms of hormone-induced alterations in gene transcription. In order to determine the effect *in vivo* of steroids on gene transcription in the chick oviduct, it appeared necessary to monitor all of the parameters involved in RNA synthesis. Second, in order to study the effect of steroid–receptor complexes on gene transcription, it was necessary to develop a quantitative *in vitro* transcription system (M. J. Tsai *et al.*, 1975). The procedure was adopted from studies carried out in prokaryotic systems and allows measurement of RNA chain initiation sites in chromatin.

The initiation of RNA synthesis can be divided into two basic processes. First, RNA polymerase binds randomly and reversibly to DNA to form a series of nonspecific complexes. However, after sufficient time and at a proper temperature, RNA polymerase binds proximal to an initiation region and forms a stable binary complex with DNA (Sippel and Hartman, 1970; Zillig *et al.*, 1970). This complex has undergone a transition involving the local destabilization of the DNA duplex structure and is now capable of rapidly initiating an RNA chain (Travers and et al., 1973). The second process is the actual initiation step in which RNA polymerase catalyzes the formation of the first phosphodiester bond between two nucleoside triphosphates.

The existence of stable RNA polymerase-DNA initiation complexes was elucidated through the use of the drug rifampicin (Hartman et al., 1967; Umezawa et al., 1968). Rifampicin is a competitive inhibitor of RNA synthesis, which acts prior to the formation of the first phosphodiester bond, but which has no effect on RNA chain elongation. RNA chain initiation by RNA polymerase bound to DNA in a stable initiation complex is so rapid that it can occur in the presence of the drug (Hinkle and Chamberlin, 1972). The fraction of RNA polymerase in stable complexes can be determined following the simultaneous addition of a mixture of rifampicin and the four ribonucleoside triphosphates (Chamberlin and Ring, 1972). RNA polymerase molecules that are free in solution or randomly bound to DNA will be inhibited by rifampicin. Under these conditions, reinitiation of RNA transcription will be completely inhibited and, thus, each RNA polymerase at a stable initiation site can synthesize one and only one RNA chain. By measuring the number of RNA chains made, the rifampicin challenge assay provides a method for quantitating the number of RNA polymerase initiation sites for a given template.

1. *The Rifampicin-Challenge Assay*

In order to test for the formation of stable RNA polymerase-DNA initiation complexes, increasing amounts of E. coli RNA polymerase (0–15 μg) were preincubated with a fixed amount of chick oviduct chromatin (5 μg) at 37°C for 15 minutes. The binary complexes were challenged by the addition of rifampicin (40 μg/ml) together with ribonucleoside triphosphates and allowed to synthesize RNA in the presence of heparin (200 μg/ml) for an additional 15 minutes at 37°C (M. J. Tsai et al., 1975; Cox, 1973). The number of RNA chains synthesized was determined from the amount and length of the RNA chains produced. The number of chains is equivalent to the number of initiation sites at which RNA polymerase was bound. By adding increasing amounts of RNA polymerase to a fixed amount of template, the total number of available initiation sites was determined from the saturation level of RNA synthesis (M. J. Tsai et al., 1975; S. Y. Tsai et al., 1975; Schwartz et al., 1975).

As described in Fig. 1, progesterone administration to immature chicks causes very slight changes in the oviduct unless the gland has first been differentiated by estrogen treatment. If this primary stimulation of the gland by estrogen is discontinued after differentiation has occurred, a subsequent (secondary) injection with progesterone mimics the estrogen effect

(Palmiter, 1973). Ovalbumin synthesis along with other processes is initiated again. This secondary stimulation with progesterone was studied as a beginning to measurement of the *in vitro* effects of purified receptors.

Estrogen-treated chicks were withdrawn from hormone treatment for 12 days and then restimulated with a single injection of progesterone (2.0 mg). Oviduct chromatin was isolated following secondary stimulation and assayed by the rifampicin-challenge technique to determine the number of RNA chain initiation sites. As shown in Table IV, withdrawn chromatin had about 8600 RNA initiation sites per picogram of DNA. Following a single injection of progesterone, a rapid increase in the number of initiation sites was found. Within a half-hour of hormone treatment, the number of initiation sites had nearly doubled to a level of 15,900 sites. After 1 hour of progesterone stimulation, a maximum of 23,000 initiation sites was detected. Thereafter, the number of initiation sites declined. During this time of intense transcriptional activity, the RNA chain propagation rate *in vitro* and the number average chain length of the RNA product did not vary significantly from the values seen for withdrawn oviduct chromatin. Therefore, the progesterone-induced increase in chromatin transcription in the oviduct was mainly due to a modulation in the number of available RNA polymerase initiation sites.

The stimulation was dependent upon the progesterone dose and was not further increased by a concomitant dose of estrogen. Thus, many of the progesterone and estrogen-responsive sites in the chromatin appeared to be identical in this specialized endocrine state.

TABLE IV

Effect of Progesterone Administration *in Vivo* on Chromatin RNA Initiation Sites[a]

Hours after progesterone administration[b]	Size of RNA product (nucleotides)	Initial elongation rate (nucleotides/sec)[c]	pmoles of RNA chains initiated per 5 μg chromatin[d]	Initiation sites per pg DNA
0	820	7.2	0.072	8,600
0.5	730	7.0	0.132	15,900
1	750	7.8	0.191	23,000
2	750	6.7	0.134	16,100
6	800	8.0	0.123	14,800
24	750	8.0	0.112	13,500

[a] From Schwartz *et al.*, 1976.

[b] Chicks were stimulated 12 days with estrogen, withdrawn for 10 days, and then injected with 2.0 mg of progesterone.

[c] Initial elongation rate determined for first minute of chain propagation.

[d] Amount of initiated chains calculated from total nucleotides incorporated at the transition point of RNA polymerase titration curves (M. J. Tsai *et al.*, 1975), assuming the new RNA contained 25% UMP. Average chain size assumed to be 770 nucleotides.

TABLE V

Effect of Progesterone Administration *in Vivo* on Levels of Ovalbumin mRNA Content of Withdrawn Chick Oviduct

Hours after progesterone administration	Number of molecules of mRNA$_{ov}$ per tubular gland cell
0	10
4	1200
10	2400
24	5400

[a] From Schwartz *et al.*, 1976.
[b] Progesterone was administered to withdrawn chicks (2 mg each) and animals killed, mRNA extracted, and assayed for mRNA ovalbumin by the method of Harris *et al.* (1975).

B. Assay of Ovalbumin mRNA Induction by Hybridization

A parallel study of this kind was done to monitor the product of a single hormone-responsive gene (Harris *et al.*, 1973). Ovalbumin mRNA is induced by estrogen in the gland *in vivo* (Woo *et al.*, 1975; Monohan *et al.*, 1976a). Extremely sensitive probes for this process have been developed, using radioactive complementary DNA (^{3}H-cDNA) synthesized *in vitro* from purified ovalbumin mRNA (Harris *et al.*, 1973; Monahan *et al.*, 1976b). The cDNA$_{ov}$ can be used in hybridization experiments to detect mRNA$_{ov}$ in amounts as little as 1 molecule per 100 cells.

Using this assay, progesterone was tested for its ability to induce ovalbumin mRNA following *in vivo* administration of the hormone. As shown in Table V, there was a dramatic increase in the number of mRNA$_{ov}$ molecules per cell after progesterone administration. Second, the time course for induction of ovalbumin mRNA was quite similar to that for total RNA initiation sites shown in Table IV. We concluded that this system could be used as a model for progesterone regulation of gene expression.

IV. EFFECT OF PURIFIED PROGESTERONE–RECEPTOR COMPLEXES *IN VITRO* ON CHROMATIN GENE TRANSCRIPTION

Nuclear uptake studies of receptor–hormone complexes *in vivo* (Anderson *et al.*, 1973; S. Y. Tsai *et al.*, 1975) and *in vitro* (Buller *et al.*, 1975a,b) had strongly indicated by correlation a role for the receptors in control of gene expression. However, due to the complexities of the system and the large number of contaminating enzyme activities in crude receptor preparations (Buller et al., 1976a; Moudgil and Toft, 1976; Schrader and O'Malley, 1977), these studies did not constitute a proof of receptor function.

A. Assay of Chromatin RNA Initiation Sites

With the availability of the *in vitro* chromatin transcription assay and of purified receptors, it was possible to test directly the effect of the receptor–hormone complexes on RNA synthesis in a cell-free system. *In vivo* progesterone administration caused a change in RNA initiation sites within 30 minutes. Therefore, if receptors mediated the process directly we would expect to see a rapid effect of receptor addition. To test this, we added intact, purified receptor–hormone complexes to the reconstituted cell-free system which contained the following purified components: progesterone–receptor complex, *E. coli* RNA polymerase, ribonucleotides, cofactors, heparin, and chromatin from withdrawn chicks (Schwartz et al., 1976).

1. Chromatin Titration with Receptor Complexes

A fixed concentration of withdrawn oviduct chromatin (5 µg) was preincubated with increasing quantities of purified progesterone–receptor complex (up to 1.1×10^{-8} M) for 30 minutes at 22°C. The intact 6 S receptors were purified by a modification of the affinity chromatography procedure described above (Kuhn et al., 1975). Receptors were first bound by preincubation with chick oviduct chromatin for 30 min at 22°C. The chromatin–receptor complexes were next incubated for an additional 30 minutes with a saturating concentration of RNA polymerase (15 µg) to allow for the formation of stable initiation complexes. Finally, rifampicin, heparin, and nucleotides were added for a 15-minute period of RNA synthesis. Figure 11 shows results of the titration experiments; RNA initiation sites increased in a receptor dose-dependent manner. The half-maximal stimulation occurred at a receptor concentration of 5×10^{-9} M. Saturation was reached at about 12×10^{-9} M receptors. This half-saturation value is indistinguishable from the K_{diss} determined for receptor binding to oviduct nuclei (Buller et al., 1975b) and to chromatin (Jaffe et al., 1975) as expected if the binding reaction is indeed related to receptor function in RNA synthesis. In addition, the incubation time required for maximal effect of receptors on chromatin was about 40 minutes (Buller et al., 1976b), the same as the time required for chromatin–receptor binding to reach a maximum (Jaffe et al., 1975).

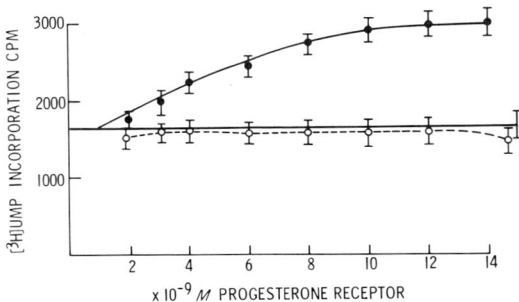

Fig. 11. Stimulation of oviduct chromatin RNA initiation sites by purified progesterone–receptor complexes. Cytosol used for affinity chromatography purification was either processed as described in the text (●———●) to prepare intact receptor 6 S dimers or was first complexed with nonradioactive progesterone (○--------○) to block receptor adsorption to the affinity resin. In the latter case, no receptors were retained by the column nor eluted from it. Both affinity column eluates were tested in the rifampicin challenge assay described in the text. Oviduct chromatin (5 μg DNA per point) was incubated with varying concentrations of receptor preparations for 30 minutes at 22°C. Then *E. coli* RNA polymerase (15 mg) was added in 100 μg/ml bovine serum albumin and 1 μmole of $MnCl_2$ and incubated for another 30 minutes at 22°C. After this preincubation period, RNA synthesis was begun by addition of 37.5 nmole each of ATP, GTP, CTP, and UTP, plus 10 μCi of [³H]UTP, 10 μg rifampicin, 0.1 μmole potassium phosphate, and 200 μg heparin. After 15 minutes incubation at 37°C, aliquots were spotted on DEAE filters (Whatman DE-81), and the filters were dropped into cold 0.5 M K_xPO_4 pH 9.0. The filters were washed and counted for ³H. Radioactive progesterone does not adsorb to the filters under these conditions. Chromatin without receptors added gave incorporation at the level shown by the solid line. Receptor concentration in the preparation not blocked by cold hormone was such that 50 μl in the assay was about 5×10^{-9} M receptor. From Schwartz *et al.*, 1976.

2. Characteristics of the Stimulatory Process

To test whether the receptor–hormone complexes were responsible for the stimulation, a second experiment was carried out. Crude progesterone receptors in cytosol were complexed with hormone before incubation with the steroid-affinity resin used in purification. With their progesterone sites already occupied by ligand, the receptor–hormone complexes in the cytosol were not retained by the resin. However, if the RNA stimulation was caused by a nonreceptor contaminant, the contaminant should not have been affected by progesterone pretreatment and should have still appeared in the affinity column eluate. As shown in Fig. 11, the precoupled receptor preparation did not contain any detectable receptor–hormone complexes and, significantly, did not stimulate RNA initiations in chromatin.

Since crude receptor preparations contain an enzyme polynucleotide polymerase which is template-independent (Buller *et al.*, 1976a), we tested the receptor-stimulated RNA reaction for its sensitivity to a variety of control conditions shown in Table VI. This table shows that RNA synthesized in the presence of receptor and chromatin was completely dependent upon template and inhibited by actinomycin D. Furthermore, none of the components alone contained significant synthetic activity and, hence, neither the chromatin, polymerase, or receptor was contaminated with other enzymes which were capable of incorporating [^{3}H]UTP into acid insoluble material. In these experiments, the progesterone receptor preincubated with chromatin in the presence of *E. coli* RNA polymerase increased RNA synthesis 50% over control values. With the addition of α-amanitin, a potent inhibitor of eukaryotic RNA polymerase II, there was little effect on the progesterone receptor-directed stimulation of RNA transcription. Thus, the stimulation of RNA synthesis also was not due to the activation of endogenous RNA polymerase which could have been a contaminant in chromatin preparations. Moreover, Table VI also shows that the increased RNA synthesis was dependent upon the native structure of the hormone–receptor complex, since neither free progesterone nor boiled receptor was effective in stimulating RNA synthesis.

3. *Requirements for Hormone on Receptor Proteins*

We also tested the requirement for hormone on the receptor proteins. Partially purified aporeceptors were prepared by a series of ion-exchange steps to about 500-fold purification. Half of the preparation was complexed

TABLE VI
Requirements for Receptor Stimulation of Chromatin RNA Initiation Sites[a]

Components added to assay	[^{3}H]UMP incorporated (cpm)[b]	Percent activity
Background		
RNA polymerase only (15 μg)	230	8
Polymerase plus progesterone–receptor complex (10^{-8} M)	400	14
Chromatin alone (5 μg as DNA)	200	7
Control		
Chromatin plus RNA polymerase	2730	100
Chromatin plus boiled receptor	2860	105
Chromatin plus 10^{-8} M free progesterone	2430	89
Experimental		
Chromatin plus polymerase plus 10^8 M receptor complexes	4100	150
Plus α-amanitin (10 μg)	3740	137
Plus actinomycin D (10 μg)	320	12

[a] From Schwartz *et al.*, 1976.
[b] Rifampicin challenge assay carried out as described in Table IV and legend of Fig. 11.

with progesterone, and half was not. In experiments not shown, the complexes stimulated chromatin initiation sites, whereas aporeceptors did not (Buller et al., 1976b). Thus, the stimulation of [^{3}H]UMP incorporation is due to a chromatin template-dependent process which is directly mediated by intact progesterone–receptor complexes.

In experiments not shown here, the same effects were observed using RNA polymerase II from hens; thus, the event appears independent of the source of polymerase. Measurement of RNA chain elongation rates and average RNA chain sizes synthesized *in vitro* in the presence of receptor showed that when RNA sites increased from 10,000/pg DNA to 15,000/pg, there was no increase in any of the other parameters (Schwartz et al., 1976). Thus, the effect of receptors appeared to be on the RNA chain initiation step.

4. *Alternative Assay Using Incorporation of* $\gamma[^{32}P]GTP$ *into RNA 5′-Termini*

Another assay of RNA chain initiation has also been used. Since each RNA chain begins with a triphosphate, incorporation of $\gamma[^{32}P]GTP$ into RNA (Maitra and Hurwitz, 1965) is also an index of chain starts. When this assay was used, the incorporation of $\gamma[^{32}P]GTP$ into 5′-termini increased by 50% in the presence of saturating amounts of receptor–hormone complexes (Schwartz et al., 1976). Thus, by this assay as well, purified receptors enhanced RNA initiation sites *in vitro*.

The kinetics of receptor binding to nuclei and to chromatin have been examined (Jaffe et al., 1975; Buller et al., 1975b). At 22°C, the binding reaction is nearly complete by 30 minutes. This time course was also observed for the receptor stimulation of RNA chain initiations to reach a maximum (Schwartz et al., 1976; Buller et al., 1976b).

B. Tissue Specificity

Previous studies have demonstrated a quantitative tissue specificity for binding of oviduct progesterone receptor complexes to nuclei and to chromatin (Spelsberg et al., 1971; Schrader et al., 1972; O'Malley et al., 1971; Buller et al., 1975a). It was of interest to investigate the ability of the receptor to stimulate RNA initiation sites in various chromatins. Figure 12 shows results of receptor titration of three different chick chromatins. Figure 12 also shows that the receptor effect was greatest on oviduct chromatin. At saturating levels of receptor, there was an increase of 4700 initiation sites per picogram of DNA in oviduct chromatin, but only 750 and 300 additional receptor-induced sites in liver and erythrocyte chromatin, respectively. It, thus, appears that the progesterone receptor-mediated effect is at

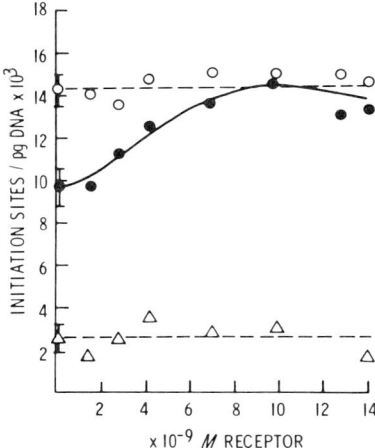

Fig. 12. Tissue specificity of receptor effect on RNA initiation sites in chromatin. Rifampicin challenge assay was used on 5 μg of chromatins (as DNA) from oviduct (●———●), liver (O--------O), and erythrocyte (△--------△). Purified 6 S receptor–hormone complexes added as shown here in the protocol described in Fig. 11 and in the text. Initiation sites determined from specific activity of [^{3}H]-UMP incorporated and number average chain length. An oviduct cell contains 1.3 μg DNA per haploid genome. From Schwartz et al., 1976.

least partly dependent on the presence of tissue-specific proteins in the oviduct chromatin. We hypothesize that these proteins are related to the nonhistone chromosomal proteins that convey quantitative tissue specificity for receptor binding and comprise a vital part of the chromatin "acceptor sites" for steroid hormone–receptor binding (Spelsberg et al., 1971).

C. Stimulation *in Vitro* of Ovalbumin mRNA Synthesis from Oviduct Chromatin

The foregoing experiments strongly support our hypothesis that receptor–hormone complexes function by direct regulation of RNA initiation in chromatin. Since progesterone can induce ovalbumin in withdrawn chicks, it was conceivable that the purified progesterone receptors could induce the ovalbumin gene in isolated oviduct chromatin. Such a demonstration would strongly reaffirm the notion that the *in vitro* receptor–chromatin interaction mimics the events *in vivo*. We have previously reported that chromatin from withdrawn chick oviduct was a poor template for the *in vitro* synthesis of ovalbumin mRNA (Harris et al., 1976). However, within 2 hours after a single injection of estrogen to withdrawn chicks, oviduct chromatin was capable of supporting the synthesis of ovalbumin mRNA sequences (Harris *et al.*, 1976; Tsai *et al.*, 1976). Ovalbumin mRNA synthesis required addition of RNA polymerase and was only detected in the chromatin prepared from progesterone-stimulated oviducts. These results implied that the ovalbumin gene in chromatin is inaccessible to RNA polymerase or "repressed" following hormone withdrawal and prior to hormonal stimulation. In contrast, stimulation by steroid hormones alters the chromatin template of the oviduct target cells in such a manner that the ovalbumin gene is open or available to be transcribed by RNA polymerase.

To extend these studies further, we then asked whether the purified progesterone receptor complex could directly stimulate the transcription of the ovalbumin gene in a cell-free system. The results of this experiment are shown in Table VII. Bulk amounts of RNA were synthesized from both withdrawn chromatin and from withdrawn chromatin incubated in the presence of progesterone receptor (1×10^{-8} M). Both RNA preparations were assayed for complementary sequences to ^{3}H-cDNA$_{ov}$ by the hybridization assay of Young *et al.* (1974). The RNA synthesized in the presence of receptor–hormone complex contained at least a 10-fold enrichment of mRNA sequences as compared to that found in untreated, withdrawn chromatin controls. It, thus, appears that a steroid–receptor complex may act directly on chromatin to enhance the number of initiation sites for RNA synthesis, leading to the synthesis of specific mRNA's for induced proteins.

D. Differential Activity of Receptor Subunits on Chromatin Transcription *in Vitro*

As discussed in an earlier section of this article, the progesterone receptor is a dimer composed of A and B subunits that have different and unique properties. The intact dimer (6 S) is located in the cytoplasm of the target cell in the absence of hormone stimulation and translocates to the nuclear

TABLE VII
Receptor Stimulation of Ovalbumin mRNA from Oviduct Chromatin *in Vitro*

Progesterone receptor added	RNA synthesized (μg)	pg of mRNA$_{ov}$ synthesized ($\times 10^{-3}$)	Percent mRNA$_{ov}$ in RNA	pg mRNA$_{ov}$ per μg DNA
None	125	1.9	0.0015	4.8
10^{-8} M	135	20	0.015	50

[a] From Schwartz *et al.*, 1976.

[b] Withdrawn oviduct chromatin (400 μg per tube) was preincubated with receptor for 30 minutes at 22°C. Then bulk RNA was synthesized at 22°C in absence of rifampicin. RNA was extracted with phenol and assayed for ovalbumin mRNA sequences by the procedure of Harris *et al.* (1975).

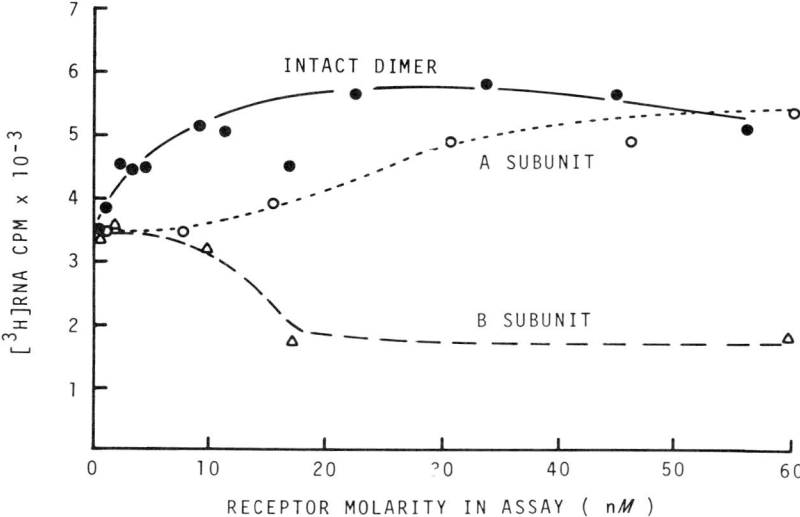

Fig. 13. Comparison of purified intact receptor A–B dimers with isolated A or B subunits. Effect of each on RNA initiation sites oviduct chromatin. Assay was done as described in Figs. 11 and 12, except 10 μg chromatin DNA per point. From Schrader et al., 1977c.

compartment upon administration of progesterone. Both the A and B subunits bind a molecule of hormone. The B subunit binds to the nonhistone protein–DNA complexes of oviduct chromatin, but not to pure DNA, while the A subunit binds to pure DNA, but poorly to chromatin. Accordingly these observations have led to the suggestion that the A subunit could be the actual gene regulatory protein and the B subunit could specify where the A protein is to localize. In the absence of the B component of the dimers, the A subunit alone should encounter difficulty in locating the specific initiation sites (genes) it is to regulate, while the B subunit alone should be totally inactive as a transcriptional stimulant.

To test these ideas, we prepared partially purified receptor subunits as well as intact A–B complexes and tested their activity in the chromatin transcription RNA initiation site assay (Buller et al., 1976b). The results are shown in Fig. 13. The intact receptor 6 S complexes stimulated RNA initiation sites in a saturable fashion, with a half maximal effect at 5×10^{-9} M receptor. When the individual subunits were tested, the B protein did not stimulate, even though the isolated protein binds to chromatin (Schrader et al., 1977a). At very high concentrations, the B protein became inhibitory in some experiments. The significance of this observation has not yet been established. The isolated A subunits, on the other hand, were incapable of stimulating transcription at low concentrations, but became active at high concentrations. The experiment was not carried out to high enough concentrations to determine if the A protein effect was saturable. Nor does the experiment indicate whether the sites induced by A are the same as those induced by the intact dimers. This determination must be done using hybridization probes to measure complexity of the new RNA's.

Finally, the requirements for 6 S receptor dimer were tested by comparing the effectiveness of intact complexes with a dissociated mixture of A and B. RNA initiation sites increased when saturating amounts of the dimer were used, but not when the A + B mixture was used. For reasons not clear at this time, we are unable to reconstitute active dimers from purified A and B; thus, in this experiment no 6 S receptors reformed in the mixture. We conclude from this experiment that the two subunits cannot act together unless coupled into the dimer form.

V. A PROPOSED MODEL FOR STEROID HORMONE REGULATION OF GENE TRANSCRIPTION

1. *Cytoplasmic Events*

The studies described above demonstrate a direct effect of receptor–hormone complexes on RNA initiation sites in target cell chromatin. Thus, our studies in the future will deal extensively with the mechanism by which this regulation occurs. In an attempt to formulate a working hypothesis for this work, we have proposed the scheme outlined in Fig. 14. Steroids enter target cells, probably by simple diffusion (Peck *et al.*, 1973) and bind to cytoplasmic receptor dimers. These 6 S dimers are presumably the physiological form in which receptors exist in the cell (Chamness and McGuire, 1972; Schrader *et al.*, 1975a). Based upon the dissociability of receptor aggregates during dialysis (see Fig. 3), we expect there is a low molecular weight coupling factor involved in their interaction. The nature of the factor is unknown, except that it may be the same factor as that which affects the elution of receptor subunit A from DEAE–cellulose (Schrader *et al.*, 1977b).

An unforeseen feature of this receptor dimer model is the requirement of two bound progesterone molecules per functional dimer, one on each subunit. Since receptors for estrogen in rat uterus also undergo a second-order association to produce 5 S molecules (Notides and Nielsen, 1974; Yamamoto, 1974), it is likely that this is a general feature of all steroid receptor systems.

Hormone binding to the intact complexes causes several changes in the receptor. There is as yet no known conformational change. However, at least three changes occur. First, hormone on the B subunit causes

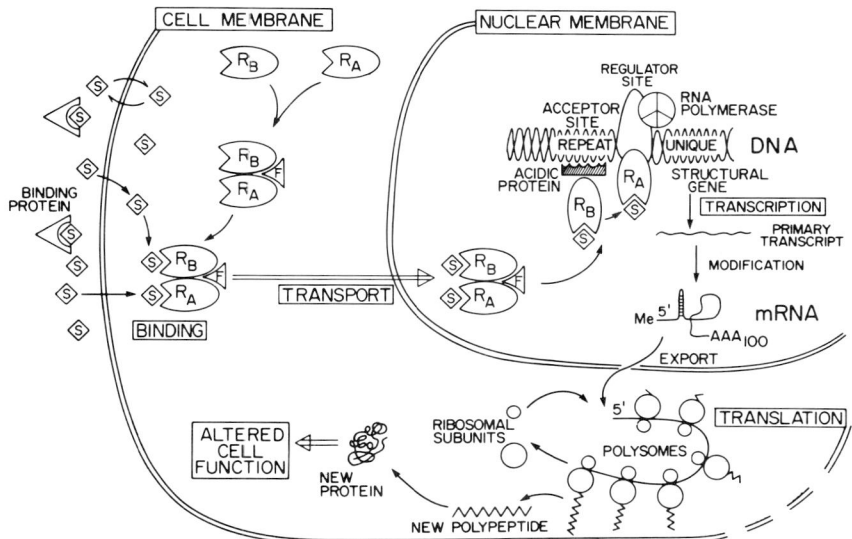

Fig. 14. Proposed model for steroid hormone effects on gene expression. Model details are discussed in the text; based upon chick oviduct progesterone receptor studies. R_B, receptor B subunit; R_A, receptor A subunit; F, low molecular weight coupling factor involved in subunit assembly; s, steroid. From Buller et al., 1976b.

expression of a chromatin acceptor–protein binding site (Schrader et al., 1972). Second, this chromatin affinity results in a net translocation of receptors to the nucleus, where the receptors bind to the chromatin (Buller et al., 1975b). It should be pointed out that the commonly held belief that receptors only enter the nucleus when complexed with progesterone has no experimental proof; the aporeceptors may, in fact, be everywhere in the cell, but only are retained by nuclei during isolation if hormone is present. The third effect of hormone is to render the receptor dimer metastable, as described in Figs. 4 and 5. This is not a complete loss of A–B interaction, however: sucrose-gradient centrifugation of the 6 S receptor–hormone complexes can be done.

2. Nuclear Events

The mechanism of transport of receptors through the nuclear membrane has not been studied adequately. From the effect of temperature on transport rates (Buller et al., 1975a,b) and of studies of receptor binding directly to isolated nuclear envelopes (Conn et al., 1977), it is not clear that a specific carrier mechanism exists. However, interesting studies of the involvement of ATP and inhibitors on nuclear uptake (Lohman and Toft,

1975) suggest the involvement of an energy-dependent or enzymatic step in uptake.

Following translocation to the cell nuclear compartment, the receptor dimers are envisioned to interact with the acceptor sites, which are target-cell specific, and present in limited numbers. These acceptors consist of the DNA complexed with specific nonhistone chromosomal proteins (Spelsberg et al., 1971, 1972, 1976). These we presume to be located proximal to each gene destined to be regulated by the receptors. Thus, the acceptors may serve as "flags" in the genome to attract the receptors to the proper genes. It will be interesting in the future to see whether these acceptors are, indeed, located in the interspersed middle-repetitive sequences of DNA, proposed as putative regulatory regions as described by Britten and Davidson (1969). Because of the B protein's putative role in directing the complexes to the proper loci, we have termed B the "specifier" subunit (O'Malley et al., 1973).

The model shows a single receptor interacting at an acceptor site. However, if the region is composed of repeated DNA an acceptor site may have multiple receptor-binding loci in it. This would have the advantage of enhancing the probability of a successful association between receptors and the gene in question. Second, such an arrangement would allow different genes to be activated at different rates or durations, merely due to differences in redundancy of their individual acceptor regions. It is interesting that Webster and co-workers (1976) recently reported that some acceptor regions may be masked in chromatin. Acceptor site redundancy might then be itself regulated at each gene by the degree of masking.

Following binding of the dimer to an acceptor site, the metastable A-B complex, itself devoid of DNA-binding activity (Fig. 6), may dissociate spontaneously to liberate the DNA-binding A protein in close proximity to the regulatory region of the gene. The A protein can then interact with the DNA, undergo some search process, and ultimately cause some change in the gene that allows its transcription by RNA polymerase. The model shown envisions the A protein acting at a specific locus as a positive regulatory element, analogous to the catabolite activator protein system in *E. coli* (Riggs et al., 1971). Two important criteria would need to be met for this analogy to hold: (a) the A protein might bind to specific DNA sequences, and (b) it may act as an unwinding protein, destabilizing the DNA sufficiently to allow formation of stable polymerase-DNA complexes. At the present time, our information on these points is insufficient to draw conclusions; the model remains a speculative, if attractive one.

A persistent problem in drawing analogies between the function of receptors and prokaryotic models is that of interaction between receptors and "nonoperator" DNA. How can the receptors search the enormous genome for a few thousand specific loci? The nature of the receptor dimer may well provide a clue to this mechanism. Since the DNA-binding site on the A subunit is occluded, no such interactions with incorrect DNA regions are to be expected until a receptor dissociation occurs. Since the B proteins already have been shown to have chromatin-binding specificity, the A proteins may, in fact, only search a small fraction of the genome, thus greatly improving the probability of a correct DNA interaction.

Finally, after initiation of a transcript, the receptors may dissociate from hormone and become nonfunctional, or probably may reside for some period of time in a functional state. The problems of receptor cycling and turnover are not considered further in the model. The messenger RNA output of each gene is probably processed, capped, and exported to the polysomes for translation. We feel on the basis of *in vitro* transcription studies (Schwartz *et al.*, 1976) that these RNA's probably are not functioning as informational regulators within the chromatin. Rather, the model predicts positive transcriptional control by the receptors.

3. *Expected Stoichiometry*

By comparing estimates of the number of acceptor sites for receptors and the number of RNA sites induced, some picture of the overall stoichiometry of hormone action can be obtained as shown in Table VIII. The numbers shown are crude estimates, probably with errors on the order of ±50%. However, grossly different techniques were used for each measurement. It is interesting to speculate from these data that the most likely stoichiometry is that each receptor-acceptor site is associated with an RNA initiation site

TABLE VIII
Stoichiometry of Hormone-Dependent Genetic Events in Chick Oviduct

Parameter	Method	No. per cell	Reference
Cytoplasmic progesterone receptors	Hormone titration	35,000	Sherman *et al.*, 1970
Nuclear acceptor sites	Receptor titration	25,000	Buller *et al.*, 1975a
Chromatin acceptor sites	Receptor titration	6,000	Jaffe *et al.*, 1975
RNA chain initiation sites[a]	Progesterone *in vivo*	14,000	Schwartz *et al.*, 1976
	Progesterone *in vitro*	9,400	Schwartz *et al.*, 1976
Poly(A)-RNA sequence[a] complexity	cDNA-poly(A) RNA back hybridization	11,000[b]	Monahan *et al.*, 1976b
Percent unique-sequence[a] DNA expressed	Nuclear RNA-excess hybridization	14,000[b]	Liarakos *et al.*, 1973

[a] The background of constitutive species not controlled by hormone has been subtracted.

[b] Determined for estrogen activity.

which, in turn, is associated with a single gene. Further analyses of this type will be forthcoming with the advent of purified hormone-responsive genes for study of these processes *in vitro*.

REFERENCES

Anderson, J. N., Peck, E. J., Jr. and Clark, J. H. (1973). *Endocrinology* **92**, 1488.
Britten, R. J., and Davidson, E. H. (1969). *Science* **165**, 349–357.
Buller, R. E., and O'Malley, B. W. (1976). *Biochem. Pharmacol.* **25**, 1–12.
Buller, R. E., Toft, D. O., Schrader, W. T., and O'Malley, B. W. (1975a). *J. Biol. Chem.* **250**, 801–808.
Buller, R. E., Schrader, W. T., and O'Malley, B. W. (1975b). *J. Biol. Chem.* **250**, 809–818.
Buller, R. E., Schwartz, R. J., and O'Malley, B. W. (1976a). *Biochem. Biophys. Res. Commun.* **69**, 106–113.
Buller, R. E., Schwartz, R. J., Schrader, W. T., and O'Malley, B. W. (1976b). *J. Biol. Chem.* **251**, 5178–5186.
Chamberlin, M. J., and Ring, J. (1972). *J. Mol. Biol.* **70**, 221–237.
Chamness, G. C., and McGuire, W. L. (1972). *Biochemistry* **11**, 2466–2472.
Chan, L., Means, A. R., and O'Malley, B. W. (1973). *Proc. Natl. Acad. Sci. U.S.A.* **70**, 1870.
Clark, J. H., Peck, E. J., Jr., Schrader, W. T., and O'Malley, B. W. (1976). *Methods Cancer Res.* **12**, 367–417.
Comstock, J. P., Rosenfeld, G. C., O'Malley, B. W., and Means, A. R. (1972). *Proc. Natl. Acad. Sci. U.S.A.* **69**, 2377.
Conn, P. M., Schrader, W. T., and O'Malley, B. W. (1977). *Endocrinology* (submitted for publication).
Coty, W. A., Schrader, W. T., and O'Malley, B. W. (1977). *J. Biol. Chem.* (submitted for publication).
Cox, R. F., Haines, M., and Carey, N. (1973). *Eur. J. Biochem.* **32**, 513.
Cox, R. F. (1973). *Eur. J. Biochem.* **39**, 49–61.
Hansen, P. E., Johnson, A., Schrader, W. T., and O'Malley, B. W. (1976). *J. Steroid Biochem.* **7**, 723–732.
Harris, S. E., Means, A. R., Mitchell, W. M., and O'Malley, B. W. (1973). *Proc. Natl. Acad. Sci. U.S.A.* **70**, 3776–3780.
Harris, S. E., Rosen, J. M., Means, A. R., and O'Malley, B. W. (1975). *Biochemistry* **14**, 2072.
Harris, S. E., Schwartz, R. J., Tsai, M. J., O'Malley, B. W., and Roy, A. K. (1976). *J. Biol. Chem.* **251**, 524–529.
Hartmann, H., Nonikel, K. O., Knüsel, F., and Nüesh, J. (1967). *Biochim. Biophys. Acta* **145**, 843–844.
Hinkle, D. C., and Chamberlin, M. J. (1972). *J. Mol. Biol.* **70**, 157–185.
Jaffe, R. C., Socher, S. H., and O'Malley, B. W. (1975). *Biochim. Biophys. Acta* **399**, 403–419.
Jensen, E. V., and De Sombre, E. R. (1974). *Vitam. Horm. (N.Y.)* **32**, 89–127.
Kuhn, R. W., Schrader, W. T., and O'Malley, B. W. (1975). *J. Biol. Chem.* **250**, 4220–4228.
Kuhn, R. W., Schrader, W. T., Coty, W. A., Conn, P. M., and O'Malley, B. W. (1977). *J. Biol. Chem.* **252**, 308–317.
Liarakos, C. D., Rosen, J. M., and O'Malley, B. W. (1973). *Biochemistry* **13**, 2809.

Lill, H., Lill, U., Sippel, A., and Hartmann, G. (1970). *In* "RNA Polymerase and Transcription" (L. G. Silvestri, ed.), Lepetit Colloq., p. 55. North-Holland Publ., Amsterdam.
Lohman, P. H., and Toft, D. O. (1975). *Biochem. Biophys. Res. Commun.* **67**, 8–15.
Maitra, U., and Hurwitz, J. (1965). *Proc. Natl. Acad. Sci. U.S.A.* **54**, 815–822.
Means, A. R., Comstock, J. P., Rosenfeld, G. C., and O'Malley, B. W. (1972). *Proc. Natl. Acad. Sci. U.S.A.* **69**, 1146.
Monahan, J. J., Harris, S. E., and O'Malley, B. W. (1976a). *J. Biol. Chem.* **251**, 3738–3748.
Monahan, J. J., Harris, S. E., Woo, S. L. C., Robertson, D. L., and O'Malley, B. W. (1976b). *Biochemistry* **15**, 223–233.
Moudgil, V. K., and Toft, D. O. (1976). *Proc. Natl. Acad. Sci. U.S.A.* **73**, 3443–3447.
Norris, J. S., and Kohler, P. O. (1976). *Science* **192**, 898–900.
Notides, A. C., and Nielsen, S. (1974). *J. Biol. Chem.* **249**, 1866–1873.
O'Malley, B. W., and McGuire, W. L. (1968). *Proc. Natl. Acad. Sci. U.S.A.* **60**, 1527.
O'Malley, B. W., and Means, A. R. (1974). *Science* **183**, 610–620.
O'Malley, B. W., and Schrader, W. T. (1972). *J. Steroid Biochem.* **3**, 617–629.
O'Malley, B. W., McGuire, W. L., Kohler, P. O., and Korenman, S. G. (1969). *Recent Prog. Horm. Res.* **25**, 105–160.
O'Malley, B. W., Toft, D. O., and Sherman, M. R. (1971). *J. Biol. Chem.* **246**, 1117–1122.
O'Malley, B. W., Spelsberg, T. C., Schrader, W. T., Chytil, F., and Steggles, A. W. (1972). *Nature (London)* **235**, 141–144.
O'Malley, B. W., Schrader, W. T., and Spelsberg, T. C. (1973). *In* "Receptors for Reproductive Hormones" (B. W. O'Malley and A. R. Means, eds.), pp. 174–196. Plenum, New York.
Palmiter, R. D. (1973). *J. Biol. Chem.* **248**, 8260.
Peck, E. J., Jr., De Liberio, J., Richards, R., and Clark, J. H. (1973). *Biochemistry* **12**, 4596–4603.
Rhoads, R. E., McKnight, G. S., and Schimke, R. T. (1971). *J. Biol. Chem.* **246**, 7407.
Riggs, A., Reiness, G., and Zubay, G. (1971). *Proc. Natl. Acad. Sci. U.S.A.* **68**, 1222.
Rosenfeld, G. C., Comstock, J. P., Means, A. R., and O'Malley, B. W. (1972). *Biochem. Biophys. Res. Commun.* **46**, 1695–1703.
Schrader, W. T. (1975). *In* "Methods in Enzymology" (B. W. O'Malley and J. G. Hardman, eds.), Vol. 36, pp. 187–211. Academic Press, New York.
Schrader, W. T., and O'Malley, B. W. (1972). *J. Biol. Chem.* **247**, 51–59.
Schrader, W. T., and O'Malley, B. W. (1977). *Biochem. Biophys. Res. Commun.* (submitted for publication).
Schrader, W. T., Toft, D. O., and O'Malley, B. W. (1972). *J. Biol. Chem.* **241**, 2401–2407.
Schrader, W. T., Buller, R. E., Kuhn, R. W., and O'Malley, B. W. (1974). *J. Steroid Biochem.* **5**, 989–999.
Schrader, W. T., Heuer, S. H., and O'Malley, B. W. (1975a). *Biol. Reprod.* **12**, 134–142.
Schrader, W. T., Socher, S. H., and Buller, R. E. (1975b). *In* "Methods in Enzymology" (B. W. O'Malley and J. G. Hardman, eds.), Vol. 36, pp. 292–313. Academic Press, New York.
Schrader, W. T., Kuhn, R. W., and O'Malley, B. W. (1977a). *J. Biol. Chem.* **252**, 299–307.
Schrader, W. T., Coty, W. A., Smith, R. G., and O'Malley, B. W. (1977b). *Ann. N.Y. Acad. Sci.* **286**, 64–80.
Schrader, W. T., Kuhn, R. W., Buller, R. E., Schwartz, R. J., and O'Malley, B. W. (1977c). *In* "Receptors in Pharmacology" (J. R. Smythies, ed.). Dekker, New York (in press).
Schwartz, R. J., Tsai, M. J., Tsai, S. Y., and O'Malley, B. W. (1975). *J. Biol. Chem.* **250**, 5175.

Schwartz, R. J., Kuhn, R. W., Buller, R. E., Schrader, W. T., and O'Malley, B. W. (1976). *J. Biol. Chem.* **251**, 5166–5177.

Sherman, M. R., Corvol, P. L., and O'Malley, B. W. (1970). *J. Biol. Chem.* **245**, 6068–6096.

Sherman, M. R., Atienza, S. B. P., Shansky, J. R., and Hoffman, L. M. (1974). *J. Biol. Chem.* **249**, 5351–5363.

Sherman, M. R., Tuazon, F. B., Diaz, S. C., and Mither, L. K. (1976). *Biochemistry* **15**, 980–989.

Sica, V., Parikh, I., Nola, E., Puca, G. A., and Cuatrecasas, P. (1973). *J. Biol. Chem.* **248**, 6543–6558.

Sippel, A. E., and Hartman, G. R. (1970). *Eur. J. Biochem.* **16**, 152–157.

Smith, H. E., Smith, R. G., Toft, D. O., Neergand, J. R., Burrows, E. P., and O'Malley, B. W. (1974). *J. Biol. Chem.* **249**, 5924–5932.

Spelsberg, T. C., Steggles, A. W., and O'Malley, B. W. (1971). *J. Biol. Chem.* **246**, 4188–4197.

Spelsberg, T. C., Steggles, A. W., Chytil, F., and O'Malley, B. W. (1972). *J. Biol. Chem.* **247**, 1368–1374.

Spelsberg, T. C., Mitchell, W. M., Chytil, F., Wilson, E. M., and O'Malley, B. W. (1973). *Biochim. Biophys. Acta* **312**, 765–768.

Spelsberg, T. C., Pikler, G. M., and Webster, R. A. (1976). *Science* **194**, 197–199.

Stancel, G. M., Leung, K. M. T., and Gorski, J. (1973). *Biochemistry* **12**, 2130–2136.

Travers, A., Baillie, D. L., and Pedersen, S. (1973). *Nature (London), New Biol.* **243**, 161–163.

Tsai, M. J., Schwartz, R. J., Tsai, S. Y., and O'Malley, B. W. (1975). *J. Biol. Chem.* **250**, 5165–5174.

Tsai, S. Y., Tsai, M. J., Schwartz, R. J., Kalimi, M., Clark, J. H., and O'Malley, B. W. (1975). *Proc. Natl. Acad. Sci. U.S.A.* **72**, 4228–4232.

Tsai, S. Y., Harris, S. E., Tsai, M. J., and O'Malley, B. W. (1976). *J. Biol. Chem.* **251**, 4713–4721.

Umezawa, H., Mizumo, S., Uamasaki, H., and Hitta, K. (1968). *J. Antibiot.* **21**, 234–235.

Webster, R. A., Pikler, G. M., and Spelsberg, T. C. (1976). *Biochem. J.* **156**, 409.

Woo, S. L. C., Rosen, J. M., Liarakos, C. D., Choi, Y. C., Busch, H., Means, A. R., and O'Malley, B. W. (1975). *J. Biol. Chem.* **250**, 7027–7039.

Yamamoto, K. R. (1974). *J. Biol. Chem.* **249**, 7068–7075.

Young, B. D., Harrison, P. R., Gilmour, R. S., Birnie, G. D., Hell, A., Humphries, S., and Paul, J. (1974). *J. Mol. Biol.* **84**, 555–568.

Zillig, W., Zechel, D., Rabussay, Schachner, M., Sethi, V. S., Palm, P., Heil, A., and Seifert, W. (1970). *Cold Spring Harbor Symp. Quant. Biol.* **35**, 47–58.

9

Studies on the Cytoplasmic Glucocorticoid Receptor and Its Nuclear Interaction in Mediating Induction of Tryptophan Oxygenase Messenger RNA in Liver and Hepatoma

PHILIP FEIGELSON,
LEELAVATI RAMANARAYANAN-MURTHY,
AND PAUL D. COLMAN

I.	Introduction	226
II.	Glucocorticoid Receptor	227
	A. Physical and Chemical Properties of the Glucocorticoid Receptor	228
	B. Stereospecificity of Steroid Binding to the Receptor	230
	C. Properties of the Steroid–Receptor Complex: Transformation to a Nuclear Binding Complex	232
III.	Metabolic Effects of Glucocorticoids	238
IV.	Control of Specific Species of mRNA by Glucocorticoids	238
V.	Glucocorticoidal Control of the mRNA for Tryptophan Oxygenase in Hepatomas	243
VI.	Interaction of the Receptor with Nuclear Components	246
VII.	Conclusions	247
	References	248

I. INTRODUCTION

A cell's genetic information is encoded in the base sequences of the nucleotides that constitute its DNA. This information is selectively utilized when the cell transcribes certain portions of these nucleotide sequences generating complementary strands of RNA, which, in turn, are translated into the primary sequences of amino acids that form the individual proteins. In embryonic development, a single fertilized egg gives rise to a vast variety of differential cells with specialized proteins and functions; yet the DNA in each of the specialized cell types is apparently identical. In general, less than 10% of the total genetic information is expressed within any eukaryotic cell. Quantitative and even qualitative control over the cellular enzymes and other proteins being synthesized are exerted by specific hormones. The important role played by steroid hormones in development and physiological regulation in animals has led investigators over the past few decades to attempt to unravel and understand the molecular mechanisms involved in their function. Several studies have shown that steroid hormones, including the glucocorticoids, bind with high affinity to specific receptor proteins in the target cell cytoplasm. The glucocorticoid-receptor complex has been shown to undergo an alteration to an "activated" state that has high affinity for chromosomal sites within the cell nucleus. This glucocorticoid-receptor interaction with the genome accompanies and is presumed to be responsible for the cellular responses characteristic of the hormone in its target tissues. Furthermore, the receptor proteins promise to be useful in elucidating genetic control mechanisms and to serve as probes to explore the organization and structure of the eukaryotic chromosomes.

Considerable information exists concerning the cellular and metabolic alterations evoked by glucocorticoid hormones acting upon responsive tissues. Extensive efforts are under way, devoted to gaining understanding of the molecular processes underlying these hormonally induced alterations. Over the past few years, every possible control mechanism has been advocated, including transcriptional control, translational control, and hormone-controlled cytoplasmic and nuclear receptors and changes in enzyme and mRNA stabilities. The recent and ongoing rapid developments in molecular biology have provided interesting concepts and hypotheses concerning gene expression and its control. New experimental tools that allow direct measurements of cellular parameters, such as measurement of specific species of mRNA, have allowed us to distinguish between these hypotheses.

The present model explaining glucocorticoid hormone action proposes the following sequence of events: (a) the hormone enters the target cell; (b) within the target cell the hormone interacts with its receptor; (c) the cytoplasmic receptor, when complexed with the hormone, translocates into the nucleus; (d) these events precede and lead to subtle alterations in the pattern of gene transcription; and (e) the altered enzyme or other protein levels which ensue effectuate the hormonally evoked cellular and physiological responses. Using the biochemical techniques presently available, the first three of these processes have been confirmed. All findings to date with respect to the glucocorticoid hormones are compatible with the fourth and fifth postulates as well. However, it must be recognized that detailed understanding of these processes still remains to be established. Ongoing investigations toward understanding the molecular mechanisms involved are focused upon the chemical nature of the cytoplasmic receptor, particularly with respect to its molecular structure, which enables specific interaction with the steroid hormone and chromatin, the chemistry of the changes in the cytoplasmic steroid–receptor complex as it undergoes "activation," the processes underlying translocation of the activated cytoplasmic receptor into the nucleus, identification of the specific nuclear sites with which it interacts, particularly with respect to the role of the chromosomal proteins, and of specific base sequences within DNA, a clarification of the molecular events which subsequently ensue in the nucleus, enabling putatively specific hormonally regulated gene transcription, a description of the processing of the gene transcript and its ultimate cytoplasmic translation into the hormonally induced enzyme protein. This article reviews studies of our laboratory, attempting to elucidate the biochemical processes by which the glucocorticoids regulate hepatic enzyme levels.

II. GLUCOCORTICOID RECEPTOR

It is generally accepted that hormones exert their physiological effects following complex formation with specific target cell proteins. In the case of steroids, as originally described for estrogen (Jensen and Jacobson, 1962), these proteins are soluble cytoplasmic components of target tissues capable of interacting with high affinity and stereospecificity with the biologically active steroid. The existence of soluble, intracellular proteins which bind other steroid hormones, i.e., progesterone, aldosterone, dihydrotestosterone, have since been documented (Tomkins *et al.,* 1969; Feldman *et al.,* 1972; Jensen and De Sombre, 1973; O'Malley and Means, 1974; King and Mainwaring, 1974). Intracellular proteins that bind their hormones with high affinity and stereospecificity and which participate in the biochemical processes leading to biologically meaningful alterations in cellular function may be considered to be "hormone receptors."

Rat liver contains three soluble proteins which bind natural glucocorticoids (Beato and Feigelson, 1972). One of these cytosol proteins is identical with serum transcortin, also known as corticosteroid-binding globulin (CBG). Another liver cytosol protein, the "B" protein, also binds the natural glucocorticoids and cross-reacts with antibodies prepared to serum transcortin, and is likely to be structurally related to it (Koblinsky, 1973). Like many other serum proteins, transcortin is synthesized in the liver and is released into the plasma (Westphal, 1971). It is not known whether the B protein, which is immunologically related to transcortin, is a precursor of or is derived from transcortin or whether it has another biosynthetic origin. Both transcortin and the B protein bind naturally occurring glucocorticoids, such as corticosterone and hydrocortisone, but neither bind the synthetic fluorinated glucocorticoids, such as dexamethasone and triamcinolone, compounds which are highly potent glucocorticoids *in vivo*.

There is a third protein present in hepatic cytosol, which binds the natural glucocorticoids and which also has very high affinity for the highly active synthetic 9α-fluorinated glucocorticoids. Several lines of evidence testify that it is this third cytoplasmic protein that is the glucocorticoid receptor which serves the physiological function of mediating glucocorticoidal action. It is believed to be the biologically significant glucocorticoid receptor by virtue of the following four observations:

1. It has specific high affinity saturable binding for natural, as well as synthetic, biologically active glucocorticoids (Koblinsky *et al.*, 1972). Beato Kalimi and Feigelson, 1972).

2. As a steroid–receptor complex it undergoes a time-and-temperature-dependent calcium ion enhanced "activation" enabling its binding to nuclei, chromatin, and stripped DNA (Kalimi *et al.*, 1975).

3. Both *in vivo* and *in vitro* its subcellular translocation from the cytoplasm to the nucleus is a function of its saturation with glucocorticoid (Beato *et al.*, 1974); and

4. Time-course and steroid dosage experiments *in vivo* indicate parallel saturation of steroid receptor with hormonal induction of rat liver tryptophan–oxygenase catalytic activity (Beato *et al.*, 1972) and hormonally induced specific mRNA level (Schutz *et al.*, 1972, 1973).

A. Physical and Chemical Properties of the Glucocorticoid Receptor

Unlike transcortin, which in sucrose density-gradient centrifugation sediments at 4 S independently of ionic strength, the hepatic dexamethasone-binding protein sediments in low salt gradients primarily as a 7 S complex which reverts reversibly to the lighter 4 S species in the presence of 0.3 M NaCl. A similar salt-dependent dissociation is demonstrable by gel-filtration chromatography of the dexamethasone-binding protein through Sephadex G-200. A comparable and presumably identical dexamethasone-binding protein exists in other glucocorticoid-responsive tissues, such as kidney and thymus, and to a much lesser extent in spleen, lung, heart, and testis (Beato and Feigelson, 1972).

A summary of the physical characteristics and molecular properties for the three glucocorticoid-binding components from rat liver cytosol is presented in Table I (Koblinsky et al., 1972).

The sensitivity of transcortin, the B protein, and the receptor to various degradative enzymes is summarized in Table II. It can be seen that nucleases, lipase, collagenase, hyaluronidase, and neuraminidase do not affect these steroid-binding components, whereas all the proteases tested caused a marked reduction in specific steroid-binding capacities (Koblinsky et al., 1972), thus indicating that the glucocorticoid receptor is a protein with no other detectable functional moieties.

Presented in Table III are the equilibrium association constants and derived thermodynamic parameters for the three glucocorticoid-binding proteins of rat liver. Furthermore, at all temperatures studied, the binding of cortisol to transcortin and to the B protein was accompanied by a negative change in entropy, while binding of dexamethasone to the receptor results in a positive entropy change. This difference in the entropy contribution to the free energy of binding indicates that the receptor interacts differently with glucocorticoids than to transcortin and the B protein (Koblinsky et al., 1972). It has been previously reported (Westphal, 1971) that the binding of cortisol to serum transcortin is accompanied by a nega-

TABLE I

Physical Parameters of Glucocorticoid-Binding Proteins of Rat Liver Cytosol and Serum Transcortin[a]

Physical parameter	Liver transcortin	B protein	Serum transcortin	Receptor protein	
				0.1 μ	0.3 μ
Stokes radius (a) (Å)	29.7	36.7	36.6	45	39
Sedimentation coefficient ($s_{20,w}$)	4.1	4.2	4.2	7.0	4.1
Partial specific volume (v_{20}) (ml/g)	0.729	0.729	0.723		
Molecular weight (MW) $\times 10^{-3}$	51.3	64.1	62.6	200	66.0
Frictional ratio (f/f_0)	1.11	1.28	1.29		1.35
Isoelectric point	5.1	4.3			

[a] From Koblinsky et al., 1972.

TABLE II

Effects of Hydrolytic Enzymes upon Glucocorticoid-Binding Proteins of Rat Liver Cytosol[a]

Enzymatic pretreatment	[³H]Cortisol bound (%)		[³H]Dexamethasone bound (%)
	Transcortin	B protein	Receptor
None	100	100	100
Deoxyribonuclease	100	100	110
Ribonuclease	100	100	109
Pronase	3	0.5	43
Papain	83	50	7
Trypsin	14	2	1
Chymotrypsin	8	3	0
Neuraminidase (*Vibrio cholerae*)	92	115	108
Neuraminidase (*Clostridium perfringens*)			85
Hyaluronidase			78
Collagenase	71	100	82
Lipase	103	86	104

[a] From Koblinsky et al., 1972.

tive entropy change, which is consistent with what we observe for hepatic transcortin and the B protein. It is interesting to note that the binding of various steroids to serum albumin demonstrates a positive entropy change similar to that for dexamethasone-binding to the receptor. An explanation for this positive entropy change, associated with steroid binding, may be the displacement of relatively ordered protein-bound water from the receptor steroid-binding site.

B. Stereospecificity of Steroid Binding to the Receptor

Competition binding experiments employing a wide spectrum of steroid analogues lead to the following conclusions governing stereospecificity of

TABLE III

Thermodynamic Parameters of Glucocorticoid Binding to Rat Liver Cytosol Proteins[a]

Sample	Steroid	$K_9 \times 10^8$	ΔG (kcal/mole)	ΔH (kcal/mole)	ΔS (cal/mole)
Receptor	[³H]Dexamethasone	7.3	−11.0	−6.1	18.0
Transcortin	[³H]Corticosterone	30.2	−11.8	−23.7	−43.4
B protein	[³H]Corticosterone	9.6	−11.2	−19.2	−29.1

[a] From Koblinsky, 1973.

the receptor's binding site for glucocorticoids (Koblinsky, 1973):

1. The planar structure of the α,β-unsaturated ketone in the A ring is essential for steroid binding to all three hepatic cortisol-binding components.

2. Aromatization of the A ring, with loss of the 3-keto moiety, imparting planarity to the A ring, prevents steroid binding to transcortin, the B protein, and the receptor. The introduction of a single, double bond between C-1 and C-2 in the A ring, reduces considerably the binding to both transcortin and the B protein while enhancing steroid binding to the receptor. Examples of this kind of substitution are in prednisolone and prednisone.

3. Substitutions on the alpha-side of the steroid decreases or eliminates binding to transcortin and the B protein, while enhancing the affinity of the steroid for the receptor. Such polar groups as 9α-F or 14α-OH inhibits the binding to transcortin; even the insertion of a hydrophobic methyl group into the 6α-position decreased the affinity to both transcortin and the B protein. These same substitutions, however, enhance binding to the receptor.

4. The 17α-OH appears nonessential for binding to these three hepatic proteins. Its presence on the alpha-side actually decreases the affinity for all steroids tested, including cortisol, 17α-OH progesterone, and cortexalone.

5. The substitution of the 11β-OH function by a ketone group, as in cortisone, interferes with the binding to all three proteins. Complete elimination of the 11-oxyfunction imparts a greater loss in affinity to the receptor protein than to transcortin or the B protein.

6. The oxidation state of the oxygen atoms in the side chain is more important for the binding of glucocorticoids to the glucocorticoid receptor than it is for steroid binding to transcortin or the B protein. For example, substitution of the C-20 keto group with a hydroxyl group or oxidation of the C-21 OH to an aldehyde completely eliminates binding to the receptor but still allows considerable binding to transcortin. However, substituting a methyl group for the C-21 hydroxyl, as with 11β-OH progesterone, does not greatly affect binding to any of the three proteins. Acetylation at C-21 interfers more markedly with the binding to the receptor protein than to transcortin and the B protein. Esterification of the C-21 hydroxyl with succinate resulting in a charged side chain still allows binding to transcortin and the B protein, while it eliminates binding to the receptor.

In summary, the competition analysis reviewed above indicates that the binding of glucocorticoid to transcortin and the B protein most likely involves hydrophobic interaction with the α-side, while the glucocorticoid receptor interacts with the β-side of the steroid, requiring the 3-keto, the 11β-OH, and the α-ketol $C_{20,21}$ side chain (Koblinsky, 1973).

C. PROPERTIES OF THE STEROID–RECEPTOR COMPLEX: TRANSFORMATION TO A NUCLEAR BINDING COMPLEX

As indicated above, a variety of studies have demonstrated that the receptor protein of hepatic cytosol has high affinity and stereospecificity to glucocorticoid hormones, both natural and synthetic. The degree of saturation *in vivo* of this cytoplasmic receptor by steroid coincides with its inducing effects upon tryptophan oxygenase and tyrosine aminotransferase (Beato *et al.*, 1972).

The glucocorticoid–receptor complex from hepatoma will bind to free DNA (Baxter *et al.*, 1972). Comparable results with estrogen and aldosterone receptors have demonstrated that a temperature-dependent process is required to convert those steroid–receptor complexes to the form capable of interacting with DNA (Gorski *et al.*, 1968); Anderson and Liao, 1968). As depicted in Fig. 1 (Kalimi *et al.*, 1975), a similar phenomenon is manifested

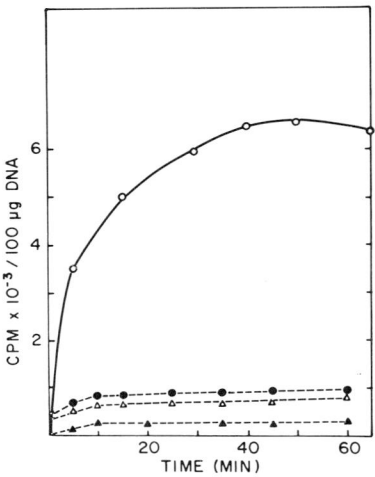

Fig. 1. Activation of [^{3}H]triamcinolone–receptor complex enabling its binding to DNA–cellulose. Each time point represents the extent of binding of [^{3}H]triamcinolone–receptor complex to DNA–cellulose at 0°C; ▲--------▲ represents the binding of free steroid alone; ●--------● represents binding after cytosol is preincubated with triamcinolone at 0°C for 30 minutes; △--------△ represents binding after cytosol alone was preincubated at 20°C for 30 minutes, then cooled to 0°C, and [^{3}H]triamcinolone was added; ○————○ represents the binding of cytosol–[^{3}H]triamcinolone preincubated at 20°C for 30 minutes (Kalimi *et al.*, 1975).

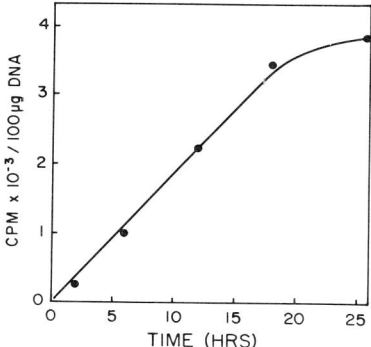

Fig. 2. The slow, low temperature activation of steroid–receptor complex (Kalimi *et al.*, 1975).

by the hepatic glucocorticoid–receptor complex. This study indicates that when the receptor is allowed to become saturated with triamcinolone at 0°C, the resulting steroid–receptor complex will not bind to DNA at this low temperature. However, if the steroid–receptor complex formed at 0°C, is briefly warmed to 20°C and then recooled to 0°C, it will now bind to DNA–cellulose at 0°C. Controls demonstrate that preheating either the cytosol alone or the steroid alone does not impart the capability to bind to DNA. Thus, at 20°C, an activation or transformation of the steroid–receptor complex occurs, enabling it to bind to DNA or as shown elsewhere to nuclei (Kalimi *et al.*, 1973).

If the steroid–receptor complex is kept at 0°C for several hours, its slow conversion to the activated state can be demonstrated, as seen in Fig. 2. Addition of millimolar levels of calcium to the steroid–receptor complex dramatically accelerates this low-temperature activation (Fig. 3).

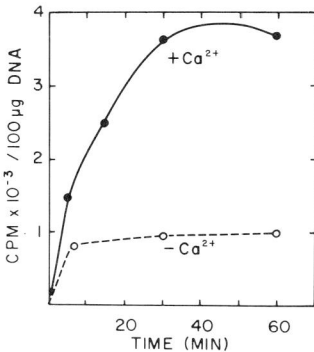

Fig. 3. Effect of Ca^{2+} upon the time course of activation of hormone–receptor complex at low temperature (Kalimi *et al.*, 1975).

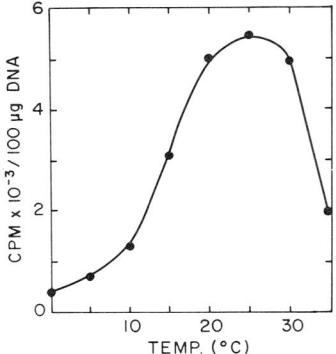

Fig. 4. Temperature dependence of the activation of the glucocorticoid-receptor complex (Kalimi *et al.*, 1975).

Figure 4 demonstrates the effect of temperature, in the absence of calcium, on the activation of the steroid-receptor complex. It is evident that under these *in vitro* conditions, the temperature which gives the maximum activation is 25°C, and that at higher temperatures, denaturation of the steroid-receptor complex occurs.

The chemical nature of the activation process remains obscure. As seen in Fig. 5, the unactivated hormone-receptor complex sediments indistinguishably from the activated complex. At low ionic strength, both complexes sediment as approximately 7-8 S species, and at high ionic strength as 3-4 S species. For both the unactivated and activated steroid-receptor complexes, increasing the ionic strength brings about a reversible dissociation of the complex to the form with lower sedimentation velocity.

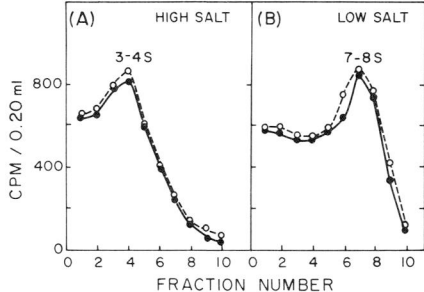

Fig. 5. Sucrose density-gradient centrifugation of unactivated and thermally activated rat liver cytosol hormone-receptor complexes at low and high ionic strengths; ●———● and ○---------○ represent unactivated and activated cytosol hormone-receptor complexes, respectively (Kalimi *et al.*, 1975).

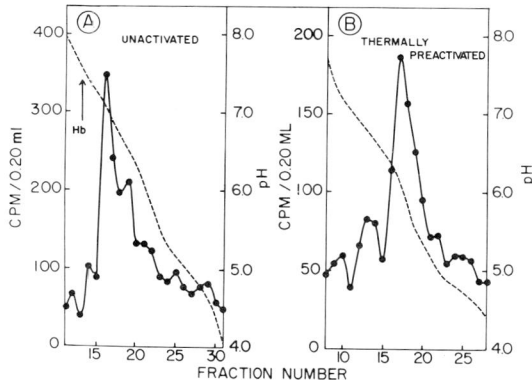

Fig. 6. Isoelectric profiles of unactivated and activated [^{3}H]triamcinolone–receptor complexes (Kalimi et al., 1975).

The isoelectric points of the unactivated and activated steroid–receptor complexes were measured. As shown in Fig. 6, the unactivated complex has an isoelectric point of 7.1, whereas the thermally activated complex manifests a marked downward shift in its isoelectric point to a pI of 6.1. It remains uncertain whether a temperature-dependent conformational change of the steroid–receptor complex occurs or whether a calcium-activated cytoplasmic enzyme covalently modifies the protein of the steroid–receptor complex. Whatever its precise chemical nature, the transformation irreversibly endows the steroid–receptor complex with the ability to bind to nuclei or to stripped DNA. It is of interest to note that, as shown in Table IV, activation of the steroid–receptor complex also increases its ability to bind to the synthetic negatively charged resin, phosphocellulose, as well as to DNA. Activation does not result, however, in loss of the ability of the

TABLE IV

Binding of Unactivated and Thermally Activated [^{3}H]Triamcinolone–Receptor Complexes to Cationic and Anionic Cellulose Matrices[a]

Matrix	Nonactivated cytosol	Activated cytosol
	cpm	cpm
DNA–cellulose	390	5282
Phosphocellulose	215	2800
DEAE–cellulose	3884	3163

[a] From Kalimi et al., 1975.

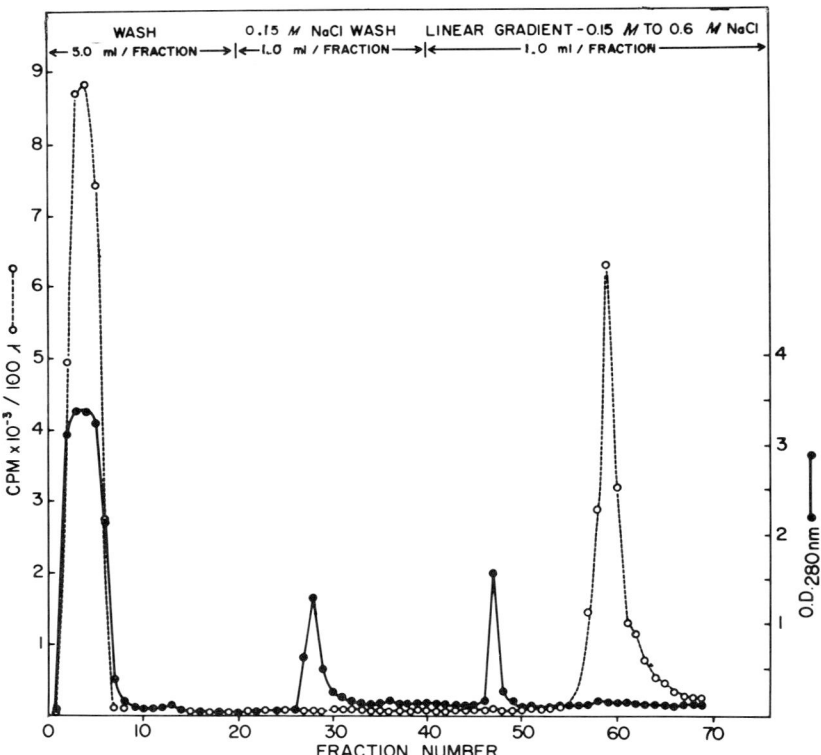

Fig. 7. Receptor purification by gradient elution on phosphocellulose chromatography of the retained thermally activated steroid–receptor complex (Colman and Feigelson, 1976).

complex to bind to positively charged DEAE–cellulose. Thus, the steroid–receptor complex contains regions with negatively charged groups, enabling its binding to DEAE–cellulose. Activation may result in the generation of positively charged domains on the steroid–receptor complex, which enables its binding to DNA, chromatin, nuclei, and phosphocellulose.

A rapid procedure for the purification of the hepatic glucocorticoid receptor has been developed which exploits the observation that "activation" of this complex enables it to bind to anionic substances such as DNA and phosphocellulose (Colman and Feigelson, 1976). The procedure consists of two phosphocellulose columns operated in sequence. After forming glucocorticoid–receptor complex at 0°C, passage through the first column removes from unfractionated cytosol all basic proteins that adhere to the immobilized phosphate residues; the unactivated steroid–receptor complex elutes in the flow-through of this first column. This steroid–receptor complex is then thermally activated and applied to a second phosphocellulose column where it is now retained, washed, and eluted by a salt gradient. As shown in Fig. 7, fractions may be obtained containing purified glucocorticoid–receptor complex with undetectably low levels of contaminating protein. This simple procedure is capable of purifying the steroid–receptor complex many thousandfold.

Quantitative studies have compared the ability of the activated steroid–receptor complex to bind to double-stranded (native) and single-stranded (denatured) DNA at low ionic strength. The degree of saturation of a given amount of DNA affixed to cellulose was measured as a function of the concentration of activated steroid–receptor complex. As shown in Fig. 8 (Feigelson et al., 1975), nanomolar levels of the activated steroid–receptor complex bind to and saturate DNA–cellulose. The degree of saturation is very similar for double-stranded native DNA and thermally denatured single-stranded DNA. Part B of the same figure depicts the same data presented as Scatchard plots; the descending slopes indicate an affinity constant K_a of 1×10^9 M^{-1}. The unusual ascending portion of this curve may be interpreted as indicating cooperative binding of the ligand. Cooperativity in this sense implies that the binding of a few molecules of steroid–receptor complex to the DNA facilitates the binding of further molecules of steroid–receptor complex. Whether this is an artifact of the *in vitro* system, or whether it reflects a fundamental property of the interaction of the steroid–receptor complex with DNA, is uncertain.

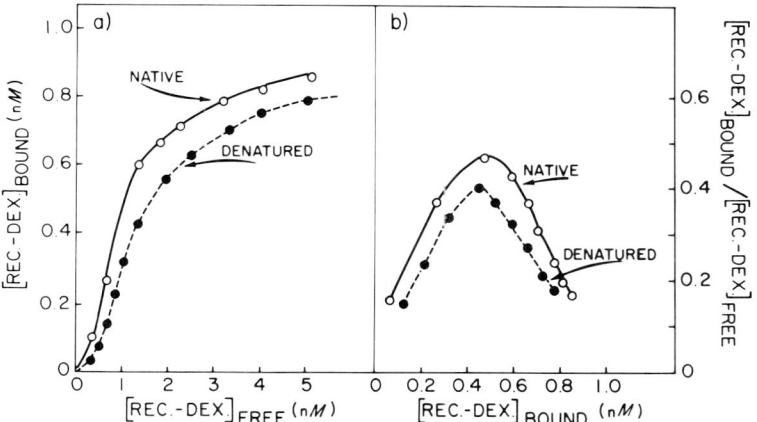

Fig. 8. Binding of activated receptor–dexamethasone complex (R-D) to native (O———O) and denatured (●--------●) rat liver DNA–cellulose (Feigelson et al., 1975).

III. METABOLIC EFFECTS OF GLUCOCORTICOIDS

One of the earliest indications of the biologic activity of the glucocorticoids was the stimulation of gluconeogenesis *in vivo* and in liver slices (Long *et al.*, 1940; Koepf *et al.*, 1941). This physiological effect is partly a consequence of the glucocorticoids acting on lymphoid tissue and muscle, resulting in the breakdown of their cellular proteins into amino acids. These amino acids are transported through the blood to the liver, where they undergo transamination and deamination. The amino groups are converted to urea and excreted. The α-keto moieties of the glucogenic amino acids enter carbohydrate metabolism and are converted by gluconeogenesis to hepatic glycogen or blood glucose. In addition, the glucocorticoids act directly on hepatocytes, causing gluconeogenesis (Long *et al.*, 1940); (Haynes, 1965) and induce elevated levels of certain enzymes involved in amino acid metabolism e.g., tryptophan oxygenase and tyrosine transaminase (Kenney and Flora, 1961; P. Feigelson *et al.*, 1962; Goldstein *et al.*, 1962; Baxter and Tomkins, 1970). Immunochemical titrations indicate that hormonal increases of hepatic enzyme activity are accompanied by increased enzyme protein levels (Feigelson and Greengard, 1962; Kenney, 1962). This was followed by the demonstration that the hormone selectively increases the *in vivo* (Schimke *et al.*, 1964) and *in vitro* (Gramer *et al.*, 1968) rates of labeled amino acid incorporation into the inducible enzymes and not into total hepatic protein. In addition, pretreatment of animals (Greengard and Acs, 1962) or hepatoma cells (Peterkofsky and Tomkins, 1967) with actinomycin D or puromycin or cycloheximide prevents enzyme induction by these steroids, demonstrating that glucocorticoids, in a transcriptionally dependent process, selectively increase the rate of synthesis of certain hepatic enzymes.

IV. CONTROL OF SPECIFIC SPECIES OF mRNA BY GLUCOCORTICOIDS

The participation of RNA in several capacities during protein synthesis motivated our early studies into the effects of glucocorticoids on the biosynthesis of RNA during the course of hormonal induction of hepatic enzymes. It was shown that radioactive precursor incorporation into liver RNA is markedly stimulated following cortisol administration (P. Feigelson *et al.*, 1960; M. Feigelson *et al.*, 1962). Indeed, this was probably the first isotopic indication of increased gene transcription evoked by a hormone. The time course of this stimulation in RNA metabolism parallels that of the induction of tryptophan oxygenase by the hormone (Feigelson and Feigelson, 1965). Further studies indicated hormonally increased rates of synthesis of both ribosomal (Hanoune and Feigelson, 1969) and total uracil-rich mRNA *in vivo* (Yu and Feigelson, 1969).

Selected regions of the genome are transcribed by RNA polymerase II into the nuclear precursors of the various messenger RNA's. The heterogeneous nuclear RNA's are processed by hydrolytic cleavage, base modification, and adenylation. They are then transported to the cytoplasm, where as mRNA they act as templates for protein synthesis. Effects of sex steroids upon rates of transcription (Chan *et al.*, 1973), and stabilization (Palmiter and Carey, 1974) of the messenger RNA have been proposed. It has also been proposed that glucocorticoids may modulate the action of a hypothetical cytoplasmic repressor of messenger RNA (Tomkins *et al.*, 1969). To distinguish between certain of these hypotheses, we measured the level of messenger RNA for one hormonally inducible protein, tryptophan oxygenase, to determine whether the increased rate of synthesis of this enzyme protein following hormonal administration was due to a rise in the tissue levels of its functional messenger RNA or to a hormonally mediated increased translational efficiency of a fixed level of this messenger RNA. To answer this question, it was necessary to develop an assay for the messenger RNA for tryptophan oxygenase. Total hepatic messenger RNA was partially purified by binding its poly(A) sequences (Kitos *et al.*, 1972;

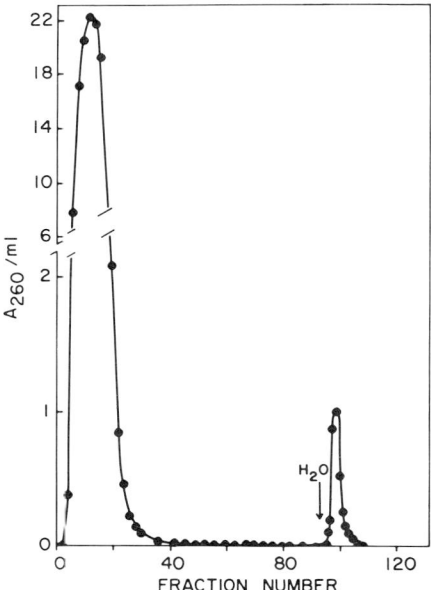

Fig. 9. Chromatography on cellulose of polysomal RNA (Schutz *et al.*, 1972).

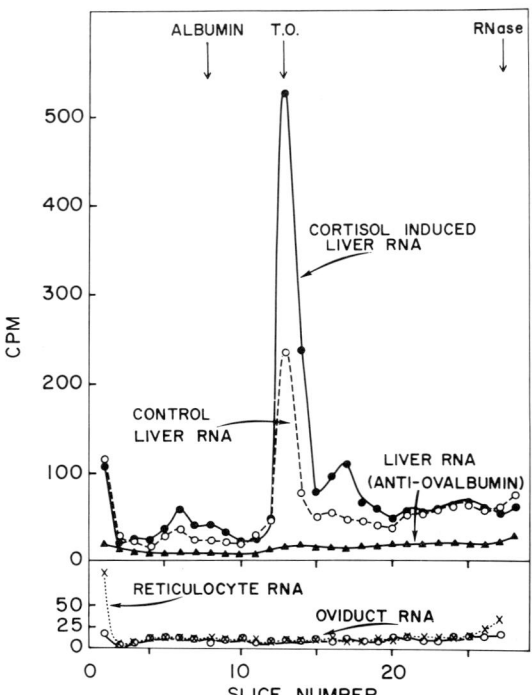

Fig. 10. SDS–gel electrophoresis of *in vitro* synthesized tryptophan oxygenase. The mRNA-dependent translational synthesis of tryptophan oxygenase. Upper panel: proteins directed by liver mRNA from uninduced animals (O---------O) and by liver mRNA from animals that had received hydrocortisone (●———●) were precipitated with carrier tryptophan oxygenase and antitryptophan oxygenase. Another sample stimulated by liver mRNA from induced animals was precipitated with chicken ovalbumin and antiovalbumin (▲———▲). Lower panel: proteins directed by cellulose-purified mRNA from rabbit reticulocytes (X---------X) and RNA from chicken oviducts (O———O) were precipitated with carrier tryptophan oxygenase and anti-tryptophan oxygenase. Arrows indicate the position of proteins used as internal markers in the sodium dodedyl sulfate–acrylamide gel electrophoresis. (Schutz *et al.*, 1973).

Schutz *et al.*, 1972), enabling its separation from other species of cellular RNA (Fig. 9). At high ionic strength, ribosomal RNA and transfer RNA do not bind to cellulose. Lowering the ionic strength elutes about 2% of the total RNA, which was shown by poly(U) hybridization and translational activity to consist of poly(A) containing messenger RNA (Sippel *et al.*, 1974). Microgram levels of messenger RNA prepared in this manner from rat liver, when added to a modified cell-free Krebs II ascites system (Mathews and Rosner, 1970), led to the incorporation of tritiated leucine into the protomeric units tryptophan oxygenase. The mRNA preparations were incubated for 1 hour in the fortified Krebs' ribosomal system. After incubation, ribosomes and polysomes were removed by centrifugation, and the supernatant containing the newly synthesized radioactive polypeptides was collected. Nascent tryptophan oxygenase was isolated from the released chains by immunoprecipitation with carrier tryptophan oxygenase and monospecific anti-tryptophan oxygenase, followed by SDS–polyacrylamide gel electrophoresis of the solubilized immunoprecipitate. The gels were stained for protein, enabling identification of various protein markers which had been added, sliced, and the radioactivity determined by liquid scintillation techniques. A radioactive peak was observed, as shown in Fig. 10, at the gel position corresponding to 43,000 daltons, which is the molecular weight of both subunits of tryptophan oxygenase. Thus, the radioactivity which appears on the gel at this position is coded for by hepatic mRNA, is immunoprecipitated by specific antibodies to tryptophan oxygenase, and has a molecular weight which corresponds to the molecular weight of the protomeric units of hepatic tryptophan oxygenase (Schutz et al., 1973). We infer that we are measuring the messenger RNA-dependent synthesis of tryptophan oxygenase.

It is known that after the administration of an inducing dose of steroid, synthesis of the inducible enzymes is enhanced for a few hours and then

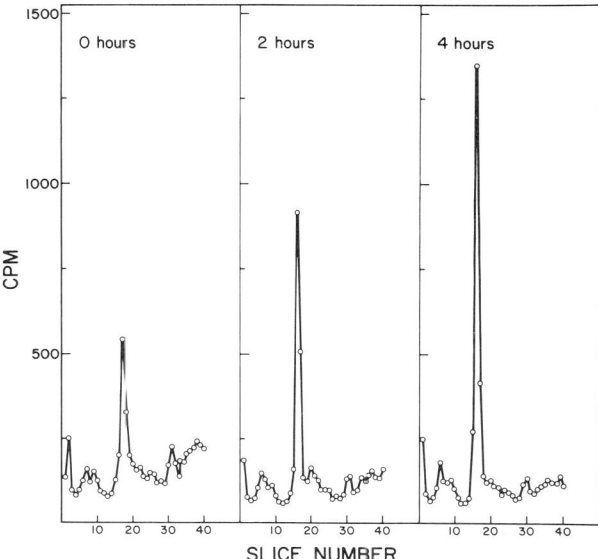

Fig. 11. Sodium dodecyl sulfate–polyacrylamide electrophoresis of tryptophan oxygenase synthesized *in vitro* (Schutz et al., 1975).

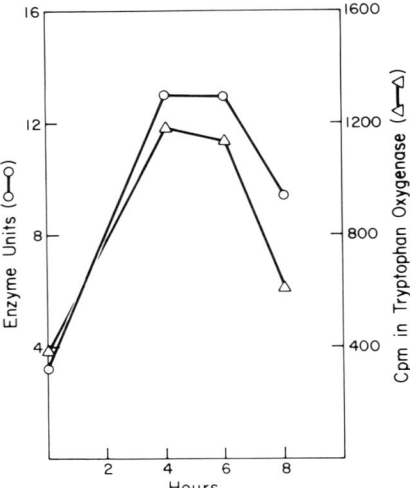

Fig. 12. Comparison of tryptophan oxygenase catalytic activity with mRNA levels for tryptophan oxygenase in the livers of rats as a function of time after interperitoneal administration of hydrocortisone (Schutz et al., 1975).

returns to control levels. Estimation of the level of functional mRNA for tryptophan oxygenase in livers of animals during the induction and deinduction phases indicate that during the period of increasing enzyme synthesis, the level of the mRNA for tryptophan oxygenase is proportionately increased. During deinduction, when the enzyme level falls, the mRNA level also decreases (Figs. 11 and 12). To confirm and extend these studies, the level of the mRNA for tryptophan oxygenase and inducible enzyme activities were compared at a fixed induction time following administration

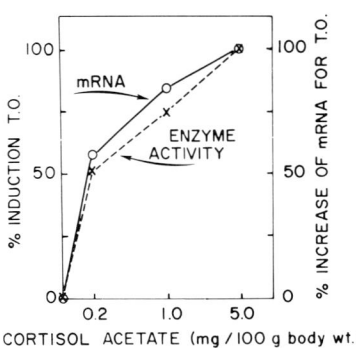

Fig. 13. Hepatic tryptophan oxygenase (T.O.) catalytic activity and mRNA concentration as a function of inducing dose of hydrocortisone (Schutz et al., 1975).

of increasing doses of steroid. The rise in enzyme activity, reflecting an increased rate of synthesis of the enzyme *in vivo*, is accompanied by a parallel increase in the level of the mRNA active in coding for tryptophan oxygenase as measured *in vitro* (Fig. 13). The data are now convincing that glucocorticoids augment the rate of synthesis of hepatic tryptophan oxygenase by elevating the tissue level of its functionally active messenger RNA (Schutz et al., 1975).

V. GLUCOCORTICOIDAL CONTROL OF THE mRNA FOR TRYPTOPHAN OXYGENASE IN HEPATOMAS

When normal cells undergo malignant transformation, alterations in enzymatic and other protein patterns occur. These alterations may be the appearance of new proteins (Abelev, 1971), e.g., the carcinofetal antigens, or the deletion of preexistent proteins, enzymes, or specialized cellular functions. Furthermore, quantitative alterations in the relative proportions of enzymes and isoenzymic species (Weinhouse, 1972), as well as aberrant responsiveness to hormonal regulators have all been reported when normal tissues become neoplastic. The following studies were conducted to gain insight as to how the genes coding for the synthesis of specific enzyme proteins, such as tryptophan oxygenase, are expressed and regulated in normal and malignant cells.

We prepared total messenger RNA from host livers and hepatomas of animals bearing Morris hepatoma tumors and from host livers and hepatomas of Morris hepatoma-bearing animals that had received an inducing dose of cortisol 4 hours prior to sacrifice. As shown in Table V, 60 μg of poly(A)-containing hepatic messenger RNA from the control tumor-bearing animals led, in 60 minutes, to the incorporation of more than 5 million cpm of tritiated leucine into the total protein synthesized in this translational system. Approximately 25% of this total incorporation existed as released chains, of which 337 cpm of [^{3}H]leucine were incorporated into tryptophan oxygenase subunits. An identical amount of hepatic mRNA derived from hepatoma-bearing animals which received hydrocortisone 4 hours prior to sacrifice coded for three times as much incorporation into nascent tryptophan oxygenase. In contrast, the mRNA isolated from the hepatomas of control and hormone-treated animals did not show any incorporation into tryptophan oxygenase subunits, indicating the absence of detectable levels of this specific mRNA species in the hepatomas of control and hormone-treated animals. It is of interest to note that the hepatic mRNA and hepatoma mRNA of control and hormone-treated animals do not cause detectably different rates of amino acid incorporation into the total protein,

TABLE V
The Levels of the Catalytic Activity and the Messenger RNA for Tryptophan Oxygenase in Host Liver and Hepatoma

Tissue	Treatment	Tryptophan oxygenase catalytic activity (μmole of kynurenine/hour/g of liver)	Heterogeneous assay of mRNA-$(A)_x$			
			Total protein (cpm × 10^6)	Total released chains (cpm × 10^6)	cpm	Tryptophan oxygenase % of total protein synthesis
Host liver 7793	None	3.1	5.39	1.35	337	0.025
Host liver 7793	Hydrocort.	10.6	5.85	1.89	931	0.069
Hepatoma 7793	None	Undetectable	5.42	1.90	Undetectable	—
Hepatoma 7793	Hydrocort.	Undetectable	5.89	1.35	Undetectable	—
Host liver 5123C	None	4.9	4.74	1.31	253	0.019
Host liver 5123C	Hydrocort.	15.8	5.51	1.45	504	0.034
Hepatoma 5123C	None	Undetectable	3.86	1.24	Undetectable	—
Hepatoma 5123C	Hydrocort.	Undetectable	4.41	1.34	Undetectable	—
Host liver 5123D	None	4.5	3.81	1.25	261	0.020
Host liver 5123D	Hydrocort.	18.0	4.36	1.36	453	0.032
Hepatoma 5123D	None	Undetectable	5.29	1.71	Undetectable	—
Hepatoma 5123D	Hydrocort.	Undetectable	6.14	1.91	Undetectable	—

[a] From Ramanarayanan-Murthy et al., 1976.

nor into the total released chains. It is only after one has succeeded in separating the protomeric units of tryptophan oxygenase from the total hepatic protein synthesized that one can detect the hepatic hormonal elevation into tryptophan oxygenase. Hepatoma mRNA from either control or hormone-treated animals did not code for detectable amino acid incorporation into tryptophan oxygenase. On the basis of this functional assay for messenger RNA, we infer that the level of functional mRNA for tryptophan oxygenase approximates 0.03% and 0.10% of the total hepatic mRNA activity in control and hormone-treated animals, respectively (Fig. 14). The level of functional mRNA for tryptophan oxygenase in hepatoma is undetectably low in control and hormone-treated animals. The deletion of this mRNA species from these hepatomas could ensue from several causes: (a) the genes for tryptophan oxygenase in hepatoma may have been cytogenetically deleted during the malignant transformation; (b) the genes for tryptophan oxygenase in hepatoma may be present but are repressed, i.e., not transcriptionally expressed; or (c) the tryptophan oxygenase gene may be transcribed, but there may be impaired processing of this gene transcript to functionally active mRNA. Experiments to distinguish between these alternatives are under way.

The lack of tryptophan oxygenase in hepatoma and its failure to be induced by glucocorticoids prompted investigations on the qualitative and quantitative nature of the functional glucocorticoid receptor in the hepatomas. Our studies indicated that hepatoma cytosol contains approx-

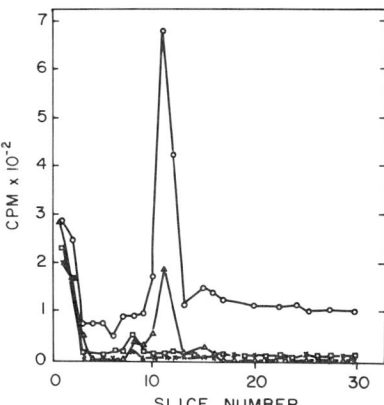

Fig. 14. Evaluation of the synthesis *in vitro* of tryptophan oxygenase protomers by mRNA derived from host livers and 7793 Morris hepatomas; (▲———▲) from control host liver mRNA; (□———□) from control tumor RNA; (○———○) from hydrocortisone induced host-liver mRNA; (X———X) from hydrocortisone induced tumor mRNA (Ramanarayanan-Murthy *et al.*, 1976).

TABLE VI
Glucocorticoid Receptor Activity in Liver and Morris Hepatoma Cytosols[a]

Source of cytosol	Specific-bound [^{3}H]triamcinolone (cpm/mg protein)	Nonspecific binding (%)
Host liver	2286	25
Morris hepatoma 7793	2339	17

[a] From Ramanarayanan-Murthy et al., 1976.

imately 200 fmoles of receptor per milligram of protein, making it comparable with host liver cytosol (Table VI). Also, incubation of purified nuclei with hepatoma cytosol receptor–steroid complex yielded no significant difference in nuclear uptake when compared with host liver cytosol receptor–steroid complex (Table VII); furthermore, hepatoma-derived steroid–receptor complex bound, as well as host liver steroid–receptor complex, to stripped rat liver DNA (Table VIII). Thus, the inability of these hepatomas to respond to glucocorticoids does not seem to be due to the absence of the glucocorticoid receptor or to any detectable impaired functional interaction with either hepatoma or hepatic nuclei (Ramanarayanan-Murthy et al., 1976).

VI. INTERACTION OF THE RECEPTOR WITH NUCLEAR COMPONENTS

The pioneering studies of Mueller and his colleagues on RNA and protein synthesis very early linked estrogen action with gene expression (Mueller et

TABLE VII
The Binding of Liver and Morris Hepatoma Cytoplasmic Glucocorticoid Receptor Complexes to Homologous and Heterologous Nuclei[a]

	[^{3}H]TA–host liver receptor complex		[^{3}H]TA–hepatoma receptor complex	
Source of nuclei	Specific-bound [^{3}H]TA (cpm/mg DNA)	Nonspecific binding (%)	Specific-bound [^{3}H]TA (cpm/mg DNA)	Nonspecific binding (%)
Host liver	57,371	38	77,214	22
Morris hepatoma 7793	67,143	18	72,814	18

[a] From Ramanarayanan-Murthy et al., 1976.
[b] [^{3}H]TA–triamcinolone acetonide (specific activity 16 Ci/mmole).

TABLE VIII

The Binding of Liver and Morris Hepatoma Cytoplasmic Glucocorticoid Receptor Complexes to Rat Liver DNA–Cellulose

Source of cytosol	Specific-bound [^{3}H]TA (cpm/100 μg DNA)	Nonspecific binding (%)
Host liver	7090	7.8
Morris hepatoma 7793	6966	9.7

^{a} From Ramanarayanan-Murthy et al., 1976.
^{b} [^{3}H]TA–triamcinolone acetonide (specific activity 16 Ci/mmole).

al., 1958). The microbial analogy of a repressor–gene interaction was quickly absorbed into the concept of steroid hormone action. This has led to a search for the specific components or acceptors that bind the hormone–receptor complex in the nucleus. Our recent studies demonstrate that brief treatment of rat liver nuclei with DNase I, causing them to lose about 10% of the nuclear DNA, results in a loss of about 80% of their capacity to bind glucocorticoid–receptor complex at low ionic strength. Thus, the steroid–receptor complex binds to a small portion of the genome, which is readily sensitive to DNase I.

VII. CONCLUSIONS

It has been experimentally demonstrated that the glucocorticoid hormone, after entering the cell, interacts with a receptor protein in the cytosol to form a glucocorticoid–receptor complex; this complex undergoes activation of unknown molecular nature, rendering it capable of entry into the nucleus, where it interacts with specific sites on the genome. It is also now established that a rise in the tissue level of functionally active specific mRNA for tryptophan oxygenase accompanies and is responsible for the hormonally induced, increased rate of synthesis of this enzyme (Feigelson et al., 1975). What can not be definitively excluded at the present time are glucocorticoidal effects upon mRNA levels, which may be mediated through selective alterations in processing or transport of specific mRNA species. However, the most likely interpretation of the data on hand is that steroid hormones mediate a steroid–receptor–genomic interaction which accelerates transcription of a relatively small number of specific genes. Each unique structural gene, which codes for a specific protein, represents less than one part in a million of the total base pairs in the mammalian genome. The majority of the receptor molecules found in the nucleus may be bound nonspecifically to unmodulatable portions of the genome. A fundamental question, which remains to be answered, is how the great selectivity in receptor action is achieved in spite of a less selective receptor binding to nuclei. Our recent studies indicate the existence of two types of receptor binding sites on the genome: the DNase I-sensitive binding sites and the DNase I-resistant binding sites. The physiological import of these two types of binding sites is under current investigation.

It has been shown that the loss in the ability of hepatomas to synthesize the hormonally modulatable hepatospecific proteins, tryptophan oxygenase and α_{2u}-globulin, is due to the deletion of these two specific messenger RNA species. Thus, selective alteration in gene expression may accompany the neoplastic transformation.

ACKNOWLEDGMENT

These studies were supported in part by NIH Grants CA 02332 and CRTY 05011 from the National Cancer Institute.

REFERENCES

Abelev, G. I. (1971). *Adv. Cancer Res.* **14**, 295.
Anderson, K. M., and Liao, S. (1968). *Nature (London)* **219**, 277.
Baxter, J. D., and Tomkins, G. M. (1970). *Proc. Natl. Acad. Sci. U.S.A.* **65**, 709.
Baxter, J. D., Rousseau, G. G., Benson, M. C., Garcea, R. L., Ito, J., and Tomkins, G. M. (1972). *Proc. Natl. Acad. Sci. U.S.A.* **69**, 1892.
Beato, M., and Feigelson, P. (1972). *J. Biol. Chem.* **247**, 7890.
Beato, M., Kalimi, M., and Feigelson, P. (1972). *Biochem. Biophys. Res. Commun.* **47**, 1464.
Beato, M., Kalimi, M., Beato, W., and Feigelson, P. (1974). *Endocrinology* **94**, 377.
Chan, L., Means, A. R., and O'Malley, B. W. (1973). *Proc. Natl. Acad. Sci. U.S.A.* **70**, 1870.
Colman, P. D., and Feigelson, P. (1976). *Mol. Cell. Endocrinol.* **5**, 33.
Feigelson, M., and Feigelson, P. (1965). *Adv. Enzyme Regul.* **3**, 11.
Feigelson, M., Gross, P., and Feigelson, P. (1962). *Biochim. Biophys. Acta* **55**, 495.
Feigelson, P., and Greengard, O. (1962). *J. Biol. Chem.* **237**, 3714.
Feigelson, P., Feigelson, M., and Greengard, O. (1960). *Proc. Int. Congr. Endocrinol., 1st, 1960* p. 823.
Feigelson, P., Feigelson, M., and Greengard, O. (1962). *Recent Prog. Horm. Res.* **18**, 491.
Feigelson, P., Beato, M., Colman, P., Kalimi, M., Killewich, L. A., and Schutz, G. (1975). *Recent Prog. Horm. Res.* **31**, 213.
Feldman, D., Funder, J. W., and Edelman, I. (1972). *Am. J. Med.* **53**, 545.
Goldstein, L., Stella, E. J., and Knox, W. E. (1962). *J. Biol. Chem.* **237**, 1723.
Gorski, J., Toft, D., Shyamalä, G., Smith, D., and Notides, A. (1968). *Recent Prog. Horm. Res.* **24**, 45.
Granner, D. K., Hayashi, S., Thompson, E. B., and Tomkins, G. M. (1968). *J. Mol. Biol.* **35**, 291.

Greengard, O., and Acs, G. (1962). *Biochim. Biophys. Acta* **61**, 652.
Hanoune, J., and Feigelson, P. (1969). *Biochim. Biophys. Acta* **199**, 214.
Haynes, R. C., (1965). *Adv. Enzyme Regul.* **3**, 111.
Jensen, E. V., and De Sombre, J. (1973). *Science* **182**, 126.
Jensen, E. V., and Jacobson, H. I. (1962). *Recent Prog. Horm. Res.* **18**, 387.
Kalimi, M., Beato, M., and Feigelson, P. (1973). *Biochemistry* **12**, 3365.
Kalimi, M., Colman, P. D., and Feigelson, P. (1975). *J. Biol. Chem.* **250**, 1080.
Kenney, F. T. (1962). *J. Biol. Chem.* **237**, 3495.
Kenney, F. T., and Flora, R. M. (1961). *J. Biol. Chem.* **236**, 2699.
King, R. J. B., and Mainwaring, W. I. P. (1974). "Steroid Cell Interactions." Univ. Park Press, Baltimore, Maryland.
Kitos, P. A., Saxon, G., and Amos, H. (1972). *Biochem. Biophys. Res. Commun.* **47**, 1246.
Koblinsky, M. (1973). Ph.D. Dissertation, Columbia University, New York.
Koblinsky, M., Beato, M., Kalimi, M., and Feigelson, P. (1972). *J. Biol. Chem.* **247**, 7897.
Koepf, G. H., Horn, H. W., Giremmill, C. L., and Torn, C. W. (1941). *Am. J. Physiol.* **135**, 175.
Long, C. N. H., Katzin, B., and Frey, E. G. (1940). *Endocrinology* **26**, 309.
Mathews, M. B., and Rosner, A. (1970). *Eur. J. Biochem.* **17**, 328.
Mueller, G. C., Herranen, A. M., and Jervell, K. F. (1958). *Recent Prog. Horm. Res.* **14**, 95.
O'Malley, B. W., and Means, A. R. (1974). *Science* **183**, 610.
Palmiter, R. D., and Carey, N. H. (1974). *Proc. Natl. Acad. Sci. U.S.A.* **71**, 2357.
Peterkofsky, B., and Tomkins, G. M. (1967). *J. Mol. Biol.* **30**, 49.
Ramanarayanan-Murthy, L., Colman, P. D., and Feigelson, P. (1976). *Cancer Res.* **36**, 3594.
Schimke, R. T., Sweeney, E. W., and Berlin, C. M. (1964). *Biochem. Biophys. Res. Commun.* **15**, 214.
Schutz, G., Beato, M., and Feigelson, P. (1972). *Biochem. Biophys. Res. Commun.* **49**, 680.
Schutz, G., Beato, M., and Feigelson, P. (1973). *Proc. Natl. Acad. Sci. U.S.A.* **70**, 1218.
Schutz, G., Killewich, L., Chen, G., and Feigelson, P. (1975). *Proc. Natl. Acad. Sci. U.S.A.* **72**, 1017.
Sippel, A. E., Stavrianopoulos, J., Schutz, G., and Feigelson, P. (1974). *Proc. Natl. Acad. Sci. U.S.A.* **71**, 4635.
Tomkins, G. M., Gelehrter, J. D., Granner, D., Martin, D., Jr., Samuels, H. H., and Thompson, E. B. (1969). *Science* **166**, 1474.
Weinhouse, S. (1972). *Cancer Res.* **32**, 2007.
Westphal, U. (1971). "Steroid-Protein Interactions," Monogr. Endocrinol., Springer-Verlag, Berlin and New York.
Yu, F. L., and Feigelson, P. (1969). *Biochem. Biophys. Res. Commun.* **35**, 499.

10

Regulation of Gene Expression by Glucocorticoid Hormones: Studies of Receptors and Responses in Cultured Cells

JOHN D. BAXTER AND ROBERT D. IVARIE

I.	Introduction	252
II.	Glucocorticoid Hormone Receptors	254
	A. Evidence for Their Involvement in Glucocorticoid Responses and Comparisons with Other Glucocorticoid-Binding Proteins	254
	B. Subcellular Localization of Glucocorticoid Receptors	255
	C. Physical and Binding Characteristics of the Receptors	255
	D. Quantitative Relations between Steroid Binding by the Receptor and the Glucocorticoid Response in Cultured Cells	256
III.	The Domain of Response to Glucocorticoid Hormones	258
	A. General Presence of Glucocorticoid Hormone Receptors and Responsiveness in Mammalian Tissues	258
	B. Glucocorticoid Action in Cultured Hepatoma Cells	258
	C. Regulation of Growth Hormone Production by Cultured Pituitary Cells	261
	D. Glucocorticoid Killing of Cultured Lymphoma Cells	261
IV.	Agonists, Partial Agonists, and Antagonists: Comparisons of Actions in Various Systems	262
V.	Structure–Activity Relations: Nature of the Receptor-Binding Site	263
VI.	Mechanism of Agonist and Antagonist Steroid Action: Allosteric Model for Steroid Hormone Action	265
VII.	Activation of the Receptor–Glucocorticoid Complex	268
	A. Studies in Cell-Free Systems	268
	B. Studies with Intact Cells	269
VIII.	Return of the Receptor to the Cytosol: The First Step in Deinduction	270

IX. Nuclear Binding of Receptor–Glucocorticoid Complexes 271
   A. Acceptor Capacity in the Cell 272
   B. Cell-Free Nuclear Binding 273
   C. The Glucocorticoid Receptor as a DNA-Binding Protein 274
   D. The Subchromatin Localization of Receptors:
      Nuclease Digestion Studies 276
   E. Evidence for a Role of Chromatin Elements Other Than
      DNA in Acceptor Activity 277
   F. Correlation Between Receptor Binding to the Nucleus and the
      Glucocorticoid Response: The Question of "Hidden"
      High-Affinity Acceptor Sites Mediating Receptor Action ... 278
X. Genetic Approaches to the Study of Glucocorticoid
   Hormone Action 279
   A. Isolation of Glucocorticoid-Resistant Cell Lines from
      Cultured S49 Lymphoma Cells 279
   B. Phenotypic Classification and Biochemical Lesions
      Associated with Steroid Resistance 280
   C. Mechanism for the Preponderance of Receptor Defects 281
   D. Comparison of the Nature of the Resistance in S49 Cells
      with that Observed in Other Glucocorticoid-Responsive
      Systems 282
XI. Regulation of mRNA by Glucocorticoid Hormones 283
   A. Regulation of Growth Hormone mRNA 283
   B. Regulation of Tyrosine Aminotransferase mRNA 285
   C. Primary Versus Secondary Induction of Specific mRNA's by
      Glucocorticoids....................................... 285
   D. The Question of How Generally Does Glucocorticoid Action
      Occur Through Induction of Specific mRNA's 286
XII. Deinduction of the Glucocorticoid Response: Posttranscriptional
     Control of Tyrosine Aminotransferase 287
XIII. Mechanisms of Glucocorticoid Receptor Action: Parallels with
      Cyclic AMP Action in Bacteria 288
XIV. Summary 290
     References 292

I. INTRODUCTION

Glucocorticoids have been of interest in studying regulation of eukaryotic gene expression not only because they serve as a useful model, but also because of the diversity of their metabolic influences, both inhibitory and stimulatory (Baxter and Forsham, 1972; Baxter *et al.,* 1973; Baxter and Harris, 1975; Feldman *et al.,* 1972; Rousseau, 1975; Baxter, 1976; Thompson and Lippman, 1974; Yamamoto and Alberts, 1976; Yamamoto *et al.,* 1976). Furthermore, these hormones are widely used pharmacologic agents for treating numerous clinical conditions (for review, see Azarnoff, 1975; Baxter, 1974).

The study of glucocorticoid action has been greatly facilitated by the availability of systems in cell culture in which the responses to these hormones typify some of those observed in the animal. In this review, we describe some of our studies of glucocorticoid hormone action in three of these hormone-responsive systems in cell culture. Cultured hepatoma cells have been used to relate glucocorticoid–receptor interactions with the steroid effects and to study the induction of tyrosine aminotransferase and the complexity of the glucocorticoid response. Cultured lymphoma cells have provided a system for analyzing glucocorticoid-regulated catabolism and the mechanisms of steroid resistance. Cultured pituitary cells have been used to examine the influence of the glucocorticoid on a specific mRNA.

Over the past several years, the scheme of glucocorticoid hormone action depicted in Fig. 1 has emerged, which has been supported by both biochemical and genetic analyses. In general, the steroid enters the cell and binds to a cytoplasmic receptor. The resulting receptor–steroid complex is then "activated" so that it binds to the nucleus. The latter interaction influences in some way specific mRNAs whose translated products are responsible for the glucocorticoid response. These steps are similar in many ways to those which appear to operate for other classes of hormones (reviewed elsewhere in these volumes). Most of the review focuses on our

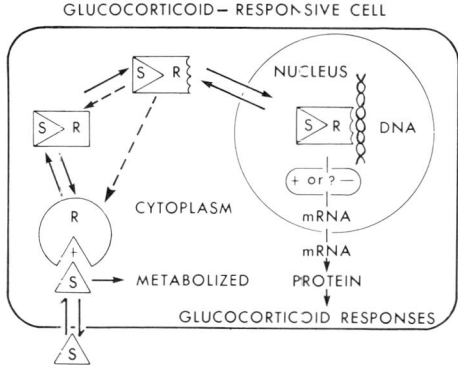

Fig. 1. Diagram of glucocorticoid-responsive cell: steps in glucocorticoid hormone action. S denotes an active, or agonist, steroid. R denotes the specific glucocorticoid receptor. The different shapes of R refer to different conformational states. The plus or minus refer to the fact that it is not clear that all of the actions on mRNA's are positive. Reprinted with permission from Baxter, 1976.

studies of these steps in glucocorticoid hormone action and on the mechanism of steroid resistance, although other work is sometimes discussed for perspective.

II. GLUCOCORTICOID HORMONE RECEPTORS

A. Evidence for Their Involvement in Glucocorticoid Responses and Comparisons with Other Glucocorticoid-Binding Proteins

The hepatoma system has been particularly helpful in establishing the correlation between glucocorticoid receptor binding and the glucocorticoid response, since induction of a specific gene product (tyrosine aminotransferase) can be easily measured and related to receptor binding. The correlations implicating the receptor in glucocorticoid hormone action have been reviewed elsewhere (Baxter et al., 1973; Rousseau, 1975; Baxter, 1976). Of particular importance here is that for agonists, the relative steroid activities for binding and induction are similar, that antagonists and partial agonists bind to the receptor in relation to their antagonist and partial agonist activities, and that inactive steroids do not bind to the receptors (Ballard et al., 1975; Baxter and Tomkins, 1970, 1971; Rousseau et al., 1972, 1973). Some of these relations are discussed below in terms of the mechanism of glucocorticoid hormone action. Strong correlations between steroid–receptor binding and the hormonal response have also been established in the lymphoma cell system (Baxter et al., 1971; Rousseau et al., 1972). Importantly, the loss of both receptor-binding activity and glucocorticoid responsiveness in this system (Baxter et al., 1971; Rosenau et al., 1972; Sibley and Tomkins, 1974b; Yamamoto et al., 1974, 1976) has strengthened the idea that the receptors mediate the glucocorticoid response.

It should be emphasized that there are many reports of binding of glucocorticoids with macromolecules which differ from these receptors and which may not be important in glucocorticoid hormone action (for review, see Baxter, 1976). In most of these cases, certain features of the binding properties of the proteins do not correlate well with the biologic response. For example, many of these proteins do not bind dexamethasone, an extremely potent glucocorticoid. In fact, studies of glucocorticoid receptors in many tissues have been greatly facilitated by the use of synthetic glucocorticoids, such as dexamethasone, because of their selective binding to the receptor. However, it is conceivable that some of the proteins which differ from the "receptors" in tissues such as liver (Beato et al., 1971), brain (McEwen et al., 1974), and kidney (Feldman et al., 1973) could have some function in hormone action, although at present there is no evidence for this.

B. Subcellular Localization of Glucocorticoid Receptors

In the absence of the hormone, the glucocorticoid receptor is found in the cytosol fraction of the cell, suggesting that the receptor is a soluble cytoplasmic protein in the cell (Baxter and Tomkins, 1971). It is possible that, intracellularly, uncomplexed receptors are distributed in both nuclei and cytoplasm, but after cellular disruption, uncomplexed receptors in the nucleus diffuse to the cytoplasmic fraction. Based on studies with mercurial reagents which inhibit steroid–receptor binding and which vary in their cellular penetration, it appears that the initial hormone–receptor contact occurs inside the cell (Levinson et al., 1972). After steroid association with the receptor, and the resulting conformational changes, half or more of the receptors are recovered tightly associated with the nuclei (Rousseau et al., 1973).

It would seem that, because of their hydrophobic nature, the steroids should readily penetrate the cell membrane. However, based on studies with other systems, several workers have suggested that transport processes are involved in glucocorticoid entry into the cell (Gross et al., 1970; Harrison et al., 1975; Rao et al., 1976). There is no evidence for or against this idea in the case of the hepatoma cells; however, the binding of dexamethasone by the hepatoma cell receptor occurs as or nearly as rapidly at 0°C or at 37°C in intact cells as it does in isolated cytosol (Baxter and Tomkins, 1971; Rousseau et al., 1973; J. D. Baxter, unpublished observations). Thus, if transport is involved in this system, it does not appear to be rate-limiting.

C. Physical and Binding Characteristics of the Receptors

The hormone–receptor interaction correspond to the reaction

$$\text{Steroid} + \text{receptor} \rightleftharpoons \text{receptor steroid complex}$$

This is suggested by two lines of data. First, a Scatchard analysis of the binding at equilibrium conforms to a single straight line, and secondly, the kinetics of association and dissociation are respectively proportional to the concentrations of the hormone and receptor, and the hormone–receptor complex (Baxter and Tomkins, 1971). In the hepatoma cell cytosol, the equilibrium dissociation constant at 0°C is around 3 nM when examined by equilibrium measurements, and around 1 nM when kinetic data are used (Baxter and Tomkins, 1971). Whether these small differences are significant is not known. In cells at 37°C, the measured binding constant is nearer to 10 nM (Baxter and Tomkins, 1970; Baxter et al., 1977).

The affinity of the receptor for the hormone may be higher when the receptor is bound in the nucleus in the activated form than when it is soluble and inactivated. This suggestion is derived from the finding that the rate of dissociation of dexamethasone from the nuclear-bound receptors (Higgins et al., 1973c) appears to be much slower than it is from the solubilized receptors (Baxter and Tomkins, 1971). However, this conclusion cannot be made with certainty, since the affinity depends on both the association and dissociation rate constants. The former cannot be measured in the case of nuclear-bound dexamethasone, since uncomplexed receptors do not bind to the nucleus.

The glucocorticoid receptor has been purified to perhaps 15-40% homogeneity (Failla et al., 1975). Very little is known about its physical properties. Binding is destroyed by proteolytic enzymes and mercurial reagents, but not by other hydrolytic enzymes (Baxter and Tomkins, 1971). Receptors in crude and purified preparations tend to aggregate (Baxter and Tomkins, 1971; Failla et al., 1975), particularly at low ionic strength. At higher ionic strength, it sediments at about 3.8 S (Baxter and Tomkins, 1971). The size and shape of the lymphoma cell receptor has been estimated by combining data from molecular-sieve chromatography and density-gradient sedimentation experiments. It appears that the receptor has a molecular weight (MW) of around 90,000 daltons and an axial ratio of 4:1 (Yamamoto et al., 1976), suggesting that the receptor is moderately asymmetrical.

D. Quantitative Relations Between Steroid Binding by the Receptor and the Glucocorticoid Response in Cultured Cells

As shown in Fig. 2, the relationship between the dexamethasone concentration required for binding to the cytosol receptor is similar to that for the induction of tyrosine aminotransferase. These data may reflect the fact that the receptor content is relatively rate-limiting in the hormonal response, i.e., if there were more receptors, the magnitude of the response might be greater. These data also argue against a major element of cooperativity in glucocorticoid agonist action. However, some cooperativity in the dose-response kinetics was suggested by Samuels and Tomkins (1970)

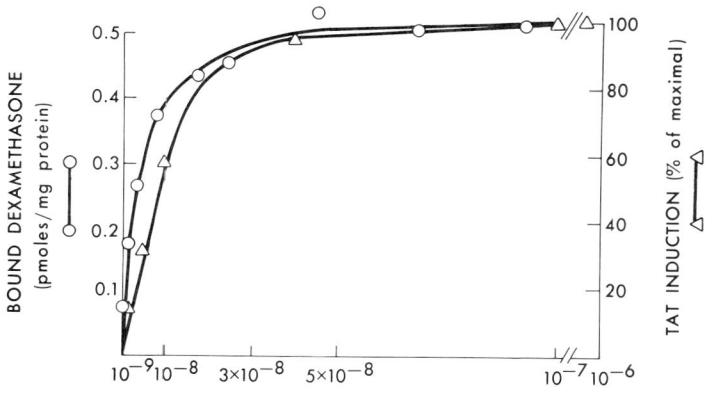

Fig. 2. Steroid binding by cytosol (O———O) and induction of tyrosine aminotransferase (TAT; △———△) at various concentrations of dexamethasone. Reprinted with permission from Baxter et al., 1973.

(and confirmed by us: G. G. Rousseau and J. D. Baxter, unpublished observations), with the use of competitive antagonists. The latter data, in fact, suggest that more than one binding subunit may be involved in the interaction.

The situation with receptor binding and lymphoid cell killing is more complex. In intact cells at 37°C we ordinarily observe half-maximal receptor binding at 25 nM dexamethasone (D. T. Matulich and J. D. Baxter unpublished observations). In our earlier studies, it appeared that there was marked killing of S49 cells at very low concentration of steroid (e.g., in the nM range) that produce only partial saturation of the receptors (Rosenau et al., 1972). This dose-response relationship for killing was also similar to that obtained when killing was measured by cloning efficiency (Sibley and Tomkins, 1974a; Sibley et al., 1974). However, more recently, Gehring et al., 1974 and A. W. Harris (personal communication) found that the dose-response curve was shifted more to the right. Thus, with lymphoid cells, the quantitative relationship between receptor binding and killing has been harder to define. This may not be surprising, since, in contrast to the case with tyrosine aminotransferase induction, the primary gene product regulated by the steroid is not known and end point measurements such as killing may reflect cumulative effects that no longer bear a direct parallel with the primary response of the steroid. In fact, the lack of a direct parallel is common in response to other classes of hormones (Lefkowitz, 1976; Levitski, 1976; Kono and Barnham, 1971).

III. THE DOMAIN OF RESPONSE TO GLUCOCORTICOID HORMONES

A. General Presence of Glucocorticoid Hormone Receptors and Responsiveness in Mammalian Tissues

As reviewed elsewhere (Baxter and Forsham, 1972; Baxter, 1976), glucocorticoids are essentially ubiquitous physiological regulators. To determine the extent to which these many tissue-specific responses could be due to primary effects on the target tissue or by secondary effects of the glucocorticoids, we examined a large number of mammalian tissues for the presence of glucocorticoid hormone receptors. It was found that the receptors are as extensively distributed in mammalian tissues (Ballard et al., 1974) as are the responses. In only rare instances, such as the immature rat uterus (Higgins et al., 1973b), were we unable to detect receptors. Thus, the case with glucocorticoids contrasts with that of all of the other classes of steroid hormones which have a much more limited distribution of target tissues.

B. Glucocorticoid Action in Cultured Hepatoma Cells

1. Induction of Tyrosine Aminotransferase

The induction of tyrosine aminotransferase by glucocorticoids in cultured hepatoma cells has been studied in detail (see below). The specific activity of this enzyme rises about 5 to 15-fold within 8–10 hours after administration of a glucocorticoid (Thompson et al., 1966). The increase in enzyme activity is fully accounted for by a similar increase in the rate of synthesis of the enzyme (Granner et al., 1970; Tomkins et al., 1972). The hormone is required for maintenance of the response; following removal of the inducing steroid, the rate of synthesis and the activity of the enzyme decay rapidly to the basal level (Thompson et al., 1966; Tomkins et al., 1966, 1969, 1972; Steinberg et al., 1975a).

2. Measurement of the Domain of Response in Cultured Hepatoma Cells

Even though there is no increase in total protein synthesis in cultured hepatoma cells, a few gene products other than tyrosine aminotransferase are also induced by glucocorticoids. These include a surface factor which promotes cell adhesiveness (Ballard and Tomkins, 1970), glutamine synthetase (under certain conditions, Kulka et al., 1972), and a phenylalanine tRNA (Stringer et al., 1974; Lippman et al., 1974). At least two activities have been reported to decrease in response to glucocorticoids:

cyclic AMP phosphodiesterase (Manganiello and Vaughn, 1972) and plasminogen activator (Wigler et al., 1975). Thus, the question has arisen of how many gene products are regulated by the steroid in these cells.

Recently, a two-dimensional gel electrophoresis method has been developed which allows an approach to questions such as this in tissue culture cells (O'Farrell, 1975a). This technique can be used to measure the rate of synthesis of over a thousand individual proteins. By pulse-labeling induced and uninduced cells and separating the labeled proteins on the gels, the number of proteins whose rate of synthesis is altered by glucocorticoids can be determined, providing that the labeling time is kept short compared to the degradation rate of the protein (Ivarie and O'Farrell, 1977). This number constitutes an indication of the *domain* of the hormonal response in these cells (Tomkins, 1975). Even though two-dimensional gels separate a large number of gene products, not all cell proteins are detected. Thus, the measured domain represents only a fraction of its total size.

Autoradiographs from induced and uninduced HTC cells after labeling for 30 minutes with [^{35}S]methionine are shown in Fig. 3. In this experiment, nine proteins showed an increase in their rates of synthesis in response to dexamethasone. One has been identified immunochemically as tyrosine aminotransferase. The identity of the other eight proteins is unknown, but they do not appear to be related to tyrosine aminotransferase, since they do not react with antiserum to the enzyme (Ivarie and O'Farrell, 1977). Two other domain proteins are probably sialoglycoproteins, as inferred from their electrophoretic properties in this system (Ivarie and O'Farrell, 1977).

Analysis of a large number of experiments of this kind using cultured hepatoma cells has revealed two general classes of glucocorticoid-affected proteins (Ivarie and O'Farrell, 1977). Class I proteins are induced almost every time they are detected and have been defined, accordingly, as the glucocorticoid domain in these cells. Increases in the rates of synthesis can be detected within 1 hour of hormonal stimulation, and the ratio of induced to control rates of synthesis for the group ranged from 3 to 10. Proteins in Class II are consistently detected, but changes in their synthetic rates are observed only infrequently. The observed changes may be actual hormonal effects, rather than a subtle artifact of the electrophoretic technique, since the gel separation of the cellular proteins is completely reproducible within a single plating and labeling of paired samples. It is notable that the only proteins having decreased rates of synthesis in response to the steroid fall into Class II. Only one protein frequently repressed (9 out of 16 experiments).

From these observations, an estimate can be made concerning the number of glucocorticoid-sensitive genes within a single target cell. If the measured domain is expressed as a fraction of the number of spots detected

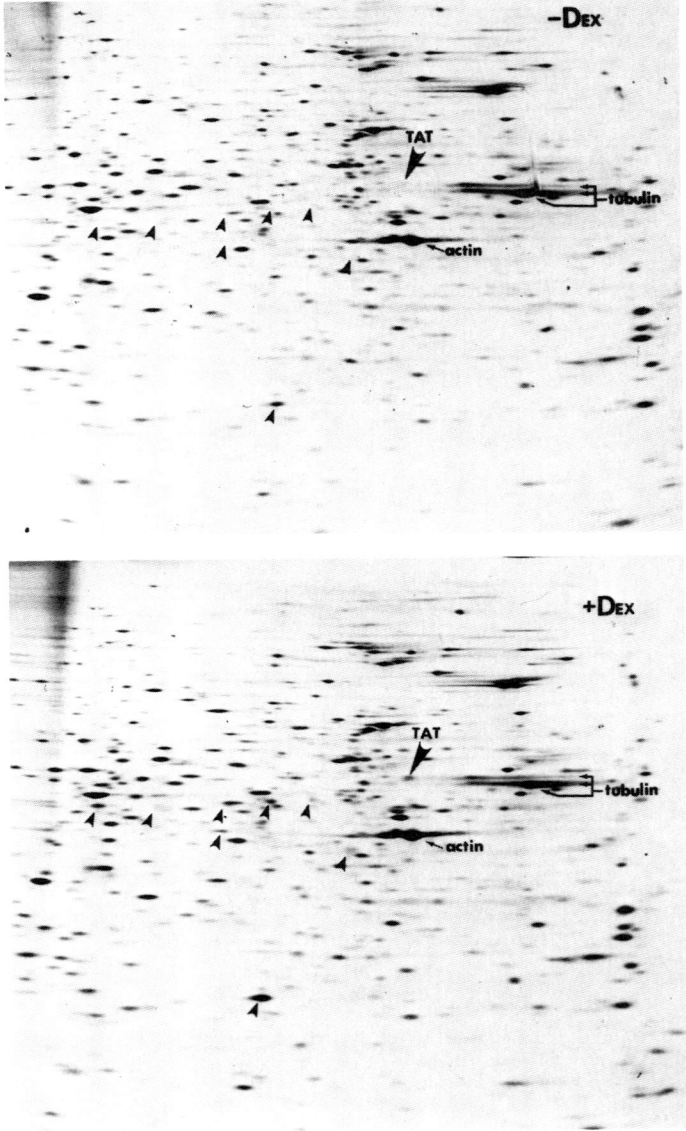

Fig. 3. Two-dimensional gel autoradiographs from induced and uninduced rat hepatoma cells. [^{35}S]methionine-labeled proteins (see text) from dexamethasone-treated (+dex, 10^{-6} M for 18 hours) and untreated cells (−dex) have been electrophoresed as described by Ivarie and O'Farrell (1977). The locations of three identified proteins, actin, tubulin, and tyrosine aminotransferase (TAT), are shown for reference. Arrows denote polypeptides whose rates of synthesis are increased by the steroid.

on a two-dimensional autoradiograph, the 0.5–1.0% of the genes actively being expressed in the cells respond to the hormone. Thus, only a small fraction of the cell's gene products respond to the inducing steroid, and the hormonal effect is highly selective and specific. Further, all induced proteins have measurable basal rates of synthesis. It would appear, therefore, that glucocorticoids control the rate of synthesis of gene products already being expressed and do not activate, for instance, transcriptionally inactive genes. In fact, modulation of expressed genes, rather than their activation, may be a general feature of glucocorticoid hormone action.

C. Regulation of Growth Hormone Production by Cultured Pituitary Cells

Cultured pituitary cells have received attention recently in terms of glucocorticoid hormone action, since the mRNA for growth hormone can be measured and shown to be under glucocorticoid control (Martial et al., 1976). As with cultured hepatoma cells, the response to glucocorticoids is relatively specific in that there is no gross stimulation of protein synthesis by the hormone. With cultured pituitary cells, preliminary analysis of the changes in a number of mRNA's in response to the steroid has also been made as an additional index of the domain of glucocorticoid hormone action (Martial et al., 1976). The proteins synthesized by mRNA from hormone-treated and control cells in a wheat germ cell-free translational system were analyzed by sodium dodecyl sulfate polyacrylamide gel electrophoresis. Again, most of the detectable proteins and, therefore, mRNA's, do not appear to be under hormonal control. However, several mRNA's, including that for pregrowth hormone (the primary translation product of growth hormone mRNA), were induced by the hormone. Thus, in these cells as well, glucocorticoids regulate a small portion of the genome. Again, the data suggest that predominantly the regulation is by modulating levels of mRNA's from genes which are already being expressed.

D. Glucocorticoid Killing of Cultured Lymphoma Cells

The gross inhibition of cellular function after glucocorticoid administration to cultured lymphoma cells may be more generally representative of the actions of these steroids in most mammalian tissues than are the stimulations observed in some tissues (for review, see Baxter and Forsham, 1972; Thompson and Lippman, 1974; Baxter, 1976). The overall domain of glucocorticoid hormone regulation in this case is a constellation of inhibitory processes, including those on transport and macromolecular synthesis, sometimes referred to as the pleiotypic response (Hershko et al., 1971). Of particular interest, some of these inhibitory responses are observed in most mammalian tissues, but it is not uncommon for other or many of the elements to be missing (Baxter, 1976). For example, in some lymphosarcoma cells that are grossly inhibited by the steroid, there is no detectable early influence on inhibiting glucose uptake (Stevens et al., 1973). In hepatic tissue, where the overall glucocorticoid response is stimulatory, inhibition of DNA synthesis can be observed (Loeb, 1976). A simple interpretation of these data is that each of these functions is independently regulated, instead of there being a single induced protein which modulates all of these processes. The receptors are probably involved in all of these effects, since glucocorticoid-resistant cells, which are apparently defective in the receptor, are not known to exhibit any of these inhibitory responses.

IV. AGONISTS, PARTIAL AGONISTS, AND ANTAGONISTS: COMPARISONS OF ACTIONS IN VARIOUS SYSTEMS

Classification of the types of steroid activity in the hepatoma system has received extensive discussion elsewhere, and a large number of steroids have been classified as agonists, antagonists, partial agonists, or inactive steroids (Samuels and Tomkins, 1970; Rousseau et al., 1972, 1973; Baxter and Forsham, 1972; Baxter et al., 1973; Rousseau, 1975; Baxter, 1976). However, two major points deserve emphasis. First, it is important to distinguish between pure antagonist and partial antagonist–partial agonist steroids. In many instances where antagonists have been employed in systems responsive to other classes of steroids, the compounds designated as antagonists are, in fact, partial agonists (Clark et al., 1976). The latter, when given alone, induce some of the same functions as the natural steroid, even though they may inhibit the latter's response to some extent. By contrast, antagonists do not elicit any response when given alone, but if present in adequate concentration may inhibit the response by an agonist. A failure to consider this distinction can lead to confusion, particularly about the comparative aspects of the mechanism of antagonist action.

The second point concerns variations in the classification of certain steroids, depending on the systems which are examined. Whereas optimal agonists in one system generally tend to be optimally active in others, consistency is not seen with the partial agonists and antagonists (for review, see Baxter, 1976). For example, progesterone has been found to have almost pure antagonist activity in cultured hepatoma cells (Rousseau et al., 1972) and in the mouse mammary tumor system (Ringold et al., 1975), whereas it is almost an optimal agonist in the cultured mouse lymphoma cells (Rosenau et al., 1972) and in mouse thymocytes (Munck and Wira, 1971).

11-Deoxycortisol (cortexolone) is almost an antagonist in mouse thymocytes (Munck and Wira, 1971; Turnell et al., 1974), but is a strong partial agonist in cultured hepatoma cells (Samuels and Tomkins, 1970). The reasons for these differences are not clear, but the receptors themselves, or intracellular factors which influence them, may differ in the various tissues.

V. STRUCTURE-ACTIVITY RELATIONS: NATURE OF THE RECEPTOR-BINDING SITE

The discovery of the antiinflammatory properties of the adrenal steroids led to one of the more intensive investigations in pharmaceutical industry history of the effects of structural modifications of a compound on biological activity (for review, see Baxter, 1976). The hope was to obtain steroids having even greater antiinflammatory properties with reduced effects on other glucocorticoid-regulated functions. This was not achieved. However, a number of cortisol analogues were obtained which gave as great a response as cortisol, but at a lower dose. In fact, the only qualitative improvement in the more potent synthetic glucocorticoids over the naturally occurring cortisol was that the former, for the most part, exhibited relatively less mineralocorticoid activity (Liddle, 1959). Thus, these steroids appear to be more specific for the glucocorticoid receptor than cortisol.

Cultured cells have been particularly useful for elucidating the mechanism of the influences of structural modifications on glucocorticoid potency. Most of the data obtained from intact animals do not distinguish whether the effect is due to metabolism of the analogue, an influence on receptor affinity, or a qualitative change in the steroid's classification. By comparing binding and biologic data from cultured hepatoma cells with observations in the animal, a reasonable account has been made of the mechanism of the various structural influences. For example, dexamethasone administered to the animal is about 32 times more potent than cortisol (Ballard et al., 1975). A major reason for this increased potency is that dexamethasone has an approximately eightfold higher affinity for the receptor than cortisol (Rousseau et al., 1972). The remainder of the difference appears to be due to the slower clearance of dexamethasone than cortisol (Ballard et al., 1975).

Figure 4 shows the structure of cortisol and certain modifications of it which result in more potent agonist or antagonist activity. The presence of a double bond between positions one and two on the steroid molecule, and/or the addition of of a fluoride moiety on position nine increase the affinity of the steroid for the receptor (Baxter and Tomkins, 1971; Rousseau et al.,

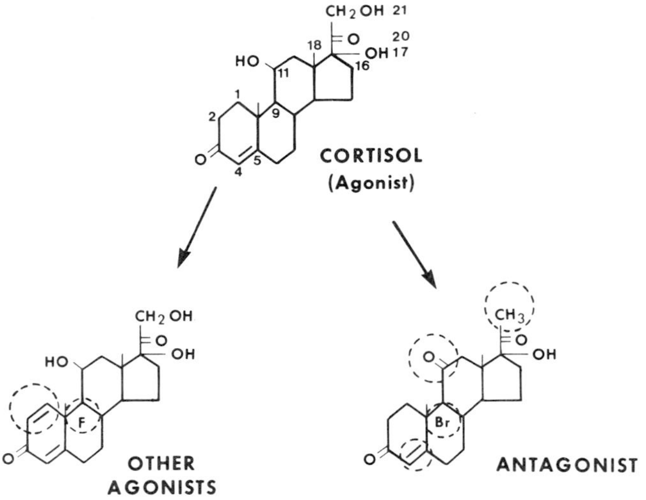

Fig. 4. Structure of cortisol and modifications which result in more potent agonist or antagonist activity.

1972; Ballard *et al.*, 1975). If the double bond at position 4-5 is reduced to the α-configuration, a very large substituent is introduced at position 9 (e.g., a bromo group instead of a fluoro group), a keto group is made at position 11, or the 21-position is methylated, the resulting steroid tends to have more antagonist or partial agonist activity than the parent reference compound. These latter substitutions are ordinarily associated with a lower or with an unchanged receptor affinity. It must be stressed that these are general influences, and the existence of one particular substituent does not always allow a precise prediction of the activity of the steroid.

Measurements of the apparent equilibrium dissociation constant as a function of temperature suggest that the enthalpy and entropy of the binding decrease with increasing temperature (Wolff *et al.*, 1976). These data are explained by the hypothesis that the steroid–receptor binding forces are hydrophobic, and displacement of water molecules upon binding is a major driving force in the reaction. Based on the temperature dependence of the association rate constant, the energy of activation has been calculated at 12 kcal/mole and the entropy of the activation at 14 e.u. The latter also suggests a hydrophobic driving force for formation of the transition state for binding (Wolff *et al.*, 1976). From experimentally determined hydrophobicities of several steroids and the relation between the surface area of proteins and their contribution to hydrophobic binding, it appears likely that both sides of the steroid are enveloped by the receptor (Wolff *et al.*, 1976).

In support of this idea is the finding that there is good (but not exact) correspondence between the surface area of the substituent added and the increase in free energy of the binding (Wolff *et al.*, 1976). Since the net difference in free energy between hydrogen bonding of protein with water and hydrogen bonding of the steroid with protein may be small, it is unlikely that hydrogen bonding contributes much to the net driving force of the reaction; hydrogen bonds are important, however, as lack of the ability to form them may result in less free energy change (Wolff *et al.*, 1976). Thus, the C-3 and C-20 ketones and the C-11 and C-21 hydroxyl groups markedly enhance binding (Baxter and Tomkins, 1971; Rousseau *et al.*, 1972; Ballard *et al.*, 1975), and some hydrogen bond donors and acceptors respectively must be present in the receptor near those sites on the steroid.

To understand the contribution of the individual substituents in binding, we made a number of comparisons of the free energies of binding of steroid pairs which differed in only one substituent (Wolff *et al.*, 1976). This allowed a determination of the free energy of binding of the individual substituent. The data have indicated that the free energy group increments are roughly additive and independent such that they have been of some usefulness in predicting the affinity of the steroids for the receptor in cases where the binding constants are unknown. However, we found that the affinity in general can be much more accurately determined by examining the effect of substitution on the structure of the steroid molecule in greater detail. From these analyses, four parameters have emerged as being major contributors: A-ring conformation, surface area, size of the individual substituents and specific polar interactions (such as those due to the presence of 11β-hydroxy group). Using these parameters, we obtained a mathematical relationship that has allowed an accurate prediction of the affinity of steroids for the receptor. This type of approach enhances the ability to predict affinity from structure and should be more generally applicable for systems responsive to other classes of ligands.

VI. MECHANISM OF AGONIST AND ANTAGONIST STEROID ACTION: ALLOSTERIC MODEL FOR STEROID HORMONE ACTION

Based on the fact that various steroids act as agonists or antagonists in hepatoma cells, Samuels and Tomkins proposed that glucocorticoids exert an allosteric effect on the receptor (Fig. 5), which is important for its biologic function. This model has subsequently received direct experimental support from several lines of investigation (Baxter and Tomkins, 1970; Rousseau *et al.*, 1972, 1973, 1975). We found that, like agonists, suboptimal

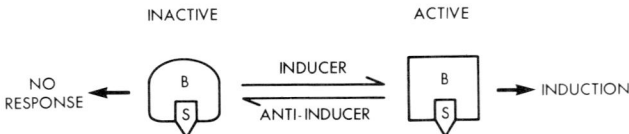

Fig. 5. Allosteric model for steroid hormone action. Inactive and active refer to the different conformational states of the receptor. The active state promoted by inducers (or agonists) results in the biologic response (induction). The inactive state, favored by anti-inducer (antagonist) binding, does not result in a biologic response. Reprinted from Baxter, 1976.

and anti-inducer steroids bind to the receptors and can inhibit the binding of agonists. The inhibition was competitive, suggesting that both classes of compounds bind to the same molecule. Further, the inhibition of binding by agonists could be quantitatively correlated with the inhibition of induction. Thus, it appears that antagonists act by binding to the receptor and preventing the binding of agonists.

The studies by Rousseau *et al.* (1972, 1973, 1975) provided further indications about the influence of agonists and antagonists on the receptor and the mechanism of antagonism. Thus, whereas agonist–receptor complexes bind to the nuclei in whole cells, antagonist–receptor complexes do not (Fig. 6). In addition, binding of agonist–receptor complexes to DNA is much

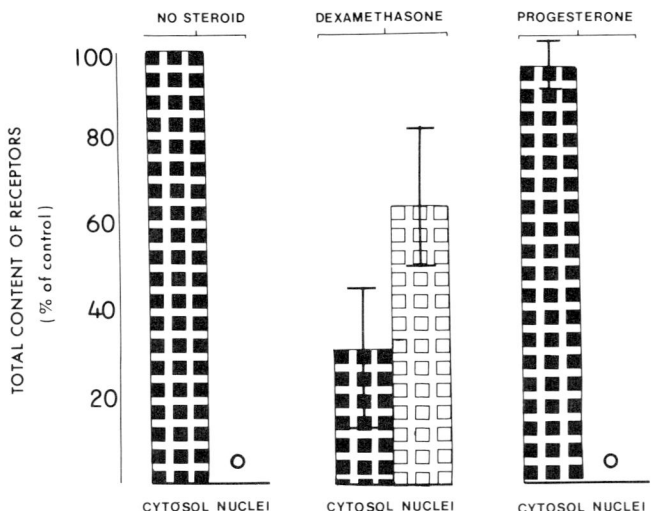

Fig. 6. Effects of an agonist (dexamethasone) and antagonist (progesterone) on the subcellular distribution of glucocorticoid receptors in cultured hepatoma cells. Data taken from Rousseau *et al.*, 1973; reprinted from Baxter, 1976.

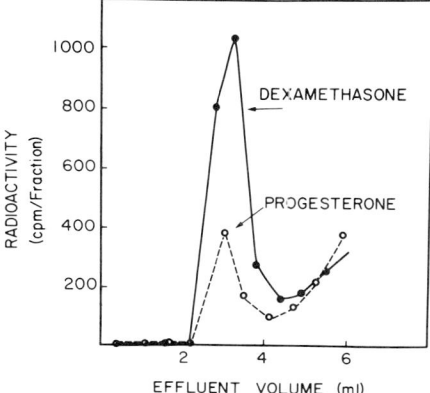

Fig. 7. Agonist–receptor complexes bind to DNA more than antagonist–receptor complexes. Shown is the elution profile in the excluded fraction of an agarose gel in which the DNA–receptor complexes elute separated from receptors not bound by DNA. In this experiment, receptor–dexamethasone (agonist) or receptor–progesterone (antagonist) complexes were incubated with DNA prior to filtration. Data taken from Rousseau et al., 1975.

stronger than is binding of antagonist–receptor complexes (Fig. 7). Agonist–receptor complexes are more stable to heat denaturation than are uncomplexed receptors or antagonist–receptor complexes (Rousseau et al., 1972). Thus, the important conformational effect of the steroid is to influence the receptor so that it can bind to the nucleus. Antagonists occupy the same receptor but do not promote the changes in the receptor necessary for nuclear binding.

The biologic properties of the partial agonists can be most easily explained by the allosteric model formulated by Rubin and Changeux (1966), assuming nonexclusive binding. The proposal is that allosteric ligands can bind to both "active" and "inactive" conformational states of the receptor. The extent to which a steroid is an agonist is determined by the extent to which it influences receptors to be in the active state. After partial agonist binding, some receptors are in each state, and, therefore, a suboptimal quantity of receptors are available for eliciting the subsequent steps in the response. Binding data (Rousseau et al., 1973) provide support for this idea. We found that the partial agonist deoxycorticosterone, which at maximally effective concentrations induces tyrosine aminotransferase by about a third that of an optimal agonist, such as dexamethasone, also results in about a third as much nuclear binding as the agonist.

The model developed in the glucocorticoid system may also apply for other steroid-responsive systems. In subsequent studies, Marver et al. (1974) found that mineralocorticoid receptors complexed with an antimineralocorticoid (spironolactone) do not bind to the nuclear chromatin. In other systems, the data are not as clear because of the problem of partial agonist–partial antagonist activity. For example, cortexolone (11-deoxycortisol) is an antagonist with respect to glucose uptake in thymocytes and promotes some nuclear binding of the receptor (Wira and Munck, 1974). However, this steroid has some albeit weak, agonist activity on uridine transport (Turnell et al., 1974). Thus, this partial agonist activity (which may be undetectable when glucose uptake is examined) predicts the small amount of nuclear binding that is observed. Similarly, in estrogen-responsive systems, some antiestrogens promote receptor binding to the nucleus, but these compounds also have agonist activities (Clark et al., 1976). Of course, there may be mechanisms for antagonist action other than those occurring through the allosteric influence on the receptor.

VII. ACTIVATION OF THE RECEPTOR–GLUCOCORTICOID COMPLEX

A. Studies in Cell-Free Systems

Following cell-free binding of an active steroid to the receptor, there must be a change enhanced by temperature, salt, and dilution before the complex can associate with nuclei (Baxter et al., 1972; Higgins et al., 1973a; Rousseau et al., 1975). The change has been termed "activation" and is analogous to the "transformation" of the estrogen receptor (Jensen and De Sombre, 1972). For example, when active steroids bind to the receptors at low ionic strength at 0°C, the resulting complexes do not bind to nuclei. However, raising the ionic strength or the temperature generates complexes that bind to nuclei even at low ionic strength and temperature. Thus, the activation step results in an increase in the receptor's affinity for nuclei. These procedures also stimulate receptor binding to chromatin or DNA. An unanswered question is whether the activation of the receptors is the same as, or the consequence of, the allosteric changes discussed in the section above.

Aside from the finding that the activation exposes a nuclear binding site on the receptor, changes in physical properties of the receptors accompanied by this reaction are poorly understood. As mentioned earlier, the rate of dissociation of the steroid may be slower from activated than from inactivated receptors. The receptor sediments in low ionic strength buffers around 6 S (Baxter and Tomkins, 1971), and this 6 S form does not bind to the nucleus. Receptors extracted from the nucleus (Higgins et al., 1973c) or obtained after a salt treatment that results in activation sediment around 4

S (J. D. Baxter, unpublished observations). However, receptors can be obtained such that only a portion of them are activated as measured by their capability of binding to isolated nuclei, even though all of them sediment around 4 S (J. D. Baxter, unpublished observations). Therefore the 6 S to 4 S conversion, although associated with activation, may not be the activating event, and the 4 S form, although necessary, does not appear to be sufficient for activation. These observations suggest that activation is due to some change in the 4 S form of the receptor which does not affect its sedimentation.

B. Studies with Intact Cells

Most studies of activation have been with cell-free systems. Since the cell ordinarily functions under conditions (37°C and salt concentrations near 0.15 M) which markedly favor activation, it might be questioned whether activation is an important reaction in the cell. Although an unambiguous answer to this question is not available, it appears that (a) activation does occur in the cell and, (b) only a portion of the cytosol receptor–steroid complexes are activated.

The data in Fig. 8 suggest that activation can occur in the cell. If cells are incubated with the hormone at 0°C, cytosol binding can reach maximal levels (Levinson et al., 1972; Rousseau et al., 1973) at a time when there is essentially no nuclear binding. Once the temperature is raised to 37°C, nuclear binding occurs very rapidly. Therefore, there is a temperature-dependent step in the cell distal to hormone–receptor complex formation that is required for nuclear binding. This temperature-dependent step is probably not nuclear binding, since binding of activated receptor–glucocorticoid complexes by isolated nuclei progresses rapidly at 0°C (Baxter et al., 1972; Higgins et al., 1973a). Although activation can be demonstrated by first binding at 0°C as shown in Fig. 9, under ordinary induction conditions at 37°C nuclear binding occurs so quickly that activation cannot, kinetically, be rate limiting.

The suggestion that some of the intracellular receptors not bound to chromatin are in the inactivated form was obtained from experiments in which hormone was incubated with intact cells and the proportion of receptor steroid complexes in the cytoplasm in the activated form was quantified (Baxter et al., 1977). Under these conditions, only 40–60% of the soluble receptor–dexamethasone complexes (e.g., those not bound by the nuclei) were capable of binding to the nucleus in a subsequent cell-free binding reaction and were, therefore, in the activated form. The remaining complexes were presumably not in the activated form. Of importance is that these experiments were performed under conditions in which the complexes, once

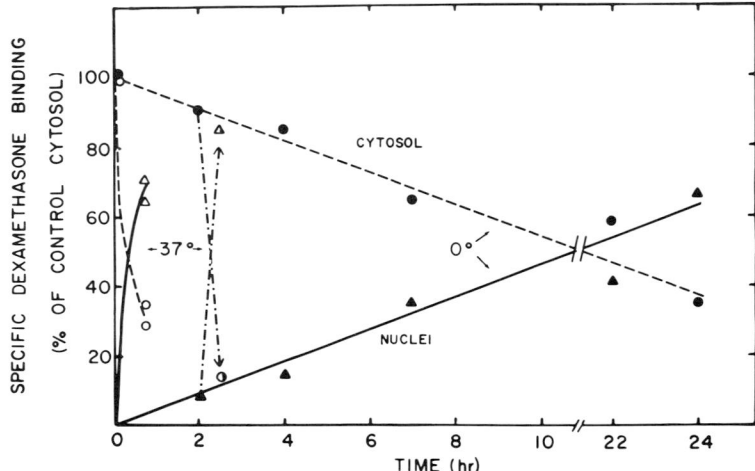

Fig. 8. Nuclear binding in the intact cell requires a temperature-dependent step. Hepatoma cells were incubated at 37°C (△, ○), at 0°C (▲, ●), or first at 0°C and then at 37°C (▲, ◐) with 50 nM [^{3}H]dexamethasone. Cultures for determination of "background" binding were incubated in parallel. Circles and triangles show the concentration of receptors of receptors in cytosol and nuclei, respectively, at the various time points. Reprinted from Rousseau et al., 1973.

activated, do not revert to the inactivated conformation (Higgins et al., 1973a). Also, as relative saturation of the receptor by the hormone occurs, the proportion of receptor–steroid complexes not bound by the nuclei in the activated form remains constant (Baxter et al., 1977). Since the amount of nuclear binding in the cell was also found to be linearly proportional to the concentration of activated receptor–dexamethasone complexes, activation may be rate-limiting in terms of determining the magnitude of nuclear binding in the cell (Baxter et al., 1977).

VIII. RETURN OF THE RECEPTOR TO THE CYTOSOL: THE FIRST STEP IN DEINDUCTION

Following removal of the hormone from the media, the steroid rapidly dissociates from its receptor, followed by a rapid return of the receptor to the cytosol (Fig. 9) and a subsequent decline in the hormonal effect (Baxter and Tomkins, 1970; Rousseau et al., 1973). Return of the receptor to the cytosol occurs even when protein and RNA synthesis are inhibited (Fig. 9). Thus, preexisting receptors, and not newly synthesized ones, are responsible for replenishing of receptors in the cytoplasm. The reaction is easily explained by assuming that when the inducer dissociates from the receptor, the steroid-induced conformational state required for nuclear binding is no longer maintained, and the receptor, therefore, simply dissociates from the nucleus. In other systems, it has been proposed that ATP is required for this return (Munck *et al.*, 1972); we have not studied this in the hepatoma system.

IX. NUCLEAR BINDING OF RECEPTOR–GLUCOCORTICOID COMPLEXES

The nuclear binding of receptor–glucocorticoid complexes has been demonstrated in intact cells (Baxter and Tomkins, 1970; Baxter *et al.*, 1971; Higgins *et al.*, 1973a; Rosenau *et al.*, 1972; Simons *et al.*, 1976). The precise nature of these nuclear binding sites or acceptors is not known. It does appear that all of the acceptor activity is located on the chromatin, as nuclear-bound receptors can be recovered bound to chromatin (S. J. Higgins, G. G. Rousseau, J. D. Baxter, unpublished observations). Isolated chromatin also binds the complexes (Simons *et al.*, 1976). DNA appears to be involved in acceptor activity and the DNA–receptor reaction simulates, in many ways, the nuclear–receptor interaction (Baxter *et al.*, 1972; Rosenau *et al.*, 1972; Yamamoto and Alberts, 1976; Yamamoto *et al.*, 1976).

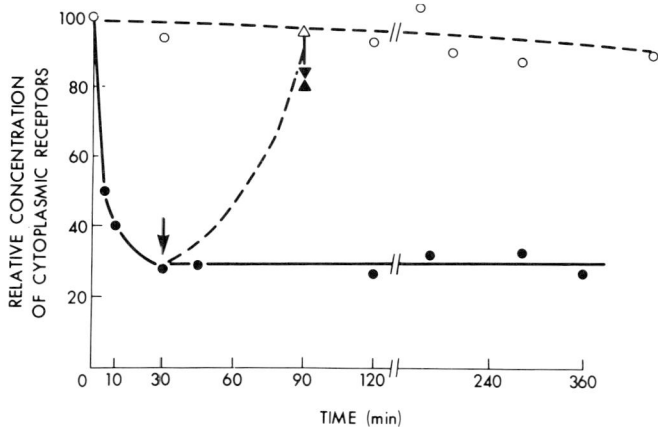

Fig. 9. Return of the hepatoma cell glucocorticoid receptor to the cytosol after removal of the steroid even when protein and RNA synthesis are inhibited. The content of cytosol receptors was monitored in control (○) and dexamethasone-treated (△, ○, ▲, ▼) cultures. At 30 minutes, dexamethasone was removed from certain cultures (△, ▲, ▼). In some of the cultures, (▲, ▼) cycloheximide (0.1 mM) and actinomycin D (5 μg/ml), respectively, were present throughout the experiment. Reprinted from Rousseau *et al.*, 1973.

A. Acceptor Capacity in the Cell

To obtain some indication of the nuclear acceptor capacity in the intact cell, nuclear binding was measured at varying intracellular concentrations of the cytoplasmic receptor–glucocorticoid complex (Baxter *et al.,* 1977). The amount of nuclear binding was linearly proportional to the cytosol receptor–steroid complex concentration, and there was no apparent saturation (Fig. 10). A Scatchard plot of the nuclear-bound over cytoplasmic-bound complexes as a function of the nuclear-bound complexes was parallel to the abscissa. These observations suggest that, as in the uterus (Williams and Gorski, 1972), the nuclear sites are far from saturated with receptor–steroid complexes at concentrations that are maximally achievable in the cell. Therefore, only a lower estimate of the nuclear acceptor capacity can be made from this type of analysis.

In parallel experiments, the relative activation of the receptors was also

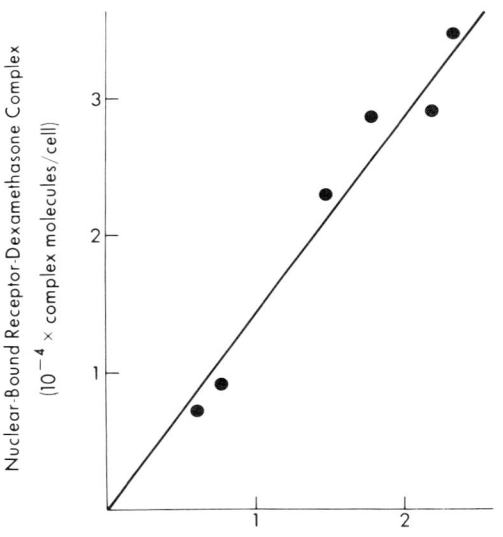

Fig. 10. Nuclear binding of receptor–dexamethasone complexes in cultured hepatoma cells as a function of the concentration of receptor–dexamethasone complexes in the cytosol (e.g., those not bound by the nuclei). Cultured hepatoma cells were incubated with varying concentrations of radioactive dexamethasone to produce increasing amounts of relative saturation of the receptors. Following the incubation, the concentration of complexes bound to the nuclei and free in the cytosol were measured by techniques similar to those described previously (Rousseau *et al.,* 1973). Reprinted from Baxter, 1976.

monitored (Baxter et al., 1977). This was a constant proportion of the cytosol receptor–steroid complex. Therefore, nuclear binding is also linearly related to the concentration of activated receptors. Assuming that the measured cytosol receptor–steroid complexes are, in fact, free in the cell, we estimate that when the receptors are saturated with steroid, the concentrations of free activated complex in the cell is around 3 nM (Baxter et al., 1977). Using this value and the idea that the acceptors are far below saturation, the average equilibrium dissociation constant (K_d) of the acceptors for binding the receptors is well above 3 nM, i.e., if the concentration of activated receptors approaches a level equivalent to the K_d, the function shown in Fig. 10 should demonstrate some tendency to reach a plateau.

B. Cell-Free Nuclear Binding

As indicated earlier, activated receptor–glucocorticoid complexes can also bind to nuclei in cell-free systems. The characteristic of the complexes bound by nuclei in the intact cell and in cell-free conditions are similar with respect to the rate of dissociation of the complexes from nuclei, the sensitivity of the complexes to release by salt, and the sedimentation properties of the extracted complexes (Higgins et al., 1973c). It would appear at this level of analysis, that the nuclear acceptors as assayed in cell-free conditions are similar to those assayed in whole cells.

Several studies using the cell-free system have been directed at determining the number of nuclear accepting sites. Higgins et al. (1973) reported that there was a limited capacity of nuclei for binding receptors. The estimation of the number of sites was in error since it came from experiments in which the receptor–steroid complex concentration was varied by adding increasing amounts of crude cytosol. The latter contains inhibitors of the nuclear-binding reaction, which vary under these experimental conditions and which are responsible for the underestimate (Higgins et al., 1973a; Simons et al., 1976). However, other data have suggested that there is a limited nuclear binding capacity. This came from the observation that receptors complexed with unlabeled steroid competed with labeled receptor–steroid complexes for nuclear binding under conditions of constant inhibitor (Higgins et al., 1973a). A further indication of specificity of this nuclear binding came from the result that glucocorticoid–receptor binding to the hepatoma nuclei was not inhibited by estrogen–receptor complexes (from uterine cytosol) under conditions in which the latter readily inhibited binding of radioactive estrogen–receptor complexes by uterine nuclei (Higgins et al., 1973b). Nevertheless, Simons et al. (1976) were later unable to reproduce some of these findings; in their studies, the relationship between nuclear binding and added receptors either in crude cytosol or in purified nuclei was found to be linear, suggesting that, at concentrations of receptor employed, there is no detectable saturation of the nuclear acceptors. Simons et al. (1976) also observed more nuclear binding than did Higgins et al. (1973a). The reasons for these discrepancies have not been resolved. However, the data of Simons et al. (1976), suggesting that in fact the nuclear accepting capacity is quite large, is more consistent with the experiments with intact cells described above. Further, the idea that the nuclei have a high capacity for accepting receptors has also received support from the observation that cell-free nuclear binding is the same whether or not the nuclei used contained receptors which had been bound in the cell (Higgins et al., 1973c).

C. The Glucocorticoid Receptor as a DNA-Binding Protein

The glucocorticoid receptor is a DNA-binding protein (Baxter et al., 1972; Rousseau et al., 1975; Simons et al., 1976; Yamamoto et al., 1974), as demonstrated by a variety of techniques. This observation provides one of the stronger lines of evidence supporting the idea that DNA is involved in acceptor activity. In fact, there is ordinarily more binding by DNA than by chromatin or nuclei (on a per milligram DNA basis) when experiments are performed at low ionic strength (Baxter et al., 1972; Rousseau et al., 1975; Simons et al., 1976). These data probably indicate that the receptor binds extensively to DNA and also that chromatin proteins may restrict the receptor's accessibility to DNA. The extensiveness of the DNA binding is also illustrated by our findings (Rousseau et al., 1975) that, even at very high receptor–dexamethasone concentrations, there is no evidence that the DNA is even approaching saturation with receptors. Although these considerations may suggest that the receptors bind anywhere there are charged polynucleotides, the available data indicate that there is some specificity to the reaction. One of the more illustrative experiments is shown in Fig. 11. There is little or no detectable binding of receptors by 23 S ribosomal RNA under conditions where marked DNA binding is observed. A further indication of specificity comes from studies with synthetic polydeoxyribonucleotides (Simons, 1977a), some of which bind receptors much less effectively than do natural DNA's. The variation in the receptor affinity for various polynucleotides suggests that multiple orders of binding affinity exist and there may be sequence-specific binding.

It is not clearly resolved whether all of the receptors can bind to DNA. Simons (1977b) has obtained evidence that only half of the receptors bind to DNA, suggesting the possibility of a mechanism analogous to that proposed

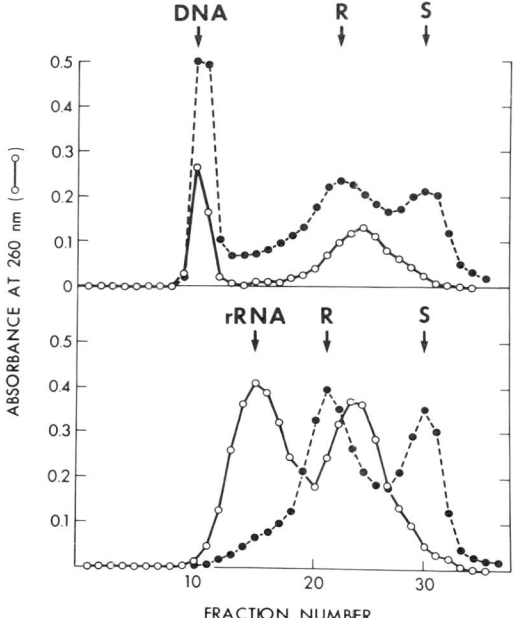

Fig. 11. Glucocorticoid receptors bind to DNA more avidly than to RNA. Shown are agarose gel elution patterns after activated glucocorticoid receptor–dexamethasone complexes are incubated with DNA (top) or rRNA (bottom). The regions of elution of DNA and rRNA receptors not bound by DNA or RNA (R) and free steroid (S) are indicated by the respective arrows. Reprinted from Rousseau et al., 1975.

in the progesterone receptor in which only half of the receptors bind to DNA and the other half bind to chromatin (O'Malley and Schrader, 1976). In conflict with this are studies by Yamamoto et al. (1976) with the lymphoma cells in which all of the receptors apparently bind to DNA.

The idea that DNA is involved in acceptor activity is further suggested by the fact that DNA binding simulates nuclear binding in several important respects. (a) Uncomplexed receptors do not bind to DNA (Rousseau et al., 1975). (b) The binding of anti-inducer–receptor complexes is much weaker than is the binding of inducer–receptor complexes (Fig. 7, Rousseau et al., 1975). (c) The activation step required for nuclear binding also stimulates DNA binding (Rousseau et al., 1975). Finally, in steroid-resistant lymphoma cells, receptor defects associated with increased or decreased nuclear binding have parallel changes in their DNA-binding properties (Yamamoto et al., 1976).

D. The Subchromatin Localization of Receptors: Nuclease Digestion Studies

The idea that DNA is involved in acceptor activity is also supported by nuclease digestion studies. When about 50% of the total DNA in chromatin is destroyed by pancreatic DNase I (Fig. 12), the chromatin's acceptor activity is also destroyed. Since this nuclease attacks DNA between the nucleosomes, as well as portions of it contained within them (Weintraub and Groudine, 1976), it is possible that the acceptors for glucocorticoid receptors (or factors required for their integrity) are present either between nucleosomes or in some of the more nuclease-sensitive portions on the cluster. For comparison, uterine nuclei which bind both estrogen and glucocorticoid receptors were digested with DNase (Higgins et al., 1973b). Whereas the enzyme destroyed glucocorticoid receptor acceptor activity, acceptors for estrogen receptors were not destroyed. These data raise the important question of whether the binding sites for estrogen receptors are fundamentally different from those of glucocorticoid receptors.

In sharp contrast to the case when acceptor activity is examined after nuclease attack, receptors already bound by nuclei are not released by a similar DNase treatment. If these receptors were bound in the nuclease-

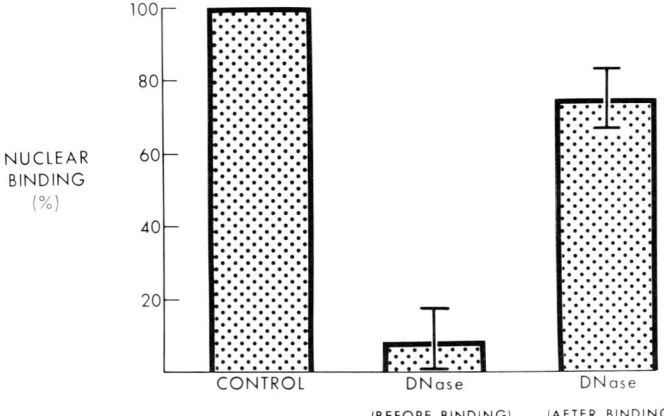

Fig. 12. Effect of DNase I on nuclear binding of receptor–glucocorticoid complexes. The first column shows cell-free binding to control nuclei not treated with DNase. The second column shows the cell-free binding to nuclei treated with DNase I (pancreatic) under conditions in which about 50% of the DNA was released with no detectable effect on nuclear morphology by light microscopy. The third column shows an experiment in which receptor–glucocorticoid complexes were first bound by nuclei, then the nuclei were treated with DNase so that a similar amount of DNA was released as in the experiment shown in the second column. Data taken from Baxter et al., 1972. Reprinted from Baxter et al., 1973.

sensitive DNA stretch between the nucleosomes, it seems likely that they would have been released. It is possible then that these receptors are bound to DNA near to or on the nucleosomes and that they protect the DNA segment to which they are bound from the digestion. As the structure of chromatin and the consequences of the nuclease digestion are being understood (Weintraub and Groudine, 1976), it may be possible to utilize data of this nature to determine more precisely the location in chromatin of the site of binding of receptor–glucocorticoid complexes.

We also studied chromatin treatment with DNase II (Levy and Baxter, 1976). A brief exposure to this endonuclease releases chromatin pieces containing about 10% of the DNA. These fragments are enriched 20-fold in nascent RNA chains, and, in this respect, the released fraction is enriched in "active" chromatin. This chromatin also contains a subset of specific DNA sequences (Gottesfeld et al., 1974). After incubating cells with dexamethasone and then treating the chromatin with the nuclease, only 10–20% of the chromatin-bound glucocorticoid receptors remained with the "transcriptionally active" chromatin. These observations may imply that the glucocorticoid receptors are extensively distributed within chromatin. However, the released pieces, although enriched for portions active in RNA synthesis, do not necessarily contain the sites where RNA synthesis is regulated. Therefore, some receptors in the inactive fraction may be involved in regulation of the response.

E. Evidence for a Role of Chromatin Elements Other than DNA in Acceptor Activity

Even though DNA is an essential factor in nuclear binding, it appears that other chromatin elements also influence acceptor activity (Simons et al., 1976). This notion is based on a comparison of the salt sensitivity and the kinetics of nuclear and DNA binding. DNA binding is much more sensitive to salt than is nuclear binding (Fig. 13). For example, at 0.15 M sodium chloride, nuclear binding is only mildly inhibited (Higgins et al., 1973c), whereas DNA binding is almost abolished (Rousseau et al., 1975). Nuclear-bound receptors dissociate more slowly than do receptors bound by purified DNA. The half-time for dissociation of receptors from nuclei is probably greater than 24 hours (Higgins et al., 1973c), whereas that from DNA is nearer to 20 minutes (Simons et al., 1976). These two lines of evidence suggest that nuclear binding is tighter than is DNA binding. Therefore, some factors in nuclei may increase the receptor's apparent affinity for DNA.

The reasons for the nuclear–DNA binding differences are not known. No clear evidence is available regarding possible specific acceptor proteins as

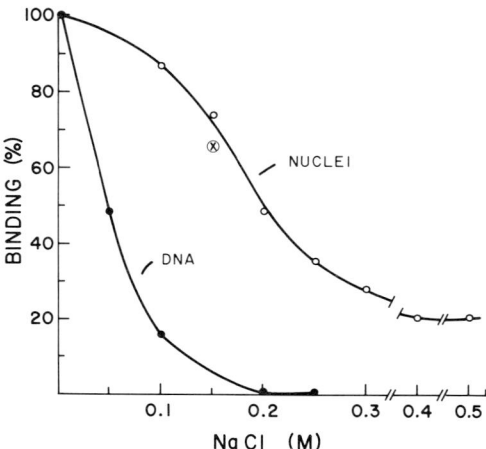

Fig. 13. Comparison of the salt sensitivity of nuclear and DNA binding. Soluble receptor–glucocorticoid complexes were activated and then incubated with DNA at various salt concentrations as indicated on the abscissa. The amount of binding was measured by agarose gel filtration. Data taken from Rousseau et al., 1975. The data for nuclear binding (○) (from Higgins et al., 1973c) were obtained by incubating nuclei containing bound receptor–glucocorticoid complexes with the salt concentrations shown on the abscissa and measuring the amount of residual binding. Shown also is the amount of nuclear binding (⊗) when the experiment was performed by incubating activated receptor–glucocorticoid complexes with nuclei at 0.15 M NaCl and then measuring the nuclear binding.

has been proposed for other systems (O'Malley and Schrader, 1976) or whether some general influence of the chromatin structure on DNA is responsible. It is possible that the apparently higher nuclear affinity is caused by the compactness of DNA in chromatin which effectively "traps" the receptor such that, when it dissociates from one location on DNA, it reassociates at other loci on DNA nearby. This type of phenomenon has received analysis with respect to other binding systems where the measured apparent affinity is higher than the actual affinity (Silhavy et al., 1975).

F. Correlation between Receptor Binding to the Nucleus and the Glucocorticoid Response: The Question of "Hidden" High-Affinity Acceptor Sites Mediating Receptor Action

The finding of a large nuclear acceptor capacity in the intact cell, a general receptor distribution in both active and inactive fractions of nuclease-sheared chromatin, and high capacity binding of purified DNA suggests that the receptor has a general affinity for DNA. These data raise the question of whether nuclear binding observed in the cell is by sites involved in the glucocorticoid response. Is all of the observed binding due to low-affinity associations of the receptor with DNA, and does this large amount of nonspecific binding hide high-affinity sites responsible for the response, but which are undetectable because of their small quantity (Yamamoto and Alberts, 1975)? We have approached this question by analyzing, in hepatoma cells, the concentrations of steroid–receptor complex required for nuclear binding and for eliciting the glucocorticoid response. By estimating the concentration of activated glucocorticoid–receptor complexes not bound by the nucleus, some limits to the proportional saturation of any hypothetical high-affinity sites can be made. For example, if nuclear acceptors were present with an equilibrium dissociation constant for the complexes of 1 pM or below, these would be essentially saturated at the 3 nM concentration of activated complex maximally achieved in the cell. In fact, even if the receptors were 10% saturated with hormone (resulting in a concentration of activated complex of 0.3 nM) such sites would still be essentially saturated with the receptors. In this event, the biologic response should be near maximal even when only 5–10% of the receptors are filled with the steroid. This is not the case. Instead, the relation between tyrosine aminotransferase induction and the relative saturation of the receptors has been found to be a linear one (Baxter *et al.*, 1977). Therefore, it is unlikely that the sites promoting induction are saturated even at maximally obtainable receptor concentrations in these cells. In fact, the linear relationship between nuclear binding and the response suggests that sites with an affinity for the receptors similar to that of the observed binding are involved in the induction. Of course, the actual shape of the dose-response curve and the actual estimate of the affinity for the receptor of the acceptor sites where the receptor acts also depends on other questions that have not been considered here, such as the number of receptors that bind at each important site, the way the interaction affects the response, and the effect of each interaction on mRNA expression. However, many of these more complex models predict cooperative or nonlinear relationships which have not been observed.

X. GENETIC APPROACHES TO THE STUDY OF GLUCOCORTICOID HORMONE ACTION

A. Isolation of Glucocorticoid-Resistant Cell Lines from Cultured S49 Lymphoma Cells

The isolation of lymphoid cell lines that do not respond to glucocorticoids has been facilitated by the strong selective pressures that can be employed since the steroid-sensitive parent lines are killed by the hormone. The major advantage in terms of genetic analysis is that a single-step isolation for steroid resistance is possible. Most of the work has been on a cell line (S49) derived from a mouse lymphoma (Horibata and Harris, 1970; Harris, 1970). These cells have also served as a model for lymphoid leukemia in man which shares the characteristics displayed in S49 cells of a high incidence of steroid resistance which is associated with detectable defects in the receptor (Lippman et al., 1973).

Steroid-resistant cells are obtained by plating steroid-sensitive cells at high densities in soft agar containing lethal concentrations of dexamethasone (Sibley and Tomkins, 1974a). The vast majority of the cells fail to form a clone; those that do grow can be picked and grown to high density for subsequent genetic and biochemical analysis. Those cells selected as steroid-resistant appear to result from a mutational event. First, all clones are completely stable showing the resistant phenotype even after a year in culture in the absence of steroid; reversion to sensitivity has not been detected (Baxter et al., 1971; Sibley and Tomkins, 1974a). Secondly, the frequency of resistance is about 3×10^{-6} per cell per generation and is increased by chemical mutagens or γ-irradiation (Sibley and Tomkins, 1974a). Thirdly, a fluctuation analysis has shown that the occurrence of resistance is a random event not induced by the selective conditions (Sibley and Tomkins, 1974a). Finally, in many cases an altered gene product, the receptor, can be demonstrated (Baxter et al., 1971; Rosenau et al., 1972; Sibley and Tomkins, 1974b; Yamamoto et al., 1976).

B. Phenotypic Classification and Biochemical Lesions Associated with Steroid Resistance

When we initially studied steroid-resistant lymphoma cells, decreased binding was found in both of the S49 steroid-resistant lines and in a line (S1AT·4TB2H) derived from another lymphoma (S1AT4) (Baxter et al., 1971). Subsequently, Sibley and Tomkins (1974a), Yamamoto et al. (1976), and Gehring and Tomkins (1974) examined a much larger number of resistant lines derived from S49 cells. By analyzing steroid-binding activity and nuclear transfer in whole cells and in cell-free systems, four classes of phenotypic variants were detected: r^- for decreased receptor-binding activity; nt^- for nuclear "transfer" deficient; nt^i for increased nuclear transfer; and d^- (deathless) associated with normal receptor and nuclear binding. There was low or no steroid-binding activity in 55% of the resistant clones, and 70–75% of them had less than 30% of the wild-type binding activity. In mixed extract experiments, lesions associated with the variant phenotypes were in the cytosol, and not the nucleus, in broken cell preparations, suggesting that the defects are in the receptor protein itself and not in some cellular factor associated with nuclei (Rosenau et al., 1972; Gehring and Tomkins, 1974; Yamamoto et al., 1976). For instance, nuclei from nt^i cells do not bind wild-type receptors more avidly than nuclei isolated from wild-type cells, and conversely, nt^i receptors show quantitatively similar transfer to nuclei from either nt^i or wild-type cells (Yamamoto et al., 1976).

Thus, these data strongly imply that steroid resistance in S49 cells is ordinarily associated with alterations in the receptor. However, the observed biochemical abnormality characterizing each phenotypic class does not demonstrate the cause of the resistance. First, many of the r^- cells have 30% as much binding activity as wild-type cells. It is likely that if these receptors were normal, some killing would be observed at steroid concentrations that saturate them. Instead, it is more likely that these receptors are defective in normal receptor function. The same holds true for nt^- cells, which transfer a significant quantity of receptors to the nucleus. In fact, nuclear binding by nt^- cell lines is, on the average, only decreased by 56% (Sibley and Tomkins, 1974b). This magnitude of nuclear binding should result in marked killing if the receptors in nt^- cells were functionally normal. Thus, receptors in these cells are probably abnormal in their function. The finding of steroid-resistant cells containing nt^i receptors also indicates that nuclear binding *per se* is not necessarily lethal, since in the cell 86–95% of these receptors bind to the nucleus. The idea that nt^- and nt^i receptors are qualitatively different than the wild-type receptors is also illustrated by the fact that, respectively, they have decreased or increased binding to nuclei or DNA (Yamamoto et al., 1976). Further, nt^i receptors sediment more slowly than wild-type receptors (Yamamoto et al., 1976). Thus, whereas defective receptor function accounts for resistance in most of the steroid-unresponsive S49 lines, the mechanisms for such defective action are not known.

From these and other considerations, it is clear that some level of specificity, in addition to hormone and nuclear binding, exists in receptor action. For example, mutant receptors may not bind to the functionally important nuclear sites or may not act properly once bound. In fact, even the d^- cells may also be resistant, due to defective receptor function, even though hormone and nuclear binding are quantitatively normal.

C. Mechanism for the Preponderance of Receptor Defects

Since defects in the receptor are obtained in all or almost all instances of S49 cell resistance, the question arises of why a substantial number of the lines are not defective in other elements of the pathway leading to death. For example, if killing were due to an induction of a lethal function, it might be expected that cells defective in it might be isolated as frequently as are cells defective in the receptor. Similarly, if several gene products other than the receptor were necessary for killing, a defect in any of these should cause resistance, and the proportion of cells which are resistant due to defective receptor function would decrease even more.

One simple explanation for this result is that the receptor gene is functionally haploid, whereas the lethal genes are diploid in their expression. In fact, recent evidence by Bourgeois and Newby (1977) suggests that this may be the case. They found that W7 cells contain twice the number of glucocorticoid receptors in S49 cells and were twice as sensitive on a dosage basis as S49 cells. Further, the earlier results of Harris (A. W. Harris, personal communication) were confirmed that the frequency of glucocorticoid resistance in W7 cells is orders of magnitude lower than in S49 cells. However, whether gene dosage figures significantly in determining the kinds of cellular variants that can be selected is not answered. Does the inability to obtain an appreciable number of steroid-resistant cell lines with normal receptor binding provide a clue to the mechanism of killing? For instance, the receptor may induce a large number of gene products, each of which is lethal to the cell. In this case, all these genes would have to mutate before any variant other than in the receptor would occur. An alternative possibility is that the receptor represses the expression of a gene product essential for cell growth. A mutation in such a gene would be lethal and never isolated. Consistent with this possibility (and discussed above) is that steroids may repress some proteins. However, against this possibility is that P. H. O'Farrell and K. R. Yamamoto (personal communication) were unable to detect, by two-dimensional gel electrophoresis, changes in the rate of synthesis of any S49 cell protein in response to dexamethasone.

D. Comparison of the Nature of Resistance in S49 Cells with that Observed in Other Glucocorticoid-Responsive Systems

Since a lot of information is available about how S49 lymphoma cells become resistant, it is of interest to know whether the pattern for steroid unresponsiveness in these cells is a general one. Resistance does follow a similar pattern in acute lymphocytic leukemia of childhood (Lippman et al., 1973) and other cases (Kaiser et al., 1974; Baxter et al., 1971; Hollander and Chiu, 1966), being almost always associated with decreased steroid binding. However, it should be noted that there are other patterns of unresponsiveness even in lymphoid cells. For example, two steroid-resistant sublines derived from another lymphoma (S1A) were markedly different. In one which had been selected for resistance, there was decreased receptor binding just like S49 r^- cells. In the other subline, which arose spontaneously, steroid resistance appeared to be inducible. These cells ceased growing for a time after exposure to the steroid, but eventually grew normally. Following withdrawal of steroid, the cells regained their steroid sensitivity. Other patterns of steroid unresponsiveness which may differ from the usual case with S49 cells are observed in developing tissues and in other types of lymphoid cells. In developing liver (Feldman, 1974) and lung (Ballard and Ballard, 1974; Giannopolous, 1975), receptors are clearly present before there is responsiveness, although, for technical reasons, the precise receptor quantity is not known (Feldman, 1974; Gianopolous, 1975). Further, there are numerous examples in lymphomic, myelomic, leukemic, and phytohemagglutin-stimulated cells where there is apparently normal steroid-binding activity and yet the cells are not inhibited by the glucocorticoid (Baxter et al., 1971; Lippman et al., 1973; Gailini et al., 1973; Gehring et al., 1972). Finally, the high frequency of resistance observed in S49 cells may not always be obtained. A. W. Harris (personal communication) has found that several thymoma cell lines (derived from the same inbred strain of mice as the S49 cells) become steroid resistant at a frequency several orders of magnitude lower than S49 cells (also confirmed by Bourgeois and Newby, 1977). These lines are of particular interest in light of the discussions in the previous sections.

XI. REGULATION OF mRNA BY GLUCOCORTICOID HORMONES

A. Regulation of Growth Hormone mRNA

As already mentioned, glucocorticoids cause an approximately fourfold increase in the rate of synthesis of growth hormone and its mRNA (Fig. 14). A cell-free translational assay has been used to monitor growth hormone mRNA activity after hormonal stimulation and during purification (Martial et al., 1977). The purified message has, in turn, been used as a template for the synthesis of a cDNA probe for use in hybridization experiments to quantify growth hormone mRNA sequences.

In a cell-free translation system from wheat germ, about four times more pregrowth hormone is synthesized from mRNA from induced than from uninduced cells. Synthesis of pregrowth hormone has been measured by immunoprecipitation of the radioactively labeled protein from a translation reaction and identified by sodium dodecyl sulfate–polyacrylamide gel electrophoresis. Of importance is that the translations are performed under conditions in which the amount of pregrowth hormone synthesized is linearly related to the amount of RNA added. Although pregrowth hormone (24,000

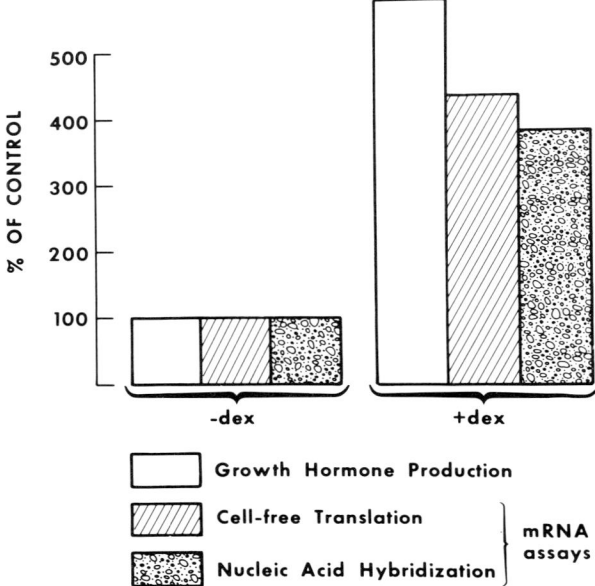

Fig. 14. Influence of dexamethasone on growth hormone production and growth hormone mRNA in cultured pituitary cells. The data shows the relative levels of growth hormone production as assayed by radioimmunoassay, and growth hormone mRNA as analyzed by either cell-free translation or cDNA–RNA hybridization. Data taken from Martial et al., 1977.

daltons) is the primary translation product of the message, the cell-free system from Krebs II ascites cells produces authentic growth hormone (19,500 daltons), provided a membrane fraction (which presumably contains an enzyme necessary for conversion of pregrowth hormone to growth hormone) is present (P. H. Seeburg, unpublished observations). Although these results imply an increase in the number of copies of growth hormone mRNA in response to glucocorticoids, the data do not exclude the possibility that only the activity or translational efficiency of preexisting mRNA is increased by structural modifications (i.e., methylation, 5′-"capping," removal of a 5′- or 3′-sequence by ribonucleolytic cleavage).

Support for the idea that the hormone-stimulated changes in growth hormone mRNA translational activity reflect changes in mRNA copy number has been obtained by hybridization data. cDNA complementary to growth hormone mRNA hybridizes more rapidly to RNA isolated from induced cells than from uninduced cells. Of note is that the increase in the rate of hybridization by RNA from hormone-treated compared to that from control cells is similar in magnitude to the increase in mRNA activity assayed by cell-free synthesis and to the increase in production of the protein by the cells. Thus, the steroid-induced increase in growth hormone production may solely be due to an increase in its mRNA content. These results are consistent with the idea that these steroids enhance the rate of growth hormone gene transcription. An indication of the specificity of this hormonal effect is obtained from the fact that the data are expressed as growth hormone mRNA per total RNA and from the sodium dodecyl sulfate–polyacrylamide gel electrophoresis analysis of the products synthesized by the cellular mRNA's in the cell-free systems as described earlier.

B. Regulation of Tyrosine Aminotransferase mRNA

The induction of tyrosine aminotransferase synthesis in hepatoma cells has, as already mentioned, been studied in considerable detail. The available data suggest that the steroid-mediated increase in the rate of tyrosine aminotransferase synthesis is due to an increase in tyrosine aminotransferase mRNA. However, the evidence for alterations in messenger concentration is indirect because it relies extensively on inhibitor studies. It is, therefore, not as conclusive as that obtained in other systems. Nevertheless, the observations in the hepatoma cell system by Tomkins and his colleagues represented some of the stronger earlier evidence that steroid hormones influence specific mRNA's.

Hence, in cultured hepatoma cells, inhibition of RNA synthesis by actinomycin D (Tomkins *et al.*, 1966, 1969) or removal of the cell nucleus by centrifugation in cytochalain B-containing medium (Ivarie *et al.*, 1974) prevents enzyme induction. In fully induced cells, there is a 10-fold increase in the number of cellular ribosomes engaged in enzyme synthesis (Scott *et al.*, 1972). A cell-free protein-synthesizing system prepared from induced cells synthesizes about 10 times more enzyme than one from uninduced cells (Beck *et al.*, 1972); all of the enzyme-specific synthesis in these extracts resides in the polysomes. From a series of experiments using inhibitors of the initiation or elongation reactions in polypeptide synthesis, it was concluded that glucocorticoids do not detectably alter the translation efficiency of tyrosine aminotransferase mRNA (Scott *et al.*, 1972; Steinberg *et al.*, 1974). A simple interpretation of all of the observations is that the inducing steroid promotes an increase in the messenger RNA for tyrosine aminotransferase.

C. Primary Versus Secondary Induction of Specific mRNA's by Glucocorticoids

A central problem in steroid hormone action has been whether the hormone acts directly on a specific gene, for instance, by enhancing its transcription (primary induction) or acts indirectly by inducing another protein (secondary induction) which, in turn, influences expression of the gene product being considered. An approach to this problem was devised by Peterkofsky and Tomkins (1968) in their studies of the steroid-mediated induction of tyrosine aminotransferase in hepatoma cells. In particular, they asked whether messenger RNA for this enzyme could accumulate in response to the hormone when protein synthesis was blocked. After treating cells with steroid and the reversible inhibitor of polypeptide synthesis, cycloheximide, removal of both steroid and inhibitor was followed by a prompt increase in enzyme activity without the usual 1–1.5 hour lag seen with hormone alone. Moreover, the rise in enzyme activity was not prevented by subsequent inhibition of RNA synthesis by actinomycin D. It appears, therefore, that the inducing steroid promotes TAT messenger RNA accumulation, even in the absence of protein synthesis. Induction of mouse mammary tumor virus RNA by glucocorticoids also occurs in the absence of protein synthesis (Ringold *et al.*, 1975), but, surprisingly, an analysis of the response by this approach has only rarely been made with other steroid-responsive systems (Palmiter *et al.*, 1976).

D. The Question of How Generally Does the Glucocorticoid Action Occur Through Induction of Specific mRNA's

In only a few cases are data available to demonstrate that glucocorticoids increase specific mRNA's. Evidence that an induction of mRNA underlies all glucocorticoid responses is based on analogy with the systems which have been analyzed in some detail, as well as a larger body of data reviewed elsewhere (Thompson and Lippman, 1974; Baxter, 1976) showing that the responses are inhibited by actinomycin D. In some cases, a glucocorticoid-regulated gene product may influence other proteins at posttranscriptional or even posttranslational levels, such that the measured gene product is certainly not under direct transcriptional control by the hormone. For example, the induction of alkaline phosphatase may be mediated by an activator of the enzyme which is induced (Cox *et al.*, 1971); thus, the induced protein may actually be the activator of the enzyme. With glucocorticoid-regulated catabolism, the inhibition of glucose uptake may require RNA synthesis (Mosher *et al.*, 1971; Young *et al.*, 1974), but it is not known whether other aspects of glucocorticoid-mediated killing in lymphoma cells are due to stimulation of mRNA. Finally, some actions of glucocorticoids occur quite rapidly (within 1 or 2 minutes; e.g., the rapid feedback inhibition by glucocorticoids of ACTH) (Dallman *et al.*, 1972; Jones *et al.*, 1974), and they may not involve transcriptional effects.

XII. DEINDUCTION OF THE GLUCOCORTICOID RESPONSE: POSTTRANSCRIPTIONAL CONTROL OF TYROSINE AMINOTRANSFERASE

Whereas RNA synthesis is necessary for the induction of tyrosine aminotransferase in cultured hepatoma cells, it is also necessary for the deinduction (Tomkins *et al.*, 1969). In fact, under certain conditions, (e.g., in cells which are deprived of serum), blocking RNA synthesis during deinduction increases enzyme activity levels ("superinduction") (Tomkins *et al.*, 1969, 1972; Thompson *et al.*, 1970, Kenny *et al.*, 1973; Steinberg *et al.*, 1975a,b).

Considerable controversy has surrounded these observations, and most of the discussion has focused on the question of whether actinomycin D blocks the decline in the induced rate of TAT synthesis, as argued by Tomkins and his colleagues (Tomkins *et al.*, 1972; Steinberg *et al.*, 1975a,b) or, alternatively, blocks enzyme degradation, as argued by Kenney *et al.* (1973). In fact, the drug affects both processes. The enzyme is degraded sufficiently rapidly in hepatoma cells (half-life of 2–3 hours), that inhibition of its turnover by the drug would also prevent its deinduction (Tomkins *et al.*, 1972). To answer this question, the rate of synthesis and degradation of the enzyme following treatment of induced cells with actinomycin D has been measured. It was found that the inhibitor has two effects on tyrosine aminotransferase: it slows the rate at which enzyme synthesis deinduces, and it reduces the rate of enzyme degradation (Steinberg *et al.*, 1975a,b). As a result, tyrosine aminotransferase activity remains at the induced level or superinduces even though enzyme production falls. The effects of enucleation on tyrosine aminotransferase are even more striking (Fan *et al.*, 1977). Removal of the nucleus from induced cells almost completely abolishes both enzyme synthesis and degradation, thereby preventing deinduction.

Although these data clearly indicate that there is posttranscriptional control of processes controlling tyrosine aminotransferase, there is no direct evidence to support the idea, initially suggested by Tomkins *et al.* (1969), that glucocorticoids have a posttranscriptional effect on regulation of the mRNA for the enzyme. An extensive analysis of the kinetics of the induction and deinduction of enzyme synthesis has favored a transcriptional mechanism of action (Steinberg *et al.*, 1975a), although a posttranscriptional mechanism could not be excluded. Regardless, the kinetic analyses placed an upper limit to the half-life of tyrosine aminotransferase RNA at 1.5 hours. Thus, if steroids controlled tyrosine aminotransferase levels strictly at the level of messenger degradation, the messenger would have to turn over with a half-life of approximately 9 minutes in the absence of the hormone and 90 minutes in the hormone's presence to generate the characteristic 10-fold induction.

XIII. MECHANISM OF GLUCOCORTICOID RECEPTOR ACTION: PARALLELS WITH CYCLIC AMP ACTION IN BACTERIA

For understanding genetic expression in eukaryotes, it is frequently useful to consider similar kinds of regulation in prokaryotes. For steroid regulation, most analogies have been made with the interreaction of the repressor of the lactose operon with DNA (Yamamoto and Alberts, 1975, 1976). However, as discussed below, the steroid system is fundamentally different from the lactose system. By contrast, another regulatory system, catabolite repression in *Escherichia coli* (Zubay, 1974), has received much less attention from a comparative point of view. Yet, this system has many properties that are similar to glucocorticoid action at both physiological and molecular biologic levels.

The similarity of the physiological influences of glucocorticoids in eukaryotic systems to those of cyclic AMP action in bacteria has been reviewed (Baxter and Forsham, 1972; Baxter, 1976). In *E. coli,* a deprivation of glucose results in a stimulation of cyclic AMP which, in turn, stimulates the metabolism of a number of sugars other than glucose (Zubay, 1974). The breakdown of these sugars results in more glucose, thereby providing an alternate source of energy for the bacterium. Thus, deprivation of glucose is the signal to seek alternate sources of energy. Similarly, in mammals, glucocorticoids decrease glucose utilization in peripheral tissues, promote catabolism of other substances which can be alternate forms of energy or gluconeogenic precursors, and stimulate glucose production (Baxter and Forsham, 1972; Baxter, 1976). Thus, glucose is a central theme in the physiology of both regulatory systems.

The two regulatory molecules are similar in that each regulates a small but, nevertheless, substantial portion of the genome. Although 0.5–1.0% of the genome in cultured hepatoma cells is affected by glucocorticoids (Ivarie and O'Farrell, 1977), the actual size may vary in different tissues. Cyclic AMP influences about 10% of the *E. coli* proteins (O'Farrell, 1975b). Further, the direction of the response is generally to induce protein synthesis, although in both cases some inhibitory influences are observed. Although the domain of response to glucocorticoids is different according to cell type, the total domain in the whole animal is quite large, being the sum of the responses in the different tissues.

At the molecular level, the binding of the regulatory ligand to its specific receptor protein and the subsequent interaction of the protein with DNA provide stronger parallels. In both cases, the interaction of the ligand with its receptor is a high affinity and reversible binding, the consequence of which is a promotion in the protein's affinity for DNA (Zubay, 1974). Antagonists exist for both binding reactions, and these prevent DNA binding (Riggs et al., 1971). Although receptor–ligand complexes associate extensively with DNA, they discriminate between RNA and DNA by binding much more tightly to the latter than to the former (Riggs et al., 1971). In the case of the CRP protein, cAMP complex binding to general DNA is not much weaker than is the binding to specific sequences of DNA (CRP promotors) at which the molecules influence specific gene transcription (Majors, 1975; Mitra and Zubay, 1975). As presented earlier in this chapter, a similar conclusion may hold for the steroid–receptor complex, although the evidence is much more indirect.

The similarities between the steroid and cAMP receptor interaction with DNA contrast with the nature of the interaction of the lac repressor with nonspecific and specific DNA sequences. With the latter, binding of the inducer to the repressor markedly decreases the repressor's affinity for specific operator sequences, yet does not alter its affinity for nonspecific DNA sequences (Lin and Riggs, 1975). As a consequence, the repressor is effectively removed from its regulatory site on the bacterial chromosome. In this respect, repressor function is different since it blocks, rather than enhances, specific gene transcription. In the presence of the inducer, the *lac* repressor is still associated with DNA, however, at nonspecific sites and not free in the cytoplasm (Lin and Riggs, 1975). Finally, the lac repressor is known to act at only one site on the bacterial chromosome, and, thus, its regulatory influence is extremely restricted. It should be noted that other operons in *E. coli* are controlled by repressors whose operator-specific binding is greatly enhanced by binding its "corepressor" or regulatory ligand (Zubay, 1974). In one case, it is thought that the repressor functions, in addition, as an activator of gene transcription, depending on the particular ligand which is bound to it (Zubay, 1974). In any case, the point is that repressor–operator interactions are fundamentally more different from steroid–receptor–DNA interactions than they are similar.

Perhaps the most important similarity between CRP and steroid receptors is the mechanism of action once bound to DNA. Thus, both apparently promote specific gene transcription, although this point has yet to be demonstrated thoroughly for steroid receptors. Although the two classes of proteins are quite similar, many questions are yet to be answered. In particular, the action of cyclic AMP in eukaryotes is fundamentally different from that in prokaryotes. In eukaryotes, cAMP works primarily through protein kinase and subsequent protein phosphorylation (Sutherland,

1972), whereas in bacteria cAMP works through the CRP protein and promotes specific gene transcription. Thus, mechanisms of protein modification as, for example, phosphorylation, acetylation, and methylation, must be considered. Further, the organization of eukaryotic chromatin may be such that very different types of influences are required to regulate transcription (Yamamoto and Alberts, 1976). However, it is still possible that steroid–receptor complexes simply promote the ability of RNA polymerase to transcribe certain regions of the genome by a mechanism analogous to that of CRP. The hope is that cell-free systems developed from higher organisms, coupled with genetically altered regulatory elements, will provide a definitive answer to the mechanism of action of the glucocorticoid hormones.

XIV. SUMMARY

In this review, we have mainly summarized results of our studies on glucocorticoid action. The responses elicited in the systems studied are diverse, but the basic molecular events in the hormone's action are similar in many respects. The glucocorticoid receptors are cytosol proteins that associate with the nucleus after binding an active steroid. The data suggest that hydrophobic interactions account for a major quantity of the free energy associated with binding, and that both sides of the steroid are enveloped by the receptor. Conformational changes may also influence the reaction to a major degree. The affinity of the steroid for the receptor can, in general, be determined from the conformation and surface area and the size and polar nature of individual substituents. There is a strong correlation between hormonal binding to the receptor and the steroid's biologic activity, with respect to agonist, as well as partial agonist and antagonist steroids. In cultured hepatoma cells, binding of the hormone to the receptor parallels the induction of tyrosine aminotransferase. However, such a quantitative relationship may not always be observed with other glucocorticoid-responsive systems. The glucocorticoid receptors are present in most mammalian tissues. The expression of a subset of specific genes in responsive cells is affected by the hormone. The gene products influenced by the hormone in a particular cell (termed its cellular domain) can be measured at the level of the proteins or their messenger RNA's. Whereas most proteins in the domain of hormonal control are induced, repression is occasionally observed. In hepatoma cells, 0.5–1.0% of the cell's gene products are induced, suggesting that a similar fraction of the expressed genes in these cells is under glucocorticoid control.

The use of antagonist steroids which competitively inhibit agonist binding to the receptor has facilitated the understanding of glucocorticoid action. Whereas agonists promote receptor binding to the nucleus, antagonist–receptor complexes do not associate with nuclei and have a reduced affinity for DNA. Several claims that antagonist–receptor complexes bind to the nucleus in many systems have been based on studies with hormones which have partial agonist activity. In any event, the biologic activities of the steroids and their influence on the receptor are most easily explained by an allosteric model in which agonist, but not antagonist, steroids cause a change in the receptor's conformation, such that it binds to the nucleus and promotes the subsequent steps in the response.

Following the binding of an active steroid to the receptor, there is a temperature and salt-dependent step, termed activation, necessary for nuclear binding. Studies in hepatoma cells suggest that activation does occur in the intact cell, as it does in cell-free systems. Whereas, on a kinetic basis, activation does not appear to be rate-limiting for the response, some of the hormone–receptor complexes in the cell apparently remain in the inactivated form, even when the receptors are saturated by the hormone. In cultured hepatoma cells, the hormone rapidly dissociates from the receptor following removal of the steroid from the medium, and, as a consequence, the receptor returns to the cytosol by a process that does not require protein or RNA synthesis. This appears to be the first step in deinduction. Thus, receptor binding to nuclei appears to be a reversible event.

Hormone–receptor complexes bind in the nucleus probably because of their DNA-binding properties. However, the receptor apparently binds more tightly to nuclei than to DNA; this may be due to some other feature of chromatin which enhances the receptor's affinity for DNA. Nuclease digestion studies suggest that receptors are extensively distributed within chromatin. The capacity of nuclei for binding receptors exceeds the cell's content of receptors. Nuclear binding and the glucocorticoid response are linearly related to the concentration of receptor–glucocorticoid complexes free in the cell. These data suggest that nuclear acceptors which have an affinity for the receptor that is similar to those responsible for the observed nuclear binding mediate the glucocorticoid response. The data argue against the idea that acceptors with an extremely high affinity for the receptor mediate the response, as they would have been saturated at much lower concentrations of receptor.

Steroid-resistant lymphoma cell lines have provided important information about receptor action; these display a variety of detectable alterations in receptor binding activity or other properties. In cases where there is decreased binding activity, these receptors must also be defective in their function. Why resistance in S49 cells due to elements other than the receptor is only rarely detected remains unexplained. However, in certain other steroid-responsive systems, changes in hormonal sensitivity are not associated with detectable alterations in the receptor.

Glucocorticoids regulate the intracellular content of specific mRNA's. Of the systems we have studied, the regulation of growth hormone mRNA is the best example in that the mRNA has been demonstrated by cell-free translation and cDNA–RNA hybridization techniques. In some cases, mRNA regulation appears to be a direct effect of the receptor, presumably on gene transcription, because mRNA accumulation can occur in the absence of protein synthesis. In the case of tyrosine aminotransferase, RNA synthesis is required for deinduction, as well as induction. Inhibition of RNA synthesis apparently results in an increased stabilization of the enzyme as well as its mRNA. Thus, there may be posttranscriptional control of this enzyme, although there is no direct evidence that the steroid influences these events. The mechanism(s) by which the hormone–receptor complex interacts with the DNA to alter specific mRNA concentrations is not known.

ACKNOWLEDGMENT

This review is dedicated to the late Gordon M. Tomkins. Much of the work described here was performed in collaboration with him or by his colleagues. We have been immeasurably influenced by his inspiration and insights.

The work was supported by NIH Grants 1-R01-AM-18878-01 and EY01785-01. John D. Baxter is an Investigator of the Howard Hughes Medical Institute. Robert Ivarie was supported by NIH Training Grant No. HL05725 from the Heart and Lung Institute.

REFERENCES

Azarnoff, D. L. (1975). *In* "Steroid Therapy" (ed.), p. 1–340, Philadelphia, Pennsylvania.
Ballard, P. L., and Ballard, R. A. (1974). *J. Clin. Invest.* **53,** 477–486.
Ballard, P. L., and Tomkins, G. M. (1970). *J. Cell Biol.* **47,** 222–234.
Ballard, P. L., Baxter, J. D., Higgins, S. J., Rousseau, G. G., and Tomkins, G. M. (1974). *Endocrinology* **94,** 998–1002.
Ballard, P. L., Carter, J. P., Graham, B. S., and Baxter, J. D. (1975). *J. Clin. Endocrinol. Metab.* **41,** 290–304.
Baxter, J. D. (1974). *J. West. Med.* **120,** 301–306.
Baxter, J. D. (1976). *Pharmacol. Ther. B.* **2,** 605–659.
Baxter, J. D., and Forsham, P. H. (1972). *Am. J. Med.* **53,** 573–589.
Baxter, J. D., and Harris, A. W. (1975). *Transplant. Proc.* **7,** 55–65.
Baxter, J. D., and Tomkins, G. M. (1970). *Proc. Natl. Acad. Sci. U.S.A.* **65,** 709–715.
Baxter, J. D., and Tomkins, G. M. (1971). *Proc. Natl. Acad. Sci. U.S.A.* **68,** 932–937.
Baxter, J. D., Harris, A. W., Tomkins, G. M., and Cohn, M. (1971). *Science* **171,** 189–191.

Baxter, J. D., Rousseau, G. G., Benson, M. C., Garcea, R. L., Ito, J., and Tomkins, G. M. (1972). *Proc. Natl. Acad. Sci. U.S.A.* **69**, 1892–1896.
Baxter, J. D., Rousseau, G. G., Higgins, S. J., and Tomkins, G. M. (1973). In "The Biochemistry of Gene Expression in Higher Organisms" (J. R. Pollack and J. W. Lee, eds.), pp. 206–224. Australia & New Zealand Book Co., Sydney.
Baxter, J. D., Matulich, D. T., Higgins, S. J., and Simons, S. S. (1977). In preparation.
Beato, M., Schmid, W., Braendle, W., Beiswig, D., and Sekeris, E. (1971). *Adv. Biosci.* **7**, 349–364.
Beck, J. P., Beck, G., Wong, K. Y., and Tomkins, G. M. (1972). *Proc. Natl. Acad. Sci. U.S.A.* **69**, 3615–3619.
Bourgeois, S., and Newby, R. F. (1977). *Cell* **11**, 423–430.
Clark, J., Baulieu, E.-E., Baxter, J. D., deCrumbrugghe, B., Jorgensen, E., Katzenellenbogen, B. S., Katzenellenbogen, J. A., Luebke, K., Moran, J., Rochefort, H. M., Sherman, M. R., and Toper, M. (1976). In "Hormone and Antihormone Action at the Target Cell" (J. H. Clark *et al.*, eds.), pp. 147–169. Dahlem Konferenzen, Berlin.
Cox, R. P., Elson, M. A., Tu, S.-H., and Griffin, M. J. (1971). *J. Mol. Biol.* **58**, 197–215.
Dallman, M. F., Jones, M. T., and Vernikos-Danellis, J. (1972). *Endocrinology* **91**, 961–968.
Failla, D., Tomkins, G. M., and Santi, D. V. (1975). *Proc. Natl. Acad. Sci. U.S.A.* **72**, 3849–3852.
Fan, W. J-W., Ivarie, R. D., and Levinson, B. L. (1976). *J. Biol. Chem.*, in press.
Feldman, D. (1974). *Endocrinology* **95**, 1219–1227.
Feldman, D., Funder, J. W., and Edelman, I. S. (1972). *Am. J. Med.* **53**, 545–560.
Feldman, D., Funder, J. W., and Edelman, I. S. (1973). *Endocrinology* **92**, 1429–1441.
Gailini, S., Minowada, J., Silvernail, P., Nussbaum, A., Kaiser, N., Resen, F., and Shimaoka, K. (1973). *Cancer Res.* **33**, 2653–2657.
Gehring, U., and Tomkins, G. M. (1974). *Cell* **3**, 301–306.
Gehring, U., Mohit, B., and Tomkins, G. M. (1972). *Proc. Natl. Acad. Sci. U.S.A.* **69**, 3124–3127.
Gehring, U., Mohit, B., and Tomkins, G. M. (1973). *Endocrinol. Proc. Int. Symp., 4th, 1972 Excerpta Med. Found. Int.* Congr. Ser. No. 273, pp. 426–432.
Giannopolous, G. (1975). *J. Steroid Biochem.* **6**, 623–631.
Gottesfeld, J. M., Garrard, W. T., Bagi, G., Wilson, R. F., and Banner, J. (1974). *Proc. Natl. Acad. Sci. U.S.A.* **71**, 2193–2197.
Granner, D. K., Thompson, E. B., and Tomkins, G. M. (1970). *J. Biol. Chem.* **245**, 1472–1478.
Gross, S. R., Aranow, L., and Pratt, W. B. (1970). *J. Cell Biol.* **44**, 103–113.
Harris, A. W. (1970). *Exp. Cell Res.* **60**, 341–353.
Harrison, R. W., Fairfield, S., and Orth, S. N. (1975). *Biochemistry* **14**, 1304–1307.
Hershko, A., Mamont, P., Shields, R., and Tomkins, G. M. (1971). *Nature (London)*, New Biol. **232**, 206–211.
Higgins, S. J., Rousseau, G. G., Baxter, J. D., and Tomkins, G. M. (1973a). *J. Biol. Chem.* **248**, 5866–5872.
Higgins, S. J., Rousseau, G. G., Baxter, J. D., and Tomkins, G. M. (1973b). *J. Biol. Chem.* **248**, 5873–5879.
Higgins, S. J., Rousseau, G. G., Baxter, J. D., and Tomkins, G. M. (1973c). *Proc. Natl. Acad. Sci. U.S.A.* **70**, 3415–3418.
Horibata, K., and Harris, A. W. (1970). *Exptl. Cell Res.* **60**, 61–77.
Hollander, N., and Chiu, Y. W. (1966). *Biochem. Biophys. Res. Commun.* **25**, 291–297.
Imperato-McGinley, J., and Peterson, R. E. (1976). *Am. J. Med.* **61**, 251–272.
Ivarie, R. D., and O'Farrell, P. H. (1977). Submitted for publication.

Ivarie, R. D., Fan, W. J.-W., and Tomkins, G. M. (1974). *J. Cell. Physiol.* **85**, 357–364.
Jensen, E. V., and De Sombre, E. R. (1972). *Annu. Rev. Biochem.* **41**, 203–230.
Jones, M. T., Tiptoft, E. M., Brush, F. R., Fergusson, D. A. N., and Neame, R. L. B. (1974). *J. Endocrinol.* **60**, 223–233.
Kaiser, N., Mitholland, R. J., and Resen, F. (1974). *Cancer Res.* **34**, 621–626.
Kenney, F. T., Lee, K. L., and Stiles, C. D. (1973). *Nature (London) New Biol.* **246**, 208–210.
Kono, T., and Barham, F. W. (1971). *J. Biol. Chem.* **246**, 6210–6216.
Kulka, R. G., Tomkins, G. M., and Crook, R. B. (1972). *J. Cell Biol.* **54**, 175–179.
Lefkowitz, R. J. (1976). *N. Engl. J. Med.* **295**, 323–328.
Levinson, B. B., Baxter, J. D., Rousseau, G. G., and Tomkins, G. M. (1972). *Science* **175**, 189–190.
Levitzki, A. (1976). In "Hormone and Anti-hormone Action at the Target Cell" (J. H. Clark *et al.*, eds.), pp. 76–86. Dahlem Konferenzen, Berlin (1976).
Levy, B., and Baxter, J. D. (1976). *Biochem. Biophys. Res. Commun.* **68**, 1045–1051.
Liddle, G. W. (1959). *Ann. N.Y. Acad. Sci.* **82**, 854–867.
Lin, S., and Riggs, A. D. (1975). *Cell* **4**, 107–111.
Lippman, M. E., Halterman, R. H., Leventhal, B. G., Perry, S., and Thompson, E. B. (1973). *J. Clin. Invest.* **52**, 1715–1725.
Lippman, M. E., Stringer, S. Y., and Thompson, E. B. (1974). *Endocrinology* **94**, 262–266.
Loeb, J. N. (1976). *N. Eng. J. Med.* **295**, 547–552.
McEwen, B. S., Denef, C. J., Gerlach, J. L., and Plapinger, L. (1974). In "The Neurosciences: Third Study Program" (F. O. Schmitt and F. G. Worden, eds.), pp. 599–619. MIT Press, Cambridge, Massachusetts.
Manganiello, V., and Vaughn, M. (1972). *J. Clin. Invest.* **51**, 2763–2767.
Majors, J. (1975). *Nature (London)* **256**, 672–674.
Martial, J. A., Baxter, J. D., Goodman, H. M., and Seeburg, P. H. (1977). *Proc. Natl. Acad. Sci. U.S.A.* **74**, 1816–1820.
Marver, D., Stewart, J., Funder, J. W., Feldman, D., and Edelman, I. S. (1974). *Proc. Natl. Acad. Sci. U.S.A.* **71**, 1431–1435.
Mitra, S., and Zubay, G. (1975). *Biochem. Biophys. Res. Commun.* **67**, 857–863.
Mosher, K. M., Young, D. A., and Munck, A. (1971). *J. Biol. Chem.* **246**, 654–659.
Munck, A., and Wira, C. (1971). *Adv. Biosci.* **7**, 301–327.
Munck, A., Wira, C., Young, D. A., Mosher, K. M., Hallahan, C., and Bell, P. A. (1972). *J. Steroid Biochem.* **3**, 567–578.
O'Farrell, P. H. (1975a). *J. Biol. Chem.* **250**, 4007–4021.
O'Farrell, P. H. (1975b). *J. Biochem. (Tokyo)* **79**, 33.
O'Malley, B. W., and Schrader, W. T. (1976). *Sci. Am.* **234**, 32–43.
Palmiter, R. D., Moore, P. B., Muwihill, E. R., and Emtage, S. (1976). *Cell* **8**, 557–572.
Peterkofsky, B., and Tomkins, G. M. (1968). *Proc. Natl. Acad. Sci. U.S.A.* **60**, 222–228.
Rao, M. L., Rao, G. S., Holler, M., Breuer, H., Schattenberg, P. J., and Slein, W. D. (1976). *Hoppe-Seyler's Z. Physiol. Chem.* **357**, 573–584.
Riggs, A. D., Reiners, G., and Zubay, G. (1971). *Proc. Natl. Acad. Sci. U.S.A.* **68**, 1222–1225.
Ringold, G. M., Yamamoto, K. R., Tomkins, G. M., Bishop, J. M., and Varmus, H. E. (1975). *Cell* **6**, 299–305.
Rosenau, W., Baxter, J. D., Rousseau, G. G., and Tomkins, G. M. (1972). *Nature (London), New Biol.* **237**, 20–24.
Rousseau, G. G. (1975). *J. Steroid Biochem.* **6**, 75–89.
Rousseau, G. G., Baxter, J. D., and Tomkins, G. M. (1972). *J. Mol. Biol.* **67**, 99–115.
Rousseau, G. G., Baxter, J. D., Higgins, S. J., and Tomkins, G. M. (1973). *J. Mol. Biol.* **79**, 539–554.

Rousseau, G. G., Higgins, S. J., Baxter, J. D., Gelfand, D., and Tomkins, G. M. (1975). *J. Biol. Chem.* **250**, 6015–6021.
Rubin, M. M., and Changeux, J. P. (1966). *J. Mol. Biol.* **21**, 265–274.
Samuels, H. H., and Tomkins, G. M. (1970). *J. Mol. Biol.* **52**, 57–74.
Scott, W. A., Shields, R., and Tomkins, G. M. (1972). *Proc. Natl. Acad. Sci. U.S.A.* **69**, 2937–2941.
Sibley, C. H., and Tomkins, G. M. (1974a). *Cell* **2**, 213–220.
Sibley, C. H., and Tomkins, G. M. (1974b) *Cell* **2**, 221–227.
Sibley, C. H., Gehring, V., Bourne, H., and Tomkins, G. M. (1974). In "Control of Proliferation in Animal Cells" (B. Clarkson and R. Baserga, eds.), pp. 115–154. Cold Spring Harbor Lab., Cold Spring Harbor, New York.
Silhavy, T. J., Szmelcman, S., Boos, W., and Schwartz, M. (1975). *Proc. Natl. Acad. Sci. U.S.A.* **72**, 2120–2124.
Simons, S. S. (1977a). *Biochem. Biophys. Acta* **496**, 349–358.
Simons, S. S. (1977b). *Biochem. Biophys. Acta* **496**, 339–348.
Simons, S. S., Martinez, H. M., Garcea, R. L., Baxter, J. D., and Tomkins, G. M. (1976). *J. Biol. Chem.* **251**, 334–343.
Steinberg, R. A., Scott, W. A., Levinson, B. B., Ivarie, R. D., and Tomkins, G. M. (1974). *Fogarty Int. Cent. Proc.* **25**, 55–82.
Steinberg, R. A., Levinson, B. B., and Tomkins, G. M. (1975a). *Cell* **5**, 29–35.
Steinberg, R. A., Levinson, B. B., and Tomkins, G. M. (1975b). *Proc. Natl. Acad. Sci. U.S.A.* **72**, 2007–2011.
Stevens, J., Stevens, Y. W., Behrens, M., and Hollander, V. P. (1973). *Biochem. Biophys. Res. Commun.* **50**, 799–806.
Stringer, S. Y., Lippman, M. E., and Thompson, E. B. (1974). *Endocrinology* **94**, 254–261.
Sutherland, E. W. (1972). *Science* **177**, 401–408.
Thompson, E. B., and Lippman, M. E. (1974). *Metab., Clin. Exp.* **23**, 159–202.
Thompson, E. B., Tomkins, G. M., and Curran, J. F. (1966). *Proc. Natl. Acad. Sci. U.S.A.* **56**, 296–303.
Thompson, E. B., Granner, D. K., and Tomkins, G. M (1970). *J. Mol. Biol.* **54**, 159–175.
Tomkins, G. M. (1975). *Science* **189**, 760–763.
Tomkins, G. M., Thompson, E. B., Hayashi, S., Gelehrter, T., Granner, D., and Peterkofsky, B. (1966). *Cold Spring Harbor Symp. Quant. Biol.* **31**, 349–360.
Tomkins, G. M., Gelehrter, T. D., Granner, D., Martin, D., Jr., Samuels, H. H., and Thompson, E. B. (1969). *Science* **166**, 1474–1480.
Tomkins, G. M., Levinson, B. B., Baxter, J. D., and Dethlefsen, L. (1972). *Nature (London) New Biol.* **239**, 9–14.
Turnell, R. W., Kaiser, N., Millholland, R. J., and Rosen, F. (1974). *J. Biol. Chem.* **249**, 1133–1138.
Weintraub, H., and Groudine, M. (1976). *Science* **193**, 848–856.
Wigler, M., Ford, J. P., and Weinstein, I. B. (1975). In "Proteins and Biological Control" (E. Reich, D. B. Rifkin, and E. Shaw, eds.), pp. 849–856. Cold Spring Harbor Lab., Cold Spring Harbor, New York.
Williams, D., and Gorski, J. (1972). *Proc. Natl. Acad. Sci. U.S.A.* **69**, 3464–3468.
Wira, C. R., and Munck, A. (1974). *J. Biol. Chem.* **249**, 5328–5336.
Wolff, M. E., Baxter, J. D., Kollman, P. A., Matulich, D. T., and Morris, J., and Lee, D. L. (1977). submitted for publication.
Yamamoto, K. R., and Alberts, B. (1975). *Cell* **4**, 301–310.
Yamamoto, K. R., and Alberts, B. (1976). *Annu. Rev. Biochem.* **45**, 721–746.

Yamamoto, K. R., Stampfer, M. R., and Tomkins, G. M. (1974). *Proc. Natl. Acad. Sci. U.S.A.* **71**, 3901–3905.

Yamamoto, K. R., Gehring, U., Stampfer, M. R., and Sibley, C. H. (1976). *Recent Prog. Horm. Res.* **32**, 3–32.

Young, D. A., Barnard, T., Mendelsohn, S., and Giddings, S. (1974). *Endocr. Res. Commun.* **1**, 63–72.

Zubay, G. (1974). *Annu. Rev. Genet.* **7**, 267–287.

11

Glucocorticoid Regulation of Mammary Tumor Virus Gene Expression

KEITH R. YAMAMOTO AND GORDON M. RINGOLD

I.	Introduction: Defining the Problems	298
	A. Demonstration of Receptor-Mediated Primary Responses	298
	B. Effects on Specific Transcripts	298
	C. Isolation of Regulated Genes	299
	D. Selection of Genetic Variants	300
	E. Steroid Regulation of Viral Genes	300
II.	Mammary Tumor Virus Genes in Murine Cells	300
	A. MTV Genes Are Endogenous in the Mouse Genome	300
	B. Glucocorticoids Stimulate MTV RNA Accumulation	301
III.	MTV RNA Induction Is a Receptor-Mediated Primary Hormone Response	302
	A. Glucocorticoid-Receptor Involvement	302
	B. MTV Induction Is a Primary Response	302
IV.	Dexamethasone Stimulates the Rate of MTV RNA Synthesis	304
	A. Kinetics of Increase in Viral RNA Concentration	304
	B. Pulse Labeling of Viral RNA	305
V.	Glucocorticoid-Responsive MTV Genes Are Mobile	307
	A. Infection of Rat Cells with MTV	307
	B. Dexamethasone Stimulates Production of Viral RNA in Infected HTC Cells	309
VI.	MTV-Infected HTC Cells Contain Unintegrated Viral DNA	311
	A. Analysis of the Molecular Forms of Unintegrated MTV DNA	311
	B. Size of the Unintegrated MTV DNA	312
	C. Cytoplasmic–Nuclear Distribution of Unintegrated Viral DNA	314
VII.	MTV Infection Alters Host Gene Response to Glucocorticoids	315
VIII.	Discussion	316
	References	319

I. INTRODUCTION: DEFINING THE PROBLEMS

There is now a wealth of data, much of it reviewed in this volume, suggesting that intracellular receptors mediate steroid responses, that steroid hormones act allosterically to increase the affinity of the receptor for binding loci in the nucleus, and that DNA is a major component of the nuclear sites. At the biochemical level, elucidation of these events was made possible by the selective labeling of receptors with high specific activity ^{3}H-steroids (Jensen and Jacobson, 1962). At the genetic level, the biologic relevance of these observations has been strongly supported by selection of several classes of mutations residing in specific properties of receptors (Sibley and Tomkins, 1974a; Yamamoto *et al.*, 1976).

Unfortunately, however, such powerful biochemical and genetic selectivity is not readily accessible for studying the molecular events that trigger the primary biologic response to steroid hormones. Hence, there is considerably less agreement about the nature and specificity of nuclear binding sites and virtually no unequivocal data concerning the biochemistry of the primary response (for review, see Katzenellenbogen and Gorski, 1975). Therefore, in this section, we briefly define some of the problems that complicate the interpretation of certain experimental approaches, and we attempt to focus on some specific requirements and strategies that may facilitate solution of these problems.

A. Demonstration of Receptor-Mediated Primary Responses

It is crucial to establish that the response under study is a primary hormone effect mediated by the intracellular receptor proteins; these considerations have recently been reviewed and discussed in detail (Yamamoto and Alberts, 1976). The experimental criteria available, while limited, are straightforward and useful: dose-response inhibition by receptor-competing ligands, rapid kinetics, and insensitivity of RNA induction to inhibition of protein synthesis. It is clear that the most readily tested systems are those in which the response can be demonstrated in a homogeneous cell population, ideally in a cloned line of cultured cells. Conversely, for responses that occur only in intact animals (e.g., ovalbumin induction; see Palmiter *et al.*, 1976), it is extremely difficult to prove that the hormonal effect is direct and receptor mediated.

B. Effects on Specific Transcripts

It seems likely that steroid responses are triggered by modulating the transcription of a few specific genes (Yamamoto and Alberts, 1976). Quantitative and qualitative changes in RNA content have been observed in various tissues and cells following steroid administration and in some cases, alterations in the intracellular concentration of specific mRNA's have been directly measured (Harris et al., 1974; McKnight et al., 1975; Ashburner et al., 1973; Parks et al., 1975; Ringold et al., 1975a,b). However, these types of experiments do not distinguish whether the hormone stimulates the rate of synthesis of the mRNA, decreases its rate of degradation, or perhaps alters its transport from nucleus to cytoplasm, thereby indirectly stabilizing it. Thus, it will be beneficial to develop systems and techniques that can differentiate the different mechanisms for affecting the intracellular concentration of the regulated transcript.

It is worth noting that it has not yet been proved in any system that steroids function by increasing the rate of synthesis of a specific mRNA. Perhaps the best evidence in favor of such a mechanism comes from the elegant cytogenetic studies of Ashburner et al. (1973) who showed that ecdysone readily induces the appearance of "puffs," indicative of transcriptional activity, at specific loci on *Drosophila* chromosomes. The assumption that steroids alter the rate of transcription is crucial to any experiment in which RNA synthesis from chromatin is monitored in attempts to mimic hormonal induction *in vitro* (Davies and Griffiths, 1973, 1974; Schwartz et al., 1975).

C. Isolation of Regulated Genes

The physical characteristics of the receptor binding sites on the genome are very poorly understood. *In vitro* binding studies are complicated by the presence of nonsaturable levels of low-affinity nonspecific binding, probably to DNA (Yamamoto and Alberts, 1974). Attempts to detect and define specific high-affinity binding are subject to several types of artifacts and have given conflicting results (Spelsberg et al., 1971; Higgins et al., 1973a,b; Chamness et al., 1974; Yamamoto and Alberts, 1975). Moreover, there is strong evidence that *in vivo*, the binding observed is of low affinity and is nonsaturable (Williams and Gorski, 1972a,b). Nevertheless, indirect data suggest that the genome may contain a few specific high-affinity sites for receptors, but that the presence of such sites is masked by the low-affinity binding (Yamamoto and Alberts, 1975). Thus, specific binding would be most easily detected and studied in the absence of the great majority of the nonspecific loci.

Taken together, these considerations imply that elucidation of the biochemical reactions at specific receptor–genome binding sites, and, indeed, the detection of these sites, would be facilitated if genetic loci under steroid regulation could be selectively purified from the remainder of the cell genome. The first progress reports describing attempts to purify a regulated gene (ovalbumin) have recently appeared (Anderson and Schimke, 1976; Woo *et al.*, 1976).

D. Selection of Genetic Variants

It is extremely difficult to establish that biochemical observations in eukaryotic systems are truly representative of events that occur *in vivo*. With prokaryotes, this correlation has been achieved by selection of mutants in the pathway of interest. Other, less rigorous criteria have been adopted where genetic tools have been unavailable (see Yamamoto and Alberts, 1976). Sibley and Tomkins (1974a,b) described procedures for the selection and characterization of stable somatic cell variants in a mouse lymphoid tissue culture cell line normally killed by glucocorticoid hormones. It will be important to pursue this approach with other hormone-responsive cell lines, especially those in which known gene products are regulated.

E. Steroid Regulation of Viral Genes

In the remainder of this report, we describe some recent experiments (many of them carried out in collaboration with H. E. Varmus and P. R. Shank, Department of Microbiology, University of California, San Francisco) concerning the regulation of mouse mammary tumor virus (MTV) genes by glucocorticoids; we concentrate especially on data that appear relevant to the points considered above. Specifically, we shall show that dexamethasone, a synthetic glucocorticoid, induces the intracellular accumulation of MTV RNA in a primary, receptor-mediated response; that the hormone specifically increases the rate of synthesis of viral RNA; that the MTV genes remain hormone responsive upon infection of cultured rat cells; that, in infected cells, some viral genes are integrated into the host genome, but that others exist free in the cell, and, thus, are amenable to purification; and, finally, that infection may alter host gene responsiveness to glucocorticoids in specific ways.

II. MAMMARY TUMOR VIRUS GENES IN MURINE CELLS

A. MTV Genes Are Endogenous in the Mouse Genome

MTV is an enveloped virus containing a single-stranded RNA genome comprised of two to three identical (or very similar) subunits of $3–3.5 \times 10^6$

dalton molecular weight (MW) (Friedrich et al., 1976). The viral envelope is acquired by budding through the cell membrane; virus production has been detected in intact animals, mammary tumor explants, and in cultured mammary tumor cells. Biologic activity is demonstrated by the appearance of mammary carcinomas or preneoplastic lesions in susceptible mice exposed to active virions (for review, see Bentvelzen, 1974).

Normal mouse cells contain multiple copies of MTV DNA covalently integrated into the genome (Varmus et al., 1972); these copies most likely represent endogenous viral genes, transmitted through the germ line as part of the normal mouse gene complement. When MTV particles infect cells, the incoming viral RNA is thought to replicate via a double-stranded DNA intermediate synthesized by the virion-associated RNA-directed DNA polymerase; this sequence of events is similar to that rigorously established for a number of other RNA tumor viruses (Temin and Baltimore, 1972). Upon infection, some of the viral DNA intermediates become covalently integrated into the host genome (Ringold et al., 1976a; and this report). In some mammary tumors that produce MTV particles, there is evidence that the tumor cells contain somewhat elevated levels of integrated viral DNA, presumably acquired via reinfection (Morris et al., 1977). Thus, uninfected nonmurine cells contain no detectable MTV genes, normal mouse tissues carry endogenous viral DNA, and mouse mammary tumor cells may contain additional exogenously derived copies.

B. Glucocorticoids Stimulate MTV RNA Accumulation

The expression of MTV genes appears to be strongly regulated at some point involving the transcript, since the intracellular concentrations of viral RNA vary widely as a complex function of tissue, host strain, and hormonal status (Varmus et al., 1973; Nandi and McGrath, 1973; Schlom et al., 1973; Bentvelzen, 1974).

A number of investigators have successfully established primary explants (Cardiff et al., 1968; McGrath, 1971; Hilgers et al., 1971), as well as continuous cell lines (Sykes et al., 1968; Lasfargues et al., 1972; Owens and Hackett, 1972), from mouse mammary tumors. To our knowledge, all mouse mammary carcinoma explants and cell lines that produce MTV in culture respond to dexamethasone by increased production of viral particles or viral RNA (McGrath, 1971; Dickson et al., 1974; Fine et al., 1974; Parks et al., 1974, 1975; Ringold et al., 1975a,b; L. J. T. Young et al., 1975). Although the evolutionary rationale for this response and the possible selective advantages for host or virus are not understood, it is striking that this mode of regulation has been conserved in various inbred mouse strains carrying MTV types that appear biologically and probably genetically distinct (Bentvelzen, 1974). This generality implies that glucocorticoid responsiveness of MTV gene expression is not an isolated occurrence, but, rather, might be a highly specific phenomenon.

Our studies with mammary tumor cells have employed GR-3A, a clonal isolate from a continuous line of mouse mammary epithelial carcinoma cells originating from a spontaneous tumor in the GR mouse strain (Mühlbock, 1965). Using the viral reverse transcriptase to synthesize DNA complementary to the MTV genome (MTV cDNA), molecular hybridization reagents for the specific and direct quantitation of the hormone inducible transcript (Parks *et al.,* 1974, 1975; Ringold *et al.,* 1975a,b) are readily prepared and extensively used in the assays described here. Thus, this system has the technical advantage of bypassing the often difficult step of mRNA isolation and purification, yet still allowing direct cDNA hybridization measurements.

III. MTV RNA INDUCTION IS A RECEPTOR-MEDIATED PRIMARY HORMONE RESPONSE

A. Glucocorticoid-Receptor Involvement

Extracts of GR-3A cells contain specific glucocorticoid receptors detectable by binding of [^{3}H]dexamethasone. This receptor activity is biochemically similar to the genetically defined receptors in mouse lymphoid cells (Yamamoto *et al.,* 1974, 1976) in its physical hormone-binding, activation, and DNA-binding characteristics (Ringold *et al.,* 1975b). Two types of experiments support the notion that these receptor proteins are involved in MTV RNA induction by dexamethasone. First, the concentration of dexamethasone required to give half-maximal induction of viral RNA ($\sim 5 \times 10^{-8}$ M) is the same as that yielding half-maximal binding of [^{3}H]dexamethasone to the receptors (Ringold *et al.,* 1975b). Second, a 500-fold excess of progesterone, a competitive inhibitor of glucocorticoid receptor-mediated responses (Rousseau *et al.,* 1972), completely abolishes the viral RNA accumulation induced by dexamethasone (Fig. 1). Analogous results and conclusions have been reported by investigators using different lines of mammary tumor cells (H. A. Young *et al.,* 1975; Shyamala and Dickson, 1976).

B. MTV Induction Is a Primary Response

In no case has it been unambiguously shown that the first event detected biochemically actually represents the primary biologic effect of a steroid

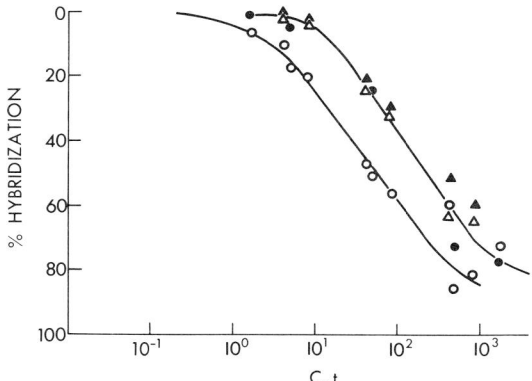

Fig. 1. Progesterone inhibition of dexamethasone-mediated induction of MTV RNA. MTV cDNA (~10^3 cpm) was annealed with increasing amounts of GR cell RNA for 16 hours at 60°C in 0.6 M NaCl. The experimental details have been described (Ringold et al., 1975b). △, RNA from untreated cells; ○, RNA from cells treated for 5 hours with 10^{-7} M dexamethasone; ▲, RNA from cells treated with 5×10^{-5} M progesterone for 5 hours. ●, RNA from cells treated with 10^{-7} M dexamethasone and 5×10^{-5} M progesterone. (From Ringold et al., 1975b.)

hormone. In fact, in several systems, there is evidence that the primary event is not being directly monitored. For example, the induction of specific proteins by glucocorticoids and estrogen is blocked by inhibitors of RNA synthesis (Peterkofsky and Tomkins, 1968; Gorski and Notides, 1969), and the estrogen-mediated induction of ovalbumin mRNA in the chick oviduct is interrupted throughout the response by some inhibitors of protein synthesis (Palmiter et al. (1976) showed that cycloheximide inhibits ovalbumin mRNA accumulation, but that another inhibitor, emetine, does not. Therefore, these authors suggested that the effect of cycloheximide might reflect its general toxicity to the animal rather than a specific requirement for protein synthesis).

Owens et al. (1973) have demonstrated that glucocorticoids have a complex role in the differentiation of secretory precursor cells in normal mammary glands. Thus, it seemed conceivable that the molecular aspects of this mechanism might also be involved in the dexamethasone-mediated effects on GR-3A cells, with MTV RNA induction occurring only as a secondary effect of the hormonal induction of cellular proteins. If this were the case, induction of MTV RNA would require ongoing protein synthesis. However, Fig. 2 shows that, when GR-3A cells are pretreated for 1 hour with cycloheximide (2 µg/ml, sufficient to inhibit ^{3}H-amino acid incorporation by 90%) and are subsequently exposed to dexamethasone for 5 hours in the continued presence of the inhibitor, MTV RNA accumulates as in the

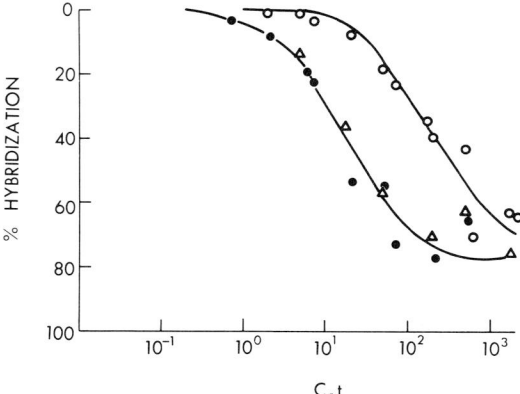

Fig. 2. Induction of MTV RNA in the presence of cycloheximide. Hybridizations were performed as described in Fig. 1. ○, RNA from untreated cells; ●, RNA from cells treated for 5 hours with 10^{-5} M dexamethasone; △, RNA from cells treated for 1 hour with 2 μg/ml cycloheximide then exposed to 10^{-5} M dexamethasone (in the continued presence of cycloheximide) for 5 hours. (From Ringold et al., 1975b.)

untreated cultures. Puromycin, another inhibitor of protein synthesis, is also unable to prevent the induction of MTV RNA; the basal levels of viral RNA are also unaffected by these inhibitors (data not shown).

In other experiments, we showed that increased levels of MTV RNA could be detected extremely rapidly after hormone addition (Ringold et al., 1975b; and see below), and that the increased accumulation of the viral transcripts is completely abolished by levels of actinomycin D which inhibit cellular RNA synthesis (Ringold et al., 1975b). Taken together, these results are consistent with the idea that dexamethasone elicits the increased accumulation of MTV RNA as a primary response.

IV. DEXAMETHASONE STIMULATES THE RATE OF MTV RNA SYNTHESIS

A. Kinetics of Increase in Viral RNA Concentration

It is well established that dexamethasone directly regulates the concentration of MTV RNA in murine mammary tumor cells. Similarly, steroids have been shown to stimulate the accumulation of specific transcripts in several other systems. In the case of MTV RNA induction in the GR-3A cells, we have shown that the hormonal effect is extremely rapid. After an apparent lag of about 15 minutes, the intracellular concentration of viral

RNA increases with a half-time of about 2.5 hours, reaching a new steady-state level (10- 20-fold over uninduced levels) by 6–7 hours (Ringold et al., 1976b). These results are consistent with a mechanism in which dexamethasone increases the rate of transcription of MTV RNA, but they do not rule out the possibility that the hormone acts solely to decrease degradation of the viral RNA.

B. Pulse Labeling of Viral RNA

A more direct approach to assessing the effect of dexamethasone on the rate of viral RNA synthesis is to pulse label RNA at various times after exposure to the hormone, and measure the fraction of labeled RNA which is virus specific. Technically, this is a difficult experiment since it requires large amounts of hybridization reagents to saturate the labeled MTV RNA in the presence of excess unlabeled viral RNA. Moreover, since the induced level of MTV RNA comprises only $\sim 0.1\%$ of the total RNA in GR-3A cells, it is essential to devise assays with low hybridization "backgrounds" relative to the levels of viral RNA that become labeled.

For our studies, [^{3}H]uridine was added to cultures at various times after dexamethasone addition; after labeling periods of 15 minutes, RNA was extracted, and labeled viral RNA was measured, using a modification of the procedure described by Smith et al. (1974) for separating DNA–RNA hybrids from RNA (E. Stavnezer and J. M. Bishop, 1977). Briefly, RNA was hybridized with unlabeled "tailed duplex" viral DNA, a product of the virus-associated reverse transcriptase (Ringold et al., 1976c), which is predominantly double-stranded viral DNA, but contains single-stranded tails complementary to viral RNA. After hybridization, the mixture is chromatographed on hydroxylapatite under conditions (8 M urea, 1% SDS, 0.2 M $Na_2PO_4^-$) in which only double-stranded DNA is bound to the matrix. Labeled RNA not hybridized to tailed duplex DNA is, thus, removed with high efficiency. Figure 3 shows the results of such an experiment and reveals that dexamethasone stimulates incorporation into viral RNA at the earliest time measured, i.e., upon simultaneous addition of hormone and [^{3}H]uridine. Furthermore, it can be seen that the new synthetic rate is achieved extremely rapidly, reaching the fully induced level by 45–60 minutes with an apparent half-time of 10–15 minutes.

These results, taken together with the kinetics of increase in viral RNA concentration (see above), strongly support the idea that dexamethasone stimulates the rate of MTV RNA synthesis. It is conceivable that the steroid additionally reduces the degradation rate of the viral transcript, since the concentration of MTV RNA increased 15-fold in the experiment shown in Fig. 3 (data not shown) while the rate of synthesis appears to have

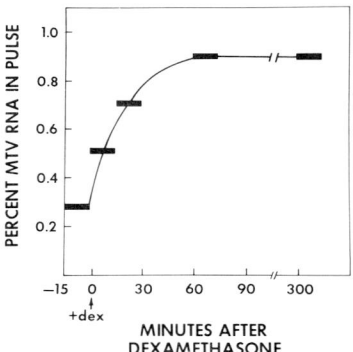

Fig. 3. Dexamethasone stimulates the rate of MTV RNA synthesis. Dexamethasone (10^{-6} M) was added to cultures of GR-3A cells at zero time. [^{3}H]uridine (750 μCi/ml) was added for 15-minute periods (37°C) at the times indicated by the bars. RNA was extracted and labeled. MTV RNA was measured according to the procedure of Stavnezer and Bishop (1977, see text); assays were performed at 60°C in the presence of 75 μg cell RNA and samples were passed twice over hydroxylapatite columns in a buffer containing 8 M urea, 1% SDS, and 0.2 M Na$_2$PO$_4^-$.

been stimulated only three- to fourfold. However, we regard results from the pulse-labeling experiments as only approximations since it is technically difficult to obtain precise measurements of the small fractions of labeled RNA hybridized; more recent experiments in which the hybridization backgrounds are further reduced suggest that the rate of MTV synthesis is stimulated by dexamethasone proportionally to the change in steady-state levels (G. M. Ringold, unpublished results).

It is worth noting that a labeling experiment of the type described does not unambiguously prove that the rate of synthesis is elevated. It is theoretically possible, for example, that dexamethasone acts solely to cause an instantaneous and drastic alteration in MTV RNA degradation by inactivating an mRNA-specific nuclease. The time-course of the response observed is extremely rapid, exhibiting virtually no detectable lag; thus, according to this scheme, the half-life of viral RNA would have to be a few minutes or less, perhaps two orders of magnitude shorter than the estimated half-lives of average poly(A)-containing cellular mRNA's (Greenberg, 1972; Singer and Penman, 1973). Such a mechanism seems somewhat unlikely, since both induction and deinduction data (not shown) imply that viral RNA has a half-life of at least 2.5 hours, assuming that synthesis is zero order and degradation is first order with respect to RNA concentration (Berlin and Schimke, 1965). Therefore, we believe that the simplest interpretation of our results is that dexamethasone leads to an increase in the rate of MTV RNA synthesis.

V. GLUCOCORTICOID-RESPONSIVE MTV GENES ARE MOBILE

A. Infection of Rat Cells with MTV

We were intrigued with the apparent generality of glucocorticoid regulation of MTV gene expression in mouse mammary cell cultures (see above). If MTV particles could be made to successfully infect nonmurine cells, it seemed that it might be possible to exploit the mobility of the viral genome to investigate the nature of the hormonal response in different host "backgrounds," and to examine the effect of newly introduced hormone responsive genes on endogenous cellular responses. Although attempts to infect cultured cells with MTV had not been generally successful, we were particularly encouraged by the experiments of Vaidya et al. (1976), who were able to use MTV isolated from mouse milk to infect mink lung and feline kidney cells. Most importantly, these workers found that dexamethasone continued to stimulate virus production in the newly infected cell populations.

We chose to infect HTC, a rat hepatoma cell line, because it contains a well-characterized glucocorticoid-receptor protein (Failla et al., 1975) and two readily assayed enzyme activities inducible with dexamethasone (Thompson et al., 1966; Kulka et al., 1972). No biologic assay is presently available to monitor infection of cultured cells by MTV; therefore, we adopted the strategy of evaluating the efficacy of infection by measuring the appearance of intracellular virus-specific nucleic acids in cells exposed to virus. Since there is considerable evidence (Vaidya et al., 1976; Morris et al., 1977) that MTV replicates via a viral DNA intermediate in a manner similar to the C-type RNA tumor viruses (Temin and Baltimore, 1972), we first tested the treated cell populations for the acquisition of MTV DNA sequences.

Approximately 2×10^5 subconfluent HTC4 cells (a subclone of HTC) were exposed to MTV produced by GR-3A cells at a ratio of 2×10^5 particles per cell. After 1 hour, the 1-ml inoculum, containing 4 μg/ml of polybrene was diluted fivefold with growth medium. Initial propagation of the cells was carried out in suspension culture to obtain sufficient numbers of cells for biochemical analysis and to remove any GR-3A cells that might have contaminated the infecting virus stock; GR-3A cells do not grow in suspension culture under the conditions used. When DNA was extracted from the infected cell population (8 weeks after exposure to virus) and from control cultures, we found by molecular hybridization that the virus-treated cultures contained large amounts of viral DNA (data not shown).

To obtain an estimate of the uniformity of infection, the cells (denoted HTC-M1) were cloned by immobilization of a single cell preparation ($\sim$100 cells/60-mm dish) in medium containing 0.3% agar. After 10–12 days, individual clones (~10^3 cells each) were removed from the agar and grown separately. In order to selectively measure the amount of viral DNA that had become stably integrated into the host cell genome, nuclei were isolated from several clonal lines grown in the absence of dexamethasone, and the DNA was fractionated according to the procedure of Hirt (1967), in which high molecular weight DNA is precipitated.

The relative level of integrated MTV DNA was estimated by annealing a constant amount of ^{32}P-labeled viral RNA with increasing amounts of the nuclear "Hirt precipitate" DNA (Fig. 4). The initial slope of these curves is proportional to the number of viral genomes present in the cellular DNA (Varmus et al., 1974). Figure 4 shows the results of such an experiment for four independently isolated clones. In the same experiment, DNA from uninfected HTC4 cells and from GR-3A cells was also annealed. GR-3A cell DNA has been shown by C_0t analysis (Britten and Kohne, 1968) to

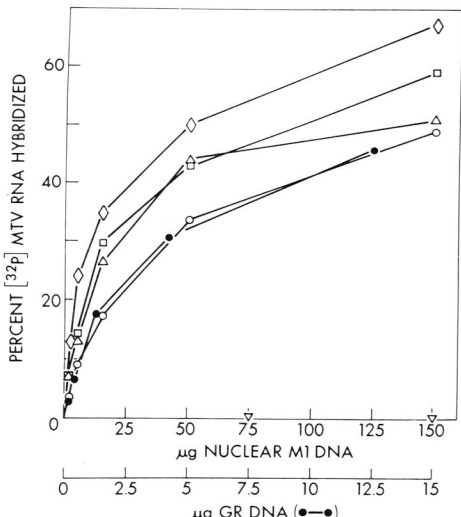

Fig. 4. MTV DNA integrated into genomes of cloned, infected HTC cells. HTC4 cells were exposed to high multiplicities of MTV, and individual subclones selected at random. Nuclei were isolated from 5×10^7 cells, and high molecular weight DNA selectively precipitated by the Hirt (1967) procedure. Hirt pellet DNA was purified and hybridized with 10^3 cpm of ^{32}P-labeled RNA in 0.6 M NaCl for 60–70 hours at 68°C. Hybridization was assayed by RNase resistance. Relative amounts of integrated viral DNA were estimated from the initial slopes of hybridization (Varmus et al., 1974), using GR DNA (50–70 copies per diploid genome; V. Morris, personal communication) as a standard; ▽———▽, uninfected HTC4 DNA; ○———○, M1.7; △———△, M1.20; □———□, M1.49; ◇———◇, M1.60; ●———● GR.

TABLE I
MTV DNA and RNA in Infected HTC Cells

Clone	Integrated MTV DNA (copies/diploid genome)	MTV RNA (copies/cell)		
		−dex	+dex	+dex/−dex
M1.7	5–10	3	3,000	1,000
M1.9	N.T.	65	13,000	200
M1.19	N.T.	25	13,000	500
M1.20	10–15	65	8,000	120
M1.46	N.T.	80	13,000	160
M1.47	N.T.	15	1,200	80
M1.49	10–15	15	3,600	240
M1.60	20	125	6,500	50
M1.62	N.T.	250	13,000	50

For DNA determinations, 5×10^7 cells were grown in the absence of dexamethasone. Nuclear DNA was prepared according to Hirt (1967), and integrated MTV DNA estimated as described in Fig. 4. For RNA determinations, RNA was extracted from cells grown in the presence or absence of 10^{-6} M dexamethasone and hybridized with MTV [^{3}H]cDNA. Conversion to copies per cell was carried out assuming $C_r t_{1/2} = 50$ to be equivalent to 5500 copies per cell (Ringold *et al.*, 1975a).

contain 50–70 copies of MTV viral sequences per diploid genome (V. Morris, personal communication). From the results shown, we conclude that all four clones were infected by MTV, and that they contain different numbers of integrated viral sequences, ranging from 5 to 10 per diploid genome in M1.7 to about 20 in M1.60 (Table I). In contrast, the uninfected HTC4 cells contain no detectable MTV DNA (Fig. 4).

B. Dexamethasone Stimulates Production of Viral RNA in Infected HTC Cells

Preliminary experiments indicated that dexamethasone increases the concentration of intracellular MTV RNA in the mass population of HTC-M1 cells (Ringold *et al.*, 1976a). Therefore, we examined the effect of the hormone on MTV RNA levels in nine cloned lines in order to estimate whether all infected cells are hormone responsive, and whether the extent of the response is identical. RNA was isolated from cells grown in the presence and absence of 10^{-6} M dexamethasone. Viral transcripts were then measured by hybridization of [^{3}H]cDNA to increasing amounts of cellular RNA. Figure 5 shows a typical result, with the extent of hybridization plotted as a function of $C_r t$ (the product of RNA concentration and time of annealing in mole-sec/liter). In the absence of dexamethasone, a basal level

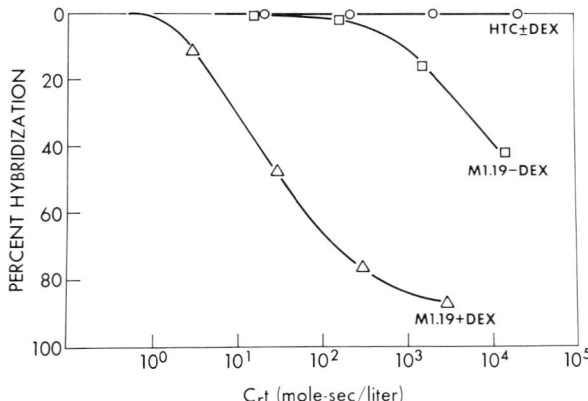

Fig. 5. MTV RNA in cloned MTV-infected HTC cells. Clones of uninfected (O———O) or infected (M1.19) HTC cells were grown in the presence (△———△) or absence (□———□) of 10^{-6} M dexamethasone. RNA was extracted, hybridized with 10^3 cpm MTV [^{3}H]cDNA, and hybrids assayed by resistance to single-strand specific nuclease S1 (Ando, 1966; Leong et al., 1972).

of MTV RNA of about 25 transcripts per cell is present in M1.19 cells; when the infected line is treated with the hormone, the intracellular RNA concentration increases about 500-fold. As expected, MTV RNA is not detectable in uninfected cells.

Table I summarizes the results of similar experiments with nine clonal lines. Several conclusions can be drawn from these data. First, the basal levels of MTV RNA present in the infected clones varies over a wide range, from 3 to 250 copies per cell. Clonal variability in MTV gene expression also occurs in mouse mammary tumor cells (Parks and Scolnick, 1973; Scolnick et al., 1976). Second, dexamethasone stimulates viral RNA accumulation in all clones, but the extent of induction and maximum steady-state levels are highly variable from clone to clone. The extent of induction ranges from 50- to 1000-fold, yielding final levels of 1,000–13,000 viral transcripts per cell. Third, the basal levels, induction ratios, and induced levels of MTV RNA are not directly related to each other or to the estimated number of viral genomes integrated.

Despite the presence of substantial quantities of viral RNA in dexamethasone-stimulated infected HTC cells, measurement of the amount of particle-associated viral RNA released into the tissue culture fluid (Ringold et al., 1975a) suggests that these cells produce only about 0.1% the amount of virus produced by GR-3A mouse mammary tumor cells. The inefficient production of viral particles is not due to a complete block of MTV protein synthesis in these cells, since viral antigens are readily detected in an indirect immunofluorescence assay employing antisera prepared against whole MTV (Ringold et al., 1976a).

VI. MTV-INFECTED HTC CELLS CONTAIN UNINTEGRATED VIRAL DNA

One interpretation of the effect of glucocorticoids on the expression of MTV RNA is that the steroid–receptor complex acts at a specific locus on the proviral DNA itself. If this were the case, it would be extremely beneficial to be able to purify viral DNA from the remainder of the host genome. At the minimum, this material would allow a direct biochemical test for the presence of such specific binding sites.

Unintegrated viral DNA has been detected in cells after infection by avian and murine C-type viruses (Guntaka et al., 1975, 1976; Gianni et al., 1975). Thus, it seemed conceivable that the MTV-infected HTC cells might also contain unintegrated viral DNA in addition to the covalently integrated sequences described above. If present, this material might be relatively easily purified for further biochemical manipulation.

A. Analysis of the Molecular Forms of Unintegrated MTV DNA

In our initial experiments, we confirmed by more rigorous procedures that the majority of the viral DNA detected in infected HTC cells is, in fact, covalently integrated into the cellular genome. When DNA from infected HTC cells was sedimented under strongly denaturing conditions (in alkaline sucrose gradients prepared in a zonal rotor; Varmus et al., 1976), we found that most of the viral DNA sedimented at 165–500 S (Ringold et al., 1976b). Since full-length viral DNA, under these conditions, sediments at either 19 S (form II/III) or 60 S (form I) (see below), we concluded that the rapid sedimentation reflects covalent linkage to high molecular weight cell DNA.

When the infected cells were grown in the presence of dexamethasone, Hirt fractionation of the DNA revealed that a substantial fraction ($\sim 30\%$) of the viral sequences remains in the supernatant with low molecular weight DNA. To assess the molecular form(s) of this viral DNA, we centrifuged DNA from the Hirt supernatant to equilibrium in cesium chloride density gradients containing propidium diiodide ($CsCl–PI_2$). Under these conditions, covalently closed circular (form I) DNA bands at a greater density than open circular (form II) and linear (form III) DNA (Hudson et al., 1969). Using forms I and II of a bacterial plasmid DNA (pML-21) as

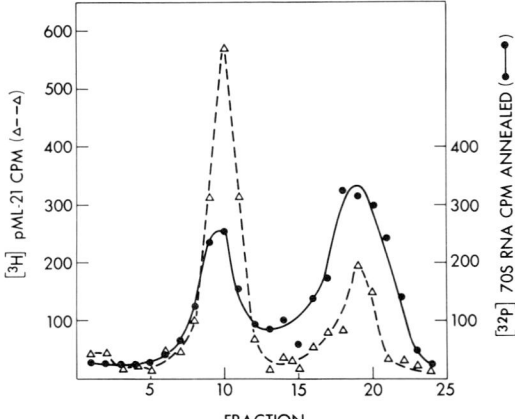

Fig. 6. Analysis of MTV DNA in CsCl-PI$_2$ gradients. Gradients contained 17.25 g of CsCl (Harshaw, Radiotracer Grade), 1.2 ml of propidium diiodide (6 mg/ml, Calbiochem), and the DNA sample in 18.3 ml of TE buffer; final density was 1.532 g/cm^3 with a dye concentration of 300 μg/ml. Gradients were centrifuged for 60–70 hours at 31,000 rpm, 20°C in the type 42.1 rotor (Beckman). Fractions were collected from the bottom, and the dye was removed by batch procedure with Dowex AG50. An aliquot of each gradient was assayed for MTV DNA by hybridization with viral [^{32}P]RNA (10^3 cpm/fraction). The extent of annealing was determined by resistance of the [^{32}P]RNA to digestion by pancreatic RNase. A ^{3}H-labeled bacterial plasmid (pML-21; △------△) was centrifuged to equilibrium in a parallel gradient to determine the banding positions of form I (fractions 8–12) and form II (fractions 16–21) DNA's.

markers in a parallel gradient, hybridization of the experimental gradient with MTV ^{32}P-RNA revealed the presence of viral DNA as form I as well as form II and/or III (Fig. 6). Based upon the relative amounts of hybridization, we estimate that form I DNA constitutes approximately 20% of the viral DNA in the Hirt supernatant, or about one to two copies per cell. We confirmed that this material is, indeed, in the closed circular form by demonstrating that it renatures with zero-order kinetics, and that nicking with DNase converts it to a completely denaturable structure (Beard and Berg, 1974) (data not shown). The viral DNA in the upper band of the CsCl–PI$_2$ gradient presumably represents the additional three to six copies of unintegrated DNA, plus one to two copies from contaminating cellular DNA.

B. Size of the Unintegrated MTV DNA

The size of the subunits of the single-stranded RNA-genome of MTV is approximately 2.5–3×10^6 daltons (35 S) (Duesberg and Cardiff, 1968), and the genome of the virus produced by GR-3A cells has a complexity of approximately 3×10^6 daltons (Friedrich *et al.*, 1976). To determine the size of MTV form I DNA in HTC-M1 cells, a portion of the DNA from the dense band of the CsCl–PI$_2$ gradient (Fig. 6) was sedimented in an alkaline sucrose gradient. As seen in Fig. 7, the majority of the viral DNA, detected by hybridization with MTV ^{32}P-RNA, sedimented at a position corresponding to an MW of approximately 6×10^6 daltons relative to pML-21, a 6.7×10^6 dalton plasmid (H. Boyer, personal communication). This result is consistent with the idea that most of the form I viral DNA represents the transcript of a single subunit of the RNA genome. Figure 7 also shows that a portion of the viral DNA (~10%) sedimented considerably slower than the bulk of the form I DNA, although faster than expected for nicked circular DNA (form II) of 6×10^6 daltons. The molecular nature of this material has not yet been further investigated.

A portion of the DNA from the upper band of the gradient shown in Fig. 6 (form II and/or III) was sedimented in an alkaline sucrose gradient and assayed for strands complementary to the viral genome ("minus" strands) and for strands with the same polarity as the viral genome ("plus" strands) by hybridization with MTV ^{32}P-RNA or ^{3}H-cDNA, respectively. We found that the minus strands sedimented as a relatively homogeneous population at approximately 17–18 S, whereas the plus strands sedimented heterogeneously from 6 to 17 S (data not shown). This pattern, similar to

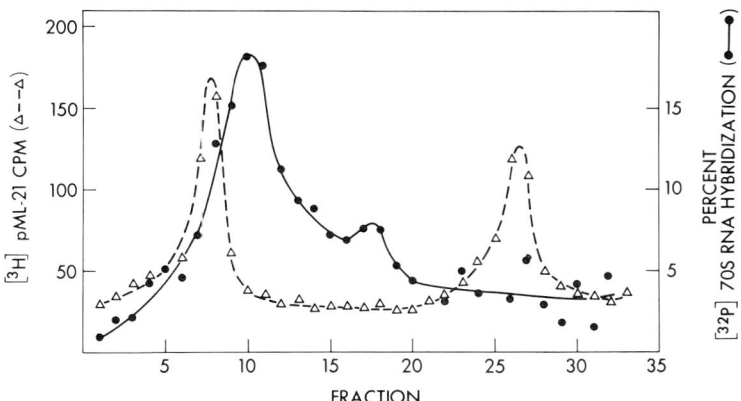

Fig. 7. Alkaline sucrose gradient sedimentation of MTV form I DNA. Five percent of the DNA from the lower band of the CsCl–PI$_2$ gradient (Fig. 6) was analyzed on a 5–20% sucrose gradient in 0.3 N NaOH, 0.7 M NaCl, and 1 mM EDTA. Centrifugation was for 11 hours in a SW 27.1 rotor at 21,000 rpm and 20°C. Fractions were collected from the bottom of the gradient and assayed for viral DNA by hybridization with MTV ^{32}P-RNA. Approximately 600 cpm of a mixture of form I and II [^{3}H]pML-21 (△------△) DNA (MW 6.7×10^6 daltons) were included in the gradient. Sedimentation is from right to left.

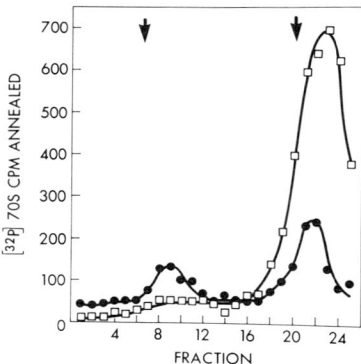

Fig. 8. Nuclear–cytoplasmic distribution of MTV DNA. HTC cells were infected at a multiplicity of 2×10^5 particles per cell and grown in the absence of dexamethasone for 15 days. Dexamethasone (10^{-6} M) was added for 60 hours and the cells were harvested and fractionated into cytoplasmic (□————□) and nuclear (●————●) fractions. Nuclear DNA was fractionated as described by Hirt (1967). The nuclear Hirt supernatant and the cytoplasmic DNA were centrifuged in alkaline sucrose gradients as described in the legend to Fig. 7. Fractions were assayed for viral DNA by hybridization with viral [^{32}P]RNA. Sedimentation is from right to left; arrows indicate the positions of [^{3}H]pML-21 DNA (form I = 65 S; form II = 19 S) centrifuged in a parallel gradient.

that seen with avian and murine C-type virus-infected cells (Varmus *et al.*, 1976; Varmus and Shank, 1976; Gianni *et al.*, 1975; Gianni and Weinberg, 1975), suggests that form II and/or III is composed of a genome-length minus strand and subgenomic length plus strands. This structure is characteristic of the product of viral RNA-dependent DNA polymerase, and is consistent with the idea that these forms might arise as a result of "reverse transcription."

C. Cytoplasmic–Nuclear Distribution of Unintegrated Viral DNA

To determine the intracellular distribution of the unintegrated MTV DNA, infected HTC cells were fractionated into cytoplasm and nuclei, and viral DNA in the nuclei was separated from the majority of cellular DNA by Hirt fractionation. Both the cytoplasmic DNA and the Hirt supernatant DNA from nuclei were analyzed in alkaline sucrose gradients (Fig. 8); the results indicate that form I viral DNA is found primarily in the nucleus, whereas the open forms of viral DNA are present in both the nucleus and the cytoplasm of infected cells.

We have recently found that the amount of unintegrated MTV DNA is increased in HTC cells by treatment with glucocorticoids (G. M. Ringold and K. R. Yamamoto, unpublished results). The cells used in this experiment had been grown for 18 days postinfection and exposed to dexamethasone for 60 hours. In contrast, the cells used in the analyses of viral DNA presented above were harvested 4 months after infection and had been exposed to dexamethasone for over 2 weeks. We are presently investigating whether the time of propagation postinfection or whether the duration of hormone treatment (or both) affect the amounts and distribution of the unintegrated viral DNA.

VII. MTV INFECTION ALTERS HOST GENE RESPONSE TO GLUCOCORTICOIDS

HTC cells display a number of specific alterations in gene expression in response to glucocorticoid hormones (R. D. Ivarie and P. H. O'Farrell, 1977). The response of the cloned line used in this study, HTC4, includes two inducible enzymatic activities: tyrosine aminotransferase (Thompson et al., 1966) and glutamine synthetase (R. D. Ivarie, unpublished; see also Kulka et al., 1972). Since infection by MTV appears functionally equivalent to addition of new hormone-responsive genes to the HTC genome, we were curious to determine whether infection affected the basal or induced expression of these "endogenous" responsive genes.

As a preliminary step, we subcloned uninfected HTC4 cells to determine the variability in the hormonal induction of tyrosine aminotransferase (TAT) and glutamine synthetase (GS). This was especially important, since Aviv and Thompson (1972) had reported that clonal isolates of their line of HTC cells displayed a 30- to 40-fold range of variability in the TAT response. Subclones of HTC4 were somewhat variable in TAT inducibility, but within a much more restricted range than observed by Aviv and Thompson. When 12 independent isolates were assayed, inducibility of TAT varied from 75 to 125% of that seen in the parental clone, while GS induction was between 60 and 140% of the HTC4 levels (Yamamoto et al., 1977). Similar results have been obtained by R. D. Ivarie and B. B. Levinson (unpublished) who surveyed TAT induction in over 250 HTC subclones.

In contrast, when MTV-infected clones were assayed, the inducibility of TAT and GS no longer followed this pattern. The results for seven clones are shown in Fig. 9; five displayed greater deviation with respect to TAT induction than observed in studies with subclones of uninfected cells; four deviated more than the controls in tests for inducibility of GS. Only in one clone (M1.49) was TAT induced to levels greater (320%) than observed in the uninfected (HTC4.1) control. In all other infected clones, the levels of

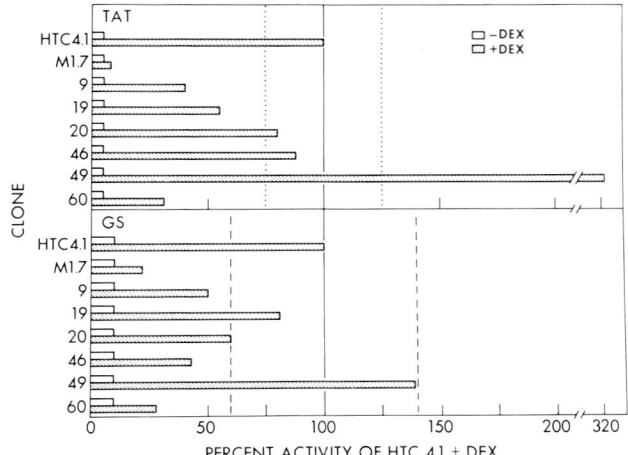

Fig. 9. TAT and GS activities in MTV infected subclones of HTC4. MTV-infected clones were grown in the presence or absence of dexamethasone, and assayed for TAT and GS activity according to Diamondstone (1966) and Kulka et al. (1972), respectively. The data shown represent the average of two to five determinations and are expressed relative to the activities in the HTC4 parental population. Dashed and dotted lines delineate the variability range for GS and TAT, respectively, as determined for uninfected cells (see text).

induction were reduced; the effect was most dramatic in M1.7, in which TAT was induced to only 8% and GS to only 22% of the levels observed in HTC4.1. Several other clones display similarly reduced induction of these enzymes following infection (J. Ring and K. R. Yamamoto, unpublished results). In no case was the basal level of either enzyme significantly affected (Fig. 9). The hormone concentration required for half-maximal induction of the enzymes in infected clones (2×10^{-8} M) is identical to that required in uninfected HTC cells (Yamamoto et al., 1977). Thus, it is improbable that the alteration in the TAT and GS responses is due to a defect in steroid uptake or receptor binding as an indirect result of membrane or intracellular changes consequent to infection.

VIII. DISCUSSION

For reasons that are not understood, the expression of murine mammary tumor virus genes appears to be strongly regulated by glucocorticoids and their corresponding receptor proteins. Using GR-3A cells, a cloned line derived from a mouse mammary carcinoma, we have shown that the elevation of viral RNA concentration is probably a direct response to the hormone which results (at least in part) from an increase in the rate of specific transcription.

Vaidya *et al.* (1976) have reported that hormone responsiveness of the MTV genes is maintained when the virus infects feline and mink cells. Likewise, our results show that dexamethasone stimulates MTV RNA accumulation in infected rat cells. Since there is considerable biochemical (Baxter *et al.*, 1972; Rousseau *et al.*, 1973) and genetic (Yamamoto *et al.*, 1974, 1976) evidence that glucocorticoid receptors interact with DNA-containing sites in the nucleus, we assume that stimulation of MTV genes occurs by a similar mechanism. However, our present results with MTV-infected HTC cells do not distinguish whether the site at which the dexamethasone receptor acts is on a segment of the viral genome (integrated or unintegrated) or on the host genome. The data do suggest, however, that some element required for the response [receptor structure, receptor binding site, viral integration site, or unknown component(s)] is likely to have been very highly conserved during the evolutionary divergence of mouse, rat, mink, and cat.

In many of the infected clones tested, the extents of hormone inducibility of TAT and GS were altered. Analysis of pulse-labeled proteins by high-resolution two-dimensional gel electrophoresis (O'Farrell, 1975) reveals very few differences in the pattern of protein synthesis after infection (R. D. Ivarie and K. R. Yamamoto, unpublished results). Furthermore, these experiments reveal that, although about 10 proteins are detectably induced by dexamethasone in HTC cells (R. D. Ivarie and P. H. O'Farrell, submitted for publication), only two or three (including one protein identified as TAT) have altered inducibility upon infection (R. D. Ivarie and K. R. Yamamoto, unpublished). The fact that only two or three of the proteins under glucocorticoid control are affected implies that the various hormone-responsive sites in these cells must differ in some way (assuming that all the responses are primary and receptor mediated; Yamamoto and Alberts, 1976).

Clearly, our data are far too preliminary to draw any conclusions about the mechanism of this effect. Indeed, we emphasize that we have not rigorously demonstrated that the presence of viral genes is required and responsible for the alterations in host gene inducibility which we observe in these subclones. Nevertheless, it is tempting to speculate that site-specific integration of the viral DNA somehow affects regulation of hormone-inducible genes, analogous, in principle, to the action of bacterial insertion elements (Bukhari *et al.*, 1977). Current studies in our laboratory are attempting to determine whether integration of viral DNA into the cellular genome is required for the alterations in TAT and GS inducibility, and whether viral genomes not responsive to dexamethasone can also produce this effect.

All of the infected cell lines described in this study had been initially exposed to extremely high concentrations of virus ($\sim 2 \times 10^5$ particles per cell) and contained multiple copies of MTV DNA stably integrated into the cell genome. Preliminary experiments indicate that when cells are exposed to lower viral multiplicities, there is a reduction in the average number of integrated proviruses (M. R. Stallcup and K. R. Yamamoto, unpublished results) and the average concentration of viral RNA (Ringold et al., 1976a). It is apparent from these studies that infection of HTC cells is extremely inefficient. It will be interesting to determine if clonal isolates from populations infected with lower concentrations of MTV contain fewer copies of integrated viral DNA; it might be beneficial to examine hormone responsiveness and the effect of infection on host gene responses in lines containing only single (or very few) integrated MTV genomes per cell.

It is intriguing that infected HTC cells contain unintegrated as well as integrated viral DNA. We have found that the unintegrated DNA, probably synthesized by the viral reverse transcriptase, is induced by dexamethasone with kinetics slightly slower than the RNA induction (K. R. Yamamoto and G. M. Ringold, unpublished results). Similar experiments with GR cells reveal no detectable unintegrated MTV DNA (G. M. Ringold, unpublished). Therefore, although viral RNA induction almost certainly begins during transcription from the integrated viral DNA, we have not ruled out the interesting possibility that dexamethasone may also regulate MTV RNA synthesis in HTC cells using the unintegrated DNA as the template. Thus, it is not clear whether unintegrated viral DNA serves any function in the hormonal response or in the life cycle of the virus. Nevertheless, since infected HTC cells can easily be grown in large numbers and since both covalently closed circular and open forms of viral DNA are maintained in these cells, it should be possible to purify MTV DNA for further biochemical analyses.

There is strong correlative evidence that the dexamethasone response of MTV genes is mediated by glucocorticoid-receptor proteins (Ringold et al., 1975b). It would be very useful in this sytem to be able to select genetic variants with defects in the receptors and in other parts of the response pathway. In addition to establishing receptor involvement *in vivo,* such variants would be valuable for *in vitro* biochemical studies of the mechanism of steroid action (for review, see Yamamoto et al., 1976). Although we have not yet selected such variants in this system, there appear to be several potential approaches. For example, it may be possible to select against the induced expression of viral antigens on the cell surface, using virus-specific antisera and complement-induced cytolysis.

To summarize, it is apparent that the glucocorticoid responsiveness of MTV genes can be exploited at several levels. Since there appears to be a direct effect on the rate of viral RNA transcription, which can be observed in homogeneous cell populations in culture, the system may ultimately be useful for attempts to reconstruct the hormonal response apparatus *in vitro*. In addition, the observation that the MTV genes retain hormonal responsiveness upon infection of nonmurine cells implies that the virus could be employed as a probe for obtaining information about the organization and regulation of "families" of genes in eukaryotic cells. Finally, the accessibility of viral DNA free from the remainder of the cell genome might aid in direct investigation of the nature of receptor-binding sites on the genome.

ACKNOWLEDGMENT

The invaluable contributions of Harold Varmus to all phases of this work are gratefully acknowledged. In addition, Peter Shank was an important collaborator in the experiments dealing with characterization of viral DNA. This work was supported by grants from the NIH, the University of California Cancer Research Coordinating Committee, the Helen Hay Whitney Foundation, and by a contract within the Virus Cancer Program of the National Cancer Institute.

REFERENCES

Anderson, J. N., and Schimke, R. T. (1976). *Cell* **7**, 331–338.
Ashburner, M., Chihara, C., Meltzer, P., and Richards, G. (1973). *Cold Spring Harbor Symp. Quant. Biol.* **38**, 655–662.
Ando, T. (1966). *Biochim. Biophys. Acta* **114**, 158–168.
Aviv, D., and Thompson, E. B. (1972). *Science* **177**, 1201–1203.
Baxter, J. D., Rousseau, G. G., Benson, M. C., Garcea, R. L., Ito, J. and Tomkins, G. M. (1972). *Proc. Natl. Acad. Sci. U.S.A.* **69**, 1892–1896.
Beard, P., and Berg, P. (1974). *Biochemistry* **13**, 2410–2413.
Bentvelzen, P. (1974). *Biochim. Biophys. Acta* **355**, 236–259.
Berlin, C. M., and Schimke, R. T. (1965). *Mol. Pharmacol.* **1**, 149–156.
Britten, R. J., and Kohne, D. E. (1968). *Science* **161**, 529–540.
Bukhari, A. I., Shapiro, J., and Adhya, S., eds. (1977). "DNA Insertion Elements, Plasmids and Episomes." Cold Spring Harbor Lab., Cold Spring Harbor, New York (in press).
Cardiff, R. D., Blair, P. B., and DeOme, K. B. (1968). *Virology* **36**, 313–317.
Chamness, G. C., Jennings, A. W., and McGuire, W. L. (1974). *Biochemistry* **13**, 327–331.
Davies, P., and Griffiths, K. (1973). *Biochem. J.* **136**, 611–622.
Davies, P., and Griffiths, K. (1974). *J. Endocrinol.* **62**, 385–400.

Diamondstone, T. I. (1966). *Anal. Biochem.* **16**, 395–401.
Dickson, C., Haslam, S., and Nandi, S. (1974). *Virology* **62**, 242–252.
Duesberg, P. H., and Cardiff, R. D. (1968). *Virology* **36**, 696–700.
Failla, D., Tomkins, G. M., and Santi, D. V. (1975). *Proc. Natl. Acad. Sci. U.S.A.* **72**, 3849–3852.
Fine, D. L., Plowman, J. K., Kelley, S. P., Arthur, L. O., and Hillman, E. A. (1974). *J. Natl. Cancer Inst.* **52**, 1881–1886.
Friedrich, R., Morris, V., Goodman, H., Bishop, J. M., and Varmus, H. E. (1976). *Virology* **72**, 330–340.
Gianni, A. M., and Weinberg, R. A. (1975). *Nature (London)* **255**, 646–648.
Gianni, A. M., Smotkin, D., and Weinberg, R. A. (1975). *Proc. Natl. Acad. Sci. U.S.A.* **72**, 447–451.
Gorski, J., and Notides, A. (1969). *In* "Biochemistry of Cell Division" (R. Baserga, ed.), pp. 57–76. Thomas, Springfield, Illinois.
Greenberg, J. R. (1972). *Nature (London)* **240**, 102–104.
Guntaka, R. V., Mahy, B. W. J., Bishop, J. M., and Varmus, H. E. (1975). *Nature (London)* **253**, 507–511.
Guntaka, R. V., Richards, O. C., Shank, P. R., Kung, H. J., Davidson, N., Fritsch, E., Bishop, J. M., and Varmus, H. E. (1976). *J. Mol. Biol.* **106**, 337–358.
Harris, S. E., Rosen, J. M., Means, A. R., and O'Malley, B. W. (1974). *J. Steroid Biochem.* **5**, 341.
Higgins, S. J., Rousseau, G. G., Baxter, J. D., and Tomkins, G. M. (1973a). *J. Biol. Chem.* **248**, 5866–5872.
Higgins, S. J., Rousseau, G. G., Baxter, J. D., and Tomkins, G. M. (1973b). *Proc. Natl. Acad. Sci. U.S.A.* **70**, 3415–3418.
Hilgers, J., Clydell-Williams, W., Myers, B., and Dmochowski, L. (1971). *Virology* **45**, 470–483.
Hirt, B. (1967). *J. Mol. Biol.* **26**, 365–369.
Hudson, B., Upholt, W. B., Devinny, J., and Vinograd, J. (1969). *Proc. Natl. Acad. Sci. U.S.A.* **62**, 813–820.
Ivarie, R. D., and O'Farrell, P. H. (1977). Submitted for publication.
Jensen, E. V., and Jacobson, H. I. (1962). *Recent Prog. Horm. Res.* **18**, 387–414.
Katzenellenbogen, B. S., and Gorski, J. (1975). *Biochem. Actions Horm.* **3**, 187–243.
Kulka, R. G., Tomkins, G. M., and Crook, R. B. (1972). *J. Cell Biol.* **54**, 175–179.
Lasfargues, E. Y., Kramarsky, B., Sarkar, N. H., Lasfargues, J.-C., and Moore, D. H. (1972). *Proc. Soc. Exp. Biol. Med.* **139**, 242–247.
Leong, J., Garapin, A.-C., Jackson, N., Fanshier, L., Levinson, W., and Bishop, J. M. (1972). *J. Virol.* **9**, 891–902.
McGrath, C. M. (1971). *J. Natl. Cancer Inst.* **47**, 455–467.
McKnight, G. S., Penequin, P., and Schimke, R. T. (1975). *J. Biol. Chem.* **250**, 8105–8110.
Mühlbock, O. (1965). *Eur. J. Cancer* **1**, 123–124.
Nandi, S., and McGrath, C. M. (1973). *Adv. Cancer Res.* **17**, 353–414.
O'Farrell, P. H. (1975). *J. Biol. Chem.* **250**, 4007–4021.
Owens, I., Vonderhaar, B., and Topper, Y. J. (1973). *J. Biol. Chem.* **248**, 472–477.
Owens, R. B., and Hackett, A. J. (1972). *J. Natl. Cancer Inst.* **49**, 1321–1332.
Palmiter, R. D., Oka, T., and Schimke, R. T. (1971). *J. Biol. Chem.* **246**, 724–737.
Palmiter, R. D., Moore, P. B., Mulvihill, E. R., and Emtage, S. (1976). *Cell* **8**, 557–572.
Parks, W. P., and Scolnick, E. M. (1973). *Virology* **55**, 163–173.
Parks, W. P., Scolnick, E. M., and Kozikowski, E. H. (1974). *Science* **184**, 158–160.

Parks, W. P., Ransom, J. C., Young, H. A., and Scolnick, E. M. (1975). *J. Biol. Chem.* **250**, 3330–3336.
Peterkofsky, B., and Tomkins, G. M. (1968). *Proc. Natl. Acad. Sci. U.S.A.* **60**, 222–228.
Ringold, G. M., Lasfargues, E. Y., Bishop, J. M., and Varmus, H. E. (1975a). *Virology* **65**, 135–147.
Ringold, G. M., Yamamoto, K. R., Tomkins, G. M., Bishop, J. M., and Varmus, H. E. (1975b). *Cell* **6**, 299–305.
Ringold, G. M., Cardiff, R., Varmus, H. E., and Yamamoto, K. R. (1977a). *Cell* **10**, 11–18.
Ringold, G. M., Yamamoto, K. R., Shank, P. R., and Varmus, H. E. (1977b). *Cell* **10**, 19–26.
Ringold, G. M., Blair, P. B., Bishop, J. M. and Varmus, H. E. (1976). *Virology* **70**, 550–553.
Rousseau, G. G., Baxter, J. D., and Tomkins, G. M. (1972). *J. Mol. Biol.* **67**, 99–115.
Rousseau, G. G., Baxter, J. D., Higgins, S. J., and Tomkins, G. M. (1973). *J. Mol. Biol.* **79**, 539–554.
Schlom, J., Michalides, R., Kufe, D., Hehlmann, R., Spiegelman, S., Bentvelzen, P., and Hageman, P. (1973). *J. Natl. Cancer Inst.* **51**, 541–551.
Schwartz, R. J., Tsai, M.-J., Tsai, S. Y., and O'Malley, B. W. (1975). *J. Biol. Chem.* **250**, 5175–5182.
Scolnick, E. M., Young, H. A., and Parks, W. P. (1976). *Virology* **69**, 148–155.
Shyamala, G., and Dickson, C. (1976). *Nature (London)* **262**, 107–112.
Sibley, C. H., and Tomkins, G. M. (1974a). *Cell* **2**, 213–220.
Sibley, C. H., and Tomkins, G. M. (1974b). *Cell* **2**, 221–227.
Singer, R. H., and Penman, S. (1973). *J. Mol. Biol.* **78**, 321–334.
Smith, M. J., Hough, B. R., Chamberlin, M. E. and Davidson, E. H. (1974). *J. Mol. Biol.* **85**, 103–126.
Spelsberg, T. C., Steggles, A. W., and O'Malley, B. W. (1971). *J. Biol. Chem.* **246**, 4188–4197.
Stavnezer, E., and Bishop, J. M. (1977). In preparation.
Sykes, J. A., Whitescarver, J., and Briggs, L., (1968). *J. Natl. Cancer Inst.* **41**, 1315–1327.
Temin, H., and Baltimore, D. (1972). *Adv. Virus Res.* **17**, 129–186.
Thompson, E. B., Tomkins, G. M., and Curran, J. F. (1966). *Proc. Natl. Acad. Sci. U.S.A.* **56**, 296–303.
Vaidya, A. B., Lasfargues, E. Y., Heubel, G., Lasfargues, J.-C., and Moore, D. H. (1976). *J. Virol.* **18**, 911–917.
Varmus, H. E., and Shank, P. R. (1976). *J. Virol.* **18**, 567–573.
Varmus, H. E., Bishop, J. M., Nowinski, R. C., and Sarkar, N. H. (1972). *Nature (London), New Biol.* **238**, 189–191.
Varmus, H. E., Quintrell, N., Medeiros, E., Bishop, J. M., Nowinski, R. C., and Sarkar, N. H. (1973). *J. Mol. Biol.* **79**, 663–679.
Varmus, H. E., Heasley, S., and Bishop, J. M. (1974). *J. Virol.* **14**, 895–903.
Varmus, H. E., Heasley, S., Linn, J., and Wheeler, K. (1976). *J. Virol.* **18**, 574–585.
Williams, D., and Gorski, J. (1972a). *Proc. Natl. Acad. Sci. U.S.A.* **69**, 3464–3468.
Williams, D., and Gorski, J. (1972b). *In* "Gene Transcription in Reproductive Tissue" (E. Diczfalusy, ed.). p. 420. Bogtrykklet Forum, Copenhagen.
Woo, S. L., Smith, R. G., Means, A. R., and O'Malley, B. W. (1976). *J. Biol. Chem.* **251**, 3868–3874.
Yamamoto, K. R., and Alberts, B. M. (1974). *J. Biol. Chem.* **249**, 7076–7086.
Yamamoto, K. R., and Alberts, B. M. (1975). *Cell* **4**, 301–310.
Yamamoto, K. R., and Alberts, B. M. (1976). *Annu. Rev. Biochem.* **45**, 721–746.
Yamamoto, K. R., Ivarie, R. D., Ring, J., Ringold, G. M., and Stallcup, M. R. (1977). Biochemical Actions of Hormones, **5**, in press.

Yamamoto, K. R., Stampfer, M. R., and Tomkins, G. M. (1974). *Proc. Natl. Acad. Sci. U.S.A.* **71,** 3901–3905.
Yamamoto, K. R., Gehring, U., Stampfer, M. R., and Sibley, C. H. (1976). *Recent Prog. Horm. Res.* **32,** 3–32.
Young, H. A., Scolnick, E. M., and Parks, W. P. (1975). *J. Biol. Chem.* **250,** 3337–3343.
Young, L. J. T., Cardiff, R. D., and Ashley, R. L. (1975). *J. Natl. Cancer Inst.* **54,** 1215–1221.

12

Biology of Mineralocorticoid Receptors

NORMAN S. ANDERSON, III, AND
DARRELL D. FANESTIL

I. Introduction 323
II. General Presence of [^{3}H]Aldosterone Receptor in Target Cells 324
III. Properties of the Cytosol Aldosterone Receptor 329
IV. Properties of the Nuclear Aldosterone Receptor 339
V. Evidence for a Receptor-Mediated Response 342
    A. Time-Course of Aldosterone Binding 342
    B. Binding of Nonmineralocorticoids to the Aldosterone Receptor 344
    C. Studies of Genetic Variants 347
References 349

I. INTRODUCTION

Beginning with the earliest observation of aldosterone accumulation in the nuclei of the toad urinary bladder (Edelman et al., 1963; Porter and Edelman, 1964), there has been substantial investigation of aldosterone binding and aldosterone receptors in specific target tissues (King and Mainwaring, 1974). Although the resultant reports are numerous and increasingly complex, final study of the mechanism of aldosterone action mediated through hormone receptors has been complicated by the lability of the aldosterone receptor (Alberti and Sharp, 1970) and presence of receptors for the structurally and biologically similar glucocorticoids (Funder et al., 1973b). Therefore, while indirect experimental evidence has suggested that actions of aldosterone are mediated through a hormone receptor, the hypothesis has not been established (Edelman, 1975).

Currently, the effects of aldosterone have been described in virtually all secretory epithelia. The tissues most extensively studied have been the kidney of the adrenalectomized rat (Edelman and Fanestil, 1970) and the urinary bladder of the toad, *Bufo marinus* (Ludens and Fanestil, 1976). Additionally, important studies of Na^+ transport have also been conducted in tissues such as gastrointestinal tract (Moll and Koczorek, 1962), sweat glands (Streeton *et al.*, 1955), salivary glands (Blair-West *et al.*, 1963; Lauler *et al.*, 1962), and anuran ventral skin and colon (Maetz *et al.*, 1958; Scheer *et al.*, 1961).

Whereas the principal physiological effects of aldosterone (Na^+ reabsorption, K^+ excretion) have been amply documented in most of these tissues, final identification of specific mineralocorticoid binding by receptors has, by necessity, been inextricably involved with studies of glucocorticoid binding (Funder *et al.*, 1973ab; Feldman *et al.*, 1973). Unequivocal identification of binding by specific receptors for aldosterone in adrenalectomized rat tissues, such as kidney (Funder *et al.*, 1973a), brain (Anderson and Fanestil, 1976), or the gastrointestinal tract (Pressley and Funder, 1975), has only been accomplished with techniques which attempt either to minimize or to quantitate binding of aldosterone to sites which have a higher affinity for glucocorticoids (Funder *et al.*, 1973a) or, conversely, to quantitate the binding of glucocorticoids to sites which have a higher affinity for aldosterone. Several laboratories have now suggested important common characteristics of the aldosterone receptor, regardless of the system studied: (a) in aldosterone responsive tissues, the aldosterone receptor has a higher affinity for mineralocorticoids than glucocorticoids; (b) the selective filling of aldosterone "sites" is accomplished at concentrations that are closely related to normal physiological levels; and (c) receptors for aldosterone bind the unmetabolized steroid.

Several excellent reviews on the action of aldosterone have been written (King and Mainwaring, 1974; Edelman and Fanestil, 1970; Ludens and Fanestil, 1976); however, in this chapter, we will concentrate principally on studies of the aldosterone receptor in the adrenalectomized rat kidney and discuss the available evidence which suggests that the physiological response to aldosterone is mediated through specific receptors located in both the cytoplasm and nuclei of mineralocorticoid-responsive cells.

II. GENERAL PRESENCE OF [³H]ALDOSTERONE RECEPTOR IN TARGET CELLS

The initial evidence of the localization of aldosterone-binding sites was provided by Edelman *et al.* (1963) in high-resolution autoradiographs of the toad bladder. In these studies, Edelman et al. (1963) observed that [^{3}H]aldosterone preferentially localized in the nucleus of cells that are actively engaged in Na$^+$ reabsorption, the toad bladder epithelial cells. Furthermore, it was shown that [^{3}H]progesterone, a steroid with little mineralocorticoid activity, did not exhibit the property of preferential localization (Porter and Edelman, 1964). Earlier findings of Davidson et al. (1962) had failed to provide evidence of specific binding of [^{3}H]aldosterone to subcellular fractions of the adrenalectomized rat kidney; however, given the conditions of isolation and analysis of the preparation that Davidson employed, it can now easily be seen that these conditions in all likelihood destroyed all receptor activity.

Following these initial studies of Edelman et al. (1963) and Porter and Edelman (1964), Sharp and Leaf (1966) examined the binding of [^{3}H]aldosterone to specific sites in the toad bladder with the use of a displacement binding technique. This method presupposes that the addition of an excess of nonradioactive steroid displaces [^{3}H]aldosterone specifically bound to receptors and does not influence the [^{3}H]aldosterone dissolved in tissue water or lipids. Sharp and Leaf (1966) demonstrated that, when toad bladder epithelial cells were incubated with 10^{-10} to 10^{-8} M of [^{3}H]aldosterone (normal physiological range), one-fifth to one-third of the [^{3}H]aldosterone bound was associated with nuclei and appeared to be specific. Perhaps the more important of the discoveries of Sharp and Leaf (1966), however, was the presence of at least two types of specific binding sites, one with high affinity for aldosterone and one with a much lower, but nevertheless physiologically important, affinity. In a contemporaneous study, Sulya et al. (1964) demonstrated that, although aldosterone readily penetrated all tissues of the adrenalectomized rat after in vivo administration of [^{3}H]aldosterone, the accumulation of [^{3}H]aldosterone was highest in those tissues specialized to promote Na$^+$ ion transport. In this study, Sulya et al. (1964) also noted the now well confirmed observation that the amount of extractable radioactive [^{3}H]aldosterone was highest in the kidney and intestinal mucosa.

Fanestil and Edelman (1966) recognized the need to study both specificity and saturability of the receptor binding and, therefore, scrutinized binding of [^{3}H]aldosterone following tissue fractionation in order to localize binding. In this important study, Fanestil and Edelman (1966) detected the greatest quantity of unmetabolized [^{3}H]aldosterone in the nuclear fraction derived from kidneys of adrenalectomized rats. Significantly, they noted that nuclear sites for [^{3}H]aldosterone in the kidney appeared to be saturated within the normal physiological range, and the accumulation was specific for mineralocorticoids (Fig. 1). Ausiello and Sharp (1968), using similar techniques of homogenization and differential centrifugation of the toad uri-

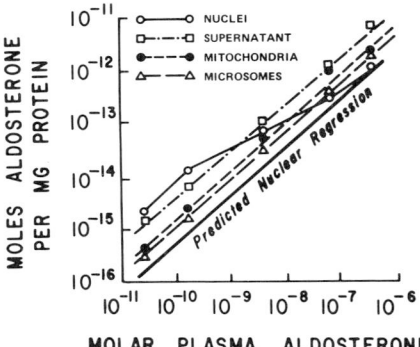

Fig. 1. The occurrence of a subcellular distribution of aldosterone in adrenalectomized rat kidney dependent on the plasma aldosterone concentration. Maximal antinaturesis was obtained with 2.78×10^{-9} moles of aldosterone, corresponding to a plasma hormone concentration of approximately 5×10^{-9} M. The predicted nuclear regression estimates nonspecific binding of [^{3}H]aldosterone (reprinted, with permission, from Fanestil and Edelman, 1966).

nary bladder, also documented specific nuclear accumulation of [^{3}H]aldosterone in the toad bladder.

This demonstration of selective accumulation of aldosterone in nuclei of rat kidney and toad bladder prompted the studies by Herman et al. (1968) and Alberti and Sharp (1969) on the extraction of the [^{3}H]aldosterone from the nucleus. Utilizing gel chromatography of a Tris extract of the nuclear fraction, Herman et al. (1968) revealed that approximately 50% of the [^{3}H]aldosterone was bound to macromolecules. In addition to extracting the intranuclear-bound [^{3}H]aldosterone, Herman et al. (1968) were also able to delineate the protein nature of the nuclear receptor. Herman et al. disclosed that the binding of [^{3}H]aldosterone to the Tris-soluble nuclear extracts could be decreased 65% by chymotrypsin and 46% by pronase, while it was virtually unaffected by deoxyribonuclease, ribonuclease, and trypsin. Further credence to observation that proteins were binding [^{3}H]aldosterone was also presented by Herman et al. (1968), who demonstrated that the nuclear receptor was sensitive to 2-(2-aminoethyl)-2-thiopseudourea p-hydroxybenzoate, an agent specific for sulfhydryl groups. As discussed in a following section, more recent studies have now revealed that at least two forms of the protein-bound [^{3}H]aldosterone can exist intranuclearly: (a) a Tris-extractable form and (b) a chromatin-bound, 0.3–0.4 M KCl extractable form (Marver et al., 1972).

As studies of the nuclear accumulation progressed, accessory studies of cytoplasmic binding of aldosterone in various tissues were initiated. Herman et al. (1968) first elicited steroid-selective protein binding in kidney cytosol both *in vivo* and *in vitro*. As Fanestil and Edelman (1966) had noted earlier with nuclear binding, the ability of various steroids to compete for [^{3}H]aldosterone binding sites in both cytosol and in nuclei was closely allied to their potency as mineralocorticoids.

The discovery of specific nuclear and cytoplasmic binding of aldosterone (Herman *et al.*, 1968; Alberti and Sharp, 1969) implied ubiquity of the aldosterone receptors in mineralocorticoid-responsive tissues. It is noteworthy, then, that consequent to the administration of 2.6×10^{-10} moles of [^{3}H]aldosterone to adrenalectomized rats, Swaneck *et al.* (1969) attained specific nuclear binding in the kidney, duodenal mucosa, spleen, liver, and brain. They (Swaneck *et al.*, 1969) noted that, although the kidney was the organ with the greatest nuclear accumulation, the duodenal mucosa and the spleen also accumulated significant amounts of [^{3}H]aldosterone. Furthermore, although other organs, such as liver and brain, exhibited lower aldosterone binding, these organs were, nevertheless, capable of "specific" binding.

It has now been shown by Duval and Funder (1974) that aldosterone binding to cytosols derived from rat liver is in all probability binding to glucocorticoid and not mineralocorticoid sites. Nevertheless, studies by Pressley and Funder (1975) in gut mucosa and by Anderson and Fanestil (1976) in the brain have extended the original findings of Swaneck *et al.* (1969) and have suggested that the binding of aldosterone to receptors in other tissues may mirror the more complete data which has accumulated for [^{3}H]aldosterone binding in the adrenalectomized rat kidney.

In their research, Pressley and Funder (1975) authenticated separate sites for mineralocorticoid and glucocorticoid binding in rat intestinal mucosa. Additionally, they offered evidence for aldosterone receptors in duodenum, jejunum, ileum, and colon but found no similar sites in the mucosa of the gastric antrum (Fig. 2). A previous study by Ballard *et al.* (1974) had also noted binding of [^{3}H]aldosterone in gut mucosa. However, they made no attempt to distinguish between mineralocorticoid and glucocorticoid binding sites.

Perhaps the most complete study of [^{3}H]aldosterone binding to a tissue other than kidney or toad bladder was conducted on the parotid gland of the rat by Funder *et al.* (1972). As the parotid has been well characterized as a mineralocorticoid target tissue (Blair-West *et al.*, 1967), it is of particular interest that in this study the characteristics of the [^{3}H]aldosterone binding were quite similar to those of the [^{3}H]aldosterone binding in rat kidney.

Currently, the available evidence suggests that specific aldosterone binding to nuclear and cytoplasmic proteins either can be or has been demonstrated in most secretory epithelia involved in the process of active Na^+ transport. However, data indicating the absence of specific aldosterone

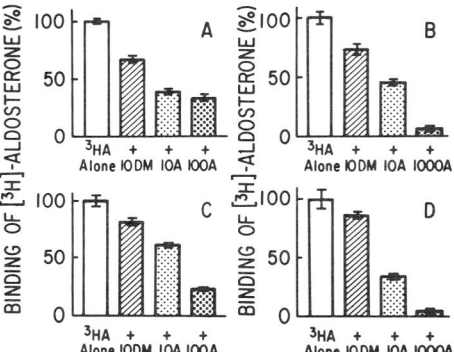

Fig. 2. Binding of [³H]aldosterone in gut mucosal cells; competition by unlabeled aldosterone and dexamethasone. Cells from duodenum (A), jejunum (B), Ileum (C), and colon (D) were incubated for 60 minutes at 4°C with [³H]A 2×10^{-9} M either alone (open bars), in the presence of tenfold unlabeled DM (hatching), in the presence of tenfold unlabeled aldosterone (fine stippling), or in the presence of 1000-fold aldosterone (coarse stippling). Each bar shows the mean ± SEM of six experimental determinations, the results being expressed as a percentage of the binding in the absence of competing unlabeled steroid (reprinted, with permission, from Pressley and Funder, 1975).

binding in tissues has also been presented by Davidson *et al.* (1962) and Duval and Funder (1974) in rat liver, Funder *et al.* (1973c) in the heart, and by our own studies with the rectal gland of the shark (J. Lewicki, N. S. Anderson, III, and D. D. Fanestil, unpublished observations, 1974). It should be emphasized that the demonstration of presence or absence of aldosterone receptors is highly dependent on several important considerations: (a) the [³H]aldosterone-binding protein in all tissues characterized, thus far, has been highly temperature labile and relatively unstable *in vitro*; (b) the level of endogenous mineralocorticoids and glucocorticoids in the experimental animal is critical in that binding of aldosterone to cells in the intact (nonadrenalectomized) animal is difficult to demonstrate, while binding to the same fractions following adrenalectomy is, as would be predicted, increased; (c) the relatively high affinity of aldosterone for glucocorticoid receptors in target tissue cells necessitates the use of criteria that determine the presence of receptors having a higher affinity for aldosterone than glucocorticoids; (d) glucocorticoid receptors, which have been described in many of these same tissues, are not as labile in a cell-free state and, thus, can be artificially selected. Therefore, studies that indicate either binding or a lack of binding of aldosterone must be performed and evaluated with these considerations in mind.

Evocations of cytosol and nuclear binding of [³H]aldosterone have contributed to the understanding of a hormone receptor-mediated response.

However, significant contributions have also been presented by investigators seeking evidence for aldosterone receptors in more specific fractions of tissue preparations. Of interest in this regard are the studies of Forte (1972), who studied [³H]aldosterone binding to renal plasma membranes and Sapirstein and Scott (1975) and Scott and Sapirstein (1975), who studied binding to mitochondrial-rich (MR) cells of the toad urinary bladder.

Forte (1972) introduced another largely unexplored concept that certain aldosterone actions may be mediated through membrane receptors. In both *in vivo* and *in vitro* studies, Forte (1972) offered that the membrane sites which bind [³H]aldosterone were selective for steroids with mineralocorticoid agonist or antagonist properties. On the basis of his investigation, Forte (1972) concluded that the binding of [³H]aldosterone to plasma membranes derived from the adrenalectomized rat kidney may be involved in the cellular mode of action.

Sapirstein and Scott (1975) and Scott and Sapirstein (1975) examined [³H]aldosterone binding to the mitochondrial-rich and granular cells of the toad urinary bladder and found increased binding of [³H]aldosterone to the MR cells (Scott and Sapirstein, 1975). They showed that, although the amount of displaceable aldosterone bound by the MR cells differed according to the month of the year, the MR cells, nevertheless, reportedly displayed the property of selectivity for mineralocorticoids. Additionally, Sapirstein and Scott (1975) were able to demonstrate mineralocorticoid/glucocorticoid selectivity of the receptor binding [³H]aldosterone by measuring the efficacy with which either deoxycorticosterone or cortisol displaced [³H]aldosterone. Their data (Sapirstein and Scott, 1975) indicated that DOCA completely displaced [³H]aldosterone from the MR cells while cortisol could only displace 24%.

While each of these studies of Forte (1972) and Sapirstein and Scott (1975) and Scott and Sapirstein (1975) requires expansion, they are nevertheless important. More recently, differential actions of aldosterone on Na^+ reabsorption (slight effect) and K^+ excretion (increased effect) were noted in a Peru strain of mice (Stewart, 1975). If binding of aldosterone can be successfully coupled to a specific cell type or another cellular organelle, it is possible that strain-related differences in aldosterone binding and actions may be more easily explained.

III. PROPERTIES OF THE CYTOSOL ALDOSTERONE RECEPTOR

Characterization of [³H]aldosterone receptors in cytosol preparations of adrenalectomized rat kidney has been principally conducted using methods which involve (a) *in vivo* administration of [³H]aldosterone to the animal with subsequent cell or subcellular fractionation, (b) whole tissue incubation with [³H]aldosterone followed by cellular and subcellular fractionation, (c) incubation of tissue slices with [³H]aldosterone followed by subcellular fractionation, (d) cell-free systems in which subcellular fractionation of tissue is followed by incubation with [³H]aldosterone, and (e) autoradiography. Of these, the tissue slice and cell-free systems of incubation with [³H]aldosterone have yielded both the greatest quantity and most useful information on the [³H]aldosterone receptor. Accordingly, the investigations that have utilized these techniques will be discussed in greatest detail, although the representative characteristics of cytosol receptors for [³H]aldosterone determined by each of the methods outlined above are presented in Table I.

Herman *et al.* (1968) were the first to expose [³H]aldosterone receptors in a cytosol fraction. In this early study, Herman *et al.* (1968) inoculated adrenalectomized rats with 2.6×10^{-10} mole of [³H]aldosterone. After 30 minutes, the kidneys were removed, homogenized, centrifuged at 100,000 g, and assayed for [³H]aldosterone binding. Additionally, they (Herman *et al.*, 1968) quantitated binding of [³H]aldosterone *in vitro* to cytosol from kidneys of untreated adrenalectomized rats. Herman *et al.* (1968) identified the cytosol binding substances as proteins by their precipitability by $(NH_4)_2SO_4$, chemical analysis which showed only trace amounts of RNA and DNA and dissociation of the receptor complex by proteolytic enzymes and sulfhydryl reagents. Notably, Herman *et al.* (1968) were able to demonstrate unquestionable specificity in that the ability of various steroids to compete for [³H]aldosterone binding closely corresponded to their potencies as mineralocorticoids.

Application of Herman's work was attempted by Robinson and Fanestil (1970), who utilized the binding of [³H]aldosterone to renal cytosols to form an assay for aldosterone by a competitive binding technique. Although they were able to measure 1.05 and 2.1×10^{-12} moles of aldosterone with coefficient of variation of only 13%, certain technical problems and the relatively high affinity of cortisol for the sites prohibited the technique from being applied to other biologic specimens.

Many investigators have since both identified (Mills *et al.*, 1972; Palem-Vliers *et al.*, 1974; Sharp and Leaf, 1966) and partially characterized (Marver *et al.*, 1972; Sharp and Leaf, 1965; Swaneck *et al.*, 1970) [³H]aldosterone binding to renal or toad urinary bladder cytosol proteins. Early experiments in our laboratory by Ludens and Fanestil (1971) determined that at least two forms of the [³H]aldosterone receptor exist *in vitro* in rat kidney cytosol. One form demonstrable in 0.3 M KCl had a molecular weight (MW) of 50,000 and the other form, present in 0.25 M sucrose, had an MW of greater than 1.5×10^6. Ludens and Fanestil (1971)

TABLE I

In Vitro Binding of [^{3}H]Aldosterone

Author	Incubation time/temp	Affinity	Competition[a]	System
Alberti and Sharp (1969)	1.5–3.0 hours/25°C	—	A ≅ SC$^+$ ≥ F DOC	Toad bladder whole cell
Anderson and Fanestil (1976)	2.5 hours/0°C	K_d = 1.5 × 10^{-9} M	A > DM > B	Adrex rat brain cell free
Forte (1972)	30 minutes/30°C	K_d ≅ 10^{-7} M	DOC ≅ prog > test > E$_2$	Adrex rat kidney membranes
Funder *et al.* (1972)	40 minutes/25°C	K_d = 1.8 × 10^{-9} M	—	Adrex rat parotid whole cell
Funder *et al.* (1973a)	20 minutes/37°C	K_d = 5 × 10^{-10} M	A > DOC > B	Adrex rat kidney whole cell
Herman *et al.* (1968)	2.0–2.5 hours/0°C	—	9αF > DOC > pred > E$_2$	Adrex rat kidney cell free
Ludens and Fanestil (1971)	3.0–3.5 hours/0°C	K_d ≅ 3.3 × 10^{-9} M	9αF > F = B > E$_2$	Adrex rat kidney cell free
Marver *et al.* (1974)	45 minutes/25°C	—	A > SC-26304 > B	Adrex rat kidney whole cell
Palem-Vliers *et al.* (1974)	1.0 hours/24°C	—	9αF > DOC > E$_2$	Adrex rat kidney whole cell
Pressley and Funder (1975)	1.0 hour/4°C	—	A > DM	Adrex rat kidney whole cell
Robinson and Fanestil (1970)	5.0 hour/4°C	K_d ≅ 8 × 10^{-9} M	9αF > F > Prog	Adrex rat kidney cell free
Rousseau *et al.* (1972)	90 minutes/0°C	K_{d_1} = 5 × 10^{-9} M	—	Adrex rat kidney cell free
Rousseau *et al.* (1972)	90 minutes/0°C	K_d = 2.5 × 10^{-8} M	DM > B > F > A	HTC cells cell free
Sapirstein and Scott (1975)	90 minutes/25°C	—	DOCA > F	Toad bladder whole cell (mitochondrial rich)
Ulmann *et al.* (1975)	30 minutes/25°C	K_{d_1} = 1.9 × 10^{-9} M	A ≫ glycyrrhetinic acid	Adrex rat kidney whole cell

[a] Abbreviations used: A, aldosterone; SC, spironolactone; F, cortisol; DOC, deoxycorticosterone; DM, dexamethasone; Prog, Progesterone; Test, testosterone; E$_2$, estradiol; 9αF, 9α-fluorocortisol; B, corticosterone; SC-26304, spirolactone; Pred, prednisolone.

also recognized that interconversion of these two forms could occur simply by the addition or removal of KCl from the incubation medium. It was noted that the two forms had virtually identical K_a's. Additionally, the patterns of binding inhibition produced by nonradioactive steroids (9α-fluorocortisol > cortisol = corticosterone > estradiol) were also identical for both forms. These two forms were, in all probability, simply interconversions of receptors and not the separate classes of receptors as was later proposed by Rousseau et al. (1972) and by Funder et al. (1973a,b) and Feldman et al. (1973). Quite possibly, the changes in ionic composition of the incubation buffer resulted in a shift in the apparent molecular weight of all (type I, type II, type III) classes of receptors.

Recently, Marver et al. (1972) inspected the sedimentation coefficients of the [^{3}H]aldosterone–protein complex and proposed that the renal cytoplasmic [^{3}H]aldosterone receptor can exist in a variety of forms as Ludens and Fanestil (1971) had shown previously. On the basis of these studies, it was concluded that the form of the isolated steroid–receptor complex was largely dictated by both ionic strength and cationic composition of the buffer applied to a sucrose density gradient. In buffers of low ionic strength, Marver found that the sedimentation coefficient of the principal cytoplasmic [^{3}H]aldosterone–receptor complex was 8.5 S. When a similar study was performed with either 0.4 M KCl or 0.4 M KCl with 6 mM CaCl$_2$, the sedimentation coefficients were 4.5 S and 3.5 S, respectively. Additionally, Marver et al. (1972) reported that, regardless of the ionic composition of the buffer, the binding of [^{3}H]aldosterone to the cytoplasmic receptor could be totally displaced with a 100-fold excess of 9α-fluorocortisol and was not precipitated by antibodies raised against whole rat serum. Therefore, she (Marver et al., 1972) judged that the multiple forms of [^{3}H]aldosterone binding demonstrated were specific and not due to contamination by plasma proteins.

Study of aldosterone binding in the adrenalectomized rat kidney and parotid by Funder et al. (1972) adduced that in each of these tissues (now agreed to be mineralocorticoid responsive), a three-step mechanism of [^{3}H]-aldosterone binding occurs. Utilizing a tissue slice system, the authors revealed time- and temperature-dependent cytosol binding followed by intranuclear and chromatin binding of [^{3}H]aldosterone. Furthermore, because cycloheximide had no effect on cytosol binding, the authors (Funder et al., 1972) speculated that either the cytosol receptors in these tissues are relatively long-lived, or, if short-lived, the biosynthesis of cytosol receptor was not impaired by the concentrations (0.1–5.0 µg cycloheximide/ml) or the time (0–30 minutes) of incubation. In a control study, Funder et al. (1972) demonstrated that 0.5 mg/ml of cycloheximide added to the kidney slices inhibited [^{3}H]leucine incorporation into cellular amino acids by 67%.

Although the kidney cytosol contained twice the concentration of [^{3}H]-aldosterone receptor compared to the parotid cytosol, the receptors from both tissues appeared to have an identical K_d (1.8 × 10^{-9} M). Notably, reexamination of this Scatchard analysis (Scatchard, 1949) data of Funder *et al.* (1972) reveals that aldosterone was binding to at least two sites. It was Rousseau *et al.* (1972), however, who first emphasized the cytoplasmic binding of [^{3}H]aldosterone to a second set of sites.

Rousseau *et al.* (1972) proposed that [^{3}H]aldosterone bound to one set of sites in cytosols derived from HTC cells and to two sets of sites in cytosols prepared from adrenalectomized kidney. Although several investigators had suggested that the [^{3}H]aldosterone was binding in tissue to separate sites with different affinity, Rousseau *et al.* (1972) distinguished binding of aldosterone to true mineralocorticoid-receptor sites from the binding of aldosterone to the now well-documented type II sites. Their data (Rousseau *et al.*, 1972) attests that the K_d of the high-affinity aldosterone sites was 5 × 10^{-9} M with a concentration of receptor sites (moles/mg protein) of 1.3 × 10^{-13}. Similarly, the K_d of the low-affinity site was 6.5 × 10^{-8} M with an N_{max} of 3.9 × 10^{-13} moles/mg protein. Rousseau *et al.* (1972) proposed, therefore, that rat kidney cytosol had at least two classes of specific aldosterone receptors of unequal capacity. He (Rousseau *et al.*, 1972) determined the higher-affinity binding sites to be mineralocorticoid receptors due to the K_d of the high-affinity site and the known physiological levels of aldosterone and postulated the low-affinity site to be a glucocorticoid site, as was later documented by Funder *et al.* (1973b).

Following his study, a most important series of articles was presented by Funder *et al.* (1973a,b) and Feldman *et al.* (1973). The authors studied *in vivo* and *in vitro* properties of the cytosol [^{3}H]aldosterone receptors and, after extensive investigation, described three classes of receptors to which aldosterone, dexamethasone, and corticosterone bound with differing affinities. They termed the separate classes of aldosterone receptor sites type I, type II, and type III. These studies performed by Funder *et al.* (1973a,b) and Feldman *et al.* (1973) both confirmed the work of Rousseau *et al.* (1972) and added several new concepts to the model. Of initial importance to Funder *et al.* (1973a) was the question of appropriate occupancy of the [^{3}H]aldosterone receptor. Given physiological plasma levels of corticosterone orders of magnitude higher than aldosterone and of deoxycorticosterone levels (DOC) at least equal to aldosterone, the question posed was the mechanism through which the high-affinity sites were "appropriately" occupied by aldosterone. In exacting experiments, Funder *et al.* (1973a) ascertained, both *in vivo* and *in vitro* in a tissue-slice system, how the needed specificity was conferred on this system.

It had previously been shown by Sandberg *et al.* (1966) and by Westphal

(1975) that the avidity with which corticosterone-binding globulin (CBG) binds these steroids is corticosterone > deoxycorticosterone ≫ aldosterone. Utilizing this knowledge, Funder *et al.* (1973a) demonstrated that the preferential binding of deoxycorticosterone (DOC) by the plasma proteins allowed increased availability of aldosterone for binding to the specific mineralocorticoid sites in the kidney. Thus, the amount of DOC bound by CBG reduced the free concentration of DOC to a level which was minimally effective as a competitor for mineralocorticoid receptors.

The question of corticosterone occupancy of the mineralocorticoid sites, however, was only partially resolved by preferential plasma binding. The normal level of corticosterone was of such a magnitude that even with the increased plasma binding, corticosterone would still be expected to occupy half of the aldosterone-receptor sites. This anomaly was then clearly accounted for by data which indicated that the type I sites have only 2% of the affinity for corticosterone, compared to aldosterone, and the type II sites have twice the affinity for corticosterone over aldosterone (Fig. 3). In a subsequent article, the type II site of aldosterone binding as originally described by Rousseau *et al.* (1972), was characterized by Funder *et al.* (1973b) as having the highest affinity for the synthetic glucocorticoid dexamethasone, and lower affinities for both corticosterone and aldosterone. Finally, the type III sites, described by Feldman *et al.* (1973), were sites with a higher affinity for corticosterone, much lower affinity for deoxycorticosterone, and limited affinity for both dexamethasone and aldosterone. In total, then, it was concluded that the type I sites were mineralocorticoid receptors (Funder *et al.*, 1973a), while the type II (Funder *et al.*, 1973b) and type III (Feldman *et al.*, 1973) sites were glucocorticoid receptors. Thus, at both lower and physiological concentrations of aldosterone, aldosterone bound principally to the type I sites (Funder *et al.*, 1973a), while at higher concentrations, it occupied an increasing number of the sites for which it had a lower affinity, namely the type II and type III sites.

These findings (Funder *et al.*, 1973a,b; Feldman *et al.*, 1973) of multiple sites for [^{3}H]aldosterone binding are consistent with many *in vivo* studies which have demonstrated that, as the plasma levels of aldosterone or deoxycorticosterone are increased, each of the mineralocorticoids have increased glucocorticoid properties, while retaining the mineralocorticoid properties (Samuels and Tomkins, 1970). Additionally, and as would be predicted from the model presented by Funder, Feldman, and Edelman, the glucocorticoids, devoid of intrinsic mineralocorticoid activity at low physiological levels, have considerable mineralocorticoid activity when administered at concentrations in excess of the normal physiological range (Cake and Litwack, 1975).

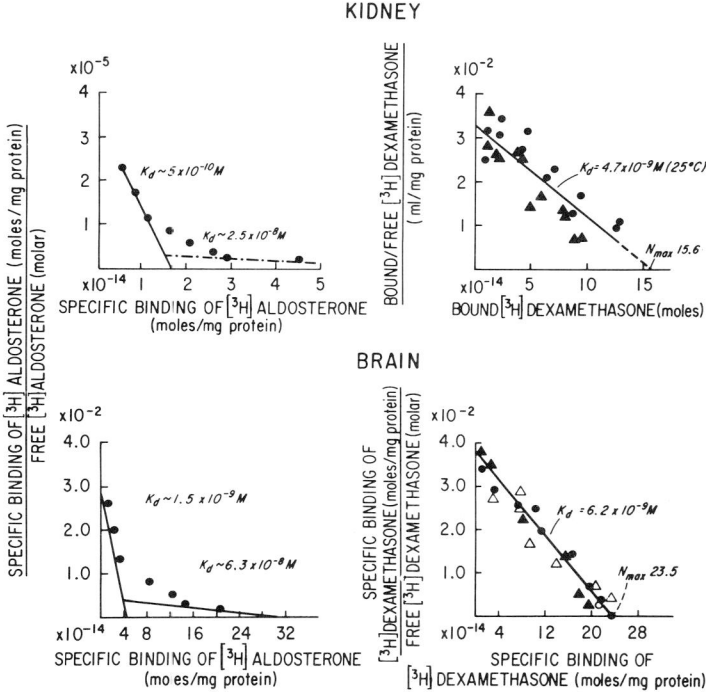

Fig. 3. Comparison of *in vitro* binding of [³H]aldosterone and [³H]dexamethasone in kidney (see Funder *et al.*, 1973a, for details) and brain (see Anderson and Fanestil, 1976, for details) analyzed by the method of Scatchard. Upper panel describes binding to cytosols prepared from renal tissue slices (reproduced, with permission from Funder *et al.*, 1973a,b). Lower panel describes binding to cytosols prepared from adrenalectomized rat brain (reproduced, with permission, from Anderson and Fanestil, 1976).

In studies conducted in our laboratory (Anderson and Fanestil, 1976), we inspected the binding of [³H]aldosterone in cytosols prepared from whole brain and noted a similarity to the multiple-receptor, multiple-affinity [³H]aldosterone binding described in the kidney (Fig. 3). Our original studies (Anderson *et al.*, 1974) of glucocorticoid binding in whole brain confirmed the work of several investigators (McEwen *et al.*, 1972; DeKloet *et al.*, 1975; (Stevens *et al.*, 1975) with regard to the type III corticosterone-type binding sites. With the use of the aldosterone antagonist spirolactone SC-9420 in our studies, we ascertained that corticosterone and dexamethasone occupy separate sites at low concentrations but that, when the level of either hormone is greatly increased, each hormone can completely inhibit the binding of the other. Ultimately, on the basis of indirect evidence provided by competition studies (Anderson and Fanestil, 1976), we further concluded that, as was originally shown in the kidney, three separate sites for aldosterone binding exist in the brain. We were not able, however, to determine whether the type I and type II sites had equal affinity for dexamethasone or whether the type II site was the only site occupied by dexamethasone. Nevertheless, the evidence suggests that in the brain aldosterone selectively binds with highest affinity to the type I site and binds with a lower affinity to the type II site (Fig. 3). Furthermore, it is quite possible that neither site discriminates for the synthetic glucocorticoid dexamethasone, i.e., each site has equal affinity for dexamethasone (Anderson and Fanestil, 1976). In view of the findings of Rousseau et al. (1972), Funder et al. (1973a,b), and our own (Anderson and Fanestil, 1976) which demonstrate multiple binding sites for aldosterone, rigorous interpretation of competition studies from early work is difficult. It has been recognized for many years that, in in vivo experimentation, steroids other than aldosterone are capable of producing mineralocorticoid or Na^+ transport effects, specifically, 11-deoxycorticosterone, 9α-fluorocortisol (agonists) (Sharp and Leaf, 1964). Conversely, certain other steroids such as the spirolactones, cortisone (Sharp and Leaf, 1964), and 11-deoxy-17α-hydroxycorticosterone (Alberti and Sharp, 1970) (antagonists) competently block the effects of mineralocorticoids. Investigators who have studied cytosol [^{3}H]aldosterone binding have demonstrated a positive correlation between mineralocorticoid properties of a steroid and its ability to displace [^{3}H]aldosterone from its receptor sites. Thus, steroids that possess mineralocorticoid activity in vivo have been reported to be the most effective competitors (Herman et al., 1968; Swaneck et al., 1970). Steroids with predominantly glucocorticoid properties are partially effective, while steroids devoid of mineralocorticoid and glucocorticoid activity, such as estradiol and dihydrotestosterone, are ineffective as competitors for [^{3}H]aldosterone binding sites, even when used at a concentration 1000-fold greater than the concentration of [^{3}H]aldosterone.

However, when investigating [^{3}H]aldosterone binding to multiple sites, it is important to consider that data derived from competition studies can be completely concentration dependent, due to the selective filling of the multiple sites. In this regard, competition studies of [^{3}H]aldosterone binding which have been performed at concentrations below or near the K_d of the type I sites have been the most useful (Funder et al., 1973a,b; Anderson and Fanestil, 1976). Our studies of the brain [^{3}H]aldosterone receptor, as shown in Table II (Anderson and Fanestil, 1976), determined that, when cytosol was labeled with 6×10^{-10} M [^{3}H]aldosterone, a level below saturation of the highest affinity component, nonradioactive aldosterone (6×10^{-10} M) was significantly more effective than dexamethasone in decreasing the

TABLE II
Percentage Binding of Tritiated Aldosterone (Aldo) and Dexamethasone (DM)

			[³H]Aldosterone		[³H]Dexamethasone	
Conc. of ³H-steroid	Competitor	N	Moles bound $\times 10^{-14}$ (mg protein)	% ± SE	Moles bound $\times 10^{-14}$ (mg protein)	% ± SE
$6 \times 10^{-10} M$	None	8	2.0	100[a]	5.8	100
	$6 \times 10^{-10} M$ Aldo	4	1.4	68.9 ± 3.8[b]	5.1	91.8 ± 2.1
	$6 \times 10^{-10} M$ DM	4	1.6	80.3 ± 3.2	4.6	83.3 ± 2.5
$6 \times 10^{-9} M$	None	8	8.4	100	22.6	100
	$6 \times 10^{-9} M$ Aldo	4	6.3	74.5 ± 4.2	14.7	65.3 ± 5.7
	$6 \times 10^{-9} M$ DM	4	5.7	67.9 ± 3.8	15.8	69.9 ± 4.3
$1.2 \times 10^{-8} M$	None	8	9.8	100	26.6	100
	$1.2 \times 10^{-8} M$ Aldo	4	5.4	55.0 ± 2.4	21.4	80.6 ± 2.0
	$1.2 \times 10^{-8} M$ DM	4	3.6	36.6 ± 3.0	11.2	41.9 ± 2.4

[a] The effect of nonradioactive aldosterone and dexamethasone on the binding of [³H]aldosterone and [³H]dexamethasone. 100% binding represents the binding of either [³H]aldosterone or [³H]dexamethasone at the appropriate concentration in the absence of any competitor.
[b] ± SEM.

amount of [³H]aldosterone bound. However, when cytosols were incubated with either $6 \times 10^{-9} M$ or $1.2 \times 10^{-8} M$ [³H]aldosterone and an equimolar amount of either nonradioactive aldosterone or nonradioactive dexamethasone, the latter was either equal to or more effective than aldosterone in decreasing the amount of [³H]aldosterone bound. From this study and a similar study with [³H]dexamethasone as the ligand, we concluded that at low concentrations ($6 \times 10^{-10} M$) of either [³H]aldosterone or [³H]dexamethasone, nonradioactive aldosterone was the more effective competitor for the [³H]aldosterone sites and nonradioactive dexamethasone was the more effective competitor for [³H]dexamethasone-binding sites. At intermediate concentrations ($6 \times 10^{-9} M$), both aldosterone and dexamethasone were equally effective in their ability to decrease [³H]aldosterone or [³H]dexamethasone bound to proteins with no apparent selectivity. Finally, at high concentrations of radioactive ligand ($1.2 \times 10^{-8} M$), dexamethasone was more effective than aldosterone in decreasing the amount of [³H]dexamethasone and [³H]aldosterone bound (Table II).

Although each property of the [³H]aldosterone receptor in tissue cytosols is important, ultimate understanding of the mechanisms and effects subsequent to the interaction of aldosterone and an aldosterone receptor can occur only after the various forms of the aldosterone receptor are purified to a considerable degree. To date, purification has not been achieved. Purification via conventional methods [such as chromatography and

$(NH_4)_2SO_4$ precipitation] is dependent upon detection of the aldosterone receptor by its association with isotopically labeled steroid. Therefore, purification is limited by the apparent instability of both cytosol and nuclear receptors (Herman et al., 1968; Robinson and Fanestil, 1970). The recently developed techniques of affinity chromatography or affinity labeling could theoretically circumvent some of the problems associated with purification of receptor. However, experimentation in our laboratory revealed certain problems inherent with both techniques which have, at least to date, prevented their successful application in the purification of the aldosterone receptor. Ludens et al. (1972a,b) defined three criteria by which the performance of a particular ligand–gel complex may be evaluated, and then used these criteria to evaluate ligand–gels in affinity chromatography of aldosterone receptor. The criteria are (a) the exposure to the ligand–gel of a preparation containing the macromolecule must remove from the preparation the biologic activity specifically associated with that macromolecule; (b) this loss of activity must be produced only by biologically specific ligands, and (c) the loss of activity must be due to a selective, reversible association between the macromolecule and the ligand–gel, such that the macromolecule of interest can be recovered free of other molecules. In the study, Ludens et al. (1972a,b) utilized deoxycorticosterone–hemisuccinate (DOC-HS) linked to aminoethyl agarose as the ligand–gel complex. Exposure of cytosol containing aldosterone-binding proteins (ABP) activity to the affinity columns resulted in the loss of ABP activity from the cytosol which satisfied the first criterion. Substitution of estriol hemisuccinate for DOC-HS in the ligand–gel complex did not result in a loss of ABP activity, which satisfied the second criterion of specificity. Although these results provided presumptive evidence that the aldosterone-binding proteins were specifically retained by the DOC-HS column, Ludens et al. (1972a,b) were unable to recover or remove aldosterone-binding activity from the column. Thus, the third criterion remained unfilled (Ludens et al., 1972b).

Agarwal (1975) has recently demonstrated multiple forms of [^{3}H]aldosterone binding by separation on a DE-52 column. The assertion that one or more of the three peaks isolated were mineralocorticoid receptors was based on evidence of [^{3}H]aldosterone and [^{3}H]corticosterone binding to specific protein peaks in kidney cytosol and the absence of specific peaks in liver cytosol incubated with each of these steroids. The methodology employed in the study of Agarwal (1975) may be of importance in initial purification of mineralocorticoid receptors. However, demonstration of competition by various nonradioactive steroids, notably aldosterone, dexamethasone, and corticosterone for each of the peaks must first be accomplished. Because the study utilized relatively high concentrations of radioactive [^{3}H]corticosterone, it may be presumed that binding to mineralocorticoid receptors did occur (Agarwal, 1975). However, further studies concerned with specificity of each peak are clearly needed to document specific mineralocorticoid receptors.

Unfortunately, detailed analysis of the influence of the interaction of aldosterone-receptor complexes with the nuclear acceptor region and final description of a mechanism whereby the complex alters nuclear function must be postponed until the aldosterone receptor can be purified to a considerable extent. Even so, indirect studies have provided impressive evidence that the formation of the aldosterone-receptor complex is necessary for the ultimate physiologic response.

IV. PROPERTIES OF THE NUCLEAR ALDOSTERONE RECEPTOR

As discussed earlier, nuclear binding of [^{3}H]aldosterone was first demonstrated in the toad bladder by means of autoradiography (Edelman et al., 1963). Fanestil and Edelman (1966) extended this early observation with in vivo experiments conducted in the kidneys of adrenalectomized rat. In these pioneering studies, they noted that unmetabolized aldosterone was binding to the nuclear fraction in a time-related manner (Fanestil and Edelman, 1966). Binding of unmetabolized aldosterone was not unexpected in that Crabbé (1961) had previously indicated that virtually all [^{3}H]aldosterone is recoverable unmetabolized after its effect on sodium transport in the toad bladder.

Equally important in the study of Fanestil and Edelman (1966) was the revelation that the nuclear binding sites were saturated within the physiological range (Fig. 1). A double reciprocal plot of their binding data over two concentration ranges indicated that two sets of nuclear-binding sites, not withstanding site saturation, were demonstrable (Fanestil and Edelman, 1966). Although they did not investigate properties of each, Fanestil and Edelman (1966) tendered data which documented: (a) selectivity of the nuclear receptors for aldosterone, in that 9α-fluorocortisol but not estradiol displaced [^{3}H]aldosterone from its nuclear sites; (b) protein nature of the nuclear receptor for DNase and RNase had no effect on the release of extracted nuclear aldosterone, while proteolytic enzymes (chymotrypsin, papain, and trypsin) accelerated the release of nuclear aldosterone (Fanestil and Edelman, 1966).

Herman et al. (1968) in a later study demonstrated that 81% of the [^{3}H]aldosterone associated with macromolecules in kidney nuclei could be extracted with 0.1 M Tris–CaCl$_2$ buffer (0.1 M Tris–HCl, 3 mM CaCl$_2$ pH

7.4). However, they were unable to elucidate the nature of the remaining 19% of aldosterone which resisted extraction. Through the addition of a 50% saturated solution of $(NH_4)_2SO_4$ to the Tris–$CaCl_2$ extracts, Herman *et al.* (1968) then partially purified the Tris–$CaCl_2$ nuclear extract. In contrast, when they attempted to isolate and partially purify nuclear complexes by chromatography on Sephadex G-50 and G-75, less of the extracted [^{3}H]aldosterone was recovered (Herman *et al.*, 1968). This finding can, however, be viewed as evidence of lability of the complex, rather than as an indication for the use of $(NH_4)_2SO_4$ in methodology, as the columns used to isolate the nuclear extracts were developed at room temperature.

Herman *et al.* (1968) also attempted direct *in vitro* labeling of the Tris–$CaCl_2$ nuclear extracts with [^{3}H]aldosterone. Although the preparation demonstrated properties of apparent specificity and a need for integrity of SH groups for binding, the possibility that cytosol contamination of the nuclear extract in this preparation contributed to the binding cannot rigorously be ruled out.

Nevertheless, the *in vivo* studies of Herman *et al.* (1968) did confirm the earlier studies of Fanestil and Edelman (1966) with regard to the selectivity of the nuclear site (9α-fluorocortisol > deoxycorticosterone > 6α-methylprednisolone > estradiol) and provided unequivocal evidence of the protein nature of the nuclear [^{3}H]aldosterone binder. That the binding substance was protein (Herman *et al.*, 1968) was ascertained by (a) chemical analysis of the Tris–$CaCl_2$ extracts; (b) dissociation of the complexes by wide-spectrum proteolytic enzymes but not by nucleases; and (c) loss of [^{3}H]aldosterone-binding activity when the complexes were treated with the sulfhydryl reagents, *p*-hydroxymercuribenzoate and 2-(2-aminoethyl)-2-thiopseudourea dihydrochloride.

A more complete extraction of the nuclear bound [^{3}H]aldosterone was ultimately achieved by Swaneck *et al.* (1970). Swaneck *et al.* (1970) were encouraged to examine [^{3}H]aldosterone binding to nuclear chromatin by the reports of other investigators (Maurer and Chalkley, 1967; Bruchovsky and Wilson, 1968) working with the nuclear binding of androgens and estrogen. Thus, the improved methodology utilized by Swaneck *et al.* (1970) in the isolation and extraction of the nuclear complexes made possible further characterization of the nuclear receptors. They recovered over half of the total nuclear content of [^{3}H]aldosterone in association with renal chromatin. Of this fraction, the majority was found to be associated with a soluble nucleohistone after passage through Sephadex G-50 (Swaneck *et al.*, 1970).

Decreased labeling of the [^{3}H]aldosterone receptor produced by various steroids mirrored the earlier work of Fanestil and Edelman (1966) and

Herman et al. (1968). However, additional steroids were added to the scheme and, thus, the pattern of inhibition was 9α-fluorocortisol > cortisol > 17β-estradiol = progesterone. As always, this was of great importance, for the ability of steroids to displace [^{3}H]aldosterone must always be accessory to their potency as mineralocorticoids in order to postulate effects of aldosterone mediated through a receptor. The aldosterone antagonist, spirolactone, at a molar ratio of 10^4:1 displaced 74% of the [^{3}H]aldosterone from renal chromatin (Swaneck et al., 1970). Importantly, this concentration of spirolactone had previously been shown to maximally inhibit the antinatriuretic effect of aldosterone (Kagawa et al., 1964b).

Properties of the nuclear [^{3}H]aldosterone receptors were most fully documented by Marver et al. (1972), who incorporated the findings of each of the previous studies and described the conditions needed for maximal nuclear accumulation. Marver et al. (1972) noted that optimum conditions are needed in the isolation of receptors for [^{3}H]aldosterone from nuclei and cytosol due to their lability. Accordingly, the conditions used in their study were: (a) low temperature, (b) pH 7–8, (c) addition of glycerol (15–30%), and (d) addition of [^{3}H]aldosterone to the suspending media (Marver et al., 1972).

Sedimentation characteristics of Tris-soluble nuclear receptors reported by Marver et al. (1972) were defined in glycerol density gradients. Marver et al. (1972) were able to demonstrate that a single peak at 3 S was diminished by aldosterone and 9α-fluorocortisol but not by 17α-isoaldosterone or 17β-estradiol. This was significant, for although many investigators had demonstrated specificity in undifferentiated nuclear extracts, Marver et al. (1972) had demonstrated the same to be true on a single peak. Additional studies indicated that the sedimentation constant of the Tris-soluble receptor, unlike the cytosol receptor, was resistant to changes in ionic strength.

In glycerol density-gradient centrifugation of the nuclear receptor extracted from chromatin with 0.3 M KCl, the species migrated as a single peak at 4 S (Marver et al., 1972). The presence of both of 3 S and 4 S receptor in the nucleus prompted additional experiments in which Marver et al. (1972) utilized rat plasma antibodies to investigate possible contamination by [^{3}H]aldosterone bound by serum proteins. Their data implied that binding to either the 3 S or 4 S receptor was not due to serum protein contaminants.

Employing this knowledge of the nuclear and cytosol receptors for aldosterone, Marver et al. (1972) examined the sequence whereby aldosterone binds to the cytosol receptor and ultimately translocates to the nucleus, where it binds to the chromatin. The results of these experiments are discussed fully in the following section.

V. EVIDENCE FOR A RECEPTOR-MEDIATED RESPONSE

A. Time-Course of Aldosterone Binding

Stimulation of sodium transport by aldosterone in both the isolated urinary bladder (Crabbé, 1961; Porter and Edelman, 1964; Sharp and Leaf, 1964) and the mammalian kidney (Barger *et al.*, 1958; Fimognari *et al.*, 1967) is characterized by a latent period of about 1 hour between exposure to the steroid and the onset of increased sodium transport. Crabbé (1961) noted that the length of the latent period was independent of the concentration of aldosterone in the bathing medium. Later, studies by Edelman *et al.* (1963) and by Sharp and Leaf (1964) confirmed this notion. Based on the assumption that a diffusion-limited delay in the onset of action would be concentration dependent, Crabbé (1961) inferred that the latent period with aldosterone was the time needed to synthesize or activate an intermediate involved in the active transport process. He substantiated this postulate when he recorded that the removal of aldosterone from the medium bathing the isolated toad bladder during the latent period did not alter the duration of the latent period or the initial rate of increase in Na^+ transport (Crabbé, 1961).

In the adrenalectomized rat, the time-course of the antinatriuretic and kaliuretic effect of a single subcutaneous injection of aldosterone is distinguished by a latent period of about 30–90 minutes between injection and the onset of the effect of urinary Na^+ and K^+ excretion (Fimognari *et al.*, 1967; Ludens *et al.*, 1967). Some have suggested that antinatriuresis precedes kaliuresis by 30–45 minutes (Morris and Davis, 1974). In any case, the maximal mineralocorticoid effect occurs 2–3 hours after administration of the hormone when little of the accumulated steroid remained in the kidney [steroid accumulation in kidney was maximal by 30 minutes, with less than 10% remaining by 2 hours (Fanestil and Edelman, 1966)]. When using urinary Na^+/K^+ ratios as an index of response, it may be shown that 2 µg aldosterone per 100 g body weight elicits 80% of the maximal response (Kirsten and Kirsten, 1972).

The relevance of cytoplasmic and nuclear binding to the time sequence of aldosterone action was evidenced in the early studies of Fanestil and Edelman (1966), Herman *et al.* (1968), and others. However, cellular reconstruction studies of Marver *et al.* (1972) on the time course of [³H]aldosterone binding provided the best time-related correlation between a receptor-mediated mechanism and the physiological response.

Marver *et al.* (1972) postulated that the interaction between the various aldosterone binding proteins was a three-step process:

Aldosterone + cytoplasmic receptor → "active" cytoplasmic complex →
Tris-soluble nuclear complex → chromatin-bound complex

This temporal sequence of events was based upon extensive investigation of the nuclear and cytoplasmic components in which cytosol binding and binding to Tris-soluble nuclear and nuclear chromatin receptors were examined after injection of 2.6×10^{-10} moles of [^{3}H]aldosterone with or without 2.6×10^{-8} M 9α-fluorocortisol. It was found (Marver et al., 1972) that (a) binding of [^{3}H]aldosterone to cytosol receptors was maximum at the earliest time point investigated (2 minutes) and declined progressively over the remaining 50 minutes; (b) both nuclear receptors (Tris-soluble and chromatin bound) reached maximum binding after 10 minutes; and (c) this was followed by a gradual parallel decrease in binding of both nuclear species over the remaining 40 minutes.

Marver et al. (1972) extended these in vivo studies with investigations employing the in vitro tissue slice system and cellular reconstitution. Under the conditions of the incubation (5.2×10^{-9} M [^{3}H]aldosterone incubated with kidney slices at 25°C) cytosol binding of [^{3}H]aldosterone was rapid and attained steady-state levels in 15 minutes. The Tris-soluble complex formed at an intermediate rate and increased over the entire 40-minute period of incubation. The chromatin-bound aldosterone was generated at the slowest rate and did not appear in appreciable quantities until after 15 minutes of incubation. Significantly, this sequence of events was altered by the temperature of incubation. In incubations performed at 0°C, both the cytosol and soluble nuclear components bound 70% of that bound at 25°C. Chromatin-bound [^{3}H]aldosterone was shown to be extremely temperature sensitive, as binding was reduced to 16% of that bound at 25°C (Marver et al., 1972).

Of crucial importance in delineating the sequence of events were reconstitution experiments in which cytosol was labeled with [^{3}H]aldosterone and then combined with unlabeled nuclear fractions at 25°C for up to 16 minutes. On a quantitative basis, Marver et al. (1972) proposed that the nuclear uptake (Tris-soluble and chromatin bound) accounted for 60% of the receptor content lost from the cytosol fraction (Fig. 4). Furthermore, they did not observe specific binding in the nuclei when the incubations were performed with (a) [^{3}H]aldosterone with no added cytosol; (b) dissociated cytosol-[^{3}H]aldosterone complexes (prepared by prewarming of cytosol to 37°C for 20 minutes) and (c) rat serum labeled with [^{3}H]aldosterone. Under identical conditions, labeled cytosol prepared in 25% glycerol, enhanced binding to the nuclei.

Marver's experimentation (Marver et al., 1972) suggested that the presence and integrity of the kidney cytosol receptor was necessary for [^{3}H]aldosterone translocation to the nucleus. Significantly, neither warming (37°C, 20 minutes) nor osmotic shock of the nuclei (0.1 M Tris 10 minutes at 0°C) prior to their incubation with labeled cytosol produced an appreci-

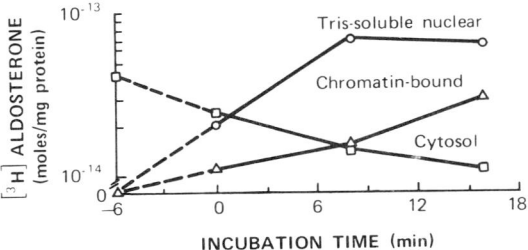

Fig. 4. Time-course of formation of nuclear [³H]aldosterone–receptor complexes in reconstituted mixtures of cytosol and nuclear fractions. Cytosols, prelabeled with [³H]aldosterone + 9 α-fluorocortisol, were mixed with washed renal nuclear fractions and incubated for various times. Times were extrapolated to −6 minutes to account for binding that occurs during processing (reprinted, with permission, from Marver et al., 1972).

able change in nuclear binding. In contrast, nuclear binding was significantly diminished when nuclei were labeled with [³H]aldosterone prior to the heat treatment (60% decrease in Tris-soluble aldosterone and a 77% decrease in chromatin-bound [³H]aldosterone). Pretreatment of isolated nuclei with DNase prior to incubation with [³H]aldosterone bound to cytosol proteins also decreased nuclear binding. Fanestil and Edelman (1966) and others (Herman et al., 1968; Swaneck et al., 1970) had shown earlier that DNase had no effect on nuclear binding after [³H]aldosterone was bound to nuclei. Thus, Marver et al. (1972) suggested correctly that either the transformation of the cytoplasmic to the nuclear form of the receptor is DNA dependent or that binding of the transformed complexes to chromatin is DNA dependent.

B. Binding of Nonmineralocorticoids to the Aldosterone Receptor

Additional indirect evidence of aldosterone mediating its physiological response through hormone receptors has also been shown in studies which have investigated the binding of compounds other than aldosterone to mineralocorticoid binding sites (Ulmann et al., 1975; Feldman and Couropmitree, 1976). An early study of Fanestil (1968) demonstrated that the mechanism of action of the aldosterone antagonist spirolactone was mediated through competitive inhibition of aldosterone binding to kidney mineralocorticoid receptors. The competitive nature of spirolactone action was originally proffered by Kagawa (1964a). Further scrutiny of the mechanism was performed with [³H]SC-26304, a potent spirolactone, by Marver et al. (1974), who found that, although cytoplasmic binding of [³H]aldosterone and [³H]SC-26304 was similar in magnitude and involved

12. Biology of Mineralocorticoid Receptors

the same set of sites, the mechanism was not simply one of competitive inhibition. When Marver et al. (1974) conducted binding studies of [³H]spirolactone in tissue slices, whole animals, and reconstituted tissue, she was not able to find nuclear accumulation of [³H]spirolactone. Thus, the mechanism of action of spirolactone was related not only to its ability to competitively displace [³H]aldosterone from renal cytoplasmic binding sites, but also to its inability to transfer to the nuclear compartment (Fig. 5). Data derived from this study (Marver et al., 1974) suggest, as have many studies, that translocation of the bound cytoplasmic complex to the nucleus is needed for the physiological response (Chu and Edelman, 1972; Lahau et al., 1973). Equally important in Marver's study was the disclosure that, although the [³H]spirolactone and [³H]aldosterone competed for the same cytoplasmic sites, they nevertheless had different sedimentation characteristics. As discussed earlier, Marver et al. (1972) reported that the [³H]aldosterone complexes sedimented at 8.5 S and 4 S in gradients with a low salt concentration

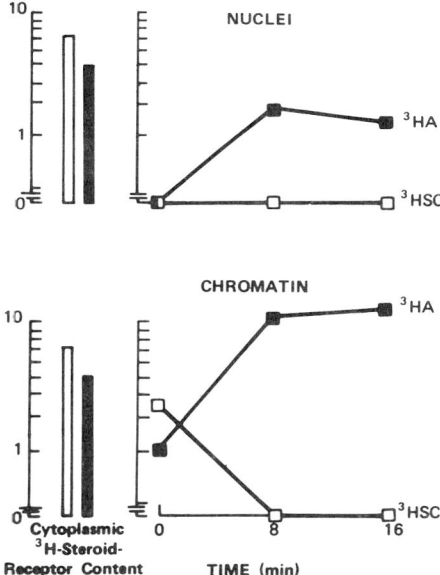

Fig. 5. Transfer of [³H]aldosterone and [³H]SC-26304–receptor complexes from cytoplasm to nuclei (upper panel) or to chromatin (lower panel). Cytoplasmic fractions from adrenalectomized rats were prelabeled with 5.2×10^{-9} M [³H]SC-26304 (³HSC) or 1.3×10^{-9} M [³H]aldosterone (³HA) ($+ 10\times$ concentration of dexamethasone each). The bars on the left indicate the specifically bound quantities in the cytoplasmic fractions. Binding to nuclei and chromatin was determined by extraction with 0.4 M KCl. These data are corrected for nonspecific binding by subtraction of the residual quantities in parallel incubations with $1000\times$ concentration of D-aldosterone (reprinted, with permission, from Marver et al., 1974).

and at 4.5 S in gradients with a high salt concentration. However, the [^{3}H]SC-26304 complexes migrated at 3 S in low salt and 4 S with high salt gradients. This apparent discrepancy of competition for the same site with different sedimentation values can be explained by using the postulate of inactive and active forms of the cytosol receptor (Samuels and Tomkins, 1970; Feldman et al., 1972). Nevertheless, an alternative hypothesis that [^{3}H]aldosterone and [^{3}H]SC-26304 induce different conformational changes of the same receptor cannot be excluded. In either case, it appears that a specific "active complex" must be formed prior to translocation to the nucleus.

Investigation of properties and mechanisms of [^{3}H]aldosterone binding have been of prime importance in delineating the physiological effects of aldosterone. Other important studies, however, have utilized substances which elicit mineralocorticoid or antimineralocorticoid responses but are unlike the mineralocorticoids in structure. Reports of various investigators (Green and Williams, 1953; Ramsay and Elliott, 1967; Revers, 1946) on the effects of certain substances or drugs on sodium retention and other mineralocorticoid or glucocorticoid effects (Opelz et al., 1973) suggested a study by Feldman and Couropmitree (1976) who analyzed the ability of various antiinflammatory agents to displace [^{3}H]aldosterone from its binding sites. Feldman and Couropmitree (1976) discovered that displacement potency for the sites was in the sequence: aldosterone > spironolactone > phenylbutazone > aspirin > indomethacin. He observed that, although the high concentration ratios were required to displace [^{3}H]aldosterone, they were, nonetheless, within the therapeutic range for phenylbutazone and aspirin. Further, he showed phenylbutazone to (a) competitively inhibit cytosol binding, (b) exhibit properties of Na^+ retention when administered to the adrenalectomized rat, (c) antagonize the action of spirolactone, and (d) prevent nuclear binding of [^{3}H]aldosterone. This research suggested that despite having nonsteroidal structures, several of the antiinflammatory drugs have intrinsic mineralocorticoid properties mediated directly or indirectly through a receptor-mediated pathway. Mineralocorticoid-like effects of the extracts of glycyrrhiza originally reported by Revers (1946), suggested a study by Ulmann et al. (1975) similar to the study by Feldman and Couropmitree (1976). Ulmann et al. noted that glycyrrhetinic acid ($\sim 10^{-4}$ M) was able to decrease the formation of [^{3}H]aldosterone–receptor complexes in both the cytoplasm and nuclei of renal tissue. Importantly, the glycyrrhetinic acid was less effective in decreasing the [^{3}H]dexamethasone binding under identical conditions and had no affinity for corticosteroid-binding globulin. Thus, Ulmann et al. (1975) deduced that, although the apparent affinity of glycyrrhetinic acid for renal mineralocorticoid receptors was low ($K_d \sim 2 \times 10^{-6}$ M), the high concentration needed for its biologic action was in agreement with the doses needed to decrease *in vitro* aldosterone binding.

C. Studies of Genetic Variants

While each of the binding studies which has been discussed is important in verifying and refining the postulate of a receptor-mediated mechanism, there is nevertheless juxtaposition of the biochemical events observed *in vitro* and physiological responses observed *in vivo*. In this regard, certain investigators have suggested that differences in binding contingent on alteration of receptor, rather than alteration of steroid, would provide stronger presumptive evidence. While evidence of this phenomenon has been provided by study of steroid-resistant variants (Hackney *et al.*, 1970; Sibley and Tomkins, 1974; Rosenau *et al.*, 1972) only recently have similar studies been pursued with the aldosterone receptor (Lassman and Mulrow, 1974; Funder *et al.*, 1974; Stewart, 1975).

The first of these studies was performed by Lassman and Mulrow who promulgated deoxycorticosterone binding in salt-sensitive hypertension (a demonstrable increase in blood pressure related to increased salt appetite after DOC administration) (Herxheimer and Woodbury, 1960) and resistant (no increased salt appetite following DOC administration) strains of rats. Their studies utilized the findings of Wolf (1967), who had noted that the increased salt appetite of the sensitive rats could be abolished by a lesion in the hypothalamus. Lassman and Mulrow, therefore, conducted experiments designed to investigate the possibility that the lack of response in the resistant rats could be explained on the basis of an alteration of the receptor for DOC in the hypothalamus. Comparison of the DOC-binding data obtained in the two strains revealed that there was a significant deficiency in the binding of DOC in the hypothalamus of the resistant strain (Lassman and Mulrow, 1974). Strain-related differences of binding in other brain areas were not adduced. Furthermore, Lassman and Mulrow (1974) indicated that the DOC-binding protein in brain was neither a classic glucocorticoid nor mineralocorticoid receptor.

Our study of [^{3}H]aldosterone binding in brain has provided evidence which now suggests the need for further evaluation of the strain-related differences presented by Lassman and Mulrow (1974). The [^{3}H]aldosterone receptor isolated from whole brain, in our study (Anderson and Fanestil, 1976), had the characteristics of a true mineralocorticoid receptor. Therefore, one must presume that the failure of Lassman and Mulrow (1974) to demonstrate a mineralocorticoid receptor was due to its binding to both mineralocorticoid and glucocorticoid sites. Additional evidence for our interpretation derives from review of the methodology employed by

Lassman and Mulrow (1974) who incubated the brain cytosols for 16 hours at 0°C. Data we generated (Anderson and Fanestil, 1976), however, indicated that after 16 hours of incubation, there was a substantial loss of binding of [^{3}H]aldosterone, while loss of [^{3}H]corticosterone binding was not as marked. It must be assumed that if the effect of DOC is mediated through the brain, a given set of receptor sites is involved. Consequently, until further research of these strain differences clearly discerns which active sites are labeled, any conclusions derived from such a study must be considered speculative.

That observed physiological differences in the salt-resistant and salt-sensitive strains of rats may not involve the renal mineralocorticoid receptor has been presented by Funder *et al.* (1974). They studied [^{3}H]aldosterone binding in the kidney of salt-sensitive and salt-resistant rats and concluded that the differences observed in the two strains were not due to differences in mineralocorticoid effector mechanisms. This inference (Funder *et al.*, 1974) was based on tissue slice studies which demonstrated that both the resistant and sensitive strains had (a) similar levels of renal cytoplasmic receptors, (b) identical dissociation constants for the cytoplasmic receptor, and (c) intact mechanisms for transfer of the receptor-steroid complex from cytoplasm to the nucleus.

Most recently, Stewart (1975) investigated the correlation between K^+, Na^+/creatinine excretion ratios and the binding of [^{3}H]aldosterone to cytosol and nuclear receptors. Two strains of mice were selected: (a) a Peru strain which was insensitive to the action of aldosterone on Na^+ and sensitized to the action of aldosterone on K^+ excretion; and (b) a CBA strain which demonstrated normal urinary Na^+ and K^+ responses following aldosterone administration. Stewart (1975) deduced that, although the binding of [^{3}H]aldosterone to receptors was higher in the CBA mice, the correlation between *in vitro* binding and the physiological effect on Na^+, K^+/creatinine excretion ratios was abolished in an F_1 backcross generation. Thus, Stewart (1975) judged that the receptor assay was not quantitatively related to the physiological response. However, when data were further evaluated to determine if a type of binding correlated with a type of physiological effect in the backcross generation, a correlation was, indeed, substantiated. The ratio of [^{3}H]aldosterone binding in the Tris-soluble nuclear fraction to that in the residual nuclear fraction correlated strongly with the ratio of the physiological effect on potassium to that of sodium (Stewart, 1975).

Of notable importance in the study of Stewart (1975) was the observation that effects of aldosterone on Na^+ reabsorption and K^+ excretion were clearly separable in the Peru strain of mice. Fimognari *et al.* (1967) and Williamson (1963) had also noted a similar dissociation between the effects of aldosterone on sodium and potassium excretion through the use of actinomycin D. The implication of each investigation is that the effect of aldosterone on potassium excretion might be mediated by a separate biochemical receptor system and that this effect is not necessarily contingent on the primary effect of aldosterone on sodium reabsorption. Clearly, more study of possible mechanisms involved in this separation of effects of aldosterone on Na^+ and K^+ excretion is warranted.

In summary, from indirect evidence, it may be inferred that specific hormone receptors intervene in hormonal actions of aldosterone. The strongest presumptive evidence has been that (a) nuclear and cytosol receptors are demonstrable in mineralocorticoid responsive tissues; (b) nuclear accumulation is saturated within the known physiological range; (c) the ability of various steroids to displace bound [^{3}H]aldosterone is closely related to their potency as mineralocorticoids; (d) spirolactone, an aldosterone antagonist, is unable to translocate to the nucleus; and (e) mineralocorticoid effects elicited by nonmineralocorticoid compounds can be explained in terms of affinity of these compounds for mineralocorticoid sites.

REFERENCES

Agarwal, M. K. (1975). *Nature (London)* **254**, 623–625.
Alberti, K. G. M. M., and Sharp, G. W. G. (1969). *Biochim. Biophys. Acta* **192**, 335–346.
Alberti, K. G. M. M., and Sharp, G. W. G. (1970). *J. Endocrinol.* **48**, 563–574.
Anderson, N. S., III, and Fanestil, D. D. (1976). *Endocrinology* **98**, 676–684.
Anderson, N. S., III, Fanestil, D. D., and Ludens, J. H. (1974). *J. Steroid Biochem.* **5**, 335.
Ausiello, D. A., and Sharp, G. W. G. (1968). *Endocrinology* **82**, 1163–1169.
Ballard, P. L., Baxter, J. D., Higgins, S. J., Rousseau, G. C., and Tomkins, G. M. (1974). *Endocrinology* **94**, 998–1002.
Barger, A. C., Berlin, R. D., and Tulenko, J. G. (1958). *Endocrinology* **62**, 804–815.
Blair-West, J. R., Brodie, A., Coghlan, J. P., Denton, D. A., Goding, J. R., and Wright, R. D. (1963). *J. Clin. Invest.* **42**, 484–496.
Blair-West, J. R., Coghlan, J. P., Denton, D. A., and Wright, R. D. (1967). *Handb. Physiol., Sect. 6: Alim. Canal* **2**, 633–664.
Bruchovsky, N., and Wilson, J. D. (1968). *J. Biol. Chem.* **243**, 5953–5960.
Cake, M. H., and Litwack, G. (1975). *Biochem. Actions Horm.* **3**, 319–390.
Chu, L. H., and Edelman, I. S. (1972). *J. Membr. Biol.* **10**, 291–310.
Crabbé, J. (1961). *J. Clin. Invest.* **40**, 2103–2110.
Davidson, E. T., Westphal, U., Williams, W. C., and Ashley, B. D. (1962). *Proc. Soc. Exp. Biol. Med.* **109**, 926–929.
DeKloet, R., Wallach, G., and McEwen, B. S. (1975). *Endocrinology* **96**, 598–609.
Duval, D., and Funder, J. W. (1974). *Endocrinology* **94**, 575–579.
Edelman, I. S. (1975). *J. Steroid Biochem.* **61**, 147–159.
Edelman, I. S., and Fanestil, D. D. (1970). *Biochem. Actions Horm.* **1**, 321–364.

Edelman, I. S., Bogoroch, R., and Porter, G. A. (1963). *Proc. Natl. Acad. Sci. U.S.A.* **50**, 1169–1177.
Fanestil, D. D. (1968). *Biochem. Pharmacol.* **17**, 2240–2242.
Fanestil, D. D., and Edelman, I. S. (1966). *Proc. Natl. Acad. Sci. U.S.A.* **56**, 872–879.
Feldman, D., and Couropmitree, C. (1976). *J. Clin. Invest.* **57**, 1–7.
Feldman, D., Funder, J. W., and Edelman, I. S. (1972). *Am. J. Med.* **53**, 545–560.
Feldman, D., Funder, J. W., and Edelman, I. S. (1973). *Endocrinology* **92**, 1429–1441.
Fimognari, G. M., Fanestil, D. D., and Edelman, I. S. (1967). *Am. J. Physiol.* **213**, 954–963.
Forte, L. R. (1972). *Life Sci.* **11**, 461–473.
Funder, J. W., Feldman, D., and Edelman, I. S. (1972). *J. Steroid Biochem.* **3**, 209–218.
Funder, J. W., Feldman, D., and Edelman, I. S. (1973a). *Endocrinology* **92**, 994–1004.
Funder, J. W., Feldman, D., and Edelman, I. S. (1973b). *Endocrinology* **92**, 1005–1013.
Funder, J. W., Duval, D., and Meyer, P. (1973c). *Endocrinology* **93**, 1300–1308.
Funder, J. W., Duval, D., Meyer, P., and Dahl, L. K. (1974). *Endocrinology* **94**, 1739–1743.
Green, J., and Williams, P. O. (1953). *Lancet* **1**, 575–577.
Hackney, J. F., Gross, S., Aronow, L., and Pratt, W. B. (1970). *Mol. Pharmacol.* **6**, 500–512.
Herman, T. S., Fimognari, G. M., and Edelman, I. S. (1968). *J. Biol. Chem.* **243**, 3849–3856.
Herxheimer, A., and Woodbury, D. M. (1960). *J. Physiol. (London)* **151**, 253–260.
Kagawa, C. M. (1964a). *Horm. Steroids, Biochem., Pharmacol., Ther. Proc. Int. Congr., 1st, 1962* Vol. 1, p. 445.
Kagawa, C. M., Bouska, D. J., Anderson, M. L., and Krol, W. F. (1964b). *Arch. Int. Pharmacodyn. Ther.* **149**, 8–24.
King, R. J. B., and Mainwaring, W. I. P. (1974). "Steroid-Cell Interactions," pp. 162–189. Univ. Park Press, Baltimore, Maryland.
Kirsten, R., and Kirsten, E. (1972). *Am. J. Physiol.* **223**, 229–235.
Lahau, M., Dietz, T., and Edelman, I. S. (1973). *Endocrinology* **92**, 1685–1699.
Lassman, M. N., and Mulrow, P. J. (1974). *Endocrinology* **94**, 1541–1546.
Lauler, D. P., Hickler, R. B., and Thorn, G. W. (1962). *N. Engl. J. Med.* **267**, 1136–1137.
Ludens, J. H., and Fanestil, D. D. (1971). *Biochim. Biophys. Acta* **244**, 360–371.
Ludens, J. H., and Fanestil, D. D. (1976). *Int. Encycl. Pharmacol. Ther.* **2**, Part B, 371–412.
Ludens, J. H., Hook, J. B., and Williamson, H. E. (1967). *Proc. Soc. Exp. Biol. Med.* **124**, 539–541.
Ludens, J. H., de Vries, J. R., and Fanestil, D. D. (1972a). *J. Biol. Chem.* **247**, 7533–7538.
Ludens, J. H., de Vries, J. R., and Fanestil, D. D. (1972b). *J. Steroid Biochem.* **3**, 193–200.
McEwen, B. S., Magnus, C., and Wallach, G. (1972). *Endocrinology* **90**, 217–226.
Maetz, J., Jard, S., and Morel, F. (1958). *C. R. Hebd. Seances Acad. Sci.* **247**, 516–518.
Marver, D., Goodman, D., and Edelman, I. S. (1972). *Kidney Int.* **1**, 210–223.
Marver, D., Stewart, J., Funder, J. W., Feldman, D., and Edelman, I. S. (1974). *Proc. Natl. Acad. Sci. U.S.A.* **71**, 1431–1435.
Maurer, H. R., and Chalkley, G. G. (1967). *J. Mol. Biol.* **27**, 431–441.
Mills, A. J., Wheldrake, J. F., and Feltham, L. A. W. (1972). *Enzymologia* **43**, 311–323.
Moll, H. C., and Koczorek, K. R. (1962). *Klin. Wochenschr.* **40**, 825–827.
Morris, D. J., and Davis, R. P. (1974). *Metab., Clin. Exp.* **23**, 473–494.
Opelz, G., Terasaki, P. I., and Hirata, A. A. (1973). *Lancet* **2**, 478–480.
Palem-Vliers, M., Genard, P., Matagne, D., and Reuter, A. (1974). *FEBS Lett.* **42**, 65–67.
Porter, G. A., and Edelman, I. S. (1964). *J. Clin. Invest.* **43**, 611–620.
Pressley, L., and Funder, J. W. (1975). *Endocrinology* **97**, 588–596.
Ramsay, A. G., and Elliott, H. C. (1967). *Am. J. Physiol.* **213**, 323–327.
Revers, F. E. (1946). *Ned. Tijdschr. Geneeskd.* **90**, 135–137.

Robinson, R. G., and Fanestil, D. D. (1970). *Karolinska Symp. Res. Methods Reprod. Endocrinol., 2nd Symp.* pp. 275–290.
Rosenau, W., Baxter, J. D., Rousseau, G. G., and Tomkins, G. M. (1972). *Nature (London)* **237**, 20–24.
Rousseau, G., Baxter, J. D., Funder, J. W., Edelman, I. S., and Tomkins, G. M. (1972). *J. Steroid Biochem.* **3**, 219–227.
Samuels, H. H., and Tomkins, G. M. (1970). *J. Mol. Biol.* **52**, 57–74.
Sandberg, A. A., Rosenthal, H., Schneider, S. L., and Slaunwhite, W. R., Jr. (1966). *Steroid Dyn., Proc. Symp., 1965* pp. 1–61.
Sapirstein, V. S., and Scott, W. N. (1975). *Nature (London)* **257**, 241–243.
Scatchard, G. (1949). *Ann. N.Y. Acad. Sci.* **51**, 660–669.
Scheer, B. T., Mumbach, M. W., and Cox, B. L. (1961). *Fed. Proc., Fed. Am. Soc. Exp. Biol.* **20**, 177.
Scott, W. N., and Sapirstein, V. S. (1975). *Proc. Natl. Acad. Sci. U.S.A.* **72**, 4056–4060.
Sharp, G. W. G., and Leaf, A. (1964). *Nature (London)* **202**, 1185–1188.
Sharp, G. W. G., and Leaf, A. (1965). *J. Biol. Chem.* **240**, 4816–4821.
Sharp, G. W. G., and Leaf, A. (1966). *Physiol. Rev.* **46**, 593–633.
Sibley, C. H., and Tomkins, G. M. (1974). *Cell* **2**, 213–220.
Stevens, W., Reed, D. J., and Grosser, B. I. (1975). *J. Steroid Biochem.* **6**, 521–527.
Stewart, J. (1975). *Endocrinology* **96**, 711–717.
Streeton, D. H. R., Conn, J. W., Louis, L. H., Fajans, S. S., Saltzer, H. S., Johnson, R. D., and Duke, A. H. (1955). *J. Lab. Clin. Med.* **46**, 957–958.
Sulya, L. L., McCaa, C. S., Read, V. H., and Bomer, D. (1964). *Nature (London)* **200**, 788–789.
Swaneck, G. E., Highland, E., and Edelman, I. S. (1969). *Nephron* **6**, 297–316.
Swaneck, G. E., Chu, L. L. H., and Edelman, I. S. (1970). *J. Biol. Chem.* **245**, 5382–5389.
Ulmann, A., Menard, J., and Corvol, P. (1975). *Endocrinology* **97**, 46–51.
Westphal, U. (1975). *Handb. Physiol., Sect. 7: Endocrinol.* **6**, 117–125.
Williamson, H. E. (1963). *Biochem. Pharmacol.* **12**, 1449–1450.
Wolf, G. (1967). *Am. J. Physiol.* **213**, 1433–1438.

13

Gonadal Steroid Receptors in Neuroendocrine Tissues

BRUCE S. McEWEN

I.	Introduction	354
II.	Estradiol	355
	A. Topography	355
	B. Properties of Estradiol Receptors	357
	C. Possibility of Sex Differences in Receptor Content	361
	D. Functioning of Estrogen Receptors in Neuroendocrine Tissues	362
III.	Testosterone	369
	A. Topography	369
	B. Tissue Uptake Studies	370
	C. Cell Nuclear Retention of Testosterone and Its Metabolites	371
	D. Properties of Androgen Receptors	372
	E. Functioning of Androgen Metabolites in Neuroendocrine Tissues	374
IV.	Progesterone	379
V.	Steroid Receptors and Sexual Differentiation of the Brain	384
	A. Aromatization	384
	B. Topography and Properties of Neonatal Estrogen-Receptor Sites	385
	C. The Fetoneonatal Estrogen-Binding Protein (fEBP) and Its Possible Protective Role	388
	D. Functional Aspects	389
VI.	Conclusion	391
	References	393

I. INTRODUCTION

One of the earliest experiments in the entire field of endocrinology is a demonstration that steroid hormones influence brain function (Berthold, 1849). Using roosters, Berthold noted, besides effects on size of comb and spurs, that castration abolished and transplantation of testes restored such characteristic behaviors as crowing, fighting, and sexual activity. Because the transplanted testes were not reinnervated but were highly vascularized, Berthold concluded that blood-borne and not neural signals were responsible for behavioral influences of the transplanted testes.

Progress in this century on hormone–brain interactions was catalyzed by discoveries that hormones directly affect neuroendocrine function and behavior. In 1957, Flerkó and Szentágothai reported that tiny bits of ovarian tissue implanted into the hypothalamus inhibit gonadotropic activity as measured by decrease in uterine weight (Flerkó and Szentágothai, 1957). Subsequently, in the early 1960's, Lisk reported similar results from hypothalamic implants of tiny amounts of crystalline estradiol (Lisk, 1960), and he and Richard Michael in England also reported that such implants could restore sexual receptivity in ovariectomized female rats and cats (Michael, 1965a; Lisk, 1967).

The notion that gonadal secretions might actually be found in brain tissue can be traced to an experiment by Steinach, who found that brain extracts from male frogs in rut would induce rut in sexually inactive males (Steinach, 1940). Actually the validity of the inference is questionable since, depending on his brain dissection technique, he may have transferred hypothalamic or pituitary hormones, as well as gonadal secretions retained by brain tissue. Direct demonstration of gonadal steroid entry into and retention by brain tissue depended upon the synthesis around 1960 of tritium-labeled steroids of high specific activity (cf. Gupta, 1960; Jensen and Jacobson, 1962; Michael, 1965a). The classical studies of Jensen's group and of many other investigators, which are summarized in this volume, indicated that target cells of many tissues accumulate and retain appropriate ^{3}H-steroids by means of intracellular binding proteins which carry the hormone into the cell nucleus and there initiate changes in RNA synthesis, leading to altered production of specific proteins and ultimately to the physiological response.

The purpose of this chapter is to summarize the current state of information for the existence of gonadal steroid receptors in brain and pituitary tissue. The discussion will include the topographic distribution of such receptors, their physical and chemical properties, and evidence that they mediate specific neuroendocrine and behavioral responses. It will also consider the role of intracellular receptors in the developmental effects of testosterone and estrogens on the sexual differentiation of the brain.

II. ESTRADIOL

A. Topography

The first recognized neural steroid hormone-binding sites were those for estradiol (for reviews, see McEwen *et al.,* 1972; Kato, 1973; Zigmond, 1975). The initial studies of the *in vivo* accumulation of [³H]estradiol revealed extremely high accumulations in pituitary as well as in uterus, and lower but substantial accumulations in the hypothalamic region of the brain. Within brain, [³H]estradiol accumulation is highest in the hypothalamus and preoptic region. A substantial proportion of tissue uptake into these brain regions and into pituitary and uterus can be prevented by concurrent administration with the [³H]estradiol of 100- or 1000-fold excesses of unlabeled 17β-estradiol, but not by similar excesses of unlabeled testosterone or 17α-estradiol. Such competition at the tissue level establishes a substantial portion of the hormone uptake as a limited-capacity phenomenon with specificity for active estrogens.

Autoradiography has provided more detailed information as to the distribution within the brain of binding sites for [³H]estradiol (Glascock and Michael, 1962; Michael, 1965a,b, 1966; Attramadal, 1965; Pfaff, 1968a; Anderson and Greenwald, 1969; Stumpf, 1968a, 1970; Warembourg, 1970a,b; Tuohimaa, 1971; Pfaff and Keiner, 1973). Neurons, rather than glial cells, appear to contain the highest concentrations of these putative receptor sites, and these neurons are concentrated within the hypophysiotropic area (medial preoptic area, anterior and medial–basal hypothalamus) and cortical and medial nuclei of amygdala (Fig. 1). Labeled cells are found to a lesser extent in the midbrain central gray matter (Pfaff and Keiner, 1973) and in spinal cord (Keefer *et al.,* 1973) and in ventral hippocampus (Pfaff and Keiner, 1973) of the female rat. Not all neurons within these areas bind estradiol, but many of the cells which do bind the hormone have an intensity of labeling comparable to that found in cells of the uterus and pituitary.

Similar patterns of estrophilic neurons, virtually identical in their distribution in the preoptic area and tuberal hypothalamus and differing somewhat in extrahypothalamic structures, have been seen among vertebrates, including fish, birds, amphibia, rodents, carnivores, and primates (see Morrell *et al.,* 1975a). This suggests an ancestral origin of the pattern

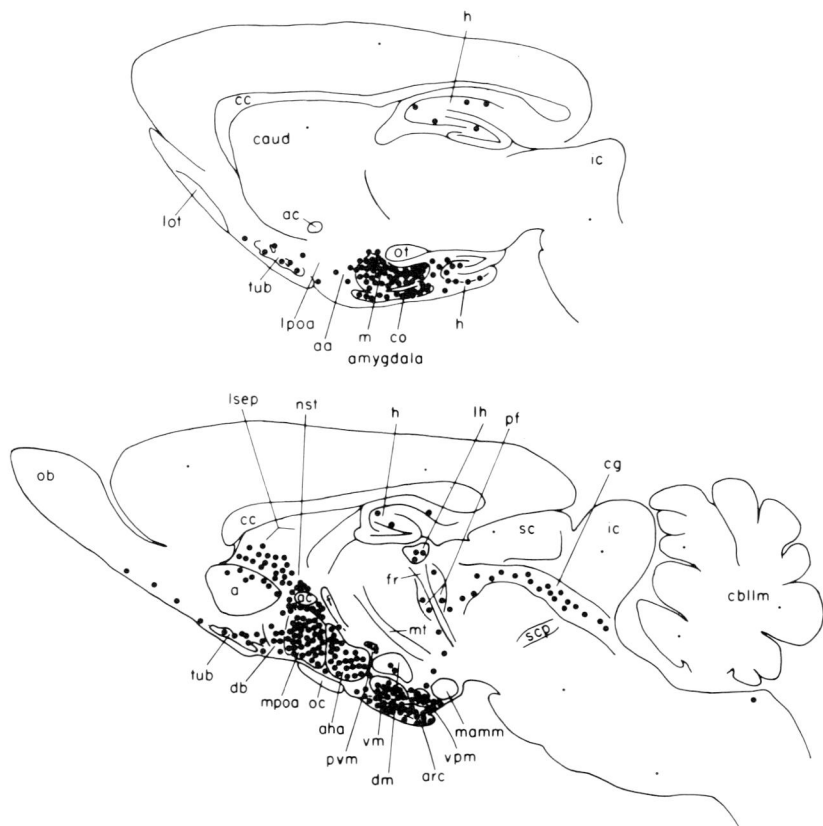

Fig. 1. Distribution of estrogen-concentrating neurons in the brain of the female rat represented schematically in two sagittal sections. Most labeled neurons could be represented in the medial plane (bottom drawing) based primarily on Fig. L740 in the atlas of Konig and Klippel (1963) and Figs. A35 and A36 in the atlas of Zeman and Innes (1963). Estradiol-concentrating neurons in the amygdala and hippocampus are represented in a more lateral plane (top drawing) based on Fig. L2590 in the atlas of König and Klippel (1963). Locations of estradiol-concentrating neurons are represented by black dots (●). Reproduced from Pfaff and Keiner (1973) by permission of the authors and The Wistar Press. Abbreviations: tub, olfactory tubercle; m,do, medial and cortical nuclei of amygdala; db, diagonal band of Broca; mpoa, medial preoptic area; aha, anterior hypothalamic area; arc, arcuate nucleus. For other abbrevations, see Pfaff and Keiner (1973, p. 142).

B. Properties of Estradiol Receptors

Cell fractionation studies of the pituitary and hypothalamus, preoptic area, and amygdala demonstrated the existence of soluble (cytosol) binding sites which resemble those found in the uterus on the basis of sedimentation rate in sucrose density gradients (approximately 8 S at low ionic strength) and specificity of binding toward active estrogens such as 17β-estradiol and diethylstilbestrol (Kahwanango et al., 1970; Eisenfeld, 1970; Mowles et al., 1971; Korach and Muldoon, 1973, 1974; Maurer, 1974; Ginsburg et al., 1974; Plapinger and McEwen, 1973; Vértes and King, 1971; Notides, 1970; Kato et al., 1970b; McGuire et al., 1973). Quantitative estimates of binding parameters indicate that the affinity for estradiol is high ($K_D \approx 1 \times 10^{-10}$ M) and similar among estrogen-sensitive tissues (see Table I). Moreover, the maximum concentration of binding sites is as much as 30 times higher in uterus and pituitary than in whole hypothalamus (Table I). In spite of similarities in sedimentation behavior, affinity constant, and hormonal specificity, it is not certain whether the estrogen-binding proteins are identical in these various estrogen target tissues.

Based on the DNA content of these tissues, the capacity of uterus and pituitary cytosol to bind [³H]estradiol corresponds to 12,000–19,000 molecules per cell (Notides, 1970; Leavitt et al., 1973), while the capacity of cytosol from the entire hypothalamus is around 2000–3000 molecules per

TABLE I
Cytosol Binding of Estradiol and DHT by Target Tissues

Tissue	Saturation binding capacity (sites/mg tissue × 10^{-8})		
	Estradiol[a] ♀[c]	DHT[b] ♀[c]	DHT[b] ♂[c]
Cortex	0.18 ± 0.03	0.68 ± 0.10	0.66 ± 0.08
Amygdala	0.83 ± 0.04	0.49 ± 0.06	0.68 ± 0.06
Hypothalamus	1.98 ± 0.12	0.80 ± 0.04	0.83 ± 0.09
Pituitary	64.6 ± 5.5	10.7 ± 0.43	4.8 ± 0.8
Uterus	61.1 ± 9.1	—	—
Ventral prostate	—	—	17.2 ± 2.7

[a] Data from Ginsburg et al. (1974).
[b] Data from Barley et al. (1975).
[c] ♀, ovaricetomized female rat; ♂, castrated male rat.

cell. These estimates are, of course, averages that do not take into account the proportion of cells in each tissue which bind the hormone.

The estradiol, which attaches to cytosol estrogen-binding sites is transferred into the cell nuclei, and substantial amounts of ^{3}H-estradiol can be recovered in isolated nuclei from these target tissues (Chader and Vilee, 1970; Zigmond and McEwen, 1970; Kato et al., 1970a; Mowles et al., 1971; Vétes and King, 1971; Friend and Leavitt, 1972; Payne et al., 1973; McEwen et al., 1975a). The relative magnitude of cell nuclear binding closely parallels the relative magnitude of cytosol "receptor" concentration in uterus, pituitary, and various brain regions. There is good agreement within the brain between autoradiographic demonstration of [^{3}H]estradiol binding and cell nuclear isolation experiments. As shown in Fig. 2 (McEwen et al., 1975a), a dissection scheme was designed to remove discrete subregions of hypothalamus, preoptic area, amygdala, and midbrain corresponding to areas having highest densities of labeling in autoradiograms (Pfaff and Keiner, 1973). Ovariectomized female rats were injected intraperitoneally with 10 μg of [^{3}H]estradiol or [^{3}H]diethylstilbestrol and sacrificed 1, 2, or 4 hours later. Cell nuclei were isolated from the abovementioned subregions and from additional brain regions such as hippocampus, cerebral cortex, and the "rest" of the hypothalamus and amygdala. (See Fig. 2 for details concerning the "rest" sample.) As shown in Fig. 3, besides pituitary, highest concentrations of radioactivity were found in basomedial hypothalamus (BMH), medial preoptic area (MPO), and corticomedial amygdala (CMA) samples. The rest sample was considerably lower than BMH and CMA, but higher than other brain regions sampled. Among the other brain regions, midbrain was highest, in agreement with autoradiographic results of Pfaff and Keiner (1973). This can be seen in Table II where nuclear binding is expressed as molecules bound per cell.

It should also be noted from Table II that the figure for pituitary is within the range of estimates quoted above from data for cytosol binding. [In uterus, it is known that 85% of the total cell-receptor capacity ends up in the cell nuclei (Williams and Gorski, 1972).] The estimates of molecules per cell in Table II for basomedial hypothalamus are higher than the estimate quoted above for whole hypothalamus, and this is, undoubtedly, a reflection of the more restricted and specific sampling procedure. Warembourg (1970b) has presented illuminating comparative data from autoradiography concerning the average number of silver grains per labeled cell in brain regions of the ovariectomized mouse after labeling with ^{3}H-estradiol. In the bed nucleus of the stria terminalis, in medial preoptic area, and in arcuate nucleus, there were 90–120 grains per labeled cell. In the amygdaloid complex and nucleus triangularis septi, there were 35–50 grains

13. Gonadal Steroid Receptors in Neuroendocrine Tissues

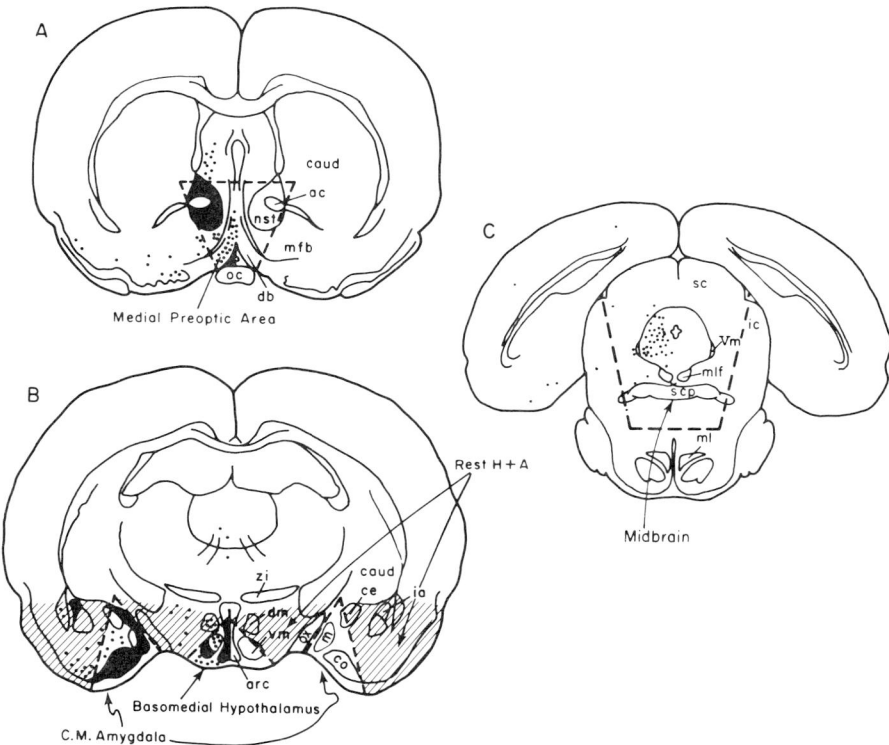

Fig. 2. Coronal planes through rat brain. Rostral–caudal positions of planes A and B are illustrated in Luine *et al.* (1974). Details of midbrain dissection (plane C) may be found in McEwen and Pfaff (1970). Broken lines delineate areas removed as medial preoptic area, basomedial hypothalamus, corticomedial amygdala, and midbrain. In B, areas adjacent to basomedial hypothalamus and corticomedial amygdala are called "Rest H plus A." The dots and the blackened areas (drawn on the left side only) indicate location of estradiol-concentrating cells found by autoradiography, and all three planes are adapted from Pfaff and Keiner (1973). Planes A and B are further modified from Luine *et al.* (1974). Reproduced from McEwen *et al.* (1975a) by permission.

per labeled cell. It must be pointed out that differences in cell size may account for some of these differences in apparent "receptor" content.

Cell nuclear-bound [^{3}H]estradiol can be extracted as a complex with protein by KCl in concentrations of 0.3 M or greater. These complexes have sedimentation coefficients in linear 5–20% sucrose density gradients run in the presence of 0.3 M salt, which are reported as 6–7 S for pituitary (Kato *et al.*, 1970a; Mowles *et al.*, 1971) and 5–7 S for hypothalamus (Vértes and King, 1971; Mowles *et al.*, 1971). According to present views derived from work on the uterus, the 5 S cell nuclear receptor may be a complex of a 4 S

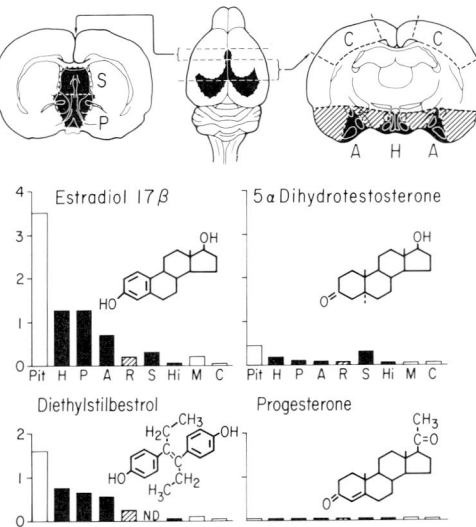

Fig. 3. Topography of cell nuclear binding of four ³H-labeled, gonadal steroids in neuroendocrine tissues of ovariectomized–adrenalectomized (OVX–ADX) rats. Samples brain regions, which were selected because they show by autoradiography high retention of [³H]estradiol (Pfaff and Keiner, 1973), are depicted at the top of the figure: P, medial preoptic area; H, basomedial hypothalamus; A, corticomedial amygdala. The rest of hypothalamus and amygdala (R) contain fewer estrophilic neurons and have been pooled in these experiments. Septum (S) and hippocampus (Hi) are also shown at the top of the figure. Other sampled tissues are pituitary (Pit), midbrain central gray (M), and cerebral cortex (C). Details of the dissection scheme and data for [³H]diethylstilbestrol [³H]DES) may be found in McEwen *et al.* (1975a). Dose of [³H]DES was 100nmoles/kg body weight. Doses of ³H-steroids were 10 nmoles/kg body weight. Survival time after tail vein infusion was 1–2 hours. Tissue was pooled from three to four rats in each experiment. For the [³H]progesterone experiment, ADX–OVX rats received two daily priming injections of 15 µg estradiol benzoate in sesame oil (see McEwen *et al.*, 1976). Reprinted from McEwen (1976) by permission.

estrogen-binding receptor subunit and an uncharacterized factor which does not bind estradiol (Notides and Nielsen, 1974; Yamamoto, 1974). The formation of this 5 S complex appears to occur more slowly in hypothalamic cell nuclei than in cell nuclei of pituitary or uterus (Linkie, 1975). However the time course of retention of total cell nuclear estradiol appears to be similar in pituitary and estrophilic regions of the brain (McEwen *et al.*, 1975a).

That the cytosol receptor is a precursor of the cell nuclear estrogen receptor may be inferred from depletion studies in which injected estradiol reduces the available brain and pituitary cytosol estradiol-binding capacity for up to 20 hours (Cidlowski and Muldoon, 1974; Lieberburg and Maclusky, unpublished). Nonsteroidal antiestrogens such as nitromifene citrate (CI628;

13. Gonadal Steroid Receptors in Neuroendocrine Tissues

Parke-Davis) prevent neural and pituitary cell nuclear and cytosol labeling by [³H]estradiol (Chazal et al., 1975; Whalen et al., 1975) and may do so, at least in the uterus, by translocating with the cytosol receptor to the cell nuclei where they are estrogenic for a brief period and then maintain the depletion of cytosol-receptor levels (Clark et al., 1974). Considerable interest now centers on the replenishment of cytosol-receptor levels that occurs after estrogen and is retarded by antiestrogen administration. The replenishment process may well involve *de novo* synthesis of receptors themselves or of factors which regenerate them (Sarff and Gorski, 1971; Glark, et al., 1974; Cidlowski and Muldoon, 1974; Whalen et al., 1975).

C. Possibility of Sex Differences in Receptor Content

Estrogen-receptor sites are present in the male rat pituitary and brain (Eisenfeld and Axelrod, 1965; Pfaff, 1968c; Anderson and Greenwald, 1969; McEwen and Pfaff, 1970; Maurer and Woolley, 1974; Vreeburg et al., 1975; Whalen and Massicci, 1975). Although neonatal androgenization of females has been reported to reduce estradiol binding in estrogen-sensitive tissues (Flerkó and Mess, 1968; Vétes and King, 1971; Plapinger, 1973; Maurer and Woolley, 1974), quantitative differences in estrogen binding between gonadectomized males and females, indicative of a natural sex difference, have been difficult to find (Maurer and Woolley, 1974; Plapinger, 1973). In

TABLE II
Estimated Cell Nuclear-Binding Capacity for Estradiol Binding *in Vivo*[a]

Tissue	Cell nuclear binding[b] (molecules/cell)
Cerebral cortex	120
Hippocampus	200
Midbrain	440
Remainder hypothalamus and amygdala	810
Corticomedial amygdala	2,850
Medial preoptic area	4,700
Basomedial hypothalamus	4,400
Pituitary	12,500

[a] Data from McEwen et al. (1975a).

[b] Cell nuclear binding was measured 2 hours after an intraperitoneal injection of 10 μg [³H]17β-estradiol into ovariectomized, adult female rats. Brain dissection is depicted in Fig. 2. Note that binding values are the average value for all cells in a particular tissue.

view of the ability of the adult rat hypothalamus and limbic brain to convert testosterone to estradiol (Naftolin *et al.,* 1972; Weisz and Gibbs, 1974a; Lieberburg and McEwen, 1975b) and because of the efficacy of estradiol in restoring male sexual behavior when injected systemically (see Pfaff, 1970) or implanted into the preoptic area of the castrated male rat (Christensen and Clemens, 1974) it is perhaps well to emphasize the similarities, rather than the possible sex differences, in neural estrogen-receptor distribution and content.

There are no sex differences in the autoradiographic patterns of estradiol and testosterone-concentrating cells in brains of an amphibian, *Xenopus laevis* (Kelley *et al.,* 1975; Morrell *et al.,* 1975b). The pattern of estradiol retention does, however, differ from that of testosterone retention in both sexes. Besides regions that concentrate radioactivity injected as either hormone (anterior preoptic area and ventral infundibular nucleus), there are areas that concentrate estradiol principally or exclusively (ventral thalamus, torus semicircularis, striatum, amygdala, and septum) and areas that concentrate testosterone exclusively (located in the medulla).

D. Functioning of Estrogen Receptors in Neuroendocrine Tissues

1. *Neural Activity*

Estrogen effects on the brain and pituitary may be measured in terms of altered neural activity, as well as altered levels of hypothalamic and pituitary hormones. Estradiol treatment of ovariectomized rats decreases the activity of neurons in the medial preoptic area and estradiol target region, and it also decreases their response to somatosensory stimuli; neurons in the basomedial hypothalamus, another estrogen target region, show increased activity as a result of estrogen treatment (Bueno and Pfaff, 1976; see Pfaff, 1977, for other references). These results fit well with the roles attributed to these two brain regions in the control of lordosis behavior. Medial preoptic lesions facilitate lordosis responding, while electrical stimulation inhibits lordosis, indicating that this area has an inhibitory effect on lordosis; lesions in the basomedial hypothalamus have the opposite effect on lordosis behavior to preoptic lesions, indicating that this area has a facilitatory effect on lordosis. Thus, estrogen treatment may have the effect of reducing inhibitory influences of the preoptic area and increasing excitatory influences of the hypothalamus (see Pfaff, 1977, for references).

Another effect of estradiol treatment of ovariectomized rats is to decrease the threshold for electrical stimuli in the preoptic area to elicit responses in the arcuate nucleus and to decrease the threshold for preoptic stimulation to increase LH secretion (Kubo et al., 1975; Everett et al., 1973). These estradiol effects appear to be due to a number of coordinated actions on components of the neuroendocrine system. First, pituitary levels of LH are highest during proestrus (see Kubo et al., 1975, for references), and this may be the result of estrogen priming. Second, hypothalamic levels of gonadotropin-releasing hormone (GnRH) are also reported to reach peak levels during proestrus, although there is some disagreement between laboratories on this point (Kalra et al., 1973; Araki et al., 1975). GnRH levels are observed to decrease after ovariectomy, however (Piacsek and Meites, 1966; Moszkowska and Kordon, 1965), indicating a relationship to ovarian secretion. Third, pituitary sensitivity to exogenous LH–RH in releasing LH is increased in female rats on the afternoon of proestrus (Rippel et al., 1973; Gordon and Reichlin, 1974; Cooper et al., 1974). It is also increased 14 or more hours after estradiol administration to ovariectomized or intact rats (Vilchez-Martinez et al., 1974a,b; Libertun et al., 1974). Finally, there is the possibility that estrogen action in the preoptic area or hypothalamus increases the efficiency of synaptic conduction, which impinges on the neurons that secrete GnRH and controls their secretory activity.

2. *Genomic Involvement*

The implied action of cell nuclear steroid hormone receptors is the regulation of genomic activity, especially the production of RNA molecules along a DNA template. According to this scheme, secondary changes in cellular protein synthesis, directed by the altered population of messenger RNA's, would be responsible for hormone effects on neuronal structure and function. We shall now consider the evidence for this mechanism in the action of estradiol on neuroendocrine tissue.

a. Temporal Aspects. A fundamental clue is timing of estrogen action. Peak estradiol levels in early proestrus precede by some hours both the LH surge and the onset of behavioral estrus. The time lag is also seen in experiments on ovariectomized rats, with lag periods of 20–30 hours for the facilitation by estrogen of lordosis responding (Green et al., 1970) and LH surge (Jackson, 1972, 1973). The duration of [^{3}H]estradiol retention on brain and pituitary cell nuclear receptors following a single, behaviorally effective dose of 10 μg appears to be less than 12 hours (McEwen et al., 1975a), and the intervening time up to the appearance of the physiological effect would seem to be due to a sequence of metabolic events initiated by the hormone, which may involve RNA and protein synthesis (see next paragraph). Thus, the estrogen effect is not that of a "stimulus," i.e., it is not required at the time the response occurs, but, rather, as a "permissive agent," increasing the probability that appropriate stimuli occurring after an induction period will elicit the response. It is important to emphasize the essential role of the appropriate stimuli (e.g., the male palpating the female's flanks, eliciting lordosis; and the endogenous biologic clock, which in the rat is entrained by the light–dark cycle, that controls ovulation), for estradiol does not by itself induce the physiological response.

b. Pharmacologic Intervention. Another important piece of evidence for genomic involvement in estrogen action is the effectiveness of an RNA synthesis inhibitor, actinomycin D, in preventing estrogen induction of lordosis responding or the LH surge. Actinomycin D must be given before estradiol to block the LH surge (Jackson, 1972, 1973) and is effective 6–12 hours, but not later, in blocking the estrogen facilitation of behavioral estrus (Terkel *et al.*, 1973; Whalen *et al.*, 1974). With respect to its neuroendocrine effects, actinomycin D has been shown both to reduce serum levels of GnRH, but not hypothalamic levels of GnRH or pituitary levels of LH; to reduce weight and RNA content of the pituitary, but not of the basomedial hypothalamus; and to attenuate LH release to electrochemical stimulation of the medial preoptic area and to exogenous LH-RH (Kalra, 1975). Thus, the action of this inhibitor may be on both the pituitary and the hypothalamus. With respect to its behavioral effects, actinomycin D, administered into the anterior hypothalamus, led to a reversible morphological alteration of nucleolar structure, the disappearance of which was correlated with the reappearance some days later of estrogen sensitivity in facilitating lordosis (Hough *et al.*, 1974). Evidence for the participation of protein synthesis in the estrogen effects on lordosis is provided by studies of intracranially applied cycloheximide, in which reversible blockade of estrogen action was again observed (Quadagno and Ho, 1975). Cycloheximide was, like actinomycin D, effective only when applied from 6 hours before estradiol to 12 hours after it.

Another piece of evidence relating directly to the cell nuclear estrogen-receptor sites is the effectiveness of antiestrogenic compounds such as clomiphene, MER-25, and CI-628 to prevent both the LH surge (Shirley *et al.*, 1968; Labhsetwar, 1970) and behavioral estrus (Meyerson and Lindström, 1968; Arai and Gorski, 1968; Komisaruk and Beyer, 1972; Whalen and Gorzalka, 1973; Södersten, 1974). These antiestrogens are known to make the receptor system unavailable to the natural estrogen (Clark *et al.*, 1974). As is the case with actinomycin D and cycloheximide, antiestrogens must be given before or shortly after estrogen treatment to be effective on behavior, or must be given on diestrus day 2 of the normal cycling female rat to block the LH surge. There is some indication of the site of action of antiestrogens on neuroendocrine function. Hypothalamic implants of an antiestrogen, tamoxifen (IC 46474), inhibit ovulation better than pituitary implants (Bainbridge and Labhsetwar, 1971; Billard and McDonald, 1973).

There are, however, some indications that antiestrogens may be weakly estrogenic in their effects on some neuroendocrine and behavioral responses, just as they are also estrogenic on some uterine responses (Callantine et al., 1966; Kang et al., 1975; Ljungkvist and Terenius, 1974). For example, like estradiol, CI-628 decreases FSH levels in OVX rats (Callantine et al., 1966); and MER-25, like estradiol benzoate, inhibits eating and reduces weight gain in female rats (Roy and Wade, 1976).

c. Neurochemical Evidence. Correlative studies of estrogen effects on pituitary and brain RNA and protein metabolism provide some evidence for altered metabolic states resulting from enhanced estrogen secretion or from estrogen administration (see Luine and McEwen, 1977). Measurements of brain and pituitary enzyme activities as a function of estrogen treatment also point to a variety of "inductive" effects on cellular metabolism. Where these effects have been examined in some detail, they appear to be the direct result of estrogen action at the receptor level, although the definitive proof of this relationship is lacking. Thus, an "inductive" neurochemical effect of estrogen may underlie a "permissive" action at the physiological level. Resolution of any paradox implicit in the juxtaposition of the terms "inductive" and "permissive" may rest on the fact that none of the neurochemical changes are increases from undetectable levels of a gene product. Rather, they appear to be increases (or decreases) in level or activity of a constituent that is already present in substantial amount in the absence of the hormonal stimulus. Modulation in the amount of these constituents might be thought of as a means of "tuning" neuronal systems, i.e., of increasing (or decreasing) the functional efficiency of specific neural circuits. For a discussion of neural circuits which are involved in the mediation of the estrogen-dependent lordosis response, the reader is referred to the work of Pfaff (Pfaff et al., 1973; McEwen and Pfaff, 1973).

With respect to biochemical changes in the pituitary related to estradiol, hypophyseal RNA levels were reported to be lowest during diestrus and to be highest in proestrus or estrus (Convey and Reece, 1969; Robinson and Leavitt, 1971). The changes in RNA concentrations were ascribed to the action of estrogen, since ovariectomy reduced concentrations of RNA in pituitary, and replacement therapy with estradiol restored normal RNA levels (Robinson and Leavitt, 1971). An excellent protein marker of estrogen action in pituitary is the enzyme glucose 6-phosphate dehydrogenase, which is the first enzyme of the pentose phosphate pathway of glucose metabolism, a pathway which is a source of reducing equivalents for reductive biosynthesis and of pentose sugars for nucleoside triphosphate and RNA synthesis (Luine et al., 1974, 1975a). This enzyme, which is also elevated by estrogen in the uterus and in the hypothalamus, is elevated in pituitary by 17β-estradiol and by diethylstilbestrol and not by 17α-estradiol or by testosterone (Luine et al., 1974). The "action spectrum" of these four steroids, thus, parallels the specificity of intracellular estrogen receptors. Estradiol elevation of G6PDH activity in pituitary is blocked by the antiestrogen, MER-25, and this action is in keeping with and, in fact, is predicted by a cell nuclear receptor action of estradiol (Luine et al., 1975a).

With respect to alterations in brain chemistry related to estradiol, there have been a number of reports of altered levels or labeling of RNA, which are somewhat conflicting, so as not to produce a coherent picture (see Luine and McEwen, 1977). One reason for this may be the high ongoing level of RNA synthesis unrelated to hormonal stimulation. Another factor is the relatively low density of estrogen-responsive cells in neural tissue. Autoradiographic studies of amino acid incorporation into protein in brain cells as a function of estrogen stimulation have presented a more coherent picture (see Luine and McEwen, 1976). It appears that estrogen-dependent increases of incorporation into proteins are restricted, for the most part, to those brain regions which contain putative estradiol receptor sites when physiological fluctuations in estrogen levels are studied, but that if estradiol is given exogenously, particularly in large amounts, other brain regions respond with an increased or decreased incorporation rate. It is presently not known whether these more widespread changes in incorporation represent alterations in the amino acid pool size, rather than altered rates of protein formation.

Studies of brain enzyme activities as a function of estrogen treatment of ovariectomized rats have pointed to effects that are, so far as is presently known, specific to receptor-containing brain regions (Luine et al., 1974, 1975a,b). Among the enzymes which change are oxidative enzymes such as glucose 6-phosphate dehydrogenase (in basomedial hypothalamus) and isocitrate and malate dehydrogenases (in basomedial hypothalamus and corticomedial amygdala). The activity of monoamine oxidase, using serotonin as substrate, is decreased by estrogen-replacement therapy in basomedial hypothalamus and corticomedial amygdala, whereas the activity of choline acetyltransferase is increased in medial preoptic area and corticomedial amygdala by estrogen treatment (Luine et al., 1975b). The activities of hypothalamic peptidases have been shown to change during the estrous cycle and are increased by estrogen replacement therapy in ovariectomized rats (Heil et al., 1971; Kuhl et al., 1974; Griffiths and Hooper,

1973, 1974). It remains to be seen whether these effects relate to the modulation of releasing-factor activities, since, in one case, the enzyme undergoing estrogen-dependent alteration inactivates LH–RF (Griffiths and Hooper, 1973, 1974).

Of primary interest in the ultimate understanding of estrogen action of sexual behavior and neuroendocrine function are the estrogen effects on neurotransmitter metabolism and action. For references concerning neurotransmitter systems and their physiological implications in reproductive function, the reader should consult Crowley and Zemlan (1977).

The actual evidence for hormonal effects at the neurochemical level is relatively scanty. First, with respect to brain catecholamines, estrogen suppression of dopamine-stimulated gonadotropin release *in vitro* in a combined median eminence–pituitary system was prevented by protein synthesis inhibitors, while stimulation by dopamine of gonadotropin release *in vivo* was shown to depend on prior estrogen priming (see McCann and Moss, 1975). In this regard, low doses of estradiol have been reported to increase the turnover of tuberoinfundibular dopamine (Fuxe *et al.*, 1969), but dopamine turnover is also reported to be reduced during proestrus (see McCann and Moss, 1975) when estrogen titers have reached their peak. Resolution of this apparent discrepancy may well depend on elucidation of the time dependency of effects of a single estradiol injection, since, as noted earlier in this section, there is a lag period between the presence of estradiol on its receptors and its physiological effects. With respect to estrogen sensitivity of basal hypothalamic dopamine, some of these dopaminergic neurons appear to contain estrogen receptors (Grant and Stumpf, 1973). Noradrenalin turnover is reported to be highest during states of high gonadotropin release, for example, during proestrus and as a result of gonadectomy (see McCann and Moss, 1975). A single estradiol injection, 56 hours before sacrifice, followed by a single progesterone injection 5 hours before sacrifice, is reported to decrease noradrenaline turnover, especially in the preoptic–anterior hypothalamic region of the rat brain, and these effects parallel the decreased gonadotropin secretion which results (Bapna *et al.*, 1971). Again, as in the case of dopamine turnover, the relationships of hormone amount and time are undoubtedly complex and beyond the scope of the present discussion. Nevertheless, it is worthwhile to note that current opinion favors a positive role for noradrenaline in the triggering of the LH surge and an inhibitory role for dopamine in prolactin secretion (see McCann and Moss, 1975). Before leaving the catecholamines, it is worthwhile to note that two studies have reported increases after gonadectomy of hypothalamic activity of tyrosine hydroxylase (TH), rate-limiting enzyme for catecholamine biosynthesis (Beattie *et al.*, 1972; Kizer *et al.*, 1974), but neither report was able to establish which gonadal steroids are involved in maintaining normal TH levels, or whether this occurs by a direct steroid action or by an indirect effect, perhaps analogous to the reserpine or stress induction of this enzyme (Thoenen *et al.*, 1969).

Second, with respect to serotonin, studies in the rat were unable to show changes in serotonin turnover in the hypothalamus following combined estradiol plus progesterone treatment in ovariectomized rats (Bapna *et al.*, 1971). However, Gradwell *et al.* (1975) reported decreased serotonin turnover (which they did not localize as to brain region) in ovariectomized-adrenalectomized rhesus monkeys as a result of either estradiol or testosterone replacement therapy. Again, it must be pointed out that the time dependence of gonadal steroid effects has not been systematically investigated in either species, nor have the regional changes in serotonin metabolism been thoroughly investigated. However, it is quite apparent that there are important gonadal steroid influences on serotonin metabolism which await elucidation.

Third, acetylcholine metabolism may be influenced by estradiol, as suggested by the observations cited earlier that choline acetyltransferase activity is increased in medial preoptic area and corticomedial amygdala of female rats by estrogen replacement therapy (Luine *et al.*, 1975b). These observations, however, must be extended to include other parameters of acetylcholine metabolism and to include a study of physiological levels of estradiol before a role for this transmitter system in the normal action of this hormone can be accepted.

d. Conclusion. The variety of possible neurochemical effects of estradiol serve to generate a working hypothesis or model of steroid hormone action on neurons. First, there are alterations in oxidative metabolism of neural tissue, and of the pituitary as well, which may provide increased amounts of energy for neuronal function, as well as providing reducing equivalents for reductive biosynthesis of lipids and pentose sugars for RNA synthesis. Second, there may be hormone-induced alterations in biosynthetic and degradative enzymes for neurotransmitters and releasing hormones. In such cases, it might be expected that part of the "inductive lag" in the manifestation of hormonal effects would be occupied by the time required for the axonal or dendritic transport of the newly synthesized enzymes. Third, there may also be hormonally induced alterations in the amount of postsynaptic receptors for neurotransmitters. At the present time the only, albeit preliminary, evidence pointing in this direction deals with the sensitivity of the pituitary to LH–RH (see earlier discussion), but future work will undoubtedly yield interesting results as techniques for quantitatively measuring these receptors become available.

III. TESTOSTERONE

A. Topography

The distribution of cells labeled by an injection of [^{3}H]testosterone (^{3}H-T) in castrated adult male rats is similar but not identical to the distribution of cells labeled by [^{3}H]estradiol (Pfaff, 1968b,c; Tuohimaa, 1971; Sar and Stumpf, 1972, 1973a; see also discussion by Zigmond, 1975). However, the intensity of cellular labeling is generally lower for [^{3}H]T than for [^{3}H]estradiol ([^{3}H]E$_2$). Highest concentrations of labeled cells are seen in the hypophysiotropic area, amygdala, and pituitary, and also in lateral septum and hippocampus. [^{3}H]T labels more cells than [^{3}H]E$_2$ in lateral septum, hippocampus, dentate gyrus, subiculum, and ventromedial nucleus, while [^{3}H-E$_{2x}$ labels more cells than [^{3}H]T in arcuate nucleus (Stumpf, 1970; Sar and Stumpf, 1937a). In the medial preoptic area, a majority of the cells are labeled by both [^{3}H]T and [^{3}H]E$_2$ (see Zigmond, 1975, for discussion). This clearly indicates overlap of responsive cells, but it may well be explained by the known conversion of [^{3}H]T to [^{3}H]E$_2$. Between 35 and 50% of cell nuclear-bound radioactivity in adult male rat limbic structures, in fact, has been identified as [^{3}H]E$_2$, following a [^{3}H]T injection (see below and Lieberburg and McEwen, 1975b). Thus, the conversion of testosterone to either E$_2$ or to 5α-reduced metabolites makes difficult the interpretation of any labeling experiment with [^{3}H]T. The pituitary is somewhat less complicated, since almost no [^{3}H]E$_2$ has been identified in cell nuclear extracts following [^{3}H]T administration (Lieberburg and McEwen, 1975b). Autoradiographic studies reveal that $\approx 15\%$ of rat pituitary cells, mostly basophils, are labeled after [^{3}H]T, while 60-80% of the cells are labeled after [^{3}H]E$_2$ (Stumpf, 1968b; Sar and Stumpf, 1973b,c).

In birds, cellular accumulation of radioactivity injected as [^{3}H]T has been reported in periventricular areas of the hypophysiotropic area (Zigmond *et al.*, 1972; Meyer, 1973). In addition, the accumulation of radioactivity after [^{3}H]T administration has been demonstrated in the midbrain of the chaffinch and zebra finch, primarily in the nucleus intercollicularis, an area from which vocalizations can be stimulated in birds (Zigmond *et al.*, 1973; Arnold *et al.*, 1976).

In an amphibian, *Xenopus laevis*, T-concentrating cells are found in anterior preoptic area and ventral infundibular nucleus, where E$_2$-

concentrating cells are also found, and in the medulla, where no labeling by E_2 is observed (Kelley et al., 1975; Morrell et al., 1975b).

B. Tissue Uptake Studies

Tissue uptake of radioactivity injected as [^{3}H]T into castrated guinea pigs and rats is highest in prostate and seminal vesicles. Concentrations of radioactivity in pituitary and neural tissues, while lower than those in accessory sex glands, are, nevertheless, equal to or higher than those in serum or plasma. Pituitary generally is highest, followed by hypothalamus and cerebral cortex, although concentrations of radioactivity among CNS structures are similar, and regional differences which are reported by one group are not always found by another (Resko et al., 1967; Roy and Laumas, 1969; McEwen et al., 1970a,b; Stern and Eisenfeld, 1971; Phuong and Sauer, 1971; Perez-Palacios et al. (1973) compared the CNS tissue uptake of ^{3}H-labeled T, 5α-dihydrotestosterone (DHT) and androstenedione and found that [^{3}H]DHT was accumulated significantly more than the other two steroids relative to cerebral cortex by pituitary and by hippocampus and midbrain tegmentum. In this connection, it should be noted that [^{3}H]DHT is detected as a metabolite of [^{3}H]T in pituitary and in brain regions (see below). Estradiol has also been detected as a T metabolite in brain tissue. (See Section III,A above and further discussion below.)

Uptake of radioactivity injected as [^{3}H]T is significantly reduced by unlabeled testosterone in pituitary and in septum and less strongly inhibited in amygdala, preoptic area, hypothalamus, and olfactory bulb (McEwen et al., 1970b; Stern and Eisenfeld, 1971). The antiandrogenic steroid, cyproterone, reduces tissue uptake of radioactivity injected as ^{3}H in pituitary, septum, preoptic area, amygdala, and hypothalamus (McEwen et al., 1970b; Stern and Eisenfeld, 1971; Sar and Stumpf, 1973d). Progesterone also reduces uptake of [^{3}H]T radioactivity in pituitary, preoptic area, and central hypothalamus (Stern and Eisenfeld, 1971; Sar and Stumpf, 1973d), and this effect may be due to inhibition of Δ^4-3-ketosteroid-5-α-reductase by progesterone, a preferred substrate, and resulting reduction of the formation of [^{3}H]DHT (Stern and Eisenfeld, 1971; Massa and Martini, 1971, 1972).

It should be noted that cyproterone is an inhibitor of the aromatizing enzyme complex of placenta (Schwarzel et al., 1973) and, thus, its effects on [^{3}H]T uptake noted above might be due in part to its ability to block [^{3}H]E_2 formation. In this connection, it was noted by McEwen et al. (1970b) that unlabeled E_2 competed as well, or better than, unlabeled T for the tissue uptake of [^{3}H]T radioactivity by preoptic area, septum, and olfactory bulb. In contrast, T competed better than E_2 for uptake of [^{3}H]T radioactivity by pituitary (McEwen et al., 1970b). These observations are consistent with the detection of [^{3}H]E$_2$ as a metabolite of [^{3}H]T in cell nuclei from limbic brain structures and failure to detect [^{3}H]E$_2$ in pituitaries of the same animals (see Section III,C).

Besides the effects noted above on uptake of [^{3}H]T radioactivity, several laboratories have reported that neonatal castration reduces the uptake of [^{3}H]T radioactivity, compared to adult castrate males, in pituitary and in all brain structures (McEwen *et al.*, 1970a), while androgen treatment of neonatal castrates selectively increases uptake of [^{3}H]T radioactivity in anterior hypothalamus, pituitary, seminal vesicles, and ventral prostate (Dixit and Niemi, 1974). Another treatment which reduces brainwide the uptake of [^{3}H]T radioactivity is hypophysectomy (McEwen *et al.*, 1970a).

C. Cell Nuclear Retention of Testosterone and Its Metabolites

The brain and pituitary possess the enzymes required for converting T to various metabolites, the functional significance of which will be discussed in Section III,D. Recent experiments in our laboratory have determined the regional distribution of tissue and cell nuclear retention of labeled metabolites produced *in vivo* from [^{3}H]T (Lieberburg and McEwen, 1975c, 1977). In all tissue homogenates from both sexes, total radioactivity was represented predominantly by [^{3}H]T (11–25%), followed by [^{3}H]DHT (8–11%), and then by a variety of other ^{3}H-androgens and [^{3}H]E$_2$ (all $\approx$6%). However, radioactivity in purified cell nuclear fractions was represented almost entirely by [^{3}H]E$_2$, DHT, and T. In nuclei from preoptic area, basomedial hypothalamus, corticomedial amygdala, and the rest of the hypothalamus, [^{3}H]E$_2$ constituted 25–80% of total nuclear radioactivity, other regions being much lower. The percentage of nuclear ^{3}H-radioactivity present as DHT was highest in pituitary (58–61%) and lower in brain regions (8–50%). Nuclear [^{3}H]T was also highest in pituitary (33–34%) and lower in brain regions.

The pattern of cell nuclear retention of [^{3}H]E$_2$ as a T metabolite differs somewhat from the pattern of cell nuclear retention of radioactivity infused as [^{3}H]E$_2$ (Lieberburg and McEwen, 1975c, 1977). [^{3}H]E$_2$ is not detected as a T metabolite in pituitary cell nuclei, even though estrogen receptors exist in this tissue in high concentrations. [^{3}H]E$_2$ as a T metabolite is particularly high in cell nuclei of corticomedial amygdala (A) of both sexes, higher than that in preoptic area (P), or in basomedial hypothalamus (H). In contrast, the cell nuclear labeling by radioactivity infused as [^{3}H]E$_2$ is higher in both POA and H than in A. These results imply that the aromatization system is absent from pituitary, a result confirmed by *in vitro* studies (Naftolin *et al.*, 1972), and especially high in the amygdala, a result also consistent with *in vitro* experiments (Weisz and Gibbs, 1974a).

The pattern of cell nuclear retention of [^{3}H]DHT as a T metabolite (Lieberburg et al., 1975c, 1976) is very similar to the pattern of cell nuclear retention of radioactivity infused as [^{3}H]DHT. This implies that the presence or absence of DHT receptors, and not the rate of DHT formation, is the limiting factor. This is consistent with the widespread distribution of 5α-reductase activity in brain and pituitary (see Fig. 4 and discussion below). A representative pattern of [^{3}H]DHT uptake is shown in Fig. 3 for cell nuclei from adrenalectomized–ovariectomized rats, which received [^{3}H]DHT 2 hours before sacrifice, and it can be seen that the labeling is highest in pituitary nuclei, followed by septum (S), H, P, A, rest of hypothalamus and amygdala (R), hippocampus (Hi), midbrain (M), and cerebral cortex (C). Cell nuclear retention of [^{3}H]DHT is less pronounced in the most heavily labeled tissues than is retention of [^{3}H]E$_2$. This indicates that there may be fewer DHT than E$_2$ receptors and also that DHT receptors may be more widespread throughout the brain than those for E$_2$. This impression is borne out by measurements of the *in vitro* saturation binding capacity of cytosols from various tissues (Table I). This data points to higher E$_2$ receptor levels in pituitary, hypothalamus, and amygdala, and higher DHT-receptor levels in cerebral cortex. Sex differences in DHT-receptor content in cytosols of amygdala and pituitary are reported by Barley *et al.* (1975) (Table I).

D. Properties of Androgen Receptors

Binding of [^{3}H]T or [^{3}H]DHT to soluble macromolecules from brain regions and pituitary of male rats has been described in a number of laboratories (Samperez *et al.*, 1969a,b, 1974; Jouan *et al.*, 1971a,b, 1973; Thieulant *et al.*, 1974a, 1975; Monbon *et al.*, 1973, 1974; Loras *et al.*, 1974; Kato and Onouchi, 1973a,b; Naess and Attramadal, 1974; Naess *et al.*, 1975a,b; Barley *et al.*, 1975). According to one laboratory, the soluble form of the "receptor" from hypothalamus and pituitary has a sedimentation rate constant of 8.6 S and a dissociation constant of 7×10^{-10} M and appears to bind DHT preferentially (Kato and Onouchi, 1973a,b). Another group reported that such molecules sediment at 6–7 S (Naess *et al.*, 1975a). In pituitary and brain, the cell nuclear form of the DHT receptor, extracted by 0.4 M KCl, has a sedimentation rate constant of 3–4 S (Lieberburg *et al.*, 1977).

Dissociation constants of binding of [^{3}H]DHT to pituitary cytosol receptors are reported to be in the range of 3.4×10^{-10} to 2.3×10^{-9} M (Kato and Onouchi, 1973a,b; Thieulant *et al.*, 1975; Naess *et al.*, 1975b; Barley *et al.*, 1975). Studies from one laboratory report of a K_d of 7.8×10^{-10} M for binding of [^{3}H]DHT by pituitary cytosol and a K_d of 2.3×10^{-9} M for binding of [^{3}H]T (Samperez *et al.*, 1974; Thieulant *et al.*, 1975). In competition experi-

TABLE III

Specificity of Pituitary Cytosol, Androgen Receptors as Revealed by Competition Studies

Steroid	Percent Competitive Effect		
	Thieulant et al.[a] (1975)	Naess et al.[b] (1975)	Barley et al.[c] (1975)
DHT (5α)[d]	100	95	90
DHT (5β)[d]	—	—	61
T	100	100	82
Cyprot. acetate[e]	—	56	82–90
$5\alpha,3\beta$-diol[f]	56	—	72
$5\alpha,3\alpha$-diol[f]	66	—	26
Progesterone	63	16	43
E_2-17β[g]	47	8	44
E_2-17α[g]	5	—	—
Androstenedione	10	—	—
Corticosterone	10	—	13
Cortisol	—	4	—

[a] $2.2 \times 10^{-9}\ M$ [³H]DHT versus $2.2 \times 10^{-7}\ M$ unlabeled steroid.

[b] $1 \times 10^{-9}\ M$ [³H]T versus concentration of unlabeled steroid required to produce a 50% competitive effect. Percent competition is based on relative concentrations required to produce 50% competition.

[c] $5 \times 10^{-9}\ M$ [³H]DHT versus $5 \times 10^{-8}\ M$ unlabeled steroid.

[d] 5α- or 5β-dihydrotestosterone.

[e] Cyproterone acetate.

[f] $5\alpha,3\beta$- or $5\alpha,3\alpha$-androstanediols.

[g] 17β- or 17α-estradiol.

ments, however, T and DHT are reported to compete almost equally well for binding of [³H]DHT in pituitary cytosol (Table III). From this information and the fact that [³H]T and [³H]DHT are both recovered from pituitary cell nuclei after *in vivo* infusion of [³H]T (Lieberburg and McEwen, 1977), it appears likely that a single class of receptors may be responsible for the binding of both hormones.

Cyproterone acetate, an antiandrogenic steroid, is reported to compete effectively with [³H]DHT for binding sites in pituitary cytosol (Table III). $5\alpha,3\beta$-Androstanediol is, likewise, an effective competitor, but the extent of competition for the T/DHT receptor by other steroids is a matter of some disagreement among laboratories (Table III). This is true, in particular, of progesterone, $5\alpha,3\alpha$-androstanediol, and 17β-estradiol. The discrepancies in reported competitive potency may be due to differences among laboratories in time allowed for binding to occur, the method of measuring binding, and the concentrations of labeled and unlabeled steroids. Whatever the reasons for the different competition results noted in Table III, studies in one laboratory showed that, under the same conditions of measurement, the cytosol T–DHT receptors from prostate, pituitary, hypothalamus, amygdala, and cerebral cortex display great similarities in binding specificity (Barley et al., 1975). Moreover, *in vivo* cell nuclear binding of [^{3}H]DHT shows identical specificity of pituitary and brain receptors with significant competition by 5α-DHT itself and by cyproterone acetate, and no competition by 5β-DHT, 3α,5α-androstanediol, or corticosterone (Lieberburg et al., 1977).

Another detailed study of the cytosol–androgen receptors of the rat pituitary gland reveals that their characteristics are very similar to those of androgen receptors from the ventral prostate, epididymis, and testis (Naess et al., 1975b). These characteristics include an isoelectric point of pH 5.8 and an extremely slow rate of dissociation of androgen from receptor at 0°C with a $t_{1/2} > 4$ days.

Besides the results noted in Table III, Fox (1975a) has shown that E_2 is an effective competitor for [^{3}H]T binding to brain cytosol and that its effect is greater at higher absolute concentrations of E_2, even when the concentration of [^{3}H]T is also increased. T is not similarly so effective in blocking ^{3}H-E_2 binding *in vitro*, although it does have some inhibitory effect at low concentrations of [^{3}H]E_2. Fox (1975a) also notes that the slight competitive effect of T for [^{3}H]E_2 binding is absent in Tfm/Y mutant mice, which also lack the capacity to bind [^{3}H]DHT and [^{3}H]T. This binding of E_2 may be a characteristic of the androgen receptor, although it is not known if the E_2-binding site on the receptor is different from the androgen-binding site.

E. Functioning of Androgen Metabolites in Neuroendocrine Tissues

The actions of testosterone in neuroendocrine tissues must be considered in terms of the actions of its two principal metabolites, DHT and estradiol, receptors for which have already been described.

1. *Dihydrotestosterone*

The 5α reduction of testosterone is catalyzed by Δ^4-3-ketosteroid-5α-reductase, EC 1.3.1.99 (Fig. 3A). The product, 17β-hydroxy-5α-androstan-3-one (5α-dihydrotestosterone, DHT), is more active than testosterone (T) in tests of growth of chick comb, rat ventral prostate, seminal vesicle, and levator ani muscle (Liao and Fang, 1969). Further reduction products of DHT, 3α- and 3β,17β-dihydroxy-5α-androstane, appear to be less potent than testosterone in the same tests (Liao and Fang, 1969). DHT is highly effective in suppressing gonadotropin release but not necessarily more so than T (Beyer et al., 1971, 1972; Feder, 1971; Davidson, 1972; Swerdloff et al., 1972; Paup et al., 1975). However, DHT is less effective than T in restoring male sexual behavior in the castrated male rat (Beyer et al., 1970a; McDonald et al., 1970; Whalen and Luttge, 1971b; Johnston and Davidson, 1972; Paup et al., 1975). The relative differences in potency between DHT and T with respect to gonadotropin secretion and sexual behavior in the male rat raise the possibility that different receptors may be involved. This will be discussed again below in connection with the aromatization of testosterone. It should be noted that the relative ineffectiveness of DHT in restoring male sexual behavior is not observed in all mammals, since DHT is highly effective in stimulating male sexual behavior in castrated male guinea pigs and rhesus monkeys (Phoenix, 1974; Alsum and Goy, 1974).

Confining the discussion to the rat, it is instructive to compare the relative amounts of T and DHT in various target tissues. Table IV summarizes the concentrations of T and DHT recovered and measured by gas–liquid chromatography from a variety of tissues of intact rats, and from plasma (Robel et al., 1973), and the proportion of [^{3}H]T and [^{3}H]DHT recovered from such tissues of castrated rats following injections of [^{3}H]T (Stern and Eisenfeld, 1971; Jouan et al., 1973; Monbon et al., 1973). It can be seen that only in seminal vesicles and prostate is the concentration of DHT (likewise the percentage of [^{3}H]DHT) higher than that of T. Significant amounts of DHT are found in pituitary and hypothalamus and kidney, but in lesser amounts than T. DHT is difficult to detect in levator ani muscle and thigh muscle, even though these tissues show an anabolic response to androgens and the former tissue is more responsive to DHT than to T (Liao and Fang,

TABLE IV
DHT and T in Rat Plasma and Tissues

Sample	DHT[a]	T[a]	DHT[b]	T[b]
Small intestine	—	—	<.2	<.2
Kidney	—	—	3.0	12.5
Parietal cortex	15[c]	38[c]	<.4	1.3
Pituitary	61	29	≤6	60.5
Hypothalamus	23	41	2.0	13.7
Thigh muscles	—	—	<0.4	2.9
Levator ani muscle	—	—	<0.2	7.9
Ventral prostate	—	—	2.8	2.0
Seminal vesicles	72	23	3.0	2.2
Plasma	7	31	<0.2	2.5

[a] Percentage of total recovered radioactivity 1 hour after i.v. [^{3}H]testosterone. Data from Stern and Eisenfeld (1971).
[b] Nanograms/gram tissue or milliliters of plasma. Data from Robel et al. (1973).
[c] Entire cerebrum.

1969). DHT, together with 3α,5α-androstanediol and androstenedione, have been detected as T metabolites in pituitary and brain of male rhesus monkeys following ventricular perfusion by [³H]T (Sholiton *et al.*, 1974).

It appears likely that DHT found in pituitary and brain tissue may have originated from 5α-reduction within that tissue. As shown in Fig. 4, there is within the brain and in pituitary tissue a distinctive pattern of *in vitro* conversion of [³H]testosterone to [³H]DHT (black bars), 3α5α-androstanediol (DIOL, gray bars), and androstenedione (white bars) (cf. Denef *et al.*, 1973, for data and references). Conversion to DHT is higher in slices of midbrain, brainstem, hypothalamus, and thalamus, and also higher in intact pituitary than in cortex, hippocampus, amygdala, pineal gland, or cerebellum. DIOL formation is high in pituitary. DIOL and androstenedione formation is lower and less differentiated among brain regions than formation of DHT. Sex differences in DHT and DIOL formation are seen in intact pituitaries (but not in brain, except for a small difference in hypothalamus), males having higher conversion rates than females (Denef *et al.*, 1973). DHT

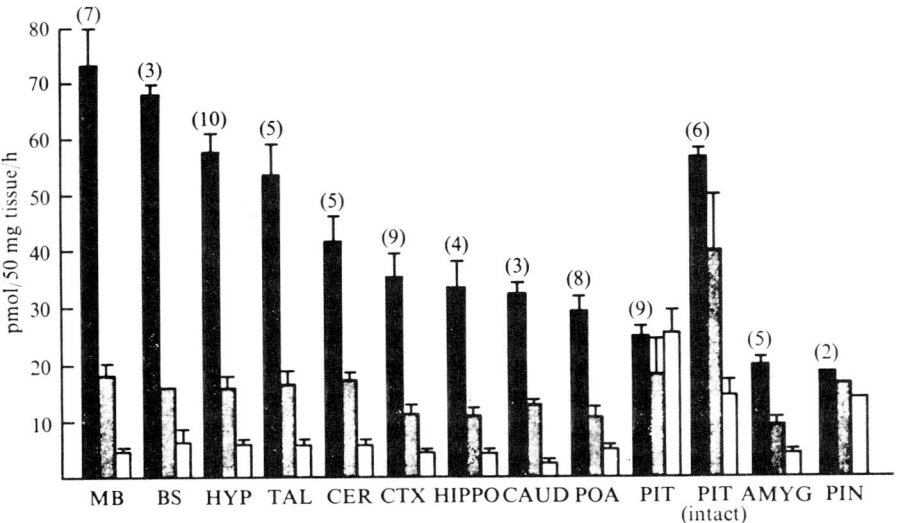

Figure 4. Regional distribution of testosterone metabolites in the brain of the adult male rat. [1,2-³H]testosterone was incubated at a concentration of 1–2 × 10⁻⁶ moles/liter with brain slices. Preparations with intact pituitary are also given. Values are means ± SEM; the number of measurements made for each mean value is given in parentheses. MB, midbrain; BS, brain stem; HYP, hypothalamus; TAL, thalamus; CER, cerebellum; CTX, parietal cortex; HIPPO, hippocampus; POA, preoptic area; CAUD, caudate nucleus; PIT, anterior pituitary; AMYG, amygdala and overlying cortex; PIN, intact pineal gland. Black bars, 5α-dihydrotestosterone, white bars, androstenedione, gray bars, 3α,5α-androstanediol. Reproduced from Denef *et al.* (1973) by permission.

and DIOL formation in pituitary increases severalfold after gonadectomy in both sexes, and the sex difference disappears (Stahl, et al., 1971; Massa et al., 1972; Thien et al., 1972, 1974; Denef et al., 1973; Thieulant et al., 1974b; Kniewald and Milkovic, 1973), but thyroidectomy and adrenalectomy are without effect on DHT formation (Denef et al., 1973). Replacement therapy with testosterone propionate prevents the postcastration rise in pituitary DHT formation in male and female rats (Denef et al., 1973; Thien et al., 1974; Kniewald and Milkovic, 1973), but estradiol benzoate (0.1 μg/100 g body weight/day) is less effective in males than testosterone propionate (Denef et al., 1973; Thien et al., 1974) and less effective in males than in females (Denef et al., 1973). In contrast to these results, high doses of estradiol benzoate (2 mg/100 g body weight/day) were found ineffective in attenuating the postcastration rise of DHT formation in female rats (Kniewald and Milkovic, 1973).

Correlations of these results to changes in gonadotropin secretion following castration and correlations between DHT formation and gonadotropin levels in postnatal development (Denef et al., 1974) have led several laboratories to propose a relationship between DHT formation and FSH secretion (Kniewald et al., 1971; Denef et al., 1973, 1974). However, one should be cautioned against equating DHT formation with the DHT responsiveness of a particular tissue (Verhoeven et al., 1974), as is illustrated by the low level of DHT in the levator ani muscle (Table III) and high responsiveness of this muscle to DHT (Liao and Fang, 1969). The discrepancies may be resolved by information regarding the presence or absence of DHT "receptors" in various tissues (see discussion below).

2. *Estradiol*

The biologic conversion of androgens to estrogens has been recognized for many years not only as the pathway for estrogen formation in the gonad and adrenal but also as an active process in placenta (for references, cf. Gual et al., 1962; Ryan, 1962). According to this work, the pathway for aromatization of ring A appears to involve hydroxylation of C-19 prior to removal of this carbon (cf. Schwarzel et al., 1973). In 1971, Naftolin and co-workers reported conversion of [^{14}C]androstenedione to estrone and estradiol by homogenates of diencephalon (and not by cerebral cortex) from 10- and 22-week human male fetuses. Subsequent work reported similar results from adult as well as fetal limbic (hypothalamus, amygdala, hippocampus) tissue from rat, rabbit, and macaque (Naftolin et al., 1971, 1972; Ryan et al., 1972; Reddy et al., 1973, 1974; Flores et al., 1973). In these studies, pituitary was consistently without significant conversion. Estrogen formation was also observed in two isolated perfused rhesus monkey brains from infused [^{3}H]androstenedione (Flores et al., 1973).

Whereas the major precursor and product in the hands of Naftolin and Ryan have been androstenedione (A) and estrone (E_1), respectively, Weisz and Gibbs (1974a) found that by using tissue fragments instead of homogenates, conversions of [7-^{3}H]testosterone to [^{3}H]estradiol (E_2) could be observed in 7-day-old female rat hypothalamus and amygdala and in 120-day-old female rat hypothalamus. Moreover, conversion rates of 0.1–0.4% (for T to E_2) and 0.2–0.8% (for A to E_1) were observed during a 1-hour incubation of tissue fragments (Weisz and Gibbs, 1974a), while Reddy et al. (1974) had reported lower conversion rates (for A to E_1) in homogenates. Both groups reported lower conversion of both T and A to estrogen in cerebral cortex than in hypothalamus or limbic structures.

The significance of aromatization of testosterone and androstenedione may well be related to reported facilitation effects of these androgens on female sexual receptivity and of estrogens on male sexual behavior. First, it has been clear since 1970 that, when given systemically, DHT is ineffective compared to testosterone in restoring sexual behavior in castrated male rats (McDonald et al., 1970; Feder, 1971; Whalen and Luttge, 1971b; Beyer et al., 1973; Beyer and Rivaud, 1973) and hamsters (Christensen et al., 1973) and marginally effective in doing so when implanted intracranially (Johnston and Davidson, 1972). However, besides testosterone, estradiol is also able to restore at least part of male sexual behavior lost following castration (Ball, 1937; Beach, 1942b; Davidson, 1969; Pfaff, 1970; Södersten, 1973; Christensen and Clemens, 1974) and 19-hydroxytestosterone, a presumed intermediate in aromatization, is also effective in doing so, even though it was without a maintenance effect on penile spines (Parrott, 1974). A particularly striking effect of microgram amounts of estradiol in mimicking an effect of milligram amounts of testosterone was reported by Fletcher and Short (1974) to be the restoration of full sexual behavior and introduction of antler changes in the castrated red deer stag (*Cervus elaphus*). Another impressive example of estrogenic effects is the demonstration that implants of estradiol in the preoptic area of castrated male rats are more effective than testosterone in restoring male copulatory activity (Christensen and Clemens, 1974). Moreover, an inhibitor of aromatization, androsta-1,4,6-triene-3,17-dione, blocks induction of male mounting behavior by testosterone but does not affect that produced by estradiol (Christensen and Clemens, 1975).

Further support for the effectiveness of estrogen in restoring components of male sexual behavior comes from reports that combined treatment of castrated male rats with estradiol benzoate and dihydrotestosterone propionate restores male copulatory behavior more effectively than either hormone alone (Baum and Vreeburg, 1973; Larsson et al., 1973a,b; Feder et al., 1974; Noble, 1974).

With respect to female mating behavior, testosterone has a significant effect in restoring lordosis responding in spayed female rats, cats, and rabbits (Beach, 1942a; McDonald et al., 1970; Beyer et al., 1970a; Whalen and Hardy, 1970; Pfaff, 1970; Beyer and Komisaruk, 1971; Södersten, 1972; McDonald and Meyerson, 1973). DHT is without effect, but 19-hydroxyandrostenedione (an estrogen precursor) is effective (Beyer et al., 1970b; Beyer and Komisaruk, 1971; McDonald and Meyerson, 1973). Further support for the conversion of androgen to estrogen in mediating female sexual receptivity is the observation that two estrogen antagonists, MER-25 and CI-628, attenuate testosterone as well as estrogen induction of lordosis responding (Whalen et al., 1972; McDonald and Meyerson, 1973). Finally, both testosterone propionate and estradiol benzoate facilitate gonadotropin secretion under conditions in which DHT propionate is without effect (Brown-Grant, 1974a).

It is important to repeat cautionary remarks made in connection with the discussion of DHT above, namely, that in species such as guinea pig (Alsum and Goy, 1974) and rhesus monkey (Phoenix, 1974), DHT is a behaviorally active androgen, and in the former case at least, estradiol is without restorative effect on male sexual behavior. Moreover, in the rat DHT has proven to have some, albeit small, effect on lordosis behavior (Beyer et al., 1971) and male copulatory behavior (Johnston and Davidson, 1972) after intracranial implantation or systemic administration (Paup et al., 1975). These results are consistent with the conclusions of Baum et al. (1974), based on effects of genital anesthetization, that DHT is not acting solely on genital sensory receptors when acting synergistically with estradiol, but rather is probably also acting centrally. A recent study by Parrott (1975) further defines the nature of the central action of aromatizable androgens by showing that these steroids, and not 5α-reduced, androgens, prevented significant increases in postejaculatory refractory period durations which follow castration. The data on Paup et al. (1975) are consistent with these observations.

It would, thus, appear that mammalian species differ in the degree to which neurons influenced by estradiol, DHT, and even by testosterone itself may be linked together into neural networks which regulate sexual behavior.

IV. PROGESTERONE

Progesterone (P), like testosterone, is likely to undergo one of a number of metabolic transformations in the brain or elsewhere in the body. Its conversion to 5β-dihydroprogesterone (5β-DHP) (Kawahara et al., 1975) and to 5α-dihydroprogesterone (5α-DHP) and 20α-dihydroprogesterone

(Massa and Martini, 1971–1972; Karavolas and Herf, 1971; Robinson and Karavolas, 1973; Cheng and Karavolas, 1973; Tabei et al., (1974) has been demonstrated to occur in vitro in pituitary and brain tissue.

Further transformation of 5α-DHP to 3α-hydroxypregnan-20-one and of 20α-hydroxyprogesterone to 20α-hydroxy-5α-pregnan-3-one and 5α-pregnane-3α,20α-diol have also been demonstrated (Robinson and Karavolas, 1973; Cheng and Karavolas, 1973; Nowak and Karavolas, 1974), but 5α-DHP appears to be the predominant metabolite in pituitary and hypothalamus (Karavolas et al., 1976).

Although differences in hypothalamic 5α-reduction in vitro exist as a function of the stage of the estrous cycle of the donor animal, estradiol priming of ovariectomized females does not significantly alter in vitro hypothalamic 5α-reduction of P (Cheng and Karavolas, 1973). 5α-DHP and its 3α-OH derivative have been reported to be active, but less so than P itself, in inducing lordosis behavior in estrogen-primed rodents (Meyerson, 1967; Whalen and Gorzalka, 1972; Wade and Feder, 1972c; Czaja et al., 1974). 5α-DHP and not 5β-DHP appears to mimic the effect of progesterone in inhibiting ovulation under rigidly defined experimental conditions in immature rats treated with PMSG (Sanyal and Todd, 1972). 20α-Dihydroxyprogesterone is effective in maintaining LH release following mating in the rabbit (Hilliard et al., 1967) and augments the effects of LRH on LH secretion by rat pituitary cells in cultures (Tang and Spies, 1975), but is without effect on lordosis behavior in the estrogen-primed rat (Whalen and Gorzalka, 1972).

Progesterone enters the brain from the blood rapidly and in large amounts (Laumas and Farooq, 1966, Seiki et al., 1968, 1969; Raisinghani et al., 1968; Whalen and Luttge, 1971a; Wade and Feder, 1972a,b; Luttge et al., 1973, 1974; Wade et al., 1973; Whalen and Gorzalka, 1974). There appears to be very little difference in the accumulation of this hormone between pituitary and various brain structures, except for a higher accumulation in midbrain and brainstem relative to forebrain structures, as shown in Fig. 5 (Seiki et al., 1968, 1969; Raisinghani et al., 1968; Whalen and Luttge, 1971a; Luttge et al., 1973, 1974; Whalen and Gorzalka, 1974; Wade and Feder, 1972a,b; Wade et al., 1973), and for a prolonged retention of [^{3}H]P radioactivity in pituitary and median eminence (Seiki et al., 1975). Estrogen priming of ovariectomized or ovariectomized–adrenalectomized animals is without effect on pituitary or neural [^{3}H]P uptake (Whalen and Luttge, 1971a; Whalen and Gorzalka, 1974; Luttge et al., 1974; Wade and Feder, 1972a). Adrenalectomy has been reported to increase in both plasma and brain levels of radioactivity remaining after [^{3}H]P injection (Whalen and Luttge, 1971a; Whalen and Gorzalka, 1974) or to have no consistent effect on retention (Luttge et al., 1974).

13. Gonadal Steroid Receptors in Neuroendocrine Tissues

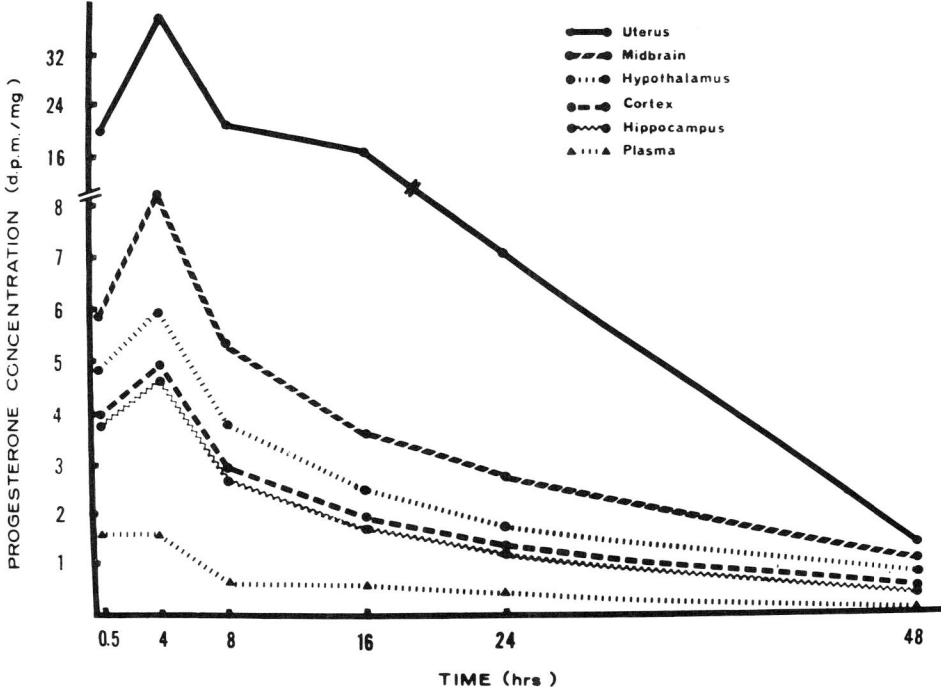

Fig. 5. Concentration of radioactivity (disint/min/mg) with the mobility of progesterone on thin-layer plates in uterus, brain tissues, and blood plasma of ovariectomized guinea pigs at several time intervals after subcutaneous injection of 40 μCi[1,2-^{3}H]progesterone in sesame oil vehicle. Reproduced from Wade and Feder (1972a) by permission.

As judged by competition experiments with unlabeled P and other steroids, there appears to be no evidence for limited capacity binding sites at the tissue level (Luttge *et al.*, 1974; Wade and Feder, 1972a). Instead, neural affinity for steroids, such as P, 20α-hydroxyprogesterone, and corticosterone in nonadrenalectomized animals, seems to be inversely related to the polarity of these steroids and seems to be positively related to the reported effectiveness of these steroids in inducing estrous behavior in estrogen-primed, gonadectomized rodents (Fig. 6; Wade and Feder, 1972b). In this connection, the guinea pig brain shows a higher uptake of P than hamster brain or rat brain, and both guinea pig and hamster brains retain P radioactivity for longer times after injection than rat brain. These species differences may be related to the differences in sensitivity to the facilitatory effects of P on estrous behavior (Wade *et al.*, 1973). It is finally of interest to note that the midbrain, a site of high accumulation of [^{3}H]P radioactivity,

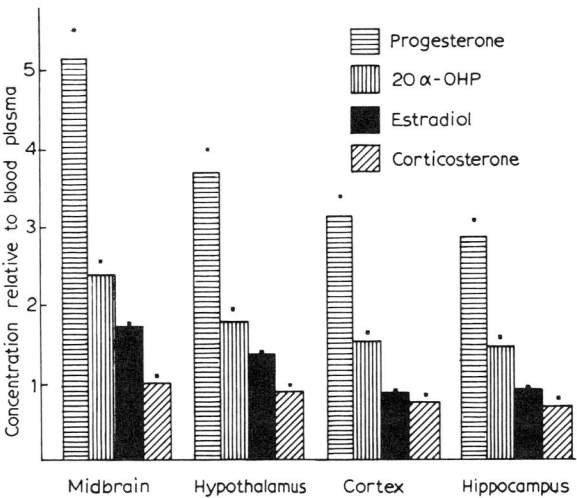

Fig. 6. Concentration of radioactivity with the mobility of progesterone, 20α-OHP, 17β-estradiol, or corticosterone on thin-layer plates relative to blood plasma in four brain regions of ovariectomized guinea pigs 4 hours after subcutaneous injection of [1,2-³H]progesterone, 1,2-[³H]20α-OHP, 6,7-³H-17β-estradiol or [1,2-³H]corticosterone, respectively, in a sesame oil vehicle. Animals injected with radioactive 17β-estradiol were pretreated with 1 mg unlabeled 17β-estradiol 15 minutes before radioisotope injection. Reproduced from Wade and Feder (1972b) by permission.

is the site of inhibition by implanted P of lordosis behavior in guinea pigs (Morin and Feder, 1974; Powers, 1972).

Attempts to saturate and, thereby, reveal limited-capacity binding sites for [³H]P, using unlabeled P, have proven uniformly unsuccessful and have tended to suggest that specific progesterone-binding sites either may not exist at all or be so few in number as to escape detection. There are, however, several pieces of evidence that tend to support the idea of limited-capacity progesterone-binding sites in brain and pituitary. First, Sar and Stumpf (1973e) have reported autoradiographic localization of binding of radioactivity injected as [³H]P in neurons of the basomedial hypothalamus of the spayed, estrogen-primed guinea pig. Unlabeled P abolishes this localization, while unlabeled cortisol is without effect. According to these authors, estrogen priming is important to see [³H]P accumulation. Similar results have been reported for cytosol binding of [³H]P in pituitary and median eminence region of spayed, estrogen-primed rats. A progesterone-saturable binding component was detected which could not be saturated by unlabeled corticosterone (Seiki and Hattori, 1973), although our laboratory could not replicate this experiment.

Second, adrenalectomy may, under some circumstances, produce an increase in tissue uptake of [³H]P in brain (see above). Not only does adrenalectomy remove one source of endogenous progesterone, it also unmasks glucocorticoid-binding sites in the brain to which progesterone is able to bind (Grosser *et al.*, 1971, 1973; McEwen *et al.*, 1976). One peculiarity about the interaction of progesterone with glucocorticoid receptors is that the progesterone does bind to glucocorticoid receptor sites *in vitro*, but, in the intact cell, it is not extensively translocated to the cell nuclei, as is the case for corticosteroids (McEwen and Wallach, 1973; McEwen *et al.*, 1976). Progesterone, in sufficiently large amounts, can, in fact, block nuclear translocation of [³H]corticosterone, and it presumably does so by occupying cytosol-receptor sites (McEwen and Wallach, 1973). Progesterone, an antiglucocorticoid in some systems, has been shown to block a number of glucocorticoid effects on thymus, chick neural retina, and hepatoma tissue culture cells (see McEwen, 1974). It is possible that P might exert some neural effects via an antiglucocorticoid action, but a major argument against this hypothesis is that glucocorticoids are normally present in large excess over circulating progesterone, thus reducing the efficacy of P as a competitive inhibitor.

The failure to adrenalectomize the guinea pigs used to study cytosol-binding sites for [³H]P in the brain and pituitary may have contributed to the failure of one report to detect any saturable binding (Atger *et al.*, 1974). In this connection, it should be noted that the adrenal produces P as well as glucocorticoids (Fajer *et al.*, 1971; Piva *et al.*, 1973; Mann and Barraclough, 1973; Shaikh and Shaikh, 1975).

It should be noted that [³H]P is not retained by highly purified pituitary or brain cell nuclei after infusion of low doses into estrogen-primed ovariectomized–adrenalectomized female rats (Fig. 3) under conditions in which comparable doses of [³H]corticosterone and [³H]dexamethasone are retained strongly by isolated nuclei (McEwen *et al.*, 1976). Published reports of cell nuclear retention of [³H]P or its metabolites are based on radioactivity in crude nuclear pellets (Robinson and Karavolas, 1973; Cheng and Karavolas, 1973) and do not necessarily indicate the presence of cell nuclear receptors. In view of the lack of conclusive evidence for such receptors and the indication of short-latency effects of P on brain EEG activity thresholds (Kawakami and Sawyer, 1959; Ramirez *et al.*, 1967), it is conceivable that P may act at the synaptic level to alter neural activity. It should be noted, however, that cycloheximide, a protein-synthesis inhibitor, has been shown to prevent progesterone-dependent postestrus refractoriness in guinea pigs (Wallen *et al.*, 1972), and actinomycin D implants in the arcuate nucleus and ventromedial hypothalamus (but not in pituitary or amygdala) block progesterone-induced LH release in testosterone-pretreated ovariectomized rats (Jackson, 1975). These observations tend to keep alive the notion that cell nuclear receptors for progesterone may actually exist in brain or pituitary.

V. STEROID RECEPTORS AND SEXUAL DIFFERENTIATION OF THE BRAIN

A. Aromatization

Sexual differentiation of the brains of mammals appears to be mediated by the secretion of testosterone from the testes during a critical period of pre- or early postnatal development (Goy, 1970). This physiological event can be mimicked by administration of testosterone during the sensitive period to females or to castrated males, and at least in two species, rat and hamster, estrogens are equally, if not more, effective compared to testosterone (Plapinger and McEwen, 1977).

The discovery by Naftolin, Ryan, and co-workers of brain enzymes capable of converting androstenedione or testosterone *in vitro* to estrone or estradiol, respectively, raises the possibility that the "aromatization" process may be obligatory, or at least significantly involved, in sexual differentiation (Naftolin *et al.*, 1971; Reddy *et al.*, 1974). The *in vitro* demonstration of aromatization established that this process is intrinsic to brain tissue, besides occurring in steroid-producing glands and the placenta. Some indication that this process occurs *in vivo* in the neonatal rat brain may be found in the work of Weisz and Gibbs (1974b). This study was replicated and extended in our laboratory to include an analysis of androgen-derived estradiol in the cell nuclear fraction. Indeed, 30–50% of the ^{3}H-radioactivity in the cell nuclear fraction from a pooled sample of limbic areas (preoptic area, amygdala) and hypothalamus of 5-day-old male or female rats was identified by extraction, chromatography, and crystallization as [^{3}H]estradiol ([^{3}H]E$_2$), whereas cerebral cortex cell nuclei contain very little [^{3}H]E$_2$ (Lieberburg and McEwen, 1975a). This enrichment is indicative of the presence of cell nuclear estrogen-receptor sites in the neonatal rat brain.

This result is consistent, moreover, with autoradiographic evidence for neuronal retention in neonatal rat hypothalamus, preoptic area, and amygdala of radioactivity injected as [^{3}H]testosterone (T) and [^{3}H]E$_2$, and with the observation that unlabeled T and E$_2$ both compete for this retention of both labeled steroids (Fig. 7; Sheridan *et al.*, 1974a,b).

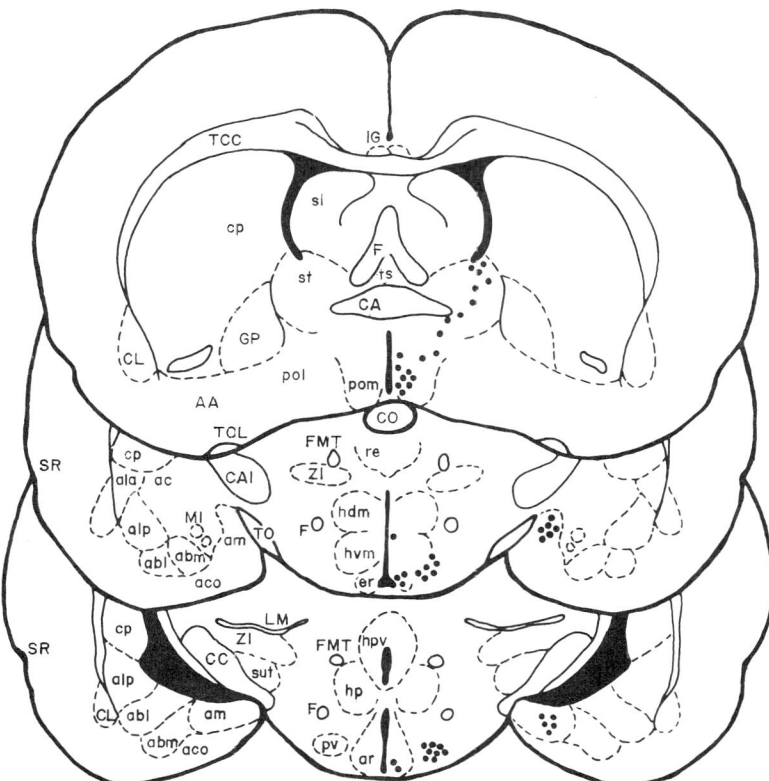

Fig. 7. Estrogen-binding neurons exist in the neonatal brain. Their topographic distribution, as obtained from dry- and thaw–mount autoradiographs after the injection of [³H]estradiol, is schematically represented in frontal cross-sections of the preoptic and central hypothalamus as well as the central amygdala. Abbreviations for the areas with dots, representing accumulation of radioactively labeled neurons: aco, n. amygdaloideus corticalis; am, n. medialis amygdalae; ar, n. arcuatus; hpv, n. periventricularis hypothelami; hvm, n. ventromedialis hypothalami, pom, n. preopticus medialis; pv, n premammillaris ventralis; st, n. interstitialis striae terminalis (for other abbreviations, see Konig and Klippel, 1963). From Sheridan et al. (1974a), by permission of J. B. Lippincott. Copyright 1974 by The Endocrine Society.

B. Topography and Properties of Neonatal Estrogen-Receptor Sites

The above-mentioned success in identifying cell nuclear estrogen-receptor sites in neonatal rat brains stands in contrast to earlier failures to demonstrate such sites with doses of [³H]E$_2$ capable of revealing such sites in adult rat brains (Plapinger and McEwen, 1973; see also Plapinger and

McEwen, 1977). In these studies, regional (i.e., hypothalamic versus cortex) differences in tissue retention of low doses of [³H]E₂ and cell nuclear retention of [³H]E₂ were not evident until the fourth postnatal week of life. It has become apparent that there are at least two explanations for these earlier results. First, as will be mentioned in the next section, the fetoneonatal estrogen-binding protein (fEBP) is apparently able to sequester small to moderate doses of [³H]17β-estradiol and to prevent this steroid, by mass action, from interacting significantly with its intracellular receptor sites. Second, the cerebral cortex contains some estrogen-receptor sites during the first 2 weeks of postnatal life (see below), and the presence of these sites tends to obscure the regional differences in binding of [³H]E₂ which are seen in the adult rat brain.

Regional cell nuclear binding at postnatal day 3 of high doses (100 nm/kg or greater) of [³H]E₂ or [³H]DES is summarized in Fig. 8. Highest binding is seen in pituitary, followed by hypothalamus, amygdala, cerebral cortex, and preoptic area. Cell nuclear binding by pooled hypothalamus, preoptic area, and amygdala (HPA), as well as by cerebral cortex cell nuclei, is

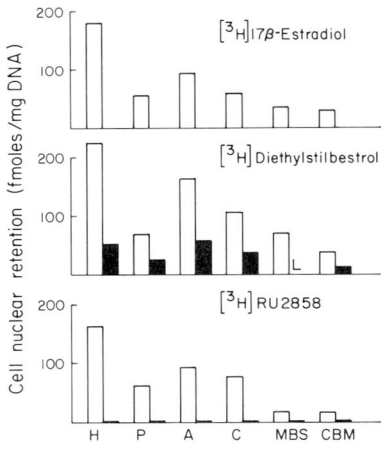

Fig. 8. Regional distribution of cell nuclear-binding sites in brains of 3-day-old female rats. [³H]Estrogens were given subcutaneously at the following doses 2 hours before sacrifice: [³H]17-β-estradiol, >100 nmoles/kg; [³H]diethylstilbestrol, >100 nmoles/kg; [³H]RU 2858, 4 nmoles/kg. Cell nuclear binding is expressed as fmoles radioactivity/mg DNA. Each panel is a single experiment with tissue pooled from four to six identically treated rats each for control and CI-628 groups. Open bars, control [³H]estrogen uptake. Black bars, 200 μg nitromifene citrate (CI-628) given 15 hours before [³H]estrogen. In the [³H]estradiol experiment there was no group receiving CI-628. L, lost sample; H, hypothalamus; P, preoptic area; A, amygdala; C, cerebral cortex, MBS, midbrain plus brain stem; CBM, cerebellum. From McEwen *et al.* (1975b) by permission.

TABLE V
Binding of Various Estrogens to Neonatal Brain Cell Nuclear Receptors and to fEBP[a]

Estrogen	Retention by nuclei	Binding to fEBP
[^{3}H]RU 2858	35	1
[^{3}H]DES	2.5	17
[^{3}H]Estradiol	1	100

[a] Based on McEwen et al. (1975b).

blocked by prior injection of a nonsteroidal antiestrogen, CI-628 (McEwen et al., 1975b), as well as by concurrent injection of unlabeled 17α-estradiol and 17β-estradiol (Maclusky and McEwen unpublished). 5α-Dihydrotestosterone, 3β,5α-androstanediol, 19-hydroxy-5α-dihydrotestosterone, and progesterone at molar ratios up to 220 times, are without significant competitive effect against [^{3}H]DES. The relatively greater effectiveness of 17α-estradiol as a competitor, compared to the 17α-isomer, may be related to the inability of the former to bind significantly to fEBP (Plapinger et al., 1973).

Otherwise, the distribution and specificity of cell nuclear estrogen retention in the neonatal rat brain are similar to those of a soluble (cytosol) binding protein recently identified by Barley and co-workers (1974) in the neonatal rat brain and by Fox (1975b) in the neonatal mouse brain. This class of macromolecules, unlike fEBP (Plapinger et al., 1973; Fox and Johnston, 1974) binds to DNA attached to cellulose (Fox, 1975b), a characteristic of intracellular steroid-receptor proteins. Moreover, these macromolecules, unlike fEBP, exhibit high affinity for the synthetic estrogen RU 2858 (Barley et al., 1974) and sediment in low ionic strength media at approximately 8 S (Fox, 1975b; MacLusky et al., 1976), properties shared by cytoplasmic estrogen receptors from the adult rat brain. Furthermore, following in vivo administration of [^{3}H]RU 2858 to neonatal animals, the levels of this cytosol protein are markedly reduced in cortex, as well as HPA, concomitant to maximal cell nuclear uptake of the labeled hormone (MacLusky et al., 1976). Thus, it seems likely that this class of macromolecules functions as a cytoplasmic receptor for the nuclear-binding mechanism.

Estrogen retention by neurons in the cerebral cortex has been detected by autoradiography (Presl et al., 1971; MacLusky et al., 1975). As noted above, the cortical estrogen receptors appear to be identical to those in HPA, with respect to sedimentation coefficient, binding specificity for various steroids, and ability to bind the antiestrogen, CI-628, and they appear to function as a precursor for the nuclear receptor. Its function remains for the moment obscure. But, owing to the absence of aromatizing activity in the cortex (Lieberburg and McEwen, 1975a), its function does not involve a response to testosterone-derived estradiol. It is possible that the cortical estrogen receptors may be responsive to estradiol secreted during the second postnatal week in both sexes (Meijs-Roelofs *et al.*, 1973; Döhler and Wuttke, 1975).

Cell nuclear binding in cerebral cortex declines to low adult levels during the third postnatal week, whereas binding in other brain regions and in pituitary changes only slightly during this period and then increases again as the animal approaches adulthood. The total cell nuclear estrogen-binding capacity of HPA on postnatal day 3 is estimated to be one-half of that observed on postnatal day 26 and only one-third of that observed in the adult female rat (Mclusky and McEwen, unpublished). Cytosol receptor content follows a developmental time course similar to that of cell nuclear binding *in vivo* (MacLusky *et al.*, 1975).

C. The Fetoneonatal Estrogen-Binding Protein (fEBP) and Its Possible Protective Role

Fetal and neonatal rat blood contains, in abundance, an estrogen-binding protein produced by the yolk sac and embryonic liver (Nunez *et al.*, 1971; Raynaud *et al.*, 1971). This protein appears to be identical to the α-fetoprotein (Uriel *et al.*, 1972; Aussel *et al.*, 1973). This fEBP has a sedimentation coefficient in sucrose density gradients of ≈4 S (Raynaud *et al.*, 1971; Plapinger *et al.*, 1973) and shows a marked preference for 17β-estradiol (E_2) over synthetic estrogens such as diethylstilbestrol (DES) or RU 2858 (Table V; see Raynaud *et al.*, 1971; Raynaud, 1973; McEwen *et al.*, 1975b) in contrast to the neonatal tissue receptor. Thus, whereas low doses of ^{3}H-E_2 are largely sequestered by fEBP and do not reach the cell nuclear receptor sites in significant amounts, comparable doses of the synthetic estrogen ^{3}H-RU 2858 do not bind to fEBP and do bind to brain cell nuclear receptor sites (Table V; see McEwen *et al.*, 1975b).

The fEBP is also found in cerebrospinal fluid and in washes of neonatal brain tissue and can, therefore, also be detected in cytosol from neonatal rat brains perfused at sacrifice to remove blood contamination (Plapinger *et al.*, 1973). This protein is immunochemically similar to fEBP from blood (Plapinger and McEwen, 1975), and its presence in brain interferes with the detection of the true cytosol receptor sites unless one uses special methodological precautions with [^{3}H]E_2 as ligand (Barley *et al.*, 1974) or uses a synthetic estrogen such as ^{3}H-RU 2858. It remains to be determined whether the presence of fEBP in brain has any significance besides the protective function ascribed to the blood fEBP (Soloff *et al.*, 1971; Uriel and de Nechaud, 1973; Plapinger *et al.*, 1973; Raynaud, 1973; McEwen *et al.*,

1975b). It is interesting to note, however, that mouse α-fetoprotein, believed to be identical to fEBP, binds to T lymphocytes (Dattwyler et al., 1975) and exerts an immunosuppressive action (Murgita and Tomasi, 1975). The involvement of estradiol in this action is unknown.

It may be predicted from the differential binding of [^{3}H]E_2 and [^{3}H]RU 2858 by fEBP and by brain receptors that the latter would be more effective than E_2 in promoting sexual differentiation of the brain (Fig. 9). Indeed this appears to be the case, and dramatically so, from recent studies of Doughty et al. (1975a). RU 2858 is also more effective than E_2 in promoting uterine growth in rats during the first 2 weeks of postnatal life when titers of fEBP are high and equally effective to E_2 when fEBP titers are low or undetectable at the end of the third postnatal week of life (Raynaud, 1973). DES, which is also a poor ligand for fEBP and which, therefore, binds better than E_2 to neonatal brain receptors, is also known to induce brain sexual differentiation (Kincl et al., 1965; Ladosky, 1967; Clemens, 1974).

Deleterious effects of estrogens are not confined to the brain. DES has been shown to induce reproductive tract abnormalities—masculine development of the reproductive tract and increased incidence of primary vaginal carcinoma—in female human children exposed to DES as fetuses (Bongiovanni et al., 1959; Herbst et al., 1972).

D. Functional Aspects

There are now three kinds of evidence pointing to the involvement of aromatization in the sexual differentiation of the rat brain. First, there is the effectiveness of estrogens as well as of testosterone in "masculinizing" the brain and the ineffectiveness of androgens such as DHT, which cannot be aromatized. DHT and its propionate are without significant masculinizing action when given to neonatal female rats as single injections in sesame oil (see Plapinger and McEwen, 1977). However, it is important to note that

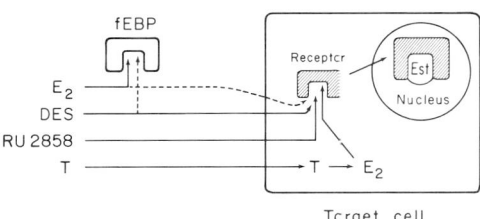

Fig. 9. Schematic diagram of the protective role of fEBP and the ability of synthetic estrogens and testosterone to bypass this mechanism. E_2, estradiol; DES, diethylstilbestrol; RU 2858, 11β-methoxyethynylestradiol; T, testosterone, Est, various estrogens in nucleus. From McEwen et al. (1975b) by permission.

a limited effect on sexual differentiation has been reported for DHT given in the form of a silastic implant under the skin of neonatal rodents, but this effect is only detected as a reduced duration of lordosis (Gerall *et al.,* 1975) and not as a reduction of the lordosis quotient (Whalen and Rezek, 1974). Second, there is the demonstrated conversion of 7-[^{3}H]testosterone to [^{3}H]estradiol, and the retention of this steroid by cell nuclei in the hypothalamus and limbic areas of the neonatal rat brain. In this connection, it is noteworthy that intrahypothalamic implants of estradiol (Döcke and Dörner, 1975), as well as testosterone (Wagner *et al.,* 1966; Nadler, 1973; Hayashi and Gorski, 1974), into neonatal female rats leads to anovulatory sterility in adult life. Third, there is the demonstration by autoradiography and by biochemical procedures of cell nuclear and soluble estrogen receptors in neonatal rat brains, with a specificity which parallels the action spectrum, in so far as it is presently known, of steroids in inducing brain sexual differentiation.

Critical experiments in proving that aromatization actually plays an important role in sexual differentiation of the brain would involve either the use of agents which block aromatization or agents which prevent access of estrogen to its intracellular receptor sites. With regard to the former approach, Clemens (1974) has reported some success in blocking the masculinizing effects of testosterone given to castrated, newborn hamsters by pentobarbital and SKF 525A, agents which may cause decreased conversion of the testosterone to estradiol. However, proof of the efficacy of these agents in blocking aromatization is currently lacking. With respect to receptor antagonists, there have been reports of success in preventing "defeminization" of female rats by giving a nonsteroidal antiestrogen, MER-25, together with testosterone propionate or RU 2858 (Doughty and McDonald, 1974; Doughty *et al.,* 1975b). There have also been three reports of failures to obtain such a blocking effect by MER-25 (Gottlieb *et al.,* 1974; Brown-Grant, 1974b; Hayashi, 1974). The reasons for these discrepancies are not clear, but it should be noted from our own experience and that of others (e.g., Ruh and Ruh, 1974) that MER-25 is not a very strong antagonist compared to a number of other antiestrogens.

It remains for future work to demonstrate whether aromatization plays a role in sexual differentiation of the brains of other species besides the rat and hamster. Recent work by Goldfoot and van der Werff Ten Bosch (1975) on the guinea pig would tend to support at least a partial role for aromatization in sexual differentiation of this species. Moreover, the recent report of Adkins (1975) with Japanese quail, indicating the effectiveness of both testosterone and estradiol injected into the egg, in demasculinizing males, suggests a possible role of aromatization in this species, for which the chromosomal sex and, therefore, the hormonally neutral sex is opposite to that of the mammal.

The recent work of Martinez-Vargas *et al.* (1975) indicates that chick embryos contain estradiol-concentrating neurons in the preoptic area and hypothalamus as early as 10 days of incubation.

The permanence of the testosterone–estrogen effects on brain sexual differentiation imply that the consequences of the hormone–receptor interaction preceding this event are different from the interaction preceding the reversible activation of adult sexual behavior or ovulation. Indeed, permanent structural alterations in the preoptic area of the rat brain appear to be one of the consequences of sexual differentiation. These alterations involve changes in the pattern of dendrites in this brain region (Greenough and Carter, 1975) and alterations in the ratio of synaptic contacts on dendritic spines to those on dendritic shafts (Raisman and Field, 1973). Studies of testosterone and estradiol effects on explants of fetal mouse hypothalamus in culture indicate that these structural changes may arise in part from an altered rate of neurite outgrowth stimulated by these two steroids (Toran-Allerand, 1976).

VI. CONCLUSION

Steroid hormone receptors are found in pituitary and brain tissue and appear to be similar to receptors in peripheral target tissues. One of the important features of these receptors in brain tissue is their discrete localization within certain brain regions which, in several instances, have been shown to respond to implanted steroid hormones and to mediate behavioral and neuroendocrine effects. Another feature of these receptors is that they appear to be involved in certain permanent, developmental changes produced by the hormone as well as in the reversible, activational effects of steroids on behavioral and neuroendocrine processes. In the case of estradiol, there is good, although not conclusive, evidence that the same kind of intracellular receptors mediate developmental effects of the hormone in neonatal life of the rat and activational effects of the hormone in adult life. The differences in the nature and permanence of these estrogen effects on the brain must involve the state of differentiation of the target neurons themselves at the time the hormone reaches them.

The genetic material, DNA, is the same in all cells of the body. However, only certain portions of the genetic information contained in the DNA are expressed during the lifetime of each cell type. Some of this information directs the events of cellular metabolism which are common to all cells.

Other information is expressed only in certain cell types. For example, only reticuloendothelial cells form hemoglobin, and only certain neurons make acetylcholine, while others make adrenalin. Other genes direct cells to adhere to other cells and form tissues. This process is of particular importance for the brain, where the connections among neurons form circuits that are responsible for the transfer of electrical messages within the brain. The process of cell differentiation, thus, involves the selective turning on of certain genes and the suppression of others. Under normal circumstances, this differentiation is irreversible for the lifetime of the tissue; i.e., blood cells do not begin to form acetylcholine, and brain cells do not begin to make hemoglobin.

Based upon this line of reasoning, we suppose that testosterone or estradiol, reaching the cell nuclei of certain hormone-sensitive differentiating neurons during the critical period for sexual differentiation of the brain, provides signals for activating certain genes and for suppressing others. By means of such a differential activation of genes, the hormone may influence the pattern of connections which these nerve cells form with other neurons and, thereby, determine the circuitry of part of the brain. Evidence for hormonal influence on patterns of neural connections was mentioned in Section V,D. Once these circuits are formed, their basic structure is no longer susceptible to the hormonal influence. Instead, during adult life, the hormone may alter the functional efficiency of these circuits, by altering the production of or sensitivity to neurotransmitters, or by influencing the oxidative metabolism of the individual hormone-sensitive neurons (see Section II,D,2). Thus, even though certain genes may be turned on in a differentiated cell, they are not necessarily fully active at all times. Their activity may, in some cases, be modulated by hormonal signals. According to this idea, estradiol which reaches the cell nuclei of adult neurons provides a signal for increasing or decreasing the activity of genes which are permanently expressed in that cell. By this means, the hormone is able to influence the functioning of developmentally fixed neural circuits which control, for example, lordosis behavior. We must now discover what chemical properties of these target neurons are essential for the appearance of this and other hormone-sensitive behavioral responses.

ACKNOWLEDGMENT

Research in the author's laboratory is supported by Research Grant NS 07080 from the United States Department of Health, Education and Welfare and by an Institutional Grant RF 70095 from The Rockefeller Foundation. The author wishes to thank Ms. Freddi Berg for editorial assistance.

REFERENCES

Adkins, E. K. (1975). *J. Comp. Physiol. Psychol.* **89**, 61–71.
Alsum, P., and Goy, R. W. (1974). *Horm. Behav.* **5**, 207–218.
Anderson, C. H., and Greenwald, S. S. (1969). *Endocrinology* **85**, 1160–1165.
Arai, Y., and Gorski, R. A. (1968). *Physiol. Behav.* **3**, 351–353.
Araki, S., Ferin, M., Zimmerman, E. A., and Vande Wiele, R. L. (1975). *Endocrinology* **96**, 644–650.
Arnold, A. P., Nottebohm, F., and Pfaff, D. W. (1976). *J. Comp. Neurol.* **165**, 487–512.
Atger, M., Baulieu, E., and Milgröm, E. (1974). *Endocrinology* **94**, 161–167.
Attramadal, A. (1965). *Proc. Int. Congr. Endocrinol., 2nd, 1964, Pt.1* Int. Congr. Ser. No. 83, pp. 612–616.
Aussel, C., Uriel, J., and Mercier-Bodard, C. (1973). *Biochimie* **55**, 1431–1437.
Bainbridge, J. G., and Labhsetwar, A. P. (1971). *J. Endocrinol.* **50**, 321–327.
Ball, J. (1937). *J. Comp. Psychol.* **24**, 135–144.
Bapna, J., Neff, N. H., and Costa, E. (1971). *Endocrinology* **89**, 1345–1349.
Barley, J., Ginsburg, M., Greenstein, B. D., MacLusky, N. J., and Thomas, P. J. (1974). *Nature (London)* **252**, 259–260.
Barley, J., Ginsburg, M., Greenstein, B. D., MacLusky, N. J., and Thomas, P. J. (1975). *Brain Res.* **100**, 383–393.
Baum, M. J., and Vreeburg, J. T. M. (1973). *Science* **182**, 283–285.
Baum, M. J., Sodersten, P., and Vreeburg, J. T. M. (1974). *Horm. Behav.* **5**, 175–190.
Beach, F. A. (1942a). *Endocrinology* **31**, 673–678.
Beach, F. A. (1942b). *Endocrinology* **31**, 679–683.
Beattie, C. W., Rodgers, C. H., and Soyka, L. F. (1972). *Endocrinology* **91**, 276–279.
Berthold, A. A. (1849). *Arch. Anat., Physiol. Wiss. Med.* **16**, 42–46.
Beyer, C., and Komisaruk, B. (1971). *Horm. Behav.* **2**, 217–225.
Beyer, C., and Rivaud, N. (1973). *Horm. Behav.* **4**, 175–180.
Beyer, C., McDonald, P., and Vidal, N. (1970a). *Endocrinology* **86**, 939–941.
Beyer, C., Vidal, N., and Mijares, A. (1970b). *Endocrinology* **87**, 1386–1389.
Beyer, C., Morali, G., and Cruz, M. L. (1971). *Endocrinology* **89**, 1158–1161.
Beyer, C., Jaffe, R. B., and Gay, V. L. (1972). *Endocrinology* **91**, 1372–1375.
Beyer, C., Larsson, K., Perez-Palacios, G., and Morali, G. (1973). *Horm. Behav.* **4**, 99–108.
Billard, R., and McDonald, P. G. (1973). *J. Endocrinol.* **56**, 585–590.
Bongiovanni, A. M., DiGeorge, A. M., and Grumbach, M. M. (1959). *J. Clin. Endocrinol. Metab.* **19**, 1004–1011.
Brown-Grant, K. (1974a). *J. Endocrinol.* **62**, 319–332.
Brown-Grant, K. (1974b). *J. Endocrinol.* **62**, 683–684.
Bueno, J., and Pfaff, D. W. (1976). *Brain Res.* **101**, 67–78.
Callantine, M. R., Humphrey, R. R., Lee, S. L., Windsor, B. L., Schottin, N. H., and O'Brien, O. P. (1966). *Endocrinology* **79**, 153–167.
Chader, G. J., and Villee, C. A (1970). *Biochem. J.* **118**, 93–97.
Chazal, G., Faudon, M., Gogan, F., and Rotsztejn, W. (1975). *Brain Res.* **89**, 245–254.
Cheng, Yi.-J., and Karavolas, H. J. (1973). *Endocrinology* **93**, 1157–1162.
Christensen, L. W., and Clemens, L. G. (1974). *Endocrinology* **95**, 984–990.
Christensen, L. W., and Clemens, L. G. (1975). *Endocrinology* **97**, 1545–1551.
Christensen, L. W., Coniglio, L. P., Paup, D. C., and Clemens, L. G. (1973). *Horm. Behav.* **4**, 223–230.
Cidlowski, J. A., and Muldoon, T. G. (1974). *Endocrinology* **95**, 1621–1629.
Clark, J. H., Peck, E. J., and Anderson, J. N. (1974). *Nature (London)* **251**, 446–448.

Clemens, L. G. (1974). *In* "Reproductive Behavior" (W. Montagna and W. A. Sadler, eds.), pp. 23–53. Plenum, New York.
Convey, E. M., and Reece, R. P. (1969). *Proc. Soc. Exp. Biol. Med.* **132**, 878–880.
Cooper, K. J., Fawcett, C. P., and McCann, S. M. (1974). *Endocrinology* **95**, 1293–1299.
Crowley, W. R., and Zemlan, F. P. (1977). *In* "Primer of Neuroendocrine Function and Behavior (N. T. Adler, ed.). Plenum, New York (*in press*).
Czaja, J. A., Goldfoot, D. A., and Karavolas, H. J. (1974). *Horm. Behav.* **5**, 261–274.
Dattwyler, R. J., Murgita, R. A., and Tomasi, T. B. (1975). *Nature (London)* **256**, 656–657.
Davidson, J. M. (1969). *Endocrinology* **84**, 1365–1372.
Davidson, J. M. (1972). *In* "Reproductive Biology" (H. Balin and S. Glasser, eds.), pp. 877–918. Excerpta Med. Found., Amsterdam.
Denef, C., Magnus, C., and McEwen, B. S. (1973). *J. Endocrinol.* **59**, 605–621.
Denef, C., Magnus, C., and McEwen, B. S. (1974). *Endocrinology* **94**, 1265–1274.
Dixit, V. P., and Niemi, M. (1974). *Endocrinol. Exp.* **8**, 39–43.
Döcke, F., and Dörner, G. (1975). *Endokrinologie* **65**, 375–377.
Döhler, K. D., and Wuttke, W. (1975). *Endocrinology* **97**, 898–907.
Doughty, C., and McDonald, P. G. (1974). *Differentiation* **2**, 275–285.
Doughty, C., Booth, J. E., McDonald, P. G., and Parrott, R. F. (1975a). *J. Endocrinol.* **67**, 419–424.
Doughty, C., Booth, J. E., McDonald, P. G., and Parrott, R. F. (1975b). *J. Endocrinol.* **67**, 459–460.
Eisenfeld, A. J. (1970). *Endocrinology* **86**, 1313–1318.
Eisenfeld, A. J., and Axelrod, J. (1965). *J. Pharmacol. Exp. Ther.* **150**, 469–475.
Everett, J. W., Krey, L. C., and Tyrey, L. (1973). *Endocrinology* **93**, 947–953.
Fajer, A. B., Holzbauer, M., and Newport, H. M. (1971). *J. Physiol. (London)* **214**, 115–126.
Feder, H. H. (1971). *J. Endocrinol.* **51**, 241–252.
Feder, H. H., Naftolin, F., and Ryan, K. J. (1974). *Endocrinology* **94**, 136–141.
Flerkó, B., and Mess, B. (1968). *Acta Physiol. Acad. Sci. Hung.* **33**, 111–113.
Flerkó, B., and Szentágothai, J. (1957). *Acta Endocrinol. (Copenhagen)* **26**, 121–127.
Fletcher, T. J., and Short, R. V. (1974). *Nature (London)* **248**, 616–618.
Flores, F., Naftolin, F., Ryan, K. J., and White, R. J. (1973). *Science* **180**, 1074–1075.
Fox, T. O. (1975a). *Proc. Natl. Acad. Sci. U.S.A.* **72**, 4303–4307.
Fox, T. O. (1975b). *Nature (London)* **258**, 441–444.
Fox, T. O., and Johnston, C. (1974). *Brain Res.* **77**, 330–336.
Friend, J. P., and Leavitt, W. W. (1972). *Acta Endocrinol. (Copenhagen)* **69**, 230–240.
Fuxe, K., Hokfelt, T., and Nilsson, O. (1969). *Neuroendocrinology* **5**, 107–120.
Gerall, A. A., McMurray, M. M., and Farrell, A. (1975). *J. Endocrinol.* **67**, 439–445.
Ginsburg, M., Greenstein, B. D., MacLusky, N. J., Morris, I. D., and Thomas, P. J. (1974). *Steroids* **23**, 773–792.
Glascock, R. F., and Michael, R. P. (1962). *J. Physiol. (London)* **163**, 38P–39P.
Goldfoot, D. A., and van der werff Ten Bosch, J. J. (1975). *Horm. Behav.* **6**, 139–148.
Gordon, J. H., and Reichlin, S. (1974). *Endocrinology* **94**, 974–977.
Gottlieb, H., Gerall, A. A., and Thiel, A. (1974). *Physiol. Behav.* **12**, 61–68.
Goy, R. W. (1970). *In* "The Neurosciences: Second Study Program" (F. O. Schmitt, ed.), pp. 196–206. Rockefeller Univ. Press, New York.
Gradwell, P. B., Everitt, B. J., and Herbert, J. (1975). *Brain Res.* **88**, 281–293.
Grant, L. D., and Stumpf, W. E. (1973). *J. Histochem. Cytochem.* 404 (Ab. #6).
Green, R., Luttge, W. G., and Whalen, R. E. (1970). *Physiol. Behav.* **5**, 137–141.
Greenough, W. T., and Carter, S. C. (1975). *Neurosci. Abstr., 5th Annu. Meet.* Abstract No. 1210, p. 789.

Griffiths, E. C., and Hooper, K. C. (1973). *Acta Endocrinol. (Copenhagen)* **74**, 41–48.
Griffiths, E. C., and Hooper, K. C. (1974). *Acta Endocrinol. (Copenhagen)* **77**, 10–18.
Grosser, B. I., Stevens, W., Bruenger, F. W., and Reed, D. J. (1971). *J. Neurochem.* **18**, 1725–1732.
Grosser, B. I., Stevens, W., and Reed, D. J. (1973). *Brain Res.* **57**, 387–395.
Gual, C., Morato, T., Hayano, M., Gut, M., and Dorfman, R. I. (1962). *Endocrinology* **71**, 920–925.
Gupta, G. N. (1960). *Diss. Abstr. Int. B* **34**, 1972 (Ph.D. Thesis, University of Chicago, Chicago, Illinois).
Hayashi, S. (1974). *Endocrinol. Jpn.* **21**, 453–457.
Hayashi, S., and Gorski, R. A. (1974). *Endocrinology* **94**, 1161–1167.
Heil, H., Meltzer, V., Kuhl, H., Abraham, R., and Taubert, H. D. (1971). *Fertil. Steril.* **22**, 181–187.
Herbst, A. L., Kurman, R. J., Scully, R. E., and Poskanzen, D. C. (1972). *N. Engl. J. Med.* **287**, 1259–1264.
Hilliard, J., Penardi, R., and Sawyer, C. H. (1967). *Endocrinology* **80**, 901–909.
Hough, J. C., Jr., Ho, K.-W., Cooke, P. H., and Quadagno, D. M. (1974). *Horm. Behav.* **5**, 367–376.
Jackson, G. L. (1972). *Endocrinology* **91**, 1284–1287.
Jackson, G. L. (1973). *Endocrinology* **93**, 887–891.
Jackson, G. L. (1975). *Neuroendocrinology* **17**, 236–244.
Jensen, E. V., and Jacobson, H. I. (1962). *Recent Prog. Horm. Res.* **18**, 387–408.
Johnston, P., and Davidson, J. M. (1972). *Horm. Behav.* **3**, 345–357.
Jouan, P., Samperez, S., Thieulant, M. L., and Mercier, L. (1971a). *C.R. Hebd. Seances Acad. Sci.* **272**, 2368–2371.
Jouan, P., Samperez, S., Thieulant, M. L., and Mercier, L. (1971b). *J. Steroid Biochem.* **2**, 223–236.
Jouan, P., Samperez, S., and Thieulant, M. L. (1973). *J. Steroid Biochem.* **4**, 65–74.
Kahwanago, I., Heinrichs, W. L., and Herrmann, W. L. (1970). *Endocrinology* **86**, 1319–1326.
Kalra, S. P. (1975). *Neuroendocrinology* **18**, 333–344.
Kalra, S. P., Krulich, L., and McCann, S. M. (1973). *Neuroendocrinology* **12**, 321–333.
Kang, Y.-H., Anderson, W. A., and deSombre, E. R. (1975). *J. Cell Biol.* **64**, 682–691.
Karavolas, H. J., and Herf, S. M. (1971). *Endocrinology* **89**, 940–942.
Karavolas, H. J., Hodges, D., and O'Brien, D. (1976). *Endocrinology* **98**, 164–175.
Kato, J. (1973). *Acta Endocrinol. (Copenhagen)* **72**, 663–670.
Kato, J., and Onouchi, T. (1973a). *Endocrinol. Jpn.* **20**, 429–432.
Kato, J., and Onouchi, T. (1973b). *Endocrinol. Jpn.* **20**, 641–644.
Kato, J., Atsumi, Y., and Muramatsu, M. (1970a). *J. Biochem. (Tokyo)* **67**, 871–872.
Kato, J., Atsumi, Y., and Inaba, M. (1970b). *J. Biochem. (Tokyo)* **68**, 759–761.
Kawahara, F. S., Berman, M. L., and Green, O. C. (1975). *Steroids* **25**, 459–463.
Kawakami, M., and Sawyer, C. H. (1959). *Endocrinology* **65**, 652–668.
Keefer, D. A., Stumpf, W. E., and Sar, M. (1973). *Proc. Soc. Exp. Biol. Med.* **143**, 414–417.
Kelley, D. B., Morrell, J. I., and Pfaff, D. W. (1975). *J. Comp. Neurol.* **164**, 47–59.
Kincl, F. A., Pi, A. F., Maqueo, M., Lasso, L. H., Oriol, A., and Dorfman, R. I. (1965). *Acta Endocrinol. (Copenhagen)* **49**, 193–206.
Kizer, J. S., Palkovits, M., Zivin, J., Brownstein, M., Saavedra, J. M., and Kopin, I. J. (1974). *Endocrinology* **95**, 799–812.
Kniewald, Z., and Milkovic, S. (1973). *Endocrinology* **92**, 1772–1775.
Kniewald, Z., Massa, R., and Martini, L. (1971). *Horm. Steroids, Proc. Int. Congr., 3rd, 1970* Excerpta Med. Found. Int. Congr. Ser. No. 219, pp. 784–791.

Komisaruk, B. R., and Beyer, C. (1972). *Horm. Behav.* **3**, 63–70.
Konig, J., and Klippel, R. A. (1963). "The Rat Brain." Williams & Wilkins, Baltimore, Maryland.
Korach, K. S., and Muldoon, T. G. (1973). *Endocrinology* **92**, 322–326.
Korach, K. S., and Muldoon, T. G. (1974). *Endocrinology* **94**, 785–793.
Kubo, K., Gorski, R. A., and Kawakami, M. (1975). *Neuroendocrinology* **18**, 176–191.
Kuhl, H., Roshiatowski, C., Oen, H., and Taubert, D. (1974). *Acta Endocrinol. (Copenhagen)* **76**, 1–14.
Labhsetwar, A. P. (1970). *J. Endocrinol.* **47**, 481–493.
Ladosky, W. (1967). *Endokrinologie* **52**, 259–261.
Larsson, K., Sodersten, P., and Beyer, C. (1973a). *Horm. Behav.* **4**, 289–300.
Larsson, K., Sodersten, P., and Beyer, C. (1973b). *J. Endocrinol.* **57**, 563–564.
Laumas, K. R., and Farooq, A. (1966). *J. Endocrinol.* **36**, 95–96.
Leavitt, W. W., Kimmel, G. L., and Friend, J. P. (1973). *Endocrinology* **92**, 94–102.
Liao, S., and Fang, S. (1969). *Vitam. and Horm. (N.Y.)* **27**, 17–90.
Libertun, C., Cooper, K. J., Fawcett, C. P., and McCann, S. M. (1974). *Endocrinology* **94**, 518–525.
Lieberburg, I., and McEwen, B. S. (1975a). *Brain Res.* **85**, 165–170.
Lieberburg, I., and McEwen, B. S. (1975b). *Brain Res.* **91**, 171–174.
Lieberburg, I., and McEwen, B. S. (1975c). *Program, Soc. Neurosc. 5th Annu. Meet.*
Lieberburg, I., and McEwen, B. S. (1977). *Endocrinology* **100**, 588–597.
Lieberburg, I., MacLusky, N. J., and McEwen, B. S. (1977). *Endocrinology* **100**, 598–607.
Linkie, D. M. (1975). *Proc. 57th Annu. Meet. Am. Endocr. Soc.*, New York, Abstract No. 33, p. 67.
Lisk, R. D. (1960). *J. Exp. Zool.* **145**, 197–207.
Lisk, R. D. (1967). *Neuroendocrinology* **2**, 197–239.
Ljungkvist, I., and Terenius, L. (1974). *Contraception* **10**, 395–405.
Loras, B., Genott, A., Monbon, M., Beucher, F., Reboud, J. P., and Bertrand, J. (1974). *J. Steroid Biochem.* **5**, 425–431.
Luine, V. N., and McEwen, B. S. (1977). In "Sexual Behavior" (R. W. Goy and D. W. Pfaff, eds.). Plenum, New York (in press).
Luine, V. N., Khylchevskaya, R. I., and McEwen, B. S. (1974). *J. Neurochem.* **23**, 925–934.
Luine, V. N., Khylchevskaya, R. I., and McEwen, B. S. (1975a). *Brain Res.* **86**, 283–292.
Luine, V. N., Khylchevskaya, R. I., and McEwen, B. S. (1975b). *Brain Res.* **86**, 293–306.
Luttge, W. G., Chronister, R. B., and Hall, N. R. (1973). *Life Sci.* **12**, 419–424.
Luttge, W. G., Wallis, C. J., and Hall, N. R. (1974). *Brain Res.* **21**, 105–115.
McCann, S. M., and Moss, R. L. (1975). *Life Sci.* **16**, 833–852.
McDonald, P. G., and Meyerson, G. J. (1973). *Physiol. Behav.* **11**, 515–520.
McDonald, P. G., Beyer, C., Newton, F., Brien, B., Baker, R., Tan, H. S., Sampson, C., Kitching, P., Greenhill, R., and Pritchard, D. (1970). *Nature (London)* **227**, 964–965.
McEwen, B. S. (1974). In "Neuroendocrinologie de l'Axe Corticotrope" (P. Dell, ed.), INSERM Colloq., Vol. 22, pp. 79–94. INSERM, Paris.
McEwen, B. S. (1976). In "Subcellular Mechanisms in Reproductive Neuroendocrinology" (F. Naftolin, K. J. Ryan and J. Davies, eds.) pp. 277–304, Elsevier, Amsterdam.
McEwen, B. S., and Pfaff, D. W. (1970). *Brain Res.* **21**, 1–16.
McEwen, B. S., and Pfaff, D. W. (1973). *Front. Neuroendocrinol.* 267–335.
McEwen, B. S., and Wallach, G. (1973). *Brain Res.* **57**, 373–386.
McEwen, B. S., Pfaff, D. W., and Zigmond, R. E. (1970a). *Brain Res.* **21**, 17–28.
McEwen, B. S., Pfaff, D. W., and Zigmond, R. E. (1970b). *Brain Res.* **21**, 29–38.

McEwen, B. S., Zigmond, R. E., and Gerlach, J. L. (1972). *Struct. Funct. Nerv. Tissue* **5**, 205–291.
McEwen, B. S., Pfaff, D. W., Chaptal, C., and Luine, V. (1975a). *Brain Res.* **86**, 155–161.
McEwen, B. S., Plapinger, L., Chaptal, C., Gerlach, J., and Wallach, G. (1975b). *Brain Res.* **96**, 400–406.
McEwen, B. S., de Kloet, R., and Wallach, G. (1976). *Brain Res.* **105**, 129–136.
McGuire, W. L., De La Garza, M., and Chamness, G. C. (1973). *Endocrinology* **93**, 810–813.
MacLusky, N., Chaptal, C., and McEwen, B. S. (1975). *Neuroscience Abstr., Soc. Neurosci., 5th Annu. Meet.* Abstract No. 682, p. 439.
MacLusky, N. J., Chaptal, C., Lieberburg, I., and McEwen, B. S. (1976). *Brain Res.* **114**, 158–165.
Mann, D. R., and Barraclough, C. A. (1973). *Endocrinology* **93**, 694–699.
Martinez-Vargas, M. C., Gibson, D. B., Sar, M., and Stumpf, W. (1975). *Science* **190**, 1307–1308.
Massa, R., and Martini, L. (1971–1972). *Gynecol. Invest.* **2**, 253–270.
Massa, R., Stupnicka, E., Kniewald, Z., and Martini, L. (1972). *J. Steroid Biochem.* **3**, 385–399.
Maurer, R. A. (1974). *Brain Res.* **67**, 175–177.
Maurer, R. A., and Woolley, D. E. (1974). *Neuroendocrinology* **16**, 137–147.
Meijs-Roelofs, H. M. A., Uilenbroek, J. T.J., de Jongs, F. H., and Welschen, R. (1973). *J. Endocrinol.* **59**, 295–304.
Meyer, C. C. (1973). *Science* **180**, 1381–1382.
Meyerson, B. J. (1967). *Endocrinology* **81**, 369–374.
Meyerson, B. J., and Lindström, L. (1968). *Acta Endocrinol. (Copenhagen)* **59**, 41–48.
Michael, R. P. (1965a). *Br. Med. Bull.* **21**, 87–90.
Michael, R. P. (1965b). *Horm. Steroids, Proc. Int. Congr., 1st, 1962* Vol. 2, pp. 469–480.
Michael, R. P. (1966). *Brain Gonadal Funct., Proc. Conf. Brain Behav., 3rd, 1963* Vol. 3, pp. 82–98.
Monbon, M., Loras, B., Reboud, J. P., and Bertrand, J. (1973). *Brain Res.* **53**, 139–150.
Monbon, M., Loras, B., Reboud, J. P., and Bertrand, J. (1974). *J. Steroid Biochem.* **5**, 417–423.
Morin, L. P., and Feder, H. H. (1974). *Brain Res.* **70**, 71–80.
Morrell, J. I., Kelley, D. B., and Pfaff, D. W. (1975a). *In* "Brain Endocrine Interactions: II. The Ventricular System" (K. Knigge *et al.*, eds.), pp. 230–256. Karger, Basel.
Morrell, J. I., Kelley, D. B., and Pfaff, D. W. (1975b). *J. Comp. Neurol.* **164**, 63–78.
Moszkowska, A., and Kordon, C. (1965). *Gen. Comp. Endocrinol.* **5**, 596–613.
Mowles, T. F., Ashkanazy, B., Mix, E., Jr., and Sheppard, H. (1971). *Endocrinology* **89**, 484–491.
Murgita, R. A., and Tomasi, T. B. (1975). *J. Exp. Med.* **141**, 269–286.
Nadler, R. D. (1973). *Neuroendocrinology* **12**, 110–119.
Naess, O., and Attramadal, A. (1974). *Acta Endocrinol. (Copenhagen)* **76**, 417–430.
Naess, O., Attramadal, A., and Aakvaag, A. (1975a). *Endocrinology* **96**, 1–9.
Naess, O., Hansson, V., Djoeseland, O., and Attramadal, A. (1975b). *Endocrinology* **97**, 1355–1363.
Naftolin, F., Ryan, K. J., and Petro, Z. (1971). *J. Clin. Endocrinol. Metab.* **33**, 368–370.
Naftolin, F., Ryan, K. J., and Petro, Z. (1972). *Endocrinology* **90**, 295–298.
Noble, R. (1974). *Horm. Behav.* **5**, 227–234.
Notides, A. C. (1970). *Endocrinology* **87**, 987–992.
Notides, A. C., and Nielsen, S. (1974). *J. Biol. Chem.* **249**, 1866–1873.

Nowak, F. V., and Karavolas, H. J. (1974). *Endocrinology* **94**, 994–997.
Nunez, E., Engelmann, F., Benassayag, C., and Jayle, M.-F. (1971). *C.R. Hebd. Seances Acad. Sci., Ser. D* **273**, 831–834.
Parrott, R. F. (1974). *J. Endocrinol.* **61**, 105–115.
Parrott, R. F. (1975). *Horm. Behav.* **6**, 99–108.
Paup, D. C., Mennin, S. P., and Gorski, R. A. (1975). *Horm. Behav.* **6**, 35–46.
Payne, A. H., Lawrence, C. C., Foster, D. L., and Jaffe, R. B. (1973). *J. Biol. Chem.* **248**, 1598–1602.
Perez-Palacios, B., Perez, A. E., Cruz, M. L., and Beyer, C. (1973). *Biol. Reprod.* **8**, 395–399.
Pfaff, D. W. (1968a). *Endocrinology* **82**, 1149–1155.
Pfaff, D. W. (1968b). *Science* **161**, 1355–1356.
Pfaff, D. W. (1968c). *Experientia* **24**, 958–959.
Pfaff, D. W. (1970). *J. Comp. Physiol. Psychol.* **73**, 349–358.
Pfaff, D. W. (1977). *In* "Primer of Neuroendocrine Function and Behavior" (N. Adler, ed.), Plenum Press (*in press*).
Pfaff, D. W., and Keiner, M. (1973). *J. Comp. Neurol.* **151**, 121–158.
Pfaff, D. W., Lewis, C., Diakow, C., and Keiner, M. (1973). *Prog. Physiol. Psychol.* **5**, 253–297.
Phoenix, C. H. (1974). *Physiol. Behav.* **12**, 1045–1055.
Phuong, N. T., and Sauer, G. (1971). *Acta Biol. Med. Ger.* **26**, 1247–1249.
Piacsek, B. E., and Meites, J. (1966). *Endocrinology* **79**, 432–439.
Piva, F., Gagliano, P., Motta, M., and Martini, L. (1973). *Endocrinology* **93**, 1178–1184.
Plapinger, L. (1973). Ph.D. Thesis, New York University, New York.
Plapinger, L., and McEwen, B. S. (1973). *Endocrinology* **93**, 1119–1128.
Plapinger, L., and McEwen, B. S. (1975). *Steroids* **26**, 255–265.
Plapinger, L., and McEwen, B. S. (1977). *In* "Biological Determinants of Sexual Behavior" (J. Hutchison, ed.). Wiley, New York (in press).
Plapinger, L., McEwen, B. S., and Clemens, L. E. (1973). *Endocrinology* **93**, 1129–1139.
Powers, J. B. (1972). *Brain Res.* **48**, 311–325.
Presl, J., Pospisil, J., and Horsky, J. (1971). *Experientia* **27**, 465–467.
Quadagno, D. M., and Ho, G. K. W. (1975). *Horm. Behav.* **6**, 19–26.
Raisinghani, K. H., Dorfman, R. I., Forchielli, E., Gyermek, L., and Genther, G. (1968). *Acta Endocrinol. (Copenhagen)* **57**, 395–404.
Raisman, G., and Field, P. M. (1973). *Brain Res.* **54**, 1–29.
Ramirez, V. D., Komisaruk, B. R., Whitmoyer, D. I., and Sawyer, C. H. (1967). *Am. J. Physiol.* **212**, 1376–1384.
Raynaud, J. P. (1973). *Steroids* **21**, 249–258.
Raynaud, J. P., Mercier-Bodard, C., and Baulieu, E. E. (1971). *Steroids* **18**, 767–788.
Reddy, V. V. R., Naftolin, F., and Ryan, K. J. (1973). *Endocrinology* **92**, 589–594.
Reddy, V. V. R., Naftolin, F., and Ryan, K. J. (1974). *Endocrinology* **94**, 117–121.
Resko, J. A., Goy, R. W., and Phoenix, C. H. (1967). *Endocrinology* **80**, 490–498.
Rippel, R. H., Johnson, E. S., and White, W. F. (1973). *Proc. Soc. Exp. Biol. Med.* **143**, 55–58.
Robel, P., Corprechot, C., and Baulieu, E. E. (1973). *FEBS Lett.* **33**, 218–220.
Robinson, J. A., and Karavolas, H. J. (1973). *Endocrinology* **93**, 430–434.
Robinson, J. A., and Leavitt, W. W. (1971). *Proc. Soc. Exp. Biol. Med.* **139**, 471–475.
Roy, E. J., and Wade, G. N. (1976). *J. Comp. Physiol. Psychol.* **90**, 156–166.
Roy, S. K., Jr., and Laumas, K. R. (1969). *Acta Endocrinol. (Copenhagen)* **61**, 629–640.
Ruh, T. S., and Ruh, M. F. (1974). *Steroids* **24**, 209–224.
Ryan, K. J. (1962). *Am. J. Obstet. Gynecol.* **84**, 1695–1713.

Ryan, K. J., Naftolin, F., Reddy, V., Flores, F., and Petro, Z. (1972). *Am. J. Obstet. Gynecol.* **114,** 454–460.
Samperez, S., Thieulant, M.-L., and Jouan, P. (1969a). *C.R. Hebd. Seances Acad. Sci.* **268,** 2965–2968.
Samperez, S., Thieulant, M.-L., Poupon, R., Duval, J., and Jouan, P. (1969b). *Bull. Soc. Chim. Biol.* **51,** 117–131.
Samperez, S., Thieulant, M.-L., Mercier, L., and Jouan, P. (1974). *J. Steroid Biochem.* **5,** 911–915.
Sanyal, M. K., and Todd, R. B. (1972). *Proc. Soc. Exp. Biol. Med.* **141,** 622–624.
Sar, M., and Stumpf, W. E. (1972). *Experientia* **28,** 1364–1366.
Sar, M., and Stumpf, W. E. (1973a). *Endocrinology* **92,** 251–256.
Sar, M., and Stumpf, W. E. (1973b). *Science* **179,** 389–391.
Sar, M., and Stumpf, W. E. (1973c). *Endocrinology* **92,** 631–635.
Sar, M., and Stumpf, W. E. (1973d). *Proc. Soc. Exp. Biol. Med.* **144,** 26–29.
Sar, M., and Stumpf, W. E. (1973e). *Science* **182,** 1266–1268.
Sarff, M., and Gorski, J. (1971). *Biochemistry* **10,** 2557–2563.
Schwarzel, W. C., Kruggel, W. G., and Brodie, H. J. (1973). *Endocrinology* **92,** 866–880.
Seiki, K., and Hattori, M. (1973). *Endocrinol. Jpn.* **20,** 111–119.
Seiki, K., Higashida, M., Imanishi, Y., Miyamoto, M., Kitagawa, T., and Kotani, M. (1968). *J. Endocrinol.* **41,** 109–110.
Seiki, K., Miyamoto, M., Yamashita, A., and Kotani, M. (1969). *J. Endocrinol.* **43,** 129–130.
Seiki, K., Hattori, M., and Karaki, M. (1975). *Endocrinol. Jpn.* **22,** 147–149.
Shaikh, A. A., and Shaikh, S. A. (1975). *Endocrinology* **96,** 37–44.
Sheridan, P. J., Sar, M., and Stumpf, W. E. (1974a). *Endocrinology* **94,** 1386–1390.
Sheridan, P. J., Sar, M., and Stumpf, W. E. (1974b). *Endocrinology* **95,** 1749–1753.
Shirley, B., Wolinsky, J., and Schwartz, N. B. (1968). *Endocrinology* **82,** 959–968.
Sholiton, L. J., Taylor, B. B., and Lewis, H. P. (1974). *Steroids* **24,** 537–547.
Södersten, P. (1972). *Horm. Behav.* **3,** 307–320.
Södersten, P. (1973). *Horm. Behav.* **4,** 247–256.
Södersten, P. (1974). *Horm. Behav.* **5,** 111–122.
Soloff, M. S., Creange, J. E., and Potts, G. O. (1971). *Endocrinology* **88,** 427–432.
Stahl, F., Poppe, I., and Dorner, G. (1971). *Acta Biol. Med. Ger.* **26,** 855–858.
Steinach, E. (1940). "Sex and Life." Viking Press, New York.
Stern, J., and Eisenfeld, A. (1971). *Endocrinology* **88,** 117–1125.
Stumpf, W. E. (1968a). *Science* **162,** 1001–1003.
Stumpf, W. E. (1968b). *Z. Zellforsch. Mikrosk. Anat.* **92,** 23–33.
Stumpf, W. E. (1970). *Am. J. Anat.* **129,** 207–217.
Swerdloff, R. S., Walsh, P. C., and Odell, W. D. (1972). *Steroids* **20,** 13–22.
Tabei, T., Haga, H., Heinrichs, W. L., and Hermann, W. L. (1964). *Steroids* **33,** 651–666.
Tang, L. K. L., and Spies, H. G. (1975). *Endocrinology* **96,** 349–356.
Terkel, A. S., Shryne, J., and Gorski, R. A. (1973). *Horm. Behav.* **4,** 377–386.
Thien, N. C., Thieulant, M. L., Samperez, S., and Jouan, P. (1972). *C.R. Hebd. Seances Acad. Sci.* **275,** 1927–1930.
Thien, N. C., Duval, J., Samperez, S., and Jouan, P. (1974). *Biochimie* **56,** 899–906.
Thieulant, M. L., Mercier, M. L., Samperez, S., and Jouan, P. (1974a). *C.R. Hebd. Seances Acad. Sci.* **278,** 2569–2572.
Thieulant, M. L., Pelle, G., Samperez, S., and Jouan, P. (1974b). *C.R. Hebd. Seances Acad. Sci.* **278,** 1281–1284.
Thieulant, M. L., Mercier, L., Samperez, S., and Jouan, P. (1975). *J. Steroid Biochem.* **6,** 1257–1260.

Thoenen, H., Mueller, R. A., and Axelrod, J. (1969). *J. Pharmacol. Exp. Ther.* **169**, 249–254.
Toran-Allerand, C. D. (1976). *Brain Res.* **106**, 407–412.
Tuohimaa, P. (1971). *In* "Basic Actions of Sex Steroids on Target Organs" (P. O. Hubinot, F. Leroy, and P. Galand, eds.), pp. 208–214. Karger, Basel.
Uriel, J., and de Nechaud, B. (1973). *In* "Alpha-Fetoprotein and Hepatoma" (H. Hirai and T. Miyaji, eds.), pp. 35–47. Univ. Park Press, Baltimore, Maryland.
Uriel, J., de Nechaud, B., and Dupiers, M. (1972). *Biochem. Biophys. Res. Commun.* **46**, 1175–1180.
Verhoeven, G., Lambergits, G., and deMoor, P. (1974). *J. Steroid Biochem.* **5**, 93–100.
Vétes, M., and King, R. J. B. (1971). *J. Endocrinol.* **51**, 271–282.
Vilchez-Martinez, J. A., Arimura, A., Debeljuk, L., and Schally, A. V. (1974a). *Endocrinology* **94**, 1300–1303.
Vilchez-Martinez, J. A., Arimura, A., and Schally, A. V. (1974b). *Proc. Soc. Exp. Biol. Med.* **146**, 859–862.
Vreeburg, J. T. M., Schretlen, P. J. M., and Baum, M. J. (1975). *Endocrinology* **97**, 969–977.
Wade, G. N., and Feder, H. H. (1972a). *Brain Res.* **45**, 525–543.
Wade, G. N., and Feder, H. H. (1972b). *Brain Res.* **45**, 545–554.
Wade, G. N., and Feder, H. H. (1972c). *Physiol. Behav.* **9**, 773–775.
Wade, G. N., Harding, C. F., and Feder, H. H. (1973). *Brain Res.* **61**, 357–367.
Wagner, J. W., Erwin, W., and Critchlow, V. (1966). *Endocrinology* **79**, 1135–1142.
Wallen, K., Goldfoot, D. A., Joslyn, W. D., and Paris, C. A. (1972). *Physiol. Behav.* **8**, 221–223.
Warembourg, M. (1970a). *C. R. Soc. Biol. Ses. Fil.* **164**, 126–129.
Warembourg, M. (1970b). *C.R. Hebd. Seances Acad. Sci.* **270**, 152–154.
Weisz, J., and Gibbs, C. (1974a). *Endocrinology* **94**, 616–620.
Weisz, J., and Gibbs, C. (1974b). *Neuroendocrinology* **14**, 72–86.
Whalen, R. E., and Gorzalka, B. B. (1972). *Horm. Behav.* **3**, 221–226.
Whalen, R. E., and Gorzalka, B. B. (1973). *Physiol. Behav.* **10**, 35–40.
Whalen, R. E., and Gorzalka, B. B. (1974). *Endocrinology* **94**, 214–223.
Whalen, R. E., and Hardy, D. F. (1970). *Physiol. Behav.* **5**, 529–533.
Whalen, R. E., and Luttge, W. E. (1971a). *Brain Res.* **33**, 147–155.
Whalen, R. E., and Luttge, W. E. (1971b). *Horm. Behav.* **2**, 117–125.
Whalen, R. E., and Massicci, J. (1975). *Brain Res.* **89**, 255–264.
Whalen, R. E., and Rezek, D. L. (1974). *Horm. Behav.* **5**, 125–128.
Whalen, R. E., Battie, C., and Luttge, W. G. (1972). *Behav. Biol.* **7**, 311–320.
Whalen, R. E., Gorzalka, B. B., deBold, J. F., Quadagno, D. M., Kan-Wha Ho, G., and Hough, J. C., Jr. (1974). *Horm. Behav.* **5**, 337–343.
Whalen, R. E., Martin, J. V., and Olsen, K. L. (1975). *Nature (London)* **258**, 742–743.
Williams, D., and Gorski, J. (1972). *Proc. Natl. Acad. Sci. U.S.A.* **69**, 3454–3468.
Yamamoto, K. R. (1974). *J. Biol. Chem.* **249**, 7068–7075.
Zeman, W., and Innes, J. R. M. (1963). "Craigie's Neuroanatomy of the Rat." Academic Press, New York.
Zigmond, R. E. (1975). *Handb. Psychopharmacol.* **5**, 239–328.
Zigmond, R. E., and McEwen, B. S. (1970). *J. Neurochem.* **17**, 889–899.
Zigmond, R. E., Stern, J., and McEwen, B. S. (1972). *Gen. Comp. Endocrinol.* **18**, 450–453.
Zigmond, R. E., Nottebohm, F., and Pfaff, D. W. (1973). *Science* **179**, 1005–1007.

14

Hormones and Their Receptors in Breast Cancer

WILLIAM L. McGUIRE, GARY C. CHAMNESS,
KATHRYN B. HORWITZ, AND DAVID T. ZAVA

I.	Introduction	402
II.	Prolactin	403
	A. Rat Mammary Tumors	403
	B. Human Breast Cancer	404
	C. Mechanism of Prolactin Dependence	406
III.	Estrogen	409
	A. Localization of Estrogens in Responsive Tumors	410
	B. Measurement of Estrogen Receptor	410
	C. Rat Mammary Tumors as a Model System	411
	D. Estrogen Receptor in Human Breast Tumors	412
	E. Antiestrogens	414
	F. Systemic Approaches to Reducing Estrogen Production	416
IV.	Progesterone	417
	A. Clinical Effects in Breast Cancer	417
	B. Subcellular Metabolism of Progesterone	418
	C. Progesterone Receptors	420
	D. Progesterone Interrelationship with Other Steroid Hormones	422
	E. Progesterone Receptors in Human Breast Cancer	424
V.	Glucocorticoids	425
VI.	Androgens	427
	A. Androgens in Mammary Carcinoma	428
VII.	Summary and Conclusions	431
	References	431

I. INTRODUCTION

The human mammary gland is sensitive to a number of hormones, among which estrogen and prolactin exert, perhaps, the most dramatic effects. It would be reasonable to predict that tumors arising by malignant transformation of mammary gland cells might retain these hormone controls. The first actual demonstration of hormone control of breast cancer was made 80 years ago, when regression of metastatic tumors was produced by ovariectomy (Beatson, 1896a,b). Unfortunately, only 30% of tumors are responsive. Most of these tumors will respond equally to adrenalectomy or hypophysectomy (Dao, 1972), so that the hormones primarily responsible for tumor growth are not individually identified. These responsive tumors are therefore classified simply as "hormone dependent."

Normal target tissues including mammary gland contain specific receptors for hormones: cytoplasmic proteins for the steroids, and cell surface receptors for polypeptides. These receptor sites are responsible for the initial interaction between the hormone and the cell, and function to trigger the biochemical chain of events characteristic for the particular hormone. Hormone-dependent tumors also contain receptors, but it now appears that independent, or autonomous, tumors often may not (McGuire *et al.*, 1974).

Consequently, it has been proposed that when malignant transformation occurs, the cell may retain all or only part of the normal population of receptor sites. If the cell retains the receptor sites, its growth and function like those of the normal cell are potentially capable of being regulated by the hormonal environment. If the cell loses the receptors as a consequence of its malignant transformation, it is no longer recognized as a target cell by circulating hormones, and endocrine control is abolished.

This implies that the presence of specific receptors in mammary tumor tissue may indicate hormone dependence, and identify the 30% of breast cancer patients who will actually benefit from endocrine therapy.

In this report, we will review the role of several hormones and their receptors in breast cancer tissues and examine mechanisms of control, as well as providing pathophysiological correlation whenever possible. Most of the studies on hormone-dependent breast carcinoma employ animal models, particularly carcinogen-induced rat mammary tumors which regress after endocrine ablative surgery. The methods of induction and ablation, the histology, endocrine aspects, and various enzyme systems of these tumors have been extensively reviewed (Huggins *et al.*, 1961; Dao, 1964; Archer and Orlando, 1968; Hilf *et al.*, 1971). Certain transplantable rat mammary tumor lines have also provided useful models for understanding the endocrinology of breast cancer (Kim *et al.*, 1963; MacLeod *et al.*, 1964; Gullino *et al.*, 1972).

II. PROLACTIN

A. Rat Mammary Tumors

Prolactin may be the single most important hormone in rat mammary tumor growth (Meites, 1972; Pearson et al., 1972; Smithline et al., 1975):

1. Procedures or agents that stimulate prolactin secretion enhance tumor growth.

(a). Prolactin alone is able to reactivate tumor growth, at least for a short term, after ablation of the ovaries, adrenals, and pituitary gland (Pearson et al., 1969; Nagasawa and Yanai, 1970).

(b). Administration of the tranquilizer perphenazine, which stimulates prolactin secretion (Bogden et al., 1974), increases the number and size of tumors in adrenalectomized–ovariectomized rats (Pearson et al., 1969).

(c). Lesions in the median eminence of the tuber cinereum stimulate release of prolactin and inhibit release of all other pituitary hormones (Meites et al., 1963). Such lesions cause a considerable increase in the size and number of tumors (Clemens et al., 1968; Klaiber et al., 1969). Estradiol benzoate implants into the median eminence of tumor-bearing rats also raise blood prolactin levels over controls and significantly increase the size and number of tumors (Nagasawa and Meites, 1970). These effects of prolactin have been reviewed (Meites et al., 1972).

2. Procedures or agents that diminish prolactin secretion or effectiveness inhibit tumor growth.

(a) Daily administration of antiprolactin antiserum causes tumor regression in 50% of dimethylbenzanthracene (DMBA)-induced tumor-bearing rats, whereas treatment with normal rabbit serum treatment results in only a 13% tumor regression (Butler and Pearson, 1971). Similar results have been reported with antiadenohypophysis serum (Pierpaoli and Sorkin, 1972).

(b) Ergot alkaloids inhibit prolactin secretion, probably by direct action on both pituitary and hypothalamus (Lu, 1971; Wuttke et al., 1971). DMBA mammary tumor growth is inhibited in rats treated with ergot alkaloids (Heuson et al., 1970; Cassell et al., 1971; Stähelin et al., 1971), as is the growth of spontaneous mammary tumors (Quadri and Meites, 1971). Complete remissions have been obtained in 62% of these rat tumors, and a majority of the regressed tumors fail to recur after cessation of treatment (Clemens and Shaar, 1972). A combination of ergocornine and reserpine designed to induce panhypopituitarism was found to be as effective as hypophysectomy in causing remission of DMBA tumors (Welsch et al., 1973). Other agents which depress serum prolactin (pargyline, L-dopa, and lysergic acid diethylamide) inhibit DMBA tumor growth, whereas haloperidol and methyldopa, which elevate serum prolactin, stimulate tumor growth (Quadri *et al.,* 1973a,b). An excellent review of the effect of ergot alkaloids on prolactin secretion and prolactin-dependent processes is available (Floss *et al.,* 1973).

Although prolactin is undoubtedly important in stimulating DMBA tumor growth, other experiments suggest that prolactin may not be solely responsible for hormone dependence. First, growth hormone is also able to stimulate mammary tumor induction in carcinogen-fed hypophysectomized rats (Young, 1961) and promote growth of established tumors following hypophysectomy (Li and Yang, 1975). Second, if DMBA-tumor-bearing rats are ovariectomized and simultaneous lesions are placed in the median eminence to increase prolactin release, the tumors grow at an accelerated pace for only 10–12 days and then regress, even though prolactin levels remain elevated (Clemens *et al.,* 1968; Sinha *et al.,* 1973). The ovarian factor responsible for maintaining tumor growth under these circumstances has not been identified. Third, pregnancy stimulates the growth of experimental tumors (Dao and Sunderland, 1959; Huggins *et al.,* 1962; McCormick and Moon, 1965), while parturition and weaning are followed by regression of a large number of these tumors. The tumor growth-promoting factor of pregnancy is probably placental lactogen (Nagasawa and Yanai, 1973). Since the maintenance of tumor size or growth during lactation depends upon the suckling stimulus and tumors regress if suckling is prevented (McCormick and Moon, 1967; McCormick, 1972), prolactin would appear to be responsible. The true situation is more complex, however, since ovariectomy blocks the stimulatory effects of endogenous or exogenous prolactin on tumor growth and injection of progesterone removes this block (McCormick and Moon, 1967). One interpretation would be that prolactin stimulation of tumor growth under these circumstances is dependent on progesterone, or, alternatively, that the high levels of progesterone, which are under prolactin control in the lactating rat (Tomogane and Yokoyama, 1975), are responsible for the tumor growth.

Finally, the recent demonstration that prolactin can alter steroid metabolism inside DMBA tumor cells provides additional evidence that part of the action of prolactin may be to modulate the direct effects of steroids on tumor cell growth and function (Miller, 1976).

B. Human Breast Cancer

We conclude from animal tumor studies that simple raising or lowering of blood prolactin levels is insufficient to explain breast tumor growth and regression, and this conclusion is supported by studies in human breast cancer. Despite considerable physiological data (Sherwood, 1971), human prolactin has only recently been conclusively shown to be an entity distinct from human growth hormone (Frantz et al., 1972b). There is no doubt that hypophysectomy causes regression of metatastic tumor (Luft et al., 1952). This could be explained by elimination of pituitary prolactin and/or growth hormone, which might be directly supporting tumor growth, or by the removal of gonadotropins and consequent lowering of estrogen and progesterone production by the ovaries, or even by the elimination of adrenocorticotropin leading to reduced adrenal synthesis of estrogen precursors, progesterone, and glucocorticoids. Early attempts to unravel these possibilities led to conflicting results. Pearson et al. (1954) correlated the degree of hypercalcuria with the growth rate of osteolytic metastases in patients with breast cancer, and using this as an index of hormonal stimulation of tumor growth, reported that bovine growth hormone (Pearson et al., 1955) and human growth hormone (Pearson and Ray, 1959) stimulated metastatic mammary carcinoma. This conclusion was not supported by Lipsett and Bergenstal (1960), who found that neither human growth hormone nor ovine prolactin stimulated calcium excretion in breast cancer patients more than in control patients. In addition, both groups (Pearson and Ray, 1959; Lipsett and Bergenstal, 1960) emphasized an important observation: following hypophysectomy, further remissions of breast cancer are not obtained with pharmacologic estrogen or androgen therapy. Furthermore, physiological doses of estrogen do not exacerbate the disease in those hypophysectomized patients who are in remission. These results suggest a central role for the pituitary in human breast tumor growth and in the response to endocrine therapy. However in other studies, the role of prolactin is less clear.

L-Dopa, which suppresses serum prolactin levels (Malarkey et al., 1971; Kleinberg et al., 1971; Friesen et al., 1972), has been administered to patients with metastatic breast cancer with variable results (Dickey and Minton, 1972; Stoll, 1972; Murray et al., 1972; Frantz et al., 1972a, 1973; Minton, 1974). Most agree that L-dopa can acutely lower prolactin levels and that relief of bone pain is frequent in patients with bone metastases. Objective tumor regression is infrequent, however, due perhaps to the incomplete or temporary nature of the prolactin suppression. It has been proposed that the relief of bone pain during L-dopa therapy be used as a simple test to predict those patients who will respond to surgical endocrine ablation, but this proposal has not yet been tested in a controlled study.

Ergot derivatives also effectively suppress prolactin levels in humans (del Pozo et al., 1972; Lemberger et al., 1974; Cleary et al., 1975; Tyson et al., 1975). Unfortunately, objective tumor regressions with these agents are rarely seen (Heuson et al., 1972a; Guerzon and Pearson, 1974; Schultz et al., 1973).

The possibility that patients with breast cancer might have higher average blood levels of prolactin has been refuted in at least four studies (Boyns et al., 1973; Wilson et al., 1974; Kwa et al., 1974; Franks et al., 1974). Nevertheless, two series did report higher prolactin levels in families with a high frequency of breast cancer (Kwa et al., 1974; Henderson et al., 1975). It has been reported that women taking reserpine (which stimulates prolactin secretion in humans) have a higher than normal incidence of breast cancer (Boston Collaborative Drug Surveillance Program, 1974; Armstrong et al., 1974; Heinomen et al., 1974). This has been challenged by two recent studies (Mack et al., 1975; O'Fallon et al., 1975). It should be noted that peak prolactin secretion occurs at night (Sassin et al., 1972, 1973), so that studies of patient populations at risk for breast cancer or with established disease may be of little value if only random daytime prolactin levels are measured.

Finally, the most disconcerting data regarding a primary role for prolactin in human breast cancer growth concern the high prolactin levels accompanying tumor regressions after pituitary stalk section. Ehni and Eckles (1959) noticed that four patients who had undergone stalk section for metastatic breast cancer lactated after the operation, though all four experienced some degree of objective tumor regression. Many years later, these important clinical observations were confirmed by actual measurement of blood levels of prolactin in patients treated with pituitary stalk section for metastatic breast cancer (Turkington et al., 1971). Of 11 such patients, eight experienced objective remissions for periods ranging from 7 months to 12 years, and five of these had elevated prolactin levels during the period of remission. Among the three who showed no objective remission, two had elevated prolactin levels. Thus, in humans as well as in animal models, the biochemical mechanism of mammary tumor regression following endocrine ablation involves more than simple alterations of the blood prolactin level.

C. Mechanism of Prolactin Dependence

Although claims of a singular role for prolactin in hormone dependence may be exaggerated, there is little doubt of prolactin's importance in stimulating several biochemical processes in mammary tissues. These processes have been extensively studied, especially with the organ culture technique, and have been reviewed recently (Turkington et al., 1973). They do not provide any direct clues about the mechanism of hormone dependence.

Other pituitary polypeptide hormones act on their respective target cells through binding to surface membrane receptors. This interaction sets off a chain of events involving generation of cyclic AMP and activation of protein kinase ultimately resulting in target cell function (Gill, 1972). It was reasonable to postulate that mammary cell surfaces also have specific receptor sites to recognize prolactin. Turkington (1970) showed that prolactin covalently linked to Sepharose (so that it theoretically could not enter cells), could still stimulate RNA synthesis in isolated mammary cells. After *in vivo* injection, radioactive prolactin was located on the surface of mammary and other target cells (Birkinshaw and Falconer, 1972; Rajaniemi *et al.*, 1974). Direct measurement of [^{125}I]prolactin binding to membrane particles from rabbit and mouse mammary gland followed (Turkington, 1971; Shiu *et al.*, 1973; Frantz *et al.*, 1974; Shiu and Friesen, 1974; Posner *et al.*, 1974b).

These findings suggested a possible explanation for hormone dependence or autonomy in breast cancer cells: the hormone-dependent tumor cell like the normal mammary cell has retained the surface receptor, whereas the autonomous cell has lost the receptor, and, hence, the ability to recognize and be regulated by prolactin (Costlow *et al.*, 1975b; Kelly *et al.*, 1974; DeSombre *et al.*, 1976; Turkington, 1974). We examined this possibility by comparing prolactin receptors in normal rat mammary tissues and in both hormone-dependent and autonomous rat mammary tumors.

Binding of [^{125}I]prolactin was first determined in tissue slices to avoid the recovery problems inherent in membrane purification procedures. Lactating mammary gland had high-affinity (K_d 2 × 10^{-9} M) saturable binding to approximately 3000 prolactin receptor sites per cell. Only rat or ovine prolactin competed for binding (Costlow *et al.*, 1974; Holcomb *et al.*, 1976).

We then studied two sublines of the transplantable rat mammary carcinoma MTW9. One of the sublines, MTW9-MD, is hormone dependent. It grows in intact rats but regresses promptly following ovariectomy. This tumor has the same number of prolactin-receptor sites as the normal mammary gland and has appreciable numbers of receptor sites for estrogen (ER). In contrast, the autonomous subline, MTW9-MA, which grows in hypophysectomized or ovariectomized rats, contained only one-sixth of the receptor sites for prolactin and estrogen found in the hormone dependent MTW9-MD (Costlow *et al.*, 1975b). These data demonstrate that receptors for prolactin can be either retained or lost during the process of malignant transformation and subsequent mammary tumor growth.

Unfortunately, tumors are not absolutely positive or negative for prolactin receptors. In DMBA tumors, a wide range is seen (Kelly *et al.*, 1974; Costlow *et al.*, 1976; DeSombre *et al.*, 1976; Holdaway and Friesen, 1976), and this has led to proposals utilizing both prolactin receptor and ER data to predict hormone responsiveness (DeSombre *et al.*, 1976). In fact, there is much experimental data which links estrogen and prolactin action.

Prolactin increases the uptake of estradiol into mammary gland explants *in vitro* (Sasaki and Leung, 1974). Furthermore, Vignon and Rochefort (1974, 1976b) have shown a prompt fall of ER in DMBA tumors regressing after ovariectomy. Prolactin injections not only stimulated the tumor to resume growth but restored the concentration of ER. The authors conclude that prolactin sensitizes the mammary tumor to estradiol by stimulating estrogen-receptor sites. Such a stimulation has recently been reported in rat liver (Chamness *et al.*, 1975). The most intriguing new development is the report of a conversion of an ovarian-nonresponsive to an ovarian-responsive mammary tumor strain by chronic stimulation of endogenous prolactin (Diamond *et al.*, 1976). It will be very important to determine whether the new tumors have acquired additional receptor sites for either estrogen or prolactin.

A recent development that may bear on the question of prolactin receptor regulation in mammary tumors comes from studies in rat liver. Independent observations show that prolactin receptors rapidly fall in liver cells following hypophysectomy and can be restored by prolactin (Posner *et al.*, 1974a, 1975; Costlow *et al.*, 1975a). Ovariectomy and thyroidectomy achieve a similar decrease in liver cell prolactin receptors, which can be restored by estradiol and thyroid hormone (Gelato *et al.*, 1975). Such a hormonal regulatory system has not yet been demonstrated for prolactin in mammary tumors, but it has been reported that placental lactogen may increase prolactin receptors in the pregnant rat mammary gland (Holcomb *et al.*, 1976).

The possible causal relationship between the loss of prolactin receptors and the loss of hormone dependence in experimental breast cancer is also complicated by the following observation. The R3230AC transplantable rat mammary carcinoma grows well in ovariectomized female rats and is, therefore, considered hormonally autonomous, yet the tumor can respond to prolactin injections by synthesizing enzymes and specific mRNA's concerned with milk protein synthesis (Turkington, 1974; Hilf *et al.*, 1967; McGuire, 1969; Nardacci and McGuire, 1976). We found a normal complement of prolactin receptor sites in this tumor (Costlow *et al.*, 1974). Clearly, in this case, autonomy arose in the presence of normal prolactin receptors and prolactin responses. One possible explanation of R3230AC's autonomy is suggested by its marked deficiency in estrogen receptor compared to hormone-dependent tumors (McGuire *et al.*, 1971, 1972a). Another explanation is that malignant transformation might sometimes unmask occluded receptors on the mammary cell surface, thereby exposing the tumor cells to stimulation by hormones which do not affect growth of normal mammary tissue. In this case, the tumors might appear autonomous to prolactin manipulation, while they are, in fact, hormone dependent but on different hormones. This situation has actually been reported in certain adrenal tumors (Schorr *et al.*, 1971).

In summary, prolactin can clearly be implicated in the growth of experimental rat mammary tumors. Its role in regulating the growth of human mammary cancer demands further study. Investigation of the events immediately following prolactin binding to receptor deserves high priority.

III. ESTROGEN

Estrogen acts directly on the normal mammary gland to promote growth and differentiation (Lyons *et al.*, 1958; Ahren and Jacobsohn, 1956; Norgren, 1967; Nagasawa and Yanai, 1971a). However, estrogen also stimulates the release of pituitary prolactin, which likewise acts upon the mammary cell (Meites and Nicoll, 1966). Since estrogen cannot support mammary tumor growth in the absence of a pituitary (Sterental *et al.*, 1963), whereas prolactin reportedly supports both normal mammary gland and mammary tumor growth in the absence of ovaries and adrenals (Pearson *et al.*, 1969; Nagasawa and Yanai, 1970), estrogen is considered by many to play only a secondary role in tumor growth and regression (Bradley *et al.*, 1976). Prolactin stimulation of tumor growth in the absence of ovarian steroids is of brief duration, however. If DMBA tumor-bearing rats are ovariectomized and simultaneous lesions are placed in the median eminence to increase prolactin release, the tumors grow at an accelerated pace for only 10–12 days and then regress, even though prolactin levels remain elevated (Clemens *et al.*, 1968; Sinha *et al.*, 1973). Furthermore, the transplantation survival of the MTW9 rat mammary tumor appears to depend on ovarian hormones (Murota and Hollander, 1971), and growth of MTW9 tumors is impaired in rats immunized with estradiol–BSA conjugates (Caldwell *et al.*, 1971). One might summarize the role of physiological estrogen levels as follows: estrogens are probably essential, but not sufficient for growth of certain mammary tumors.

On the other hand, estrogens in pharmacologic doses cause regression of mammary tumors (Pearson and Nasr, 1971). This paradoxical effect of estrogen may involve interference with the prolactin stimulation of growth, since the effect can be overcome by increasing endogenous (Nagasawa and Yanai, 1971b) or exogenous (Meites *et al.*, 1971) prolactin.

There is considerable current information on portions of the intracellular estrogen response mechanism in both rat mammary tumor systems and human breast cancer. We will now examine aspects of this mechanism and its role in endocrine control over mammary cancer cells.

A. Localization of Estrogens in Responsive Tumors

In 1959, two laboratories reported that radioactively labeled estrogen injected *in vivo* into experimental animals was localized in those organs which either respond to estrogen or excrete it (Glascock and Hoekstra, 1959; Jensen and Jacobson, 1960). Soon after, breast cancer patients scheduled for adrenalectomy to remove the source of circulating estrogens were given [^{3}H]hexestrol just prior to surgery. It was discovered that the tumor metastases of the patients responding to the adrenalectomy concentrated a larger fraction of [^{3}H]hexestrol than those of patients who failed to respond (Folca *et al.*, 1961), as if only responsive tumors behaved as estrogen target tissues. Other investigators studying the uptake of radioactive estrogens into human mammary tissue (Pearlman *et al.*, 1969; Ellis *et al.*, 1969; James *et al.*, 1971; Braunsberg *et al.*, 1973) found a correlation between the uptake of estrogen by malignant breast tissue and the response to endocrine therapy, but this correlation was not sufficiently strong to be useful for predicting response in an individual patient.

Similar results were obtained in experimental mammary carcinomas, and hormone-dependent tumors *in vitro* also took up more estrogen than autonomous tumors (King *et al.*, 1965, 1966; Mobbs, 1966, 1969; Sander and Attramadal, 1968; Terenius, 1968, 1972; Jensen *et al.*, 1967). This *in vitro* uptake could be completely inhibited by synthetic estrogen analogues, while the relatively low uptake in other tissues such as muscle could not be inhibited, indicating specificity of the uptake into tumors. From these results, Jensen proposed that the *in vitro* technique might be extended to human tumor tissue samples to predict the response to adrenalectomy. By this time, estrogen receptor had been discovered in target tissues, including tumors (Jensen and DeSombre, 1972; Gorski *et al.*, 1968; Mueller *et al.*, 1972; Bresciani *et al.*, 1969; McGuire and Julian, 1971), and appeared to be responsible for the specific uptake of estrogen by these tissues. Direct studies of the presence and role of receptor in mammary tumors followed and raised the possibility of using the presence of the receptor to predict hormone dependence.

B. Measurement of Estrogen Receptor

There are now several procedures for measurement of ER in cytosols of target tissues (McGuire *et al.*, 1975, 1977; Korenman, 1969). The receptor can be quantitated by demonstration of specific 8 S and 4 S binding of [^{3}H]estradiol on sucrose density gradients (SDG). The dextran-coated-charcoal method (DCC) is equally quantitative and less expensive. Non-receptor-bound [^{3}H]estradiol is removed from specific estradiol-bound receptor by charcoal. The binding data obtained from incubating cytosol with increasing concentrations of hormone can be plotted by the method of Scatchard to determine both the number and affinity of estrogen-binding sites.

Assays based on protamine precipitation of receptor have recently been developed to measure both free and hormone bound receptor from cytoplasmic (Chamness et al., 1975) and nuclear (Zava et al., 1976) extracts. The receptor is precipitated with protamine, then the solid phase protamine–receptor complex is incubated with radioactive estradiol. Incubation at 30° or 37°C permits exchange of any previously bound nonradioactive ligand, while at 4°C only unoccupied receptor is radiolabeled. The combination of these assays has the unique advantage of using only one basic technique to assess both free and bound estrogen receptor sites in tumor cytosol and nuclei. This procedure could prove particularly useful where premenopausal cancer patients might have high levels of plasma estrogens that would transfer cytoplasmic ER to nuclear sites, making them inaccessible to assay by SDG or DCC. Since the presence of free cytoplasmic ER in tumors now has prognostic value in helping to predict the proper type of treatment for breast cancer patients (see below), those premenopausal women who have ER masked by endogenous estrogens might not be given treatment that would be of greatest benefit.

C. Rat Mammary Tumors as a Model System

Because of many similarities to human breast cancer, DMBA-induced rat mammary tumors have been extensively studied to provide insight into the mechanism of hormonal influence in tumor growth. These tumors have complex hormonal requirements for growth (Leung and Sasaki, 1975; Bradley et al., 1976) and have ER values that range widely (DeSombre et al., 1976; Leung and Sasaki, 1975; Nomura et al., 1974). Absent or low levels of tumor ER are associated with a failure to regress after ovariectomy, whereas the majority of ER-positive tumors regress following endocrine ablative procedures. The finding of ER-positive DMBA tumors which do not respond is similar to the situation in human breast cancer and demands further study. It has been suggested (Shyamala, 1972) that the receptor might be defective in nonresponding tumors, but nuclear translocation of ER is normal in rat DMBA tumors (Vignon and Rochefort, 1976a). In addition, chromatin from autonomous rat mammary tumors is capable of binding ER under cell-free conditions (McGuire et al., 1972a,b). It is fair to summarize that in DMBA rat mammary tumors, ER may be essential to hormonally regulated growth and regression, but the mere presence of ER in a tumor does not guarantee that the tumor will behave in a hormone-dependent fashion.

D. Estrogen Receptor in Human Breast Tumors

The properties of the estrogen receptor found in hormone-dependent rat tumors have now been demonstrated in human mammary tumors as well (McGuire and De La Garza, 1973a). In ER-positive tumors, Scatchard plots of the binding data from either DCC or protamine assays usually reveal a single class of receptor sites with a very high-affinity binding component (K_d 10^{-10} M) (McGuire, 1973; McGuire and De La Garza, 1973b). The receptor sediments primarily at 8 S in low-salt sucrose gradients and 4 S in high-salt gradients (McGuire and De La Garza, 1973a).

ER values in primary tumors range from 0 to almost 1000 fmoles per milligram of cytosol protein (McGuire et al., 1975b). The wide range of values may be due to a combination of factors. First, since tumors commonly exhibit cellular heterogeneity, the ER content might vary directly with the proportion of those cells that contain cytoplasmic ER. Early reports indicated no obvious correlation between the histology of a tumor and its ability to bind E (McGuire et al., 1975). More recently, a strong association between ER and invasive lobular carcinoma has been described, while a low frequency of ER is seen in tumors with a prominent local lymphocyte reaction (Rosen et al., 1975). Second, one might suppose that contamination of a tumor specimen by normal mammary cells containing ER would give variable assay results. But this is not the case since ER cannot be readily detected in nonlactating human breast cells (Feherty et al., 1971; Korenman and Dukes, 1970; Hähnel et al., 1971). This last point has been confirmed in animal studies in which E uptake or actual ER levels are very low in virgin mammary glands, but then markedly increase during lactation (Puca and Bresciani, 1969; Wittliff et al., 1972; Shyamala and Nandi, 1972; Hseuh et al., 1973). Finally, the amount of endogenous E secreted by the patient must be considered, since endogenous E would occupy ER sites and make them unavailable for assay using conventional techniques. This may at least partially explain why the highest values for tumor ER are seen in postmenopausal patients. Exchange techniques for measuring ER occupied by endogenous E are now available (Katzenellenbogen et al., 1973; Truong et al., 1973; Daehnfeldt, 1974; Chamness et al., 1975; Zava et al., 1976).

Jensen's original suggestion that the presence of ER in a human breast tumor might indicate that the tumor is hormone dependent and will regress with appropriate endocrine manipulation (Jensen et al., 1967) has now been evaluated. A number of laboratories using a variety of techniques have assayed ER in breast tumor specimens, and data on clinical response to endocrine therapy are now available in many of these cases. On July 18–19,

1974, an international workshop was held in Bethesda, Maryland, to correlate these data (McGuire *et al.,* 1975a). Details of both ER assay procedures and clinical evaluation criteria were examined, and 436 treatment trials in 380 patients were ultimately accepted. The general pattern of results was the same for all investigators, and the collective data are summarized below.

1. Surgical Ablation (Castration, Adrenalectomy, Hypophysectomy)

Thirty-three percent of 211 treatment trials yielded objective tumor regression. Of the 94 trials in patients with zero tumor ER values, only 8 (8%) were successful, whereas 59 (55%) of the 107 trials in patients with positive tumor ER values succeeded. Patients with borderline tumor ER values had a 30% response rate.

2. Additive Therapy (Pharmacologic Doses of Estrogens, Androgens, and Glucocorticoids)

Thirty-four percent of 170 trials yielded objective tumor regressions. Of the 82 trials in patients with zero tumor ER values, 7 (8%) were successful, whereas 51 (60%) of the 85 trials in patients with positive tumor ER values succeeded.

3. Miscellaneous Therapy

Twenty-seven percent of 55 trials yielded responses to a variety of endocrine therapies including antiestrogens, aminogluthethimide, etc. Of 32 trials in patients with zero tumor ER values, 5 (16%) were successful, whereas 10 (43%) of 23 trials in patients with positive ER values succeeded.

There remains little doubt that estrogen-receptor values can be helpful in predicting the results of endocrine therapy for metastatic breast cancer. It is clear that if a patient has a zero tumor ER value the chances of tumor regression in response to endocrine therapy are minimal. A large number of patients can, thus, be spared unrewarding major endocrine ablative therapy if ER assays are performed routinely. When the tumor ER value is positive, the response to endocrine therapy is 55–60%. This single piece of evidence when coupled with available clinical prognostic factors, such as menopausal status, disease-free interval, site of dominant lesion, and especially response to previous hormonal therapies should permit the practicing oncologist to select or reject endocrine therapy with considerable confidence.

Why did 45% of the patients with positive tumor ER values not respond to endocrine therapy? Several possible reasons have been discussed. First, the role of other hormone receptors must be considered, since ER is only one part of the complex hormonal control system which influences mammary cell growth and function. The mechanism(s) by which these other hormones affect breast tumor growth must be equally important, since receptors for prolactin, progestins, and androgens have also been identified in breast tumors; these are discussed elsewhere in this review. Perhaps simultaneous analysis for these receptor proteins in addition to ER will be helpful in eliminating the 45% of those patients who have positive tumor ER values but do not respond to any type of hormonal manipulation. Second, tumors might contain a heterogeneous population of hormone-dependent and autonomous cell types and, therefore, express a mixed response to hormone therapy. Such conditions could explain why some ER-positive tumors show only partial or short-term remission before progressing to a completely autonomous condition. Third, tumors might contain defective cytoplasmic receptor proteins that prevent the induction of the incompletely known sequence of biochemical events ultimately leading to tumor regression upon hormone therapy. Defective receptor proteins have in fact been demonstrated in several experimental systems (Shyamala, 1972; Vignon and Rochefort, 1976a), but no correlations to human tumor responses have yet been made. Fourth, it has been suggested that specific nuclear acceptor sites for receptor are required for hormone action (Buller et al., 1975), and it is possible that absent or defective sites would lead to insensitivity to ER. The evidence for such sites remains controversial (Chamness et al., 1973, 1974; Shepherd et al., 1974; Clark and Peck, 1976).

E. Antiestrogens

The discovery that certain estrogen analogues could antagonize estrogen stimulation of target tissues was promptly applied to the problem of breast cancer. Growth of DMBA tumors could be inhibited by clomiphene (Schulz et al., 1969) or nafoxidine (Terenius, 1971b; DeSombre and Arbogast, 1974) or tamoxifen (Jordan and Koerner, 1976), though there exists one report of tumor growth-promoting activity of these agents (Gallez et al., 1973). Tumor induction was also prevented by nafoxidine (Heuson et al., 1972c). The ability of tamoxifen to cause regression of a DMBA tumor was highly correlated with the presence of estrogen receptor in a biopsy of that tumor (Jordan and Jaspan, 1976).

The positive results of these experiments led to clinical trials of antiestrogens for therapy of breast cancer patients. Tamoxifen was used successfully (O'Halloran and Maddock, 1974; Cole et al., 1971; Ward, 1973) as was nafoxidine (Heuson et al., 1972b, 1975; Bloom and Boesen, 1974) and clomiphene (Hecker et al., 1974). The remission rates were reported to be around 30%, the same as those achieved by other endocrine therapies. And as with other endocrine therapies, success was correlated with the presence of estrogen receptor in the patient's tumor (McGuire *et al.*, 1975a), though the correlation did not appear to be quite as good as with other endocrine therapies.

The mechanism of action of antiestrogens has been studied principally in the rat uterus. They have been found, not only to bind to the estrogen receptor (Terenius, 1971a; Rochefort *et al.*, 1972a), but to translocate this receptor into the nucleus (Clark *et al.*, 1973) and even to initiate early estrogenic responses (Katzenellenbogen and Ferguson, 1975). A complete response does not develop, however, and the cells remain for a time refractory to the action of active estrogens. Because some antiestrogens retain receptor in the nucleus for many days, in contrast to several hours for active estrogens (Clark *et al.*, 1973), this retention was at first thought to be an essential feature of their effect. More recent work has shown that some do not share this property, though apparently all fail to replenish receptor in the cytoplasm (Clark *et al.*, 1974), which may explain insensitivity to later estrogen action. Nothing is yet known of the differences between receptor–estrogen and receptor–antiestrogen complexes in the nucleus which might account for the differences in their activity.

Even less is known of antiestrogen action in human breast cancer, beyond the fact that antiestrogens bind to tumor estrogen receptor (Jordan and Koerner, 1975; Garola *et al.*, 1974) and decrease DNA synthesis in a human breast cancer cell line (Lippman and Bolan, 1975). It has been suggested that a principal effect may be the reduction of estrogen-stimulated prolactin levels (Heuson *et al.*, 1972a; Jordan *et al.*, 1975; Leung *et al.*, 1975), but this effect does not seem to be sufficient to account for the response in rat DMBA tumors (Jordan and Koerner, 1976). It is also possible that antiestrogens inhibit ovarian synthesis of estradiol. These questions are under active investigation.

Because of the protective effect of early pregnancy against development of breast cancer, combined with the increased estradiol excretion seen during pregnancy (Cole and MacMahon, 1969; MacMahon *et al.*, 1973) and low urinary excretion of estriol in breast cancer patients (Dickinson *et al.*, 1974), it has been proposed that estriol has significant anticarcinogenic properties by acting as an antiestrogen, competing with estradiol for the cytoplasmic receptor sites in mammary tissues (Lemon, 1969, 1970, 1975; Lemon *et al.*, 1971). This possibility now seems unlikely because the relatively weak binding of estriol to the receptor compared to estradiol would require large amounts of estriol to compete successfully (Korenman, 1969), while it has recently been shown that there is actually more unconjugated estradiol than estriol present during pregnancy (Loriaux *et al.*, 1972;

Lipsett, 1971). In addition, estriol itself is able to enter target cell nuclei and to induce the synthesis of an estrogen-specific protein in the rat uterus; the degree of stimulation is proportional to the amount of estriol bound to the cytoplasmic receptor and to the amount of estriol found in the nucleus (Ruh *et al.*, 1973). Finally, estriol has now been shown to be carcinogenic in mice (Rudali *et al.*, 1975). Although it is easy to criticize parts of the estriol hypothesis on theoretical grounds, the very important observations regarding the protective effect of early pregnancy on the subsequent development of breast cancer should not be ignored. With a few exceptions (Sherman and Korenman, 1974), new approaches to understanding the relevance of this observation are notably lacking.

F. Systemic Approaches to Reducing Estrogen Production

In castrated premenopausal or in postmenopausal breast cancer patients, estrogen precursors are secreted by the adrenal gland and converted to estrogens by peripheral tissues (Barlow *et al.*, 1969; Longcope, 1971; Kirschner and Taylor, 1972; Grodin *et al.*, 1973; Judd *et al.*, 1974). This has been the rationale for surgical adrenalectomy in these patients. One alternative to surgical removal of the adrenals has been to administer pharmacologic doses of glucocorticoid, thus inhibiting ACTH release and producing adrenal atrophy. This pharmacologic approach results in an overall remission rate of 25% (Lipton and Santen, 1974), which may be somewhat less than achieved by surgical adrenalectomy (Dao, 1972). This fact coupled with the severe side effects of high doses of glucocorticoids has prompted another approach to adrenal suppression. The anticonvulsive drug aminogluthethimide (AG) produces a block in steroidogenesis at an early step in the biosynthetic pathway (Dexter *et al.*, 1967; Cash *et al.*, 1967). However, reduction in cortisol production by AG causes a large compensatory increase in ACTH production, leading to adrenal steroidogenesis. The logical attempt to inhibit this AG-induced rise in ACTH by adding physiological amounts of dexamethasone (dex) to the regimen met with only limited success (Hall *et al.*, 1969; Griffiths *et al.*, 1973) until it was discovered that AG accelerates dex metabolism. Using higher doses of dex with AG (Santen *et al.*, 1974), complete adrenal suppression has been achieved for as long as 19 months, and objective tumor regression occurred in 8 of 22 patients without producing cushingoid side effects.

AG/dex treatment, thus, appears to achieve an effective nonsurgical adrenalectomy for postmenopausal breast cancer patients. The treatment also seems likely, at least in theory, to provide an alternative to ovariectomy for premenopausal patients when administered along with antiestrogens or with a gonadotropin inhibitor.

IV. PROGESTERONE

A. Clinical Effects in Breast Cancer

Because of the cyclic changes of blood estrogen and progesterone levels that occur in females and these hormones' interrelationships in regulating target tissue development and growth, it was inevitable that progesterone would be studied for its effect on breast cancer. Although progesterone itself is not a carcinogen, it may be a potent target-specific cocarcinogen for induction of mammary tumors by viral or chemical agents (Poel, 1968). The hormone has also been implicated in both tumor enhancement and tumor suppression.

That progesterone plays a role in stimulating tumor growth is suggested by the pioneering studies of Huggins et al. (1962; Huggins and Yang, 1962; Huggins, 1965). They showed that pregnancy promoted the growth of DMBA-induced rat mammary tumors. Administration of progesterone to intact rats accelerated the appearance of tumors, increased the number of tumors, and augmented the growth rate of established tumors.

Parturition and weaning are followed by regression of a large number of pregnancy-stimulated tumors (Huggins et al., 1962; Dao and Sunderland, 1959; McCormick and Moon, 1965). The principal tumor growth-promoting factors of pregnancy and lactation are probably placental lactogen (Nagasawa and Yanai, 1973) and prolactin (McCormick and Moon, 1967; McCormick, 1972), as noted previously. Ovariectomy, however, blocks the stimulatory effects of endogenous or exogenous prolactin on tumor growth, and injection of progesterone removes this block (McCormick and Moon, 1967). Either prolactin stimulation of tumors under these circumstances is dependent upon progesterone, or, alternatively, the high levels of circulating progesterone stimulated by prolactin in the lactating rat (Tomogane et al., 1975) are responsible for the tumor growth. This does not mean that progesterone alone is responsible for maintaining rat mammary tumor growth, since, in these experiments, the animals had both high prolactin levels and intact adrenal glands. On the other hand, they do suggest that progesterone plays an important physiological role in stimulating tumor growth.

In contrast to the stimulatory effects of progesterone described above, progesterone can induce rat mammary tumor regression or prevent tumor appearance, at least when combined with moderate to large doses of estrogen (Huggins et al., 1962; McCormick and Moon, 1973). In humans, too, the percentage of breast tumor regressions in response to a progesterone–estrogen combination is generally higher than with progesterone alone (Muggia et al., 1968). Postmenopausal patients with endogenous estrogen levels (presumably of adrenal origin) sufficient to cornify the vaginal mucosa have a 29% tumor remission rate with progesterone therapy, whereas patients with an atrophic vaginal smear experience only 6% remission rate with progesterone alone (Stoll, 1967a). These data would support a requirement for estrogen in progesterone-mediated tumor regression and may be due to estrogen stimulation of progesterone-receptor synthesis (see below). In fact, since moderate to large doses of estrogens alone can cause mammary tumor regression in rats (Pearson and Nasr, 1971; Nagasawa and Yanai, 1971b; Meites et al., 1971) and humans (Council on Drugs, 1960), it is necessary to ask whether addition of the progestational agent accomplishes more than the estrogen alone. The answer would seem to be yes, at least in some cases, because patients whose tumors have failed to regress following treatment with high dose estrogen alone have responded to a combination of estrogen–progesterone (Growley and MacDonald, 1965; Stoll, 1967b,c).

The mechanism by which progesterone promotes tumor regression is not clear. Large doses of synthetic progestins can cause significant lowering of serum LH and cortisol levels, suggesting that alteration of pituitary function may be involved (Sadoff and Lusk, 1974), but at least four previously hypophysectomized patients are reported to have had breast tumor regression following combinations of estrogen–progesterone (Landau et al., 1962; Kennedy, 1965). This is in contrast to the lack of tumor response to estrogens alone in hypophysectomized patients (Pearson and Ray, 1959; Lipsett and Bergenstal, 1960; Kennedy and French, 1965).

In sum, the specific mechanisms involved in progesterone-mediated breast tumor growth and regression are poorly understood. However, the hormone's metabolism, its binding to specific receptor proteins, and its effect on the actions of other steroid hormones have been extensively studied in several target tissues.

B. Subcellular Metabolism of Progesterone

Progesterone is a precursor common to estrogens, androgens, and adrenal hormones. The uptake and metabolic fates of progesterone have been extensively investigated in uteri (Bryson and Sweat, 1969; Armstrong and King, 1971; Hashimoto et al., 1968; Egert and Maass, 1974; Wiest, 1963, 1971; Collins and Jewkes, 1974), mammary gland (Lawson and Pearlman, 1964; Chatterton, 1971), and other target tissues (Podratz et al., 1974; Tabei et al., 1974; O'Malley et al., 1969; Morgan and Wilson, 1970). The results and interpretations of these studies have often been quite contradictory, for the following reasons. They have been performed in a variety of different tissues from different species under *in vivo, in vitro,* or cell-free conditions. In some cases, the progesterone concentration has been high, and, in others, it has been low. Certain studies deal with normal animals, others with pseudopregnant or pregnant animals. Metabolic patterns differ in estrogen treated versus castrated animals. It is perhaps understandable, then, that a simple representative metabolic scheme cannot be presented. Despite these limitations, certain observations are pertinent to the present discussion.

Although studies of progesterone metabolism and excretion in breast cancer patients reveal no major differences from control patients, the intracellular metabolism of progesterone by the tumor itself may be quite important. It has been shown that certain human breast tumors can synthesize progesterone from pregnenolone, which means that the tumor itself can control intracellular hormone concentration (Deshpande, 1975).

In contrast to estrogens, where intracellular metabolism does not seem to play an important regulatory role, progesterone can be extensively metabolized in a manner analogous to androgens, where testosterone is converted intracellularly to an active metabolite, dihydrotestosterone, and an inactive product, androstanediol (Bruchovsky and Wilson, 1968; Wilson, 1972). Lawson and Pearlman (1964) administered [^{3}H]progesterone as a continuous infusion and found that the mammary gland of the pregnant rat was able to concentrate tritium above plasma levels. In addition to progesterone, small amounts of 20α-hydroxypregn-4-en-3-one (20α-OHPg) were found. The pattern of metabolites varied with the endocrine status of the gland: 20α-OHPg dominated the pregnant gland, whereas ring A reduction to dihydroprogesterone (5α-DHPg) was higher in the lactating gland (Chatterton, 1971; Chatterton et al., 1969). Since estrogen priming is required for full functional expression of progesterone activity, its effect on formation of metabolites may provide a clue to their physiological role. Saffran et al. (1974) have shown that, at physiological progesterone concentrations, the effect of estrogen is to inhibit reductase activity. At high progesterone concentrations, the effect is reversed. Progesterone concentration does not affect 20α-OH steroid dehydrogenase activity, which is increased by estrogen at low or high progesterone levels.

Thus, the role of estrogen on progesterone metabolism appears to be twofold. First, it increases PgR (see below) and, thereby, reduces progesterone metabolism because the hormone is protected by receptor binding. Second, it increases the concentration of reducing enzymes, particularly 20α-OHSD, thereby increasing metabolism. The net effect of estrogen treatment is balanced between increased binding and increased degradation and the concentration of progesterone determines which effect predominates.

One serious problem in the earlier studies was that the presence and importance of an intracellular receptor for progesterone had not been appreciated. Although it is perhaps incorrect to assume that all progesterone effects must operate through a receptor mechanism, a good place to begin would be to see which metabolites in a given tissue can bind to the progesterone receptor or perhaps to some other receptor, and whether this binding correlates with biologic activity. This could give insight as to whether a certain metabolic pathway is critical to the action of the hormone or whether the pathway is primarily a means of degradation and excretion. In mammalian tissues, [^{3}H]5α-DHPg does not bind to a receptor, the unlabeled hormone does not compete for progesterone binding to PgR, and neither 5α-DHPg nor 3α-hydroxy-5α-pregnan-20-one possess progestational activity (Leavitt and Grossman, 1974; Coffey, 1973). Therefore, it appears that these metabolites serve little biologic function in mammals.

Strott (1974) has studied the chick oviduct to show which metabolites can bind to PgR in this tissue and whether this binding correlates with biologic activity. In unstimulated oviducts, essentially no bound progesterone can be found. In marked contrast to this, after estrogen stimulation 70% of protein-bound hormone is unreacted progesterone. Therefore, as in mammals, in estrogen-primed chicks, progesterone is the major bound hormone, though some 5α-DHPg is also bound. In the chick, unlike the mammal, the biologic activity of 5α-DHPg may reside in its ability to compete for progesterone binding to PgR (O'Malley and Schrader, 1972).

In the absence of evidence for a functional role of progesterone metabolites in mammals, their significance remains to be determined, and their formation may simply serve to terminate the action of progesterone. One must conclude that the capacity to elicit a progestational effect resides in the progesterone molecule itself, and that it acts without metabolic transformation, as supported by the demonstration of specific progesterone-binding proteins in a variety of target tissues and cells.

C. Progesterone Receptors

We now turn to studies of progesterone receptor (PgR) and its dependence on estrogen priming. Extensive investigations, using guinea pig uterus, unequivocally demonstrated PgR in a mammal (Faber et al., 1972b; Milgrom et al., 1973; Atger et al., 1974; Kontula et al., 1974b; Freifeld et al., 1974; Philibert and Raynaud, 1974; Feil and Bardin, 1975). The receptor migrates at 6–8 S in sucrose gradients and does not bind glucocorticoids. Uterine levels of PgR are maximum at proestrus and fall progressively during estrus and postestrus to a 16-fold lower level in diestrus. Injection of estrogen causes an eight-fold rise in PgR within 24 hours, which can be prevented by inhibition of protein or RNA synthesis.

14. Hormones and Their Receptors in Breast Cancer

The normal half-life of PgR is approximately 3–5 days, but an injection of progesterone will deplete the uterine cytoplasm of PgR within 3 hours. Evidence for nuclear translocation of PgR is available from direct biochemical and autoradiographic studies. Similar conclusions have been reached about PgR in the hamster (Leavitt and Grossman, 1974; Leavitt et al., 1974), rabbit (Faber et al., 1972a, 1973; Davies et al., 1974), mouse (Feil et al., 1972; Philibert and Raynaud, 1973), rat (Faber et al., 1972a; Feil et al., 1972; Philibert and Raynaud, 1973; Saffran et al., 1973; Hsueh et al., 1974), and human (Kontula et al., 1973; Smith et al., 1974; Young and Cleary, 1974). In the latter two species, PgR has been difficult to demonstrate reproducibly because the majority of radioactive progesterone binds in the 4 S region of the sucrose gradient, making it difficult to distinguish PgR from the corticosteroid-binding globulin. With incorporation of glycerol into buffers or gradients, the receptor complex is stabilized (Young and Cleary, 1974), and a specific, high-affinity (K_d 3–8 × 10^{-9} M) 7 S binding component is seen occasionally in myometria from women treated with estrogen (Kontula et al., 1973), in endometrium obtained from proliferative (estrogen-dominated) tissues (Young and Cleary, 1974; Pollow et al., 1974), in hyperplastic endometrium (Haukkamaa and Luukkainen, 1974), and in endometrial carcinoma (Pollow et al., 1974).

The receptor is precipitated by ammonium sulfate (Kontula et al., 1974a), and this property has been used in its purification (Smith et al., 1975). The pure receptor (which migrates as a single band of molecular weight (MW) 110,000 on SDS polyacrylamide gels) sediments at 3.7 S on sucrose gradients (after elution with hypertonic salt), has a K_d of ∼ 10^{-9} M and does not bind hydrocortisone. The purified receptor–hormone complex will bind to nuclei; the nuclear bound form also sediments at 3.7 S.

The most exhaustive studies of progesterone receptor (PgR) have been done in the estrogen-primed chick oviduct. In this tissue, administration of a single dose of progesterone *in vivo* stimulates chromatin template capacity, DNA-dependent RNA polymerase activity, and synthesis of a specific messenger RNA, culminating with induction of the specific protein avidin (O'Malley et al., 1969). Unlabeled progesterone, its active metabolites, and testosterone (a good inducer of avidin) block [^{3}H]progesterone binding to the receptor (Sherman et al., 1970). Progesterone receptor concentration is increased 20-fold by estradiol (Toft and O'Malley, 1972). The receptor has been purified to homogeneity and found to consist of two similar subunits which have distinctly different affinities for DNA and chromatin (Schrader et al., 1972).

Although the normal breast is also a target of progesterone action, virtually no information about receptor binding of the hormone exists. After injection, an apparent selective accumulation of progesterone by human breast tissue has been described (Deshpande et al., 1967a); this property seems to be lost in neoplastic tissue (Ellis et al., 1969). Terenius (1973) used charcoal-resistant radioactivity of cytosols containing [^{3}H]progesterone and excess hydrocortisone to indicate the presence of a progesterone binder in human and rat mammary carcinomas. Attempts to demonstrate receptors directly in normal mammary tissue using progesterone have been unsuccessful, despite the fact that glucocorticoid receptors (which are often difficult to distinguish from PgR) are present (Shyamala, 1973; Gardner and Wittliff, 1973a). Recent demonstration of PgR in human breast cancer will be discussed below.

This survey of PgR in various tissues fails to explain progesterone-induced regression and stimulation of experimental and human breast cancers, but it may provide important clues about the estrogen requirement for progesterone effects. Most important is the stimulation of PgR following estrogen priming. Estrogen modulation of PgR levels is probably a direct effect on the target cell and not mediated by the pituitary, since in ovariectomized, adrenalectomized, and hypophysectomized rats uterine PgR levels are restored by estradiol but not by prolactin injections (Horwitz, 1975). In addition to controlling PgR levels, the estrogen requirement for progesterone action may be due to estrogen's role in regulating progesterone metabolism.

D. Progesterone Interrelationship with Other Steroid Hormones

Progesterone may control breast tumor growth or regression in several ways. The simplest mechanism involves a direct effect of the hormone on the tumor. However, progesterone can also modify the actions of the other steroid hormones, which influence the mammary gland, and this may form the basis for interhormonal control mechanisms.

1. Estrogens

The ability of progesterone to antagonize and/or modify the action of estrogen is well documented (Hsueh et al., 1975; Bullock and Wellen, 1974). Tamoxifen and nafoxidine, two widely used antiestrogens, exhibit progesteronelike effects (Armstrong and More, 1974; Heuson et al., 1972c; Hsueh et al., 1976). Hsueh et al. (1976) have shown that after depletion of cytoplasmic ER by high-dose estrogen treatment, progesterone blocks the overshoot of ER seen during replenishment. They propose that this reduction of ER is correlated with reduced sensitivity of the uterus to estrogen. There is no evidence, however, that progesterone affects replenishment of

ER after physiological estrogen treatments or alters basal ER levels. In sum, estrogen and progesterone may exert feedback control on each other in the target tissue. Estradiol pretreatment enhances tissue sensitivity to progesterone through increased PgR levels. Progesterone, in turn, may modify cytoplasmic ER and redirect the cell's ability to respond to estradiol.

2. *Androgens*

The androgenic properties of progestins are well known, and fetal virilization can result from their use in man (Voorhess, 1967). Progestins can masculinize the reproductive tract of rat fetuses (Suchowsky and Junkmann, 1961) and can mimic androgen effects in several organs (Mowszowicz *et al.*, 1974; Fahim and Hall, 1970; Bullock *et al.*, 1975; Naqvi *et al.*, 1969). Recently, Bullock *et al.* (1975) and Mowszowicz *et al.* (1974) have demonstrated that progestins can be either synandrogenic (by potentiating androgen effects) or antiandrogenic (by inhibiting these effects), depending on the steroid structure, dose, and tissue. If androgens have similar modifying effects on progesterone actions, it may be one reason why they are effective in treatment of hormone-dependent breast cancer. Although the mechanism of androgen-induced regression of breast tumors is not known, androgens cause regressions of fetal mammary buds (Kratochwil, 1971) and may have similar effects on dedifferentiated malignant cells. It is possible that progestin-induced tumor regression is a reflection of the progestins' androgenic properties.

3. *Glucocorticoids*

By far, the most familiar model for the interaction of two differing steroids is that proposed by Rousseau *et al.* (1972) to explain the inhibitory effects of progestins and the stimulatory effects of glucocorticoids on tyrosine aminotransferase production in rat hepatoma tissue culture (HTC) cells. Competition by progestins for glucocorticoid binding has also been demonstrated in mammary carcinomas (Gardner and Wittliff, 1973b; Shyamala, 1974) and lactating mammary glands (Shyamala, 1973; Gardner and Wittliff, 1973a). Since glucocorticoids are involved in mammary gland maturation, it is possible that progestins may affect mammary tumors by modifying glucocorticoid action.

We have recently shown that MCF-7, a stable cell line derived from a human mammary carcinoma, contains receptors for progestins, androgens, glucocorticoids, and estrogens. These cells may prove useful for studying interrelationships between the binding and biologic actions of these four steroids and their role in tumor endocrine response (Horwitz *et al.*, 1975a).

E. **Progesterone Receptors in Human Breast Cancer**

As discussed previously, around 40% of human breast cancers fail to respond to endocrine therapy in spite of the presence of estrogen receptor. However, since binding to receptors is only an early step in hormone action, it is possible that, in ER+ tumors where endocrine manipulations fail, the lesion is at a later stage. An ideal marker of an endocrine-responsive tumor would, therefore, be a measurable product of hormone action, rather than the initial binding step.

Because in estrogen target tissues the synthesis of PgR depends on the action of estrogen (Freifeld et al., 1974), we investigated the possibility that PgR might be such a marker. If so, it would be expected that PgR would be rare in tumors which lack ER. The presence of PgR in tumors containing ER would indicate that the tumor is capable of synthesizing at least one end product under estrogen regulation, and that the tumor remains endocrine responsive. Conversely, the prospect of a successful response to therapy would be low in tumors with ER but no PgR.

We have used 8 S binding of the synthetic progestin $[^3H]R5020$ (Philibert and Raynaud, 1973) to identify PgR in human breast cancer tissue (Horwitz and McGuire, 1975; Horwitz et al., 1975b). We have now determined PgR and ER in 236 human mammary tumors. Of 64 ER-negative tumors, only 5 (8%) had PgR, while 107 of 172 (62%) ER positive tumors had PgR. These percentages approximate the response rate to endocrine therapy based on ER, so that this result is consistent with the hypothesis that PgR is a marker of endocrine-responsive tumors. Confirmation of this hypothesis requires direct correlation of the presence of PgR with objectively defined clinical remission. Our preliminary data is encouraging. We find that, in cases where ER is positive and PgR negative, successful response rate is very low, analogous to the response rates seen with ER-negative tumors. In contrast, if both receptors are present, remissions are seen in a larger percentage of patients than would be predicted on the basis of ER alone. However, it should be emphasized that this is very preliminary data, representing only the simplest cases in which receptor measurements were performed on a single biopsy and response to a single trial of endocrine therapy is involved.

Most questions remain unsolved. How does one interpret contradictory responses to one or more therapeutic trials? What is the effect of previous therapy on receptor levels in multiple biopsies or metastases? How do menopausal status or menstrual cycle affect PgR levels in biopsies? Is measurement of only cytoplasmic receptors an adequate representation of the total receptor content of the cell? And, in considering cytoplasmic receptors, what constitutes a positive assay for PgR? How are we to interpret the tumors which have no 8 S binding but considerable suppressible 4 S? Finally, we have shown that human breast tumor cells can contain receptors for at least four steroid hormones. How are we to incorporate androgen and glucocorticoid receptor data in estimating the response potential of a tumor?

V. GLUCOCORTICOIDS

Glucocorticoids affect a wide variety of normal tissues. In the rat mammary gland, they are required along with prolactin to support lactation (Turkington et al., 1973), and their availability limits the rate of milk production (Thatcher and Tucker, 1970a,b). Experiments with mammary gland explants have indicated that proliferation and maintenance of rough endoplasmic reticulum is a primary direct effect of the glucocorticoids in lactation (Oka and Topper, 1971). Spermidine may mediate these effects, since Oka et al. (1974) recently showed that spermidine is increased by glucocorticoids and can replace them in inducing casein and α-lactalbumin synthesis in explants; the glucocorticoid effect is abolished by specific inhibition of spermidine synthesis.

A specific receptor protein for glucocorticoids has been described in a number of target tissues. Like other steroid receptors, it appears to be localized in the cytoplasm and to be translocated to the cell nucleus after interaction with glucocorticoids (King and Mainwaring, 1974). There is little definite information on its mechanism of action. Though specific acceptor sites for binding the receptor in the nucleus have been proposed to be on the DNA of hepatoma cells (Baxter et al., 1972), receptor binding to DNA was not found to be saturable (Rousseau et al., 1974), so that other components must also be involved if such acceptor sites are actually present. A glucocorticoid binder found among the nonhistone proteins of liver nuclei has properties similar to those of the cytoplasmic receptor, suggesting that it may not be a separate component (Defer et al., 1974). The action of glucocorticoid receptor as studied in hepatoma cells has been recently reviewed (Rousseau, 1975).

In liver and hepatoma tissue, the action of the hormone-receptor complex is largely inductive, while, in lymphocytes and lymphoma cells, its action is inhibitory and ultimately leads to cell death (Munck and Wira, 1970). Most glucocorticoid-resistant cells derived from established lymphoma lines and isolated resistant human leukemic lymphoblasts are found to have lost their cytoplasmic receptors (Hollander and Chiu, 1966; Baxter et al., 1971; Lippman et al., 1973). It is interesting, however, that about 10% of resistant cell lines contain an altered receptor that cannot enter the nuclei, while another

10% have another type of nonfunctional receptor (Sibley and Tomkins, 1974; Gehring and Tomkins, 1974; Yamamoto et al., 1974). Clearly, more than one lesion can exist in the pathway from hormone binding to response.

Glucocorticoids have been used extensively in the treatment of human cancer, especially in malignancies of lymphatic origin. They have also been found to inhibit mammary tumor growth in a number of animal models, including the R3230AC (Sparks et al., 1955; Hilf et al., 1965), though paradoxically they may also be required to permit tumor induction by chemical carcinogens (Kornel, 1973) and appear to induce mouse mammary tumor virus as well (McGrath, 1971; Young et al., 1975). The effectiveness of glucocorticoids in treatment of human breast cancer was discussed earlier. It should be noted that, in a recent investigation by Pihl et al. (1975), regressions due to prednisone treatment occurred only when tumors contained ER. This would suggest that glucocorticoid therapy has features in common with ablative and other hormone therapies.

The actual mechanism of glucocorticoid-induced remission is not known. Some have assumed that the high doses normally used inhibit ACTH production and, therefore, cut off adrenal synthesis of estrogen precursors (Pihl et al., 1975). It has also been suggested that there may be a differential effect on cellular versus hormonal immune mechanisms, such that less blocking antibody is produced to interfere with cell-mediated destruction of tumor (Lipsett, 1974). Glucocorticoids may also act directly on mammary tumor cells, since specific glucocorticoid receptors have recently been found in several animal mammary tumors (Gardner and Wittliff, 1973b; Shyamala, 1974), as well as in normal lactating mammary tissue (Tucker et al., 1971; Shyamala, 1973; Gardner and Wittliff, 1973a; Turnell et al., 1974). Both DMBA and R3230AC rat tumors have receptor levels similar to those of the lactating gland, and much more receptor than virgin or pregnant gland (Gardner and Wittliff, 1973a). These rat receptors all share the same sedimentation properties, relative steroid affinities, and ability to translocate to cell nuclei (Goral and Wittliff, 1975). Virus-induced mouse mammary tumors have less receptor than lactating mouse mammary gland, but, again, the receptors are qualitatively similar (Shyamala, 1975). In human breast cancer, the occurrence and distribution of glucocorticoid receptors is not yet known, nor has any correlation yet been shown between the presence of receptors and glucocorticoid-induced remission. An exciting new development, however, is the discovery of glucocorticoid receptor in the MCF-7 cell line, which was derived from a hormone-dependent human breast tumor. Since MCF-7 cells also possess substantial levels of the receptors for estrogens, progestins, and androgens, they may prove valuable in establishing both the significance of glucocorticoid receptor and its relation-

VI. ANDROGENS

Androgens affect their target cells through a receptor mechanism similar in many ways to that described earlier for the other steroids (King and Mainwaring, 1974). Although testosterone (T) is the primary circulating androgen, there is now abundant evidence that, in a number of target tissues, including the prostate, T must be converted by the enzyme 5α-reductase (Δ^4-3-ketosteroid 5α-reductase) to dihydrotestosterone (DHT) in order to bind the androgen receptor and enter the nuclei. DHT is, in turn, metabolized by 3-ketoreductase (3-ketosteroid oxidoreductase) to androstanediols, which do not bind the DHT receptor. It has been suggested, on the basis of different *in vitro* actions of DHT and androstanediols, that the two, operating through distinct mechanisms, may both be physiologically important (Baulieu, 1970). No separate receptor for androstanediols has been identified, however. Some tissues, on the other hand, may possess a different receptor specific for T itself; the mouse kidney has very little 5α-reductase activity, so that [^{3}H]T is translocated largely unchanged to the nuclei, where it presumably is the active androgen (Bullock and Bardin, 1974). DHT is rapidly converted to androstanediols in mouse kidney cytosol, even at 4°C, so that affinity of the receptor for DHT has been difficult to evaluate (Bullock and Bardin, 1974). The 3-keto reductase reaction is reversible *in vivo,* so that the biologic activity of androstanediols in mouse kidney may be due to their conversion back to DHT (Bullock and Bardin, 1975).

The importance of T metabolism for at least some androgenic activities is emphasized by two congenital defects. The testicular feminization syndrome described in mice, rats, and humans appears to be due to a deficiency of DHT receptors (Gehring *et al.,* 1971; Attardi and Ohno, 1974; Bullock and Bardin, 1972); conversion of T to DHT by 5α-reductase appears normal in these cases (Bullock and Bardin, 1973). Another form of human inherited male pseudohermaphroditism has been described in which 5α-reductase is deficient, while T production is normal (Imperato-McGinley *et al.,* 1974). However, considerable male development of these patients at about age 12, together with the observations that 5α-reductase is very low in adult animal tissues (Mainwaring and Mangan, 1973) and that DHT receptor levels fall with age (Shain and Axelrod, 1973), suggest that conversion of T to DHT may be less significant after development is completed.

The level of DHT receptors in the rat prostate falls rapidly after castration (Jung and Baulieu, 1971). However they are restored after several days, even in adrenalectomized or hypophysectomized animals, so some factor other than a steroid or pituitary hormone may be involved in the control of receptor levels (Sullivan and Strott, 1973). Another study did not find receptor restoration 7 days after castration (Bruchovsky and Craven, 1975); however, prostate nuclei were able to take up DHT, although cytoplasmic receptor was not demonstrable. A component appearing in prostate cytosol after castration was found to interfere with DHT binding to receptor, suggesting that the observations of receptor loss after castration may be, at least in part, apparent rather than real.

Analogues which function as antiandrogens have been described. Two classes can be distinguished: one in which compounds possess progestational activity, represented by cyproterone acetate and medroxyprogesterone acetate, and a second in which there is no progestational activity, represented by flutamide, BOMT, and unesterified cyproterone. Members of both classes directly inhibit DHT binding to its receptor (Liao et al., 1974; Peets et al., 1974). Progestational antiandrogens bind to progesterone receptor as well (Terenius, 1974), which may provide a mechanism for their apparent synergism with androgens in some tissues at doses lower than those required for androgen antagonism (Mowszowicz et al., 1974).

A. Androgens in Mammary Carcinoma

Androgens cause regression of a large percentage of carcinogen-induced rat mammary tumors (Huggins et al., 1961; Furth, 1961), though this effect is reversed at extremely high androgen doses (Heise and Gorlich, 1966). A number of androgens and androgen derivatives have proved effective in treatment of human breast cancer (Cooperative Breast Cancer Group, 1964; Goldenberg et al., 1973; Volk et al., 1974). Like other endocrine therapies, androgen administration appears to be particularly useful against tumors possessing receptors for estrogen (McGuire, 1975). The actual mechanism of androgen-induced regression is not known, but from existing data at least five different hypotheses can be proposed:

1. Androgens could act directly on tumors through an androgen receptor. There is no evidence that androgen receptors are required for normal female functions, and in fact Tfm/0 mice deficient in these receptors reproduce normally, except for somewhat premature aging of the ovaries (Lyon and Glenister, 1974; Ohno et al., 1973). Nevertheless, androgens cause regression of mammary buds or mammary bud explants of

fetuses of either sex (Kratochwil, 1971). The action is prevented by cyproterone acetate (Elger and Neumann, 1966; Neumann and Elger, 1966), consistent with mediation by DHT receptor. Both DHT receptors (Wagner et al., 1973; Persijn et al., 1975; Poortman et al., 1975; Horwitz et al., 1975a; Lippman et al., 1975) and androgen-metabolizing enzymes, including 5α-reductase (Miller et al., 1973; Raith et al., 1973; Jenkins and Ash, 1972; Rose et al., 1975), have been described in human breast tumors, so that it is possible that tumor regression might also involve the DHT receptor system. An androgen-dependent transplantable mouse mammary tumor, the Shionogi 115, has been shown to possess androgen receptor (Bruchovsky and Meakin, 1973) and to metabolize T to DHT (Yamaguchi et al., 1974), although T is the principal intranuclear steroid following injections of [^{3}H]T. Since two of seven autonomous sublines of the same tumor also possessed androgen receptor, and T is translocated to the nucleus (Bruchovsky et al., 1975), it would seem that the presence of androgen receptor may be necessary but not sufficient for androgen-dependent growth behavior. In tissue culture lines derived from the Shionogi tumor, DHT was more effective in growth-promoting activity than T, but unmetabolized T was still translocated (Smith and King, 1972; Sutherland et al., 1974; Gordon et al., 1974).

2. Quadri et al. (1974) have found that high doses of prolactin can override testosterone suppression of DMBA mammary tumor growth. Since T treatment has been reported not to reduce circulating levels of prolactin (Kalra et al., 1973), it was hypothesized that androgen might somehow reduce tumor responsiveness to prolactin, perhaps by an effect on prolactin receptors. Evidence from our laboratory reveals that pharmacologic androgen administration does reduce prolactin receptor content of DMBA mammary tumors (Costlow et al., 1976). It is not clear whether this is a cause or a result of the androgen-induced tumor regression.

3. Androgens could induce mammary tumor regression by conversion to estrogens. Pharmacologic doses of estrogens do reverse tumor growth, and conversion of only 2% of the standard 1 mg testosterone propionate injection to rats would produce sufficient estradiol to induce such a regression (Meites et al., 1971). In particular, it has been shown that both breast adipose tissue and breast tumors can aromatize various steroid precursors to active estrogens (Abul-Hajj, 1975; Nimrod and Ryan, 1975). Further, both androgen- and estrogen-induced regressions share the property of being reversed by large doses of prolactin (Quadri et al., 1974; Meites et al., 1971), suggesting a parallelism in their mechanisms.

4. Alternatively, androgens may block estrogen production. Though androgen suppression of gonadotropin production and consequent cessation of ovarian function is probable, this mechanism seems unlikely to be effec-

tive in postmenopausal women. More likely would be androgen inhibition of peripheral conversion of adrenal precursors to active estrogens. Such a mechanism would be consistent with the activity of several androgens that probably cannot be converted to estrogens, and of at least one, Δ^1-testololactone, which has no known hormonal activity at all (Volk et al., 1974). This mechanism might also allow one to explain the observation that very high doses of testosterone propionate are less effective than lower doses in causing regression of DMBA tumors (Heise and Gorlich, 1966); perhaps the intermediate doses serve to block conversion of adrenal precursors, while the very high doses permit conversion of very small amounts of the injected T itself, yielding just enough estrogen to stimulate tumor growth.

5. Of particular interest is the possible direct influence of androgens on estrogen receptor. Because tumors lacking estrogen receptor fail to respond to androgen treatment (McGuire, 1975), it has been suggested that androgens may affect ER directly. At extremely high concentrations *in vitro*, T and DHT have been reported to competitively inhibit estrogen binding to ER (Rochefort et al., 1972; Ruh and Ruh, 1975; Korach and Muldoon, 1975; Schmidt et al., 1976). In addition, androstenediol, a weak androgen commonly found in human female plasma, competitively inhibits estrogen binding to ER at somewhat lower concentrations (Poortman et al., 1975). In rat uteri *in vitro*, extremely high concentrations of androgens (10^{-6} M) transfer ER to the nucleus and induce proteins normally induced only by estradiol. Androgen stimulation of induced protein can be blocked with antiestrogens but not antiandrogens (Ruh and Ruh, 1975), strongly supporting the thesis that androgens are affecting ER and not androgen receptor. Although androgens appear to be acting directly in *in vitro* systems, some controversy remains as to whether these androgen-mediated events occur *in vivo* (Schmidt et al., 1976; Rochefort, 1977).

In mammary tumors, the possibility that androgen treatment might decrease ER was suggested by Deshpande et al. (1967b), who reported that pretreatment with dromostanolone propionate decreased the amounts of injected [^{3}H]estradiol present in human breast tumors compared with control patients. A similar observation was made in rat mammary tumors (Mobbs, 1970). We have now confirmed these earlier observations by showing a decrease in cytoplasmic ER in tumors during regression after androgen therapy (Zava and McGuire, 1977). From the above, it would be reasonable to speculate that androgens either deplete ER or render it inactive, so that endogenous estrogens could no longer stimulate tumor growth.

Clearly, androgen action on normal target tissues and androgen action on tumors may not share the same mechanism. If not, discovery of the actual mechanisms could lead to design of more effective, nonvirilizing androgen analogues for use in therapy, as well as enhancing our understanding of endocrine control over mammary tumor growth.

VII. SUMMARY AND CONCLUSIONS

Breast cancer is often hormone responsive, since growth or regression of tumors can often be modulated by appropriate endocrine manipulations. Prolactin, estrogen, and progesterone appear to be the major hormones involved in regulation of breast tumor growth. Considerable insight into the mechanism of action of these hormones on tumor growth stimulation has been provided by demonstration of specific receptors for each. The inference that each hormone acts independently through its receptor to control tumor growth is belied by current studies which show that certain hormones are capable of regulating the receptor sites, metabolism, or nuclear translocation of others. This may begin to explain the complex hormonal interactions and requirements of normal and neoplastic breast tissues. Considerable progress has thus been made in understanding the basis for success of various ablative therapies.

The pharmacologic actions of estrogens, androgens, and progestins in causing breast tumor regression is much less well understood. The role of hormone-receptor sites has not been established in the mechanism of tumor regression caused by these pharmacologic therapies. Nevertheless, when estrogen receptors are absent in a tumor, we can with accuracy predict that endocrine therapies will fail, whereas when ER is present the likelihood of a successful response to pharmacologic or ablative therapy is high.

Receptor sites seem to be a common denominator and useful marker for hormone dependence or hormone responsiveness, irrespective of their actual role in the tumor regression process. Further investigations into the receptor functions should lead to new approaches in the endocrine management of patients with breast cancer.

ACKNOWLEDGMENT

This work was supported in part by the USPHS Grants CA-11378, CB-23862, and American Cancer Society Grant BC-23.

REFERENCES

Abul-Hajj, Y. J. (1975). *Steroids* **26**, 488–500.
Ahren, K., and Jacobsohn, D. (1956). *Acta Physiol. Scand.* **37**, 190–203.

Archer, F. L., and Orlando, A. (1968). *Cancer Res.* **28,** 217–224.
Armstrong, B., Stevens, N., and Doll, R. (1974). *Lancet* **2,** 672–675.
Armstrong, D. T., and King, E. (1971). *Endocrinology* **89,** 191–197.
Armstrong, E. M., and More, I. A. R. (1974). *Cytobios* **11,** 13–16.
Atger, M., Baulieu, E.-E., and Milgróm, E. (1974). *Endocrinology* **94,** 161–167.
Attardi, B., and Ohno, S. (1974). *Cell* **2,** 205–212.
Barlow, J., Emerson, K., and Saxena, B. N. (1969). *N. Engl. J. Med.* **280,** 633–637.
Baulieu, E.-E. (1970). *Ann. Clin. Res.* **2,** 246.
Baxter, J. D., Harris, A. W., Tomkins, G. M., and Cohn, M. (1971). *Science* **171,** 189–191.
Baxter, J. D., Rousseau, G. G., Benson, M. C., Garcea, R. L., Ito, J., and Tomkins, G. M. (1972). *Proc. Natl. Acad. Sci. U.S.A.* **69,** 1892–1896.
Beatson, G. T. (1896a). *Lancet* **2,** 104.
Beatson, G. T. (1896b). *Lancet* **2,** 162.
Birkinshaw, M., and Falconer, I. R. (1972). *J. Endocrinol.* **55,** 323–324.
Bloom, H. J. G., and Boesen, E. (1974). *Br. Med. J.* **2,** 7–10.
Bogden, A. E., Taylor, D. J., Kuo, E. Y. H., Mason, M. M., and Speropoulos, A. (1974). *Cancer Res.* **34,** 3018–3025.
Boston Collaborative Drug Surveillance Program. (1974). *Lancet* **2,** 669–671.
Boyns, A. R., Cole, E. N., Griffiths, K., Roberts, M. M., Buchan, R., Wilson, R. G., and Forrest, A. P. M. (1973). *Eur. J. Cancer* **9,** 99–102.
Bradley, C. J., Kledzik, G. S., and Meites, J. (1976). *Cancer Res.* **36,** 319–324.
Braunsberg, H., James, V. H. T., Irvine, W. T., Jamieson, C. W., James, F., Sellwood, R. A., Carter, A. E., and Hulbert, M. (1973). *Lancet* **1,** 163–165.
Bresciani, F., Puca, G. A., Nola, E., Salvatore, M., and Ardovino, I. (1969). *Atti Soc. Ital. Patol.* **11,** 203–224.
Bruchovsky, N., and Craven, S. (1975). *Biochem. Biophys. Res. Commun.* **62,** 837–843.
Bruchovsky, N., and Meakin, J. (1973). *Cancer Res.* **33,** 1689–1695.
Bruchovsky, N., and Wilson, J. D. (1968). *J. Biol. Chem.* **243,** 2012–2021.
Bruchovsky, N., Sutherland, D. J. A., Meakin, J. W., and Minesita, T. (1975). *Biochim. Biophys. Acta* **381,** 61–71.
Bryson, M. J., and Sweat, M. L. (1969). *Endocrinology* **84,** 1071–1075.
Buller, R. E., Schrader, W. T., and O'Malley, B. W. (1975). *J. Biol. Chem.* **250,** 809–818.
Bullock, D. W., and Wellen, G. F. (1974). *Proc. Soc. Exp. Biol. Med.* **146,** 294–298.
Bullock, L. P., and Bardin, C. W. (1972). *J. Clin. Endocrinol. Metab.* **35,** 935–937.
Bullock, L. P., and Bardin, C. W. (1973). *J. Steroid Biochem.* **4,** 139–151.
Bullock, L. P., and Bardin, C. W. (1974). *Endocrinology* **94,** 746–756.
Bullock, L. P., and Bardin, C. W. (1975). *Steroids* **25,** 107–119.
Bullock, L. P., Barthe, P. L., Mowszowicz, I., Orth, D. N., and Bardin, C. W. (1975). *Endocrinology* **97,** 189–195.
Butler, T. P., and Pearson, O. H. (1971). *Cancer Res.* **31,** 817–820.
Caldwell, B. V., Tillson, S. A., Esber, H., and Thorneycroft, I. H. (1971). *Nature (London)* **231,** 118–119.
Cash, R. R., Brough, J., Cohen, M. N., and Satoh, P. S. (1967). *J. Clin. Endocrinol. Metab.* **27,** 1239–1248.
Cassell, E. E., Meites, J., and Welsch, C. W. (1971). *Cancer Res.* **31,** 1051–1053.
Chamness, G. C., Jennings, A. W., and McGuire, W. L. (1973). *Nature (London)* **241,** 458–460.
Chamness, G. C., Jennings, A. W., and McGuire, W. L. (1974). *Biochemistry* **13,** 327–331.
Chamness, G. C., Huff, K., and McGuire, W. L. (1975). *Steroids* **25,** 627–635.

Chatterton, R. T. (1971). *In* "The Sex Steroids" (K. W. McKerns, ed.), Chapter 12. Appleton, New York.
Chatterton, R. T., Chatterton, A. J., and Hellman, L. (1969). *Endocrinology* **85**, 16–24.
Clark, J. H., and Peck, E. J. (1976). *Nature (London)* **260**, 635–637.
Clark, J. H., Anderson, J. N., and Peck, E. J. (1973). *Steroids* **22**, 707–718.
Clark, J. H., Peck, E. J., and Anderson, J. N. (1974). *Nature (London)* **251**, 446–448.
Cleary, R. E., Crabtree, R., and Lemberger, L. (1975). *J. Clin. Endocrinol. Metab.* **40**, 830–833.
Clemens, J. A., and Shaar, C. J. (1972). *Proc. Soc. Exp. Biol. Med.* **139**, 659–662.
Clemens, J. A., Welsch, C. W., and Meites, J. (1968). *Proc. Soc. Exp. Biol. Med.* **127**, 969–972.
Coffey, J. C. (1973). *Steroids* **22**, 561–566.
Cole, M. P., Jones, C. T. A., and Todd, I. D. H. (1971). *Br. J. Cancer* **25**, 270–275.
Cole, P., and MacMahon, B. (1969). *Lancet* **1**, 604–606.
Collins, J. A., and Jewkes, D. M. (1974). *Am. J. Obstet. Gynecol.* **118**, 179–185.
Cooperative Breast Cancer Group. (1964). *J. Am. Med. Assoc.* **188**, 1069–1072.
Costlow, M. E., Buschow, R. A., and McGuire, W. L. (1974). *Science* **184**, 85–86.
Costlow, M. E., Buschow, R. A., and McGuire, W. L. (1975a). *Life Sci.* **17**, 1457–1466.
Costlow, M. E., Buschow, R. A., Richert, N. J., and McGuire, W. L. (1975b). *Cancer Res.* **35**, 970–974.
Costlow, M. E., Buschow, R. A., and McGuire, W. L. (1976). *Cancer Res.* **36**, 3941.
Council on Drugs. (1960). *J. Am. Med. Assoc.* **172**, 1271–1283.
Daehnfeldt, J. L. (1974). *Proc. Soc. Exp. Biol. Med.* **146**, 159–162.
Dao, T. L. (1964). *Prog. Exp. Tumor Res.* **5**, 157–216.
Dao, T. L. (1972). *Annu. Rev. Med.* **23**, 1–18.
Dao, T. L., and Sunderland, H. (1959). *J. Natl. Cancer Inst.* **23**, 567–586.
Davies, J., Challis, J. R. G., and Ryan, K. J. (1974). *Endocrinology* **95**, 164–173.
Defer, N., Dastugue, B., and Kruh, J. (1974). *Biochimie* **56**, 1549–1557.
del Pozo, E., Brun del Re, R., Varga, L., and Friesen, H. (1972). *J. Clin. Endocrinol. Metab.* **35**, 768–771.
Deshpande, N. (1975). *J. Steroid Biochem.* **6**, 735–741.
Deshpande, N., Bulbrook, R. D., and Belzer, F. O. (1967a). *Proc. Int. Congr. Horm. Steroids, 2nd, 1966* Excerpta Med. Found. Int. Congr. Ser. No. 132, pp. 750–753.
Deshpande, N., Jensen, V., Bulbrook, R. D., Berne, T., and Ellis, F. (1967b). *Steroids* **10**, 219–232.
DeSombre, E., and Arbogast, L. Y. (1974). *Cancer Res.* **34**, 1971–1976.
DeSombre, E. R., Kledzik, G., Marshall, S., and Meites, J. (1976). *Cancer Res.* **36**, 354–358.
Dexter, R. N., Fishman, L. M., Ney, R. I., and Liddle, G. W. (1967). *J. Clin. Endocrinol. Metab.* **27**, 473–480.
Diamond, E. J., Koprak, S., Shen, S. K., and Hollander, V. P. (1976). *Cancer Res.* **36**, 77–80.
Dickey, R. P., and Minton, J. P. (1972). *Am. J. Obstet. Gynecol.* **114**, 267–269.
Dickinson, L. E., MacMahon, B., Cole, P., and Brown, J. B. (1974). *N. Engl. J. Med.* **291**, 1211–1213.
Egert, D., and Maass, H. (1974). *Acta Endocrinol. (Copenhagen)* **77**, 160–170.
Ehni, G., and Eckles, N. E. (1959). *J. Neurosurg.* **16**, 628–652.
Elger, W., and Neumann, F. (1966). *Proc. Soc. Exp. Biol. Med.* **123**, 637–640.
Ellis, F. G., Berne, T. V., Deshpande, N., Belzer, F. O., and Bulbrook, R. D. (1969). *Surg., Gynecol. Obstet.* **128**, 975–984.
Faber, L. E., Sandmann, M. L., and Stavely, H. E. (1972a). *J. Biol. Chem.* **247**, 5648–5649.
Faber, L. E., Sandmann, M. L., and Stavely, H. E. (1972b). *J. Biol. Chem.* **247**, 8000–8004.

Faber, L. E., Sandmann, M. L., and Stavely, H. (1973). *Endocrinology* **93**, 74–80.
Fahim, M. S., and Hall, D. G. (1970). *Am. J. Obstet. Gynecol.* **106**, 183–186.
Feherty, P., Farrer-Brown, G., and Kellie, A. E. (1971). *Br. J. Cancer* **25**, 697–710.
Feil, P. D., and Bardin, C. W. (1975). *Endocrinology* **97**, 1398–1407.
Feil, P. D., Glasser, S. R., Toft, D. O., and O'Malley, B. W. (1972). *Endocrinology* **91**, 738–746.
Floss, H. G., Cassady, J. M., and Robbers, J. E. (1973). *J. Pharm. Sci.* **62**, 699–715.
Folca, P. J., Glascock, R. F., and Irvine, W. T. (1961). *Lancet* **2**, 796–802.
Franks, S., Ralphs, D. N. L., Seagroatt, V., and Jacobs, H. S. (1974). *Br. Med. J.* **4**, 320–321.
Frantz, A. G., Habif, D. V., Hyman, G. A., and Suh, H. K. (1972a). *Clin. Res.* **20**, 864.
Frantz, A. G., Kleinberg, D. L., and Noel, G. L. (1972b). *Recent Prog. Horm. Res.* **28**, 527–590.
Frantz, A. G., Habif, D. V., Hyman, G. A., Suh, H. K., Sassin, J. F., Zimmerman, E. A., Noel, G. L., and Kleinberg, D. L. (1973). *In* "Human Prolactin" (J. L. Pasteels and C. Robyn, eds.), p. 273–290. Excerpta Med. Found., Amsterdam.
Frantz, W. L., MacIndoe, J. H., and Turkington, R. W. (1974). *J. Endocrinol.* **60**, 485–497.
Freifeld, M. L., Feil, P. D., and Bardin, C. W. (1974). *Steroids* **23**, 93–103.
Friesen, H., Guyda, H., Hwang, P., Tyson, J. E., and Barbeau, A. (1972). *J. Clin. Invest.* **51**, 706–709.
Furth, J. (1961). *Fed. Proc., Fed. Am. Soc. Exp. Biol.* **20**, 865–873.
Gallez, G., Heuson, J. C., and Waelbroeck, C. (1973). *Eur. J. Cancer* **9**, 699–700.
Gardner, D. G., and Wittliff, J. L. (1973a). *Biochim. Biophys. Acta* **320**, 617–627.
Gardner, D. G., and Wittliff, J. L. (1973b). *Br. J. Cancer* **27**, 441–444.
Garola, R., Levy, C. M., Vegh, I., Magin, C., Martinez, J. C., and Hecker, E. (1974). *Oncology* **30**, 105–112.
Gehring, U., and Tomkins, G. M. (1974). *Cell* **3**, 301.
Gehring, U., Tomkins, G. M., and Ohno, S. (1971). *Nature (London)* **232**, 106–107.
Gelato, M., Marshall, S., Boudreau, M., Bruni, J., and Campbell, G. A. (1975). *Endocrinology* **96**, 1292–1296.
Gill, G. N. (1972). *Metab., Clin. Exp.* **21**, 571–588.
Glascock, R. F., and Hoekstra, W. G. (1959). *Biochem. J.* **72**, 673–682.
Goldenberg, I. S., Waters, N., Ravdin, R. S., Ansfield, F. J., and Segaloff, A. (1973). *J. Am. Med. Assoc.* **223**, 1267–1268.
Goral, J. E., and Wittliff, J. L. (1975). *Biochemistry* **14**, 2944–2952.
Gordon, J., Smith, J. A., and King, R. J. B. (1974). *Mol. Cell. Endocrinol.* **1**, 259–270.
Gorski, J., Toft, D., Shyamala, G., Smith, D., and Notides, A. (1968). *Recent Prog. Horm. Res.* **24**, 45–80.
Griffiths, C. T., Hall, T. C., Saba, Z., Barlow, J. J., and Nevinny, H. B. (1973). *Cancer* **32**, 32–37.
Grodin, J. M., Siiteri, P. K., and MacDonald, P. C. (1973). *J. Clin. Endocrinol. Metab.* **36**, 207–214.
Growley, L. G., and MacDonald, I. (1965). *Cancer* **18**, 436–446.
Guerzon, P. G., and Pearson, O. H. (1974). *Clin. Res.* **22**, 632A.
Gullino, P. M., Grantham, F. H., Losonczy, I., and Berghoffer, B. (1972). *J. Natl. Cancer Inst.* **49**, 1333–1348.
Hähnel, R., Twaddle, E., and Vivian, A. B. (1971). *Steroids* **18**, 681–708.
Hall, T., Barlow, J., Griffiths, C., and Saba, Z. (1969). *Clin. Res.* **17**, 402.
Hashimoto, I., Hendricks, D. M., Anderson, L. L., and Melampy, R. M. (1968). *Endocrinology* **82**, 333–341.

Haukkamaa, M., and Luukkainen, T. (1974). *J. Steroid Biochem.* **5,** 447–452.
Hecker, E., Vegh, I., Levy, C. M., Magin, C. A., Martinez, J. C., Loureino, J., and Garola, R. E. (1974). *Eur. J. Cancer* **10,** 747–749.
Heinomen, O. P., Shapiro, S., Tuominen, L., and Turunen, M. I. (1974). *Lancet* **2,** 675–677.
Heise, E., and Gorlich, M. (1966). *Br. J. Cancer* **20,** 539–545.
Henderson, B. E., Gerkins, V., Rosario, I., Casagrande, J., and Pike, M. C. (1975). *N. Engl. J. Med.* **293,** 790–795.
Heuson, J. C., Waelbroeck-Van Gaver, C., and Legros, N. (1970). *Eur. J. Cancer* **6,** 353–356.
Heuson, J. C., Coume, A., and Staquet, M. (1972a). *Eur. J. Cancer* **8,** 155–156.
Heuson, J. C., Coume, A., and Staquet, M. (1972b). *Eur. J. Cancer* **8,** 387–389.
Heuson, J. C., Waelbroeck, C., Legros, N., Gallez, G., Robyn, C., and L'Hermite, M. (1972c). *Gynecol. Invest.* **2,** 130–137.
Heuson, J. C., Engelsman, E., Blonk-vander Wijst, J., Maass, H., Drochmans, A., Michel, J., Nowakowski, H., and Gorins, A. (1975). *Br. Med. J.* **2,** 711.
Hilf, R., Michel, I., Bell, C., Freeman, J. J., and Borman, A. (1965). *Cancer Res.* **25,** 286–299.
Hilf, R., Michel, I., and Bell, C. (1967). *Recent Prog. Horm. Res.* **23,** 229–295.
Hilf, R., Battaglini, J. W., Delmez, J. A., Cohen, N., and Rector, W. D. (1971). *Cancer Res.* **31,** 1195–1200.
Holcomb, H. H., Costlow, M. E., Buschow, R. A., and McGuire, W. L. (1976). *Biochim. Biophys. Acta* **428,** 104–112.
Holdaway, I. M., and Friesen, H. G. (1976). *Cancer Res.* **36,** 1562–1567.
Hollander, N., and Chiu, Y. W. (1966). *Biochem. Biophys. Res. Commun.* **25,** 291.
Horwitz, K. B. (1975). Doctoral Dissertation, pp. 80–85. University of Texas, Dallas, Texas.
Horwitz, K. B., and McGuire, W. L. (1975). *Steroids* **25,** 497–505.
Horwitz, K. B., Costlow, M. E., and McGuire, W. L. (1975a). *Steroids* **26,** 785–795.
Horwitz, K. B., McGuire, W. L., Pearson, O. H., and Segaloff, A. (1975b). *Science* **189,** 726–727.
Hsueh, A. J. W., Peck, E. J., and Clark, J. H. (1973). *J. Endocrinol.* **58,** 503–511.
Hsueh, A. J. W., Peck, E. J., and Clark, J. H. (1974). *Steroids* **24,** 599–611.
Hsueh, A. J. W., Peck, E. J., and Clark, J. H. (1975). *Nature (London)* **254,** 337–338.
Hsueh, A. J. W., Peck, E. J., and Clark, J. H. (1976). *Endocrinology* **98,** 438–444.
Huggins, C. (1965). *Cancer Res.* **25,** 1163–1175.
Huggins, C., and Yang, N. C. (1962). *Science* **137,** 257–262.
Huggins, C., Grand, L., and Brillantes, F. (1961). *Nature (London)* **189,** 204–207.
Huggins, C., Moon, R. C., and Morii, S. (1962). *Proc. Natl. Acad. Sci. U.S.A.* **48,** 379–386.
Imperato-McGinley, J., Guerrero, L., Gautier, T., and Peterson, R. E. (1974). *Science* **186,** 1213–1215.
James, F., James, V. H. T., Carter, A. E., and Irvine, W. T. (1971). *Cancer Res.* **31,** 1268–1272.
Jenkins, J. S., and Ash, S. (1972). *Lancet* **2,** 513–514.
Jensen, E. V., and DeSombre, E. R. (1972). *Annu. Rev. Biochem.* **41,** 203–230.
Jensen, E. V., and Jacobson, H. I. (1960). *In* "Biological Activities of Steroids in Relation to Cancer" (G. Pincus and E. P. Vollmer, eds.), p. 191. Academic Press, New York.
Jensen, E. V., DeSombre, E. R., and Jungblut, P. W. (1967). *In* "Endogenous Factors Influencing Host-Tumor Balance" (R. W. Wissler, T. L. Dao, and S. Wood, Jr., eds.), p. 15. Univ. of Chicago Press, Chicago, Illinois.
Jordan, V. C., and Jaspan, T. (1976). *J. Endocrinol.* **68,** 453–460.
Jordan, V. C., and Koerner, S. (1975). *Eur. J. Cancer* **11,** 205–206.
Jordan, V. C., and Koerner, S. (1976). *J. Endocrinol.* **68,** 305–311.

Jordan, V. C., Koerner, S., and Robison, C. (1975). *J. Endocrinol.* **65**, 151–152.
Judd, H., Judd, G. E., Lucas, W. E., and Yed, S. S. C. (1974). *J. Clin. Endocrinol. Metab.* **39**, 1020–1024.
Jung, I., and Baulieu, E. E. (1971). *Biochimie* **53**, 807–817.
Kalra, P. S., Fawcett, C. P., Krulich, L., and McCann, S. M. (1973). *Endocrinology* **92**, 1256.
Katzenellenbogen, B. S., and Ferguson, E. R. (1975). *Endocrinology* **97**, 1–12.
Katzenellenbogen, J. A., Johnson, H. J., and Carlson, K. E. (1973). *Biochemistry* **12**, 4092–4099.
Kelly, P. A., Bradley, C., Shiu, R. P. C., Meites, J., and Friesen, H. G. (1974). *Proc. Soc. Exp. Biol. Med.* **146**, 816–819.
Kennedy, B. J. (1965). *Cancer* **18**, 1551–1557.
Kennedy, B. J., and French, L. (1965). *Am. J. Surg.* **110**, 411–414.
Kim, U., Furth, J., and Yannopoulos, K. (1963). *J. Natl. Cancer Inst.* **31**, 233–259.
King, R. J. B., and Mainwaring, W. I. P. (1974). "Steroid-Cell Interactions." pp. 41–101. Univ. Park Press, Baltimore, Maryland.
King, R. J. B., Cowan, D. M., and Inman, D. R. (1965). *J. Endocrinol.* **32**, 83–90.
King, R. J. B., Gordon, J., Cowan, D. M., and Inman, D. R. (1966). *J. Endocrinol.* **36**, 139–150.
Kirschner, M. A., and Taylor, J. P. (1972). *J. Clin. Endocrinol. Metab.* **35**, 513–521.
Klaiber, M. S., Gruenstein, M., Meranze, D. R., and Shimkin, M. B. (1969). *Cancer Res.* **29**, 999–1001.
Kleinberg, D. L., Noel, G. L., and Frantz, A. (1971). *J. Clin. Endocrinol. Metab.* **33**, 873–876.
Kontula, J., Jänne, O., Luukkainen, T., and Vihko, R. (1973). *Biochim. Biophys. Acta* **328**, 145–153.
Kontula, K., Jänne, O., Luukkainen, T., and Vihko, R. (1974a). *J. Clin. Endocrinol. Metab.* **38**, 500–503.
Kontula, K., Jänne, O., Rajakakowski, E., Tanhuapaa, E., and Vihko, R. (1974b). *J. Steroid Biochem.* **5**, 39–44.
Korach, K. S., and Muldoon, T. G. (1975). *Endocrinology* **97**, 231–236.
Korenman, S. G. (1969). *Steroids* **13**, 163–178.
Korenman, S. G., and Dukes, B. A. (1970). *J. Clin. Endocrinol. Metab.* **30**, 369.
Kornel, L. (1973). *Acta Endocrinol. (Copenhagen)* **74**, Suppl. 178, 1–45.
Kratochwil, K. (1971). *J. Embryol. Exp. Morphol.* **25**, 141–143.
Kwa, H. G., De Jong-Bakker, M., Engelsman, E., and Cleton, F. J. (1974). *Lancet* **1**, 433–434.
Landau, R. L., Ehrlich, E. N., and Huggins, C. (1962). *J. Am. Med. Assoc.* **182**, 632–636.
Lawson, D. E. M., and Pearlman, W. H. (1964). *J. Biol. Chem.* **239**, 3226–3232.
Leavitt, W. W., and Grossman, C. J. (1974). *Proc. Natl. Acad. Sci. U.S.A.* **71**, 4341–4345.
Leavitt, W. W., Toft, D. O., Strott, C. A., and O'Malley, B. W. (1974). *Endocrinology* **94**, 1041–1053.
Lemberger, L., Crabtree, R., Clemens, J., Dyke, R. W., and Woodburn, R. T. (1974). *J. Clin. Endocrinol. Metab.* **39**, 579–584.
Lemon, H. M. (1969). *Cancer* **23**, 781–790.
Lemon, H. M. (1970). *Cancer* **25**, 423–435.
Lemon, H. M. (1975). *Cancer Res.* **35**, 1341–1353.
Lemon, H. M., Miller, D. M., and Foley, J. F. (1971). *Natl. Cancer Inst., Monogr.* **34**, 77–83.
Leung, B. S., and Sasaki, G. H. (1975). *Endocrinology* **97**, 564–572.
Leung, B. S., Sasaki, G. H., and Leung, J. (1975). *Cancer Res.* **35**, 621–627.
Li, C. H., and Yang, W. (1975). *Life Sci.* **15**, 761–764.
Liao, S., Howell, D. K., and Chang, T. (1974). *Endocrinology* **94**, 1205–1209.
Lippman, M. E., and Bolan, G. (1975). *Nature (London)* **256**, 592–593.

14. Hormones and Their Receptors in Breast Cancer 437

Lippman, M. E., Halterman, R., Perry, S., Leventhal, B., and Thompson, E. B. (1973). *Nature (London), New Biol.* **242,** 157–158.
Lippman, M. E., Bolan, G., and Huff, K. (1975). *Nature (London)* **258,** 339–341.
Lipsett, M. B. (1971). *Lancet* **2,** 1378.
Lipsett, M. B. (1974). *Ann. N.Y. Acad. Sci.* **230,** 489–490.
Lipsett, M. B., and Bergenstal, D. M. (1960). *Cancer Res.* **20,** 1172–1178.
Lipton, A., and Santen, R. J. (1974). *J. Clin. Endocrinol. Metab.* **39,** 1020.
Longcope, C. (1971). *Am. J. Obstet. Gynecol.* **111,** 778–781.
Loriaux, D. L., Ruder, H. J., Knab, D. R., and Lipsett, M. B. (1972). *J. Clin. Endocrinol. Metab.* **35,** 887–891.
Lu, K. (1971). *Endocrinology* **89,** 229–233.
Luft, R., Olivecrona, H., and Sjögren, B. (1952). *Nord. Med.* **47,** 351.
Lyon, M., and Glenister, P. H. (1974). *Nature (London)* **247,** 366–367.
Lyons, W. R., Li, C. H., and Johnson, R. E. (1958). *Recent. Prog. Horm. Res.* **14,** 219–254.
McCormick, G. M. (1972). *Cancer Res.* **32,** 1574–1576.
McCormick, G. M., and Moon, R. C. (1965). *Br. J. Cancer* **19,** 160–166.
McCormick, G. M., and Moon, R. C. (1967). *Cancer Res.* **27,** 626–631.
McCormick, G. M., and Moon, R. C. (1973). *Eur. J. Cancer* **9,** 483–486.
McGrath, C. M. (1971). *J. Natl. Cancer Inst.* **47,** 455–467.
McGuire, W. L. (1969). *Science* **165,** 1013–1014.
McGuire, W. L. (1973). *J. Clin. Invest.* **52,** 73–77.
McGuire, W. L. (1975). *Cancer* **36,** 638–644.
McGuire, W. L., and De La Garza, M. (1973a). *J. Clin. Endocrinol. Metab.* **36,** 548–552.
McGuire, W. L., and De La Garza, M. (1973b). *J. Clin. Endocrinol. Metab.* **37,** 986–989.
McGuire, W. L., and Julian, J. A. (1971). *Cancer Res.* **31,** 1440–1445.
McGuire, W. L., Julian, J. A., and Chamness, G. C. (1971). *Endocrinology* **89,** 969–973.
McGuire, W. L., Huff, K., Jennings, A., and Chamness, G. C. (1972a). *Science* **175,** 335–336.
McGuire, W. L., Huff, K., and Chamness, G. C. (1972b). *Biochemistry* **11,** 4562–4565.
McGuire, W. L., Chamness, G. C., and Costlow, M. E. (1974). *Metab., Clin. Exp.* **23,** 75–100.
McGuire, W. L., Carbone, P. P., Sears, M. E., and Escher, G. C. (1975a). *In* "Estrogen Receptors in Human Breast Cancer" (W. L. McGuire, P. P. Carbone, and E. P. Vollmer, eds.), pp. 1–7. Raven, New York.
McGuire, W. L., Pearson, O. H., and Segaloff, A. (1975b). *In* "Estrogen Receptors in Human Breast Cancer" (W. L. McGuire, P. P. Carbone, and E. P. Vollmer, eds.), pp. 17–30. Raven, New York.
McGuire, W. L., De La Garza, M., and Chamness, G. C. (1977). *Cancer Res.* **37,** 637–639.
Mack, T. M., Henderson, B. E., Gerkins, V. R., Arthur, M., Baptista, J., and Pike, M. C. (1975). *N. Engl. J. Med.* **292,** 1366–1371.
MacLeod, R. M., Allen, M. S., and Hollander, V. P. (1964). *Endocrinology* **75,** 249–258.
MacMahon, B., Cole, P., and Brown, J. (1973). *J. Natl. Cancer Inst.* **50,** 21–42.
Mainwaring, W., and Mangan, F. R. (1973). *J. Endocrinol.* **59,** 121–139.
Malarkey, W. B., Jacobs, L. S., and Daughaday, W. H. (1971). *N. Engl. J. Med.* **285,** 1160–1163.
Meites, J. (1972). *J. Natl. Cancer Inst.* **48,** 1217–1224.
Meites, J., and Nicoll, C. S. (1966). *Annu. Rev. Physiol.* **28,** 57–88.
Meites, J., Nicholl, C. S., and Talwalker, P. K. (1963). *Adv. Neuroendocrinol., Proc. Symp., 1961* pp. 238–288.
Meites, J., Cassell, E., and Clark, J. (1971). *Proc. Soc. Exp. Biol. Med.* **137,** 1225–1227.
Meites, J., Lu, K. H., Wuttke, W., Nagasawa, H., and Quadri, S. K. (1972). *Recent Prog. Horm. Res.* **28,** 471–526.

Milgrom, E., Thi, L., Atger, M., and Baulieu, E.-E. (1973). *J. Biol. Chem.* **248**, 6366–6374.
Miller, W. R. (1976). *Cancer Res.* **36**, 336–338.
Miller, W. R., McDonald, D., Forrest, A. P. M., and Shivas, A. A. (1973). *Lancet* **1**, 912–913.
Minton, J. P. (1974). *Cancer* **33**, 358–363.
Mobbs, B. G. (1966). *J. Endocrinol.* **36**, 409–414.
Mobbs, B. G. (1969). *J. Endocrinol.* **44**, 463–464.
Mobbs, B. G. (1970). *J. Endocrinol.* **48**, 293–294.
Morgan, M. D., and Wilson, J. D. (1970). *J. Biol. Chem.* **245**, 3781–3789.
Mowszowicz, I., Bieber, D., Chung, K., Bullock, L. P., and Bardin, C. W. (1974). *Endocrinology* **95**, 1589–1599.
Mueller, G. C., Vonderhaar, B., Kim, U. H., and Mahieu, M. L. (1972). *Recent Prog. Horm. Res.* **28**, 1–49.
Muggia, F. M., Cassileth, P. A., Ochoa, M., Flatow, F. A., Gellhorn, A., and Hyman, G. A. (1968). *Ann. Intern. Med.* **68**, 328–337.
Munck, A., and Wira, C. (1970). *Adv. Biosci.* **7**, 301–330.
Murota, S.-I., and Hollander, V. P. (1971). *Endocrinology* **89**, 560–564.
Murray, R. M. L., Mozaffarian, G., and Pearson, O. H. (1972). *In* "Prolactin and Carcinogenesis" (A. R. Boyns and K. Griffiths, eds.), pp. 158–161. Alpha Omega Alpha Publ., Cardiff, Wales.
Nagasawa, H., and Meites, J. (1970). *Cancer Res.* **30**, 1327–1329.
Nagasawa, H., and Yanai, R. (1970). *Int. J. Cancer* **6**, 488–495.
Nagasawa, H., and Yanai, R. (1971a). *Endocrinol. Jpn.* **18**, 53.
Nagasawa, H., and Yanai, R. (1971b). *Int. J. Cancer* **8**, 463–467.
Nagasawa, H., and Yanai, R. (1973). *Int. J. Cancer* **11**, 131–137.
Naqvi, E., Zarrow, M. X., and Denenberg, V. H. (1969). *Endocrinology* **84**, 669–670.
Nardacci, N. J., and McGuire, W. L. (1976). *Clin. Res.* **24**, 462A.
Neumann, F., and Elger, W. (1966). *J. Endocrinol.* **36**, 347–353.
Nimrod, A., and Ryan, K. J. (1975). *J. Clin. Endocrinol. Metab.* **40**, 367–372.
Nomura, Y., Abe, Y., and Inokuchi, K. (1974). *Gann* **65**, 523–528.
Norgren, A. (1967). *Acta Univ. Lund., Sect. 2* p. 1.
O'Fallon, W. M., Labarthe, D. R., and Kurland, L. T. (1975). *Lancet* **2**, 292.
O'Halloran, M. J., and Maddock, P. G. (1974). *J. Ir. Med. Assoc.* **67**, 38.
Ohno, S., Christian, L., and Attardi, B. (1973). *Nature (London)* **243**, 119.
Oka, T., and Topper, Y. J. (1971). *J. Biol. Chem.* **246**, 7701.
Oka, T., and Perry, J. W. (1974). *J. Biol. Chem.* **249**, 7647–7652.
O'Malley, B. W., and Schrader, W. T. (1972). *J. Steroid Biochem.* **3**, 617–629.
O'Malley, B. W., McGuire, W. L., Kohler, P. O., and Korenman, S. G. (1969). *Recent Prog. Horm. Res.* **25**, 105–160.
Pearlman, W. H., De Hertogh, R., Laumas, K. R., and Pearlman, M. R. S. (1969). *J. Clin. Endocrinol. Metab.* **29**, 707–720.
Pearson, O. H., and Nasr, H. (1971). *Horm. Steroids, Proc. Int. Congr., 3rd, 1970* Excerpta Med. Found. Int. Congr. Ser. No. 219, p. 602.
Pearson, O. H., and Ray, B. S. (1959). *Cancer* **12**, 85–92.
Pearson, O. H., West, C. D., Hollander, V. P., and Treves, N. E. (1954). *J. Am. Med. Assoc.* **154**, 234–239.
Pearson, O. H., Ray, B. S., Harrold, C. C., West, C. D., Li, M. D., McClean, J. P., and Lipsett, M. B. (1955). *Trans. Assoc. Am. Physicians* **68**, 101–111.
Pearson, O. H., Llerena, O., Llerena, L., Molina, A., and Butler, T. (1969). *Trans. Assoc. Am. Physicians* **82**, 225–238.
Pearson, O. H., Murray, R., Mozaffarian, G., and Pensky, J. (1972). *In* "Prolactin and

Carcinogenesis" (A. R. Boyns and K. Griffiths, eds.), 154–157. Alpha Omega Alpha Publ., Cardiff, Wales.
Peets, E. A., Henson, M. F., and Neri, R. (1974). *Endocrinology* **94**, 532–540.
Persijn, J. P., Korsten, C. B., and Engelsman, E. (1975). *Br. Med. J.* **2**, 503.
Philibert, D., and Raynaud, J.-P. (1973). *Steroids* **22**, 89–99.
Philibert, D., and Raynaud, J.-P. (1974). *Endocrinology* **94**, 627–632.
Pierpaoli, W., and Sorkin, E. (1972). *Nature (London)* **238**, 58–59.
Pihl, A., Sander, S., Brennhovd, I., and Olsens, S. (1975). *In* "Estrogen Receptors in Human Breast Cancer" (W. L. McGuire, P. P. Carbone, and E. P. Vollmer, eds.), pp. 193–203. Raven Press, New York.
Podratz, K. C., Munns, T. W., and Katzman, P. A. (1974). *Steroids* **24**, 775–792.
Poel, W. E. (1968). *Br. J. Cancer* **22**, 867–873.
Pollow, K., Lubbert, H., Boquoi, E., Kruezer, G., and Pollow, B. (1974). *Endocrinology* **96**, 319–328.
Poortman, J., Prenen, J. A. C., Schwarz, F., and Thijssen, J. H. H. (1975). *J. Clin. Endocrinol. Metab.* **40**, 373–379.
Posner, B. I., Kelly, P. A., and Friesen, H. G. (1974a). *Proc. Natl. Acad. Sci. U.S.A.* **71**, 2407–2410.
Posner, B. I., Kelly, P. A., Shiu, R. P. C., and Friesen, H. G. (1974b). *Endocrinology* **95**, 521–531.
Posner, B. I., Kelly, P. A., and Friesen, H. G. (1975). *Science* **188**, 57–59.
Puca, G. A., and Bresciani, F. (1969). *Endocrinology* **85**, 1–10.
Quadri, S. K., and Meites, J. (1971). *Proc. Soc. Exp. Biol. Med.* **138**, 999–1001.
Quadri, S. K., Clark, J. L., and Meites, J. (1973a). *Proc. Soc. Exp. Biol. Med.* **142**, 22–26.
Quadri, S. K., Kledzik, G. S., and Meites, J. (1973b). *Proc. Soc. Exp. Biol. Med.* **142**, 759–761.
Quadri, S. K., Kledzik, G. S., and Meites, J. (1974). *J. Natl. Cancer Inst.* **52**, 875–878.
Raith, L., Wirtz, A., Wiedemann, M., and Karl, H. J. (1973). *Acta Endocrinol. (Copenhagen)*, Suppl. **177**, 28–29.
Rajaniemi, H., Okasanen, A., and Vanha-Perttula, T. (1974). *Horm. Res.* **5**, 6–20.
Rochefort, H. (1977). *Res. Steroids* **7**, (in press).
Rochefort, H., Lignon, F., and Capony, F. (1972a). *Gynecol. Invest.* **3**, 43–62.
Rochefort, H., Lignon, F., and Capony, F. (1972b). *Biochem. Biophys. Res. Commun.* **47**, 662–676.
Rose, L. I., Underwood, R. H., Dunning, M. A., Williams, G., and Pinkus, G. S. (1975). *Cancer* **36**, 399–403.
Rosen, P. P., Menendez-Botet, C. J., Nisselbaum, J. S., Urban, J. A., Mike, V., Fracchia, A., and Schwartz, M. K. (1975). *Cancer Res.* **35**, 3187–3194.
Rousseau, G. G. (1975). *J. Steroid Biochem.* **6**, 75–89.
Rousseau, G. G., Baxter, J. D., and Tomkins, G. M. (1972). *J. Mol. Biol.* **67**, 99–115.
Rousseau, G. G., Higgins, S. J., Baxter, J. D., and Tomkins, G. M. (1974). *J. Steroid Biochem.* **5**, 935–939.
Rudali, G., Apiou, F., and Muel, B. (1975). *Eur. J. Cancer* **11**, 39–41.
Ruh, T. S., and Ruh, M. F. (1975). *Endocrinology* **97**, 1144–1150.
Ruh, T. S., Katzenellenbogen, B. S., Katzenellenbogen, J. A., and Gorski, J. (1973). *Endocrinology* **92**, 125–134.
Sadoff, L., and Lusk, W. (1974). *Obstet. Gynecol.* **43**, 262–266.
Saffran, J., Loeser, B. K., Haas, B., and Stavely, H. E. (1973). *Biochem. Biophys. Res. Commun.* **53**, 202–209.
Saffran, J., Loeser, B. K., Haas, B. M., and Stavely, H. E. (1974). *Steroids* **23**, 117–131.

Sander, S., and Attramadal, A. (1968). *Acta Pathol. Microbiol. Scand.* **74**, 169–178.
Santen, R. J., Lipton, A., and Kendall, J. (1974). *J. Am. Med. Assoc.* **230**, 1661–1665.
Sasaki, G. H., and Leung, B. S. (1974). *Res. Commun. Chem. Pathol. Pharmacol.* **8**, 409–412.
Sassin, J. F., Frantz, A. G., Weitzman, E. D., and Kapen, S. (1972). *Science* **177**, 1205–1207.
Sassin, J. F., Frantz, A. G., Kapen, S., and Weitzman, E. D. (1973). *J. Clin. Endocrinol. Metab.* **37**, 436–440.
Schmidt, W. N., Sadler, M. A., and Katzenellenbogen, B. S. (1976). *Endocrinology* **98**, 702–716.
Schorr, I., Rathnam, P., Saxena, B. B., and Ney, R. L. (1971). *J. Biol. Chem.* **246**, 5806–5811.
Schrader, W. T., Toft, D. O., and O'Malley, B. W. (1972). *J. Biol. Chem.* **247**, 2401–2407.
Schultz, K. B., Czygan, P.-J., del Pozo, E., and Friesen, H. G. (1973). *In* "Human Prolactin" (J. L. Pasteels and C. Robyn, eds.), pp. 268–271. Excerpta Med. Found., Amsterdam.
Schulz, K.-D., Haselmeier, B., and Holzel, F. (1969). *Acta Endocrinol. (Copenhagen), Suppl.* **138**, 236.
Shain, S. A., and Axelrod, L. R. (1973). *Steroids* **21**, 801–812.
Shepherd, R. E., Huff, K., and McGuire, W. L. (1974). *Endocr. Res. Commun.* **1**, 73–85.
Sherman, B. M., and Korenman, S. G. (1974). *Cancer* **33**, 1306–1312.
Sherman, M. R., Corvol, P. L., and O'Malley, B. W. (1970). *J. Biol. Chem.* **245**, 6085–6096.
Sherwood, L. M. (1971). *N. Engl. J. Med.* **284**, 774–777.
Shiu, R. P. C., and Friesen, H. G. (1974). *Biochem. J.* **140**, 301–311.
Shiu, R. P. C., Kelly, P. A., and Friesen, H. G. (1973). *Science* **180**, 968–970.
Shyamala, G. (1972). *Biochem. Biophys. Res. Commun.* **46**, 1623–1630.
Shyamala, G. (1973). *Biochemistry* **12**, 3085–3090.
Shyamala, G. (1974). *J. Biol. Chem.* **249**, 2160–2163.
Shyamala, G. (1975). *Biochemistry* **14**, 437–444.
Shyamala, G., and Nandi, S. (1972). *Endocrinology* **91**, 861–867.
Sibley, C. H., and Tomkins, G. M. (1974). *Cell* **2**, 221.
Sinha, D., Cooper, D., and Dao, T. (1973). *Cancer Res.* **33**, 411–414.
Smith, H. E., Smith, R. G., Toft, D. O., Neergaard, J. R., Burrows, E., and O'Malley, B. W. (1974). *J. Biol. Chem.* **249**, 5924–5932.
Smith, J. A., and King, R. J. B. (1972). *Exp. Cell Res.* **73**, 351–359.
Smith, R. G., Iramain, C. A., Buttram, V. C., and O'Malley, B. W. (1975). *Nature (London)* **253**, 271–272.
Smithline, F., Sherman, L., and Kolodny, H. D. (1975). *N. Engl. J. Med.* **292**, 783–792.
Sparks, L. L., Daane, T. A., Hayashida, T., Cole, R. D., Lyons, W. R., and Li, C. (1955). *Cancer* **8**, 271–284.
Stähelin, H., Burckhardt-Vischer, B., and Flückiger, E. (1971). *Experientia* **27**, 915–916.
Sterental, A., Dominguez, J. M., Weissman, C., and Pearson, O. H. (1963). *Cancer Res.* **23**, 481–484.
Stoll, B. A. (1967a). *Cancer* **20**, 1807–1813.
Stoll, B. A. (1967b). *Br. Med. J.* **1**, 150–153.
Stoll, B. A. (1967c). *Br. Med. J.* **3**, 338–341.
Stoll, B. A. (1972). *Lancet* **1**, 431
Strott, C. A. (1974). *Endocrinology* **95**, 826–837.
Suchowsky, G. K., and Junkmann, K. (1961). *Endocrinology* **68**, 341–349.
Sullivan, J. N., and Strott, C. A. (1973). *J. Biol. Chem.* **248**, 3202–3208.
Sutherland, D. J. A., Robins, E. C., and Meakin, J. W. (1974). *J. Natl. Cancer Inst.* **52**, 37–48.
Tabei, T., Haga, H., Heinrichs, W., and Herrmann, W. L. (1974). *Steroids* **23**, 651–666.
Terenius, L. (1968). *Cancer Res.* **28**, 328–337.
Terenius, L. (1971a). *Acta Endocrinol., (Copenhagen)* **66**, 431–447.

Terenius, L. (1971b). *Eur. J. Cancer* **7**, 57–64.
Terenius, L. (1972). *Eur. J. Cancer* **8**, 55–58.
Terenius, L. (1973). *Eur. J. Cancer* **9**, 291.
Terenius, L. (1974). *Steroids* **23**, 909–919.
Thatcher, W. W., and Tucker, H. A. (1970a). *Proc. Soc. Exp. Biol. Med.* **134**, 915–918.
Thatcher, W. W., and Tucker, H. A. (1970b). *Endocrinology* **86**, 237–240.
Toft, D. O., and O'Malley, B. W. (1972). *Endocrinology* **90**, 1041–1045.
Tomogane, H., Ota, K., and Yokoyama, A. (1975). *J. Endocrinol.* **65**, 155–161.
Truong, H., Geynet, C., Millet, C., Soulignac, O., Boucourt, R., Vignau, M., Torelli, V., and Baulieu, E.-E. (1973). *FEBS Lett.* **35**, 289–294.
Tucker, H. A., Larson, B. L., and Gorski, J. (1971). *Endocrinology* **89**, 152.
Turkington, R. W. (1970). *Biochem. Biophys. Res. Commun.* **41**, 1362–1367.
Turkington, R. W. (1971). *J. Clin. Endocrinol. Metab.* **33**, 210–216.
Turkington, R. W. (1974). *Cancer Res.* **34**, 758–763.
Turkington, R. W., Underwood, L. E., and Van Wyk, J. J. (1971). *N. Engl. J. Med.* **285**, 707–710.
Turkington, R. W., Majumder, G. C., Kadohama, N., MacIndoe, J. H., and Frantz, W. L. (1973). *Recent Prog. Horm. Res.* **29**, 417–455.
Turnell, R. W., Beers, P. C., and Wittliff, J. L. (1974). *Endocrinology* **95**, 1770–1773.
Tyson, J. E., Khojandi, M., Huth, J., Smith, B., and Thomas, P. (1975). *Am. J. Obstet. Gynecol.* **121**, 375–379.
Vignon, F., and Rochefort, H. (1974). *C. R. Hebd. Seances Acad. Sci.* **278**, 103–106.
Vignon, F., and Rochefort, H. (1976a). *10th Meet. Mammary Cancer, Kobe*, p. 42.
Vignon, F., and Rochefort, H. (1976b). *Endocrinology* **98**, 722–729.
Volk, H., Deupree, R. J., Goldenberg, I. S., Wilde, R. C., Carabasi, R. A., and Escher, G. C. (1974). *Cancer* **33**, 9–13.
Voorhess, M. L. (1967). *J. Pediatr.* **71**, 128–131.
Wagner, R. K., Gorlich, L., and Jungblut, P. W. (1973). *Acta Endocrinol. (Copenhagen)*, Suppl. **173**, 65.
Ward, H. W. C. (1973). *Br. Med. J.* **1**, 13–14.
Welsch, C. W., Iturri, G., and Meites, J. (1973). *Int. J. Cancer* **12**, 206–212.
Wiest, W. G. (1963). *Endocrinology* **73**, 310–316.
Wiest, W. G. (1971). *In* "The Sex Steroids" (K. W. McKerns, ed.), Chapter 10. Appleton, New York.
Wilson, J. D. (1972). *N. Engl. J. Med.* **287**, 1284–1291.
Wilson, R. G., Buchan, R., Roberts, M. M., Forrest, A. P. M., Boynes, A. R., Cole, E. N., and Griffiths, K. (1974). *Cancer* **33**, 1325–1327.
Wittliff, J. L., Gardner, D. G., Battema, W. L., and Gilbert, P. J. (1972). *Biochem. Biophys. Res. Commun.* **48**, 119–125.
Wuttke, W., Cassell, E., and Meites, J. (1971). *Endocrinology* **88**, 737–741.
Yamaguchi, K., Kasai, H., Minesita, T., Kotoh, K., and Matsumoto, K. (1974). *Endocrinology* **95**, 1424–1430.
Yamamoto, K. R., Stampfer, M. R., and Tomkins, G. M. (1974). *Proc. Natl. Acad. Sci. U.S.A.* **71**, 3901–3905.
Young, H. A., Scolnick, E. M., and Parks, W. P. (1975). *J. Biol. Chem.* **250**, 3337–3343.
Young, P. C. M., and Cleary, R. E. (1974). *J. Clin. Endocrinol. Metab.* **39**, 425–439.
Young, S. (1961). *Nature (London)* **190**, 356–357.
Zava, D. T., and McGuire, W. L. (1977). *Cancer Res.* **37**, 1608–1610.
Zava, D. T., Harrington, N. Y., and McGuire, W. L. (1976). *Biochemistry* **15**, 4292–4297.

15

Steroid-Binding Serum Globulins: Recent Results

ULRICH WESTPHAL

I.	Introduction	443
II.	Progesterone-Binding Globulin of the Pregnant Guinea Pig	445
	A. Purification and Characterization	445
	B. Conformational Changes upon Interaction with Steroids	449
	C. Fluorescence Quenching upon Interaction with Δ^4-3-Ketosteroids	451
III.	Kinetics of Steroid–Protein Interactions	458
IV.	On the Chemical Nature of the Binding Site	464
	A. Chemical Modification of α_1-Acid Glycoprotein	464
	B. Chemical Modification of Progesterone-Binding Globulin	468
	References	471

I. INTRODUCTION

Several proteins in the blood serum of humans and other mammalian species form stoichiometric complexes with steroid hormones: albumin, corticosteroid-binding globulin (CBG), testosterone–estradiol-binding globulin (TeBG), and α_1-acid glycoprotein (AAG). Whereas human serum albumin (HSA) consists of a polypeptide chain free of carbohydrate, AAG, CBG, and TeBG are glycoproteins with relatively high sugar content (Table I). The binding of the steroid hormones to the serum proteins is mediated essentially by hydrophobic forces and hydrogen bonds; noncovalent complexes are formed that are dissociable. The dissociation constant increases with rising temperature.

TABLE I
Steroid-Binding Proteins in Human Serum

Protein	MW	Carbohydrate (%)	Conc. (μM)	Binding to[a]	Association constant (μM^{-1}) 4°C	37°C
HSA	69,000	0	550	P	0.36	0.18
AAG	41,000	42	18	P	1.5	0.6
CBG	52,000	26	0.7	P	700	90
				C	520	24
TeBG	94,000	32	0.04	T	1100	350
				E	600	220
PBG[b]	88,000	71	13	P	2200	350

[a] P, progesterone; C, cortisol; T, testosterone; E, estradiol.
[b] Progesterone-binding globulin from pregnant guinea pig serum.

An inverse relationship exists between the serum concentrations of the binding proteins and their affinity for steroids. For example, the association constant of CBG for progesterone at 37°C is approximately 500 times higher than that of HSA, but there are about 800 HSA molecules for each molecule of CBG in normal blood serum. This is the reason why the participation of HSA in the binding of steroid hormones may be substantial, a fact that is often overlooked when one considers the nature of the bound and unbound portion of a steroid hormone circulating in the blood. The steroids are biologically inactive as long as they are associated with the serum proteins; they can be "activated" by dissociation to the free hormone. In this manner, a relatively large amount of steroid can be carried in an indifferent storage form and can be made available immediately at the target tissue (Westphal, 1971).

The most meaningful objective of the physicochemical study of steroid hormone interaction with proteins would be the investigation of steroid-receptor proteins (Westphal, 1961; King and Mainwaring, 1974). Unfortunately, these receptors have not been available in purified form in sufficient amounts to make such a study practical. Therefore, we have concentrated our efforts on the exploration of the chemical basis underlying the interaction of steroid hormones with serum proteins, preferably those of high affinity and specificity. Earlier results from our and other laboratories on the binding of steroids to the human proteins listed in Table I have been summarized (Westphal, 1971); additional results on HSA (Westphal and Harding, 1973), AAG (Ryan and Westphal, 1972; Kute and Westphal, 1976), CBG (Rosner and Bradlow, 1971; Chader et al., 1972; Rosner et al.,

1973, 1976; LeGaillard *et al.,* 1974, 1975, 1976), and TeBG (Mickelson and Pétra, 1975; Rosner and Smith, 1975) have been published.

Studies on CBG, the serum protein that binds progesterone in human serum with highest affinity, are handicapped by its instability to heat and acidic milieu, and by its low concentration in the blood. It was fortunate, therefore, that we discovered in the serum of the pregnant guinea pig a protein, different from CBG, that binds progesterone and certain other steroids with high affinity, and that occurs in relatively high quantity (Diamond *et al.,* 1969). The existence of such a protein was postulated by Heap (1969) in independent studies. In the present report, some recent results on this progesterone-binding globulin (PBG) will be discussed. In addition, some new findings on the chemical nature of the steroid-binding site of PBG and of AAG will be discussed.

II. PROGESTERONE-BINDING GLOBULIN OF THE PREGNANT GUINEA PIG

A. Purification and Characterization

The progesterone-binding globulin occurs in the serum of pregnant guinea pigs at the relatively high concentration of about 1.2×10^{-5} moles progesterone binding sites per liter (Burton *et al.,* 1974), corresponding to more than a milligram per milliliter. PBG has considerable stability to elevated temperature; more than 50% of the steroid-binding activity survives a 2-day exposure to 60°C (MacLaughlin and Westphal, 1974). The heat resistance is greater than that of CBG from which it can be separated (Milgrom *et al.,* 1970; Burton *et al.,* 1971). Also noteworthy is the remarkable stability toward acidic and alkaline milieu; in contrast to the lability of CBG at low pH, incubation of PBG for 48 hours at pH 2 or pH 11 results in very little inactivation (Harding *et al.,* 1974).

Purification of PBG has been reported from several laboratories (Milgrom *et al.,* 1973; Lea, 1973a; Burton *et al.,* 1974); ion exchange chromatography, gel filtration, ammonium sulfate precipitation, and electrophoresis were the principal methods applied in the initial studies. A useful simplification of the purification procedure was achieved (Stroupe and Westphal, 1975a) by taking advantage of the acid stability of PBG and its extremely low isoelectric pH of 2.8 (Harding *et al.,* 1974): chromatography at pH 4.5 of the serum over a column of sulfopropyl (SP) Sephadex, a strong cation exchanger, results in adsorption of most serum proteins except PBG which is eluted in the void volume of the column. A single run gives a PBG preparation free of albumin and of CBG, which presumably is inactivated under the acidic conditions.

The prepurified PBG preparations were subjected to affinity chromatography on columns of immobilized steroids (Cheng et al., 1976). Sepharose 4B was coupled with diaminodipropylamine to which the 17-hemisuccinate of 19-nortestosterone was then attached through a peptide bond. An equally effective affinity gel was obtained by coupling the hemisuccinate of deoxycorticosterone to the diaminodipropylamino derivative of Sepharose 4B. When PBG is applied to the affinity column, a portion of the protein is not adsorbed and is readily eluted by the starting buffer; this material does not bind progesterone. The active PBG fraction is eluted with 10 μM progesterone or 5α-pregnane-3,20-dione, steroids that have a high affinity for PBG and are, thus, able to displace the protein from the steroid–Sepharose matrix. Repetition of the affinity chromatography of the active fraction results in one peak of pure PBG; no inactive protein can be detected.

Equilibrium dialysis and Scatchard analysis of the affinity-purified PBG gave an n value of 1.03 as an average of six determinations at different temperatures. The association constant of the progesterone complex, K_a, was 2.2×10^9 M^{-1} at 4°C, 1.1×10^9 M^{-1} at 22°C, and decreased further with increasing temperature (Table II and Table V below). Determination of the molecular weight by sedimentation equilibrium ultracentrifugation (Chervenka, 1970) gave an apparent weight average molecular weight (MW) of 88,000. In agreement with previous results (Burton et al., 1974), the affinity-purified PBG was found to have the unusually high carbohydrate content of about 70%, almost one fourth of which consisted of sialic acid (Table III). The amino acid composition of affinity-purified PBG is given in Table IV.

One of the unique properties of PBG is its polydispersity. This can be readily demonstrated by dividing the glycoprotein peak, obtained by gel filtration, into two halves; the half fraction that elutes first has a higher molecular weight and a higher carbohydrate content than the later portion

TABLE II
Properties of PBG

Parameter	Value
Molecular weight	88,000; polydisperse
Isoelectric pH	2.8
Peptide content	~30%
Carbohydrate content	~70%
K_a, 4°C (progesterone)	2.2×10^9 M^{-1}
K_a, 37°C (progesterone)	3.5×10^8 M^{-1}
No. of steroid-binding sites (n)	1

TABLE III
Carbohydrate Content of Affinity-Purified PBG

Carbohydrate	%
Hexose	29.0
Hexosamine	23.5
Fucose	1.5
Sialic acid	17.0
	71.0

(Burton et al., 1974). Further subdivision by gel filtration gave active species of gradually decreasing molecular weight, forming a virtually continuous series of changing molecular sizes of PBG. This can be seen by several independent methods: Figure 1 shows an electrophoretic analysis of the size distribution of two arbitrary fractions of the polydisperse active PBG species, i.e., PBG I (MW 117,000) and PBG II (MW 78,000), in comparison with the PBG activity of unfractionated pooled serum and of serum from an individual animal. Clearly, the full range of different size species is present in the pooled serum, as well as in the serum of the individual donor; the polydispersity is, therefore, not the result of the preparative procedures or of pooling. This conclusion has been verified by sucrose-gradient centrif-

TABLE IV
Amino Acid Composition of Progesterone-Binding Globulin

Residue	Grams per 100 g polypeptide	Moles/mole PBG
Asp	10.6	22
Thr	8.1	19
Ser	5.1	14
Glu	10.8	20
Pro	4.5	11
Gly	2.2	9
Ala	3.6	12
Val	4.2	10
½ Cys	0.85	2
Met	2.2	4
Ile	2.4	5
Leu	13.3	28
Tyr	6.9	10
Phe	6.2	10
Lys	5.4	10
His	4.1	7
Arg	5.9	9
Trp	3.9	5

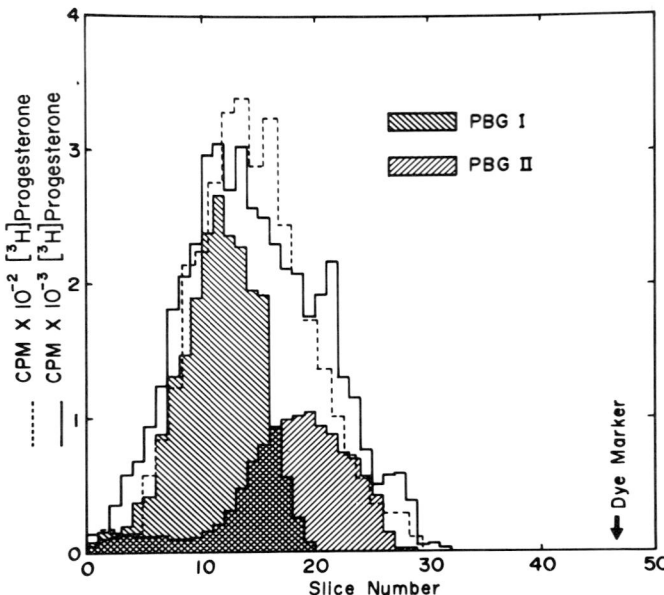

Fig. 1. Polyacrylamide gel electrophoresis of PBG labeled with [^{3}H]progesterone. Solid line, open area, pooled pregnant guinea pig serum; broken line, serum from single animal; shaded areas, PBG I and PBG II (see text). The serum of the single animal contained about 10% of the radioactivity added to the pooled serum sample. From Burton et al. (1974).

ugation analysis of six individual sera from pregnant guinea pigs (Burton et al., 1974). The polyacrylamide electrophoresis gives essentially the same result in the presence of sodium dodecyl sulfate, indicating that size and not charge is the determining factor, in concordance with the gradient sedimentation studies. Purification of PBG by affinity chromatography does not affect the polydisperse nature of this glycoprotein (Cheng et al., 1976).

It has been previously concluded (Burton et al., 1974) that the polydispersity of PBG results from the attachment of different amounts of carbohydrate to a polypeptide core of about 27,000 MW; such polypeptide–carbohydrate relationship is known for other polydisperse glycoproteins. Assuming a peptide content of about 30% and 88,000 MW for the affinity-purified PBG (Table II), a polypeptide core of about 27,000 MW can again be calculated.

The unusually high carbohydrate values for pure PBG have been obtained consistently in our laboratory. It should be noted, however, that lower amounts have been found by other investigators; Milgrom et al. (1973) reported 48.7% for their preparation, and Lea (1973a) determined only 42%. No definite explanation can be given for these dissimilarities, except for the

15. Steroid-Binding Serum Proteins

possibility that different strains of guinea pigs produce variant glycoproteins. We have eliminated differences in the purification methods as the cause of the variations of the carbohydrate content (Burton *et al.*, 1974).

B. Conformational Changes upon Interaction with Steroids

A few observations have been reported previously on the induction of conformational changes in proteins upon steroid binding. Alfsen (1963) found bovine serum albumin to become less levorotatory and more acidic upon binding testosterone. Both human and bovine serum albumin develop a difference spectrum in the aromatic absorption region when complexed with different steroids (Ryan, 1968; Ryan and Gibbs, 1970). Concerning high-affinity serum binders, rat CBG polymerizes when its ligand is removed (Chader and Westphal, 1968), and addition of steroid to the polymerized protein reverses the aggregation. This offers indirect evidence that the conformation of rat CBG is ligand dependent. Chader *et al.* (1972) made similar observations with rabbit CBG. In both of these cases, the aggregation is accompanied by reversible loss of steroid-binding affinity.

Circular dichroism spectra of PBG and of the PBG–progesterone complex are shown in Fig. 2. Compared to free PBG, the steroid complex has a

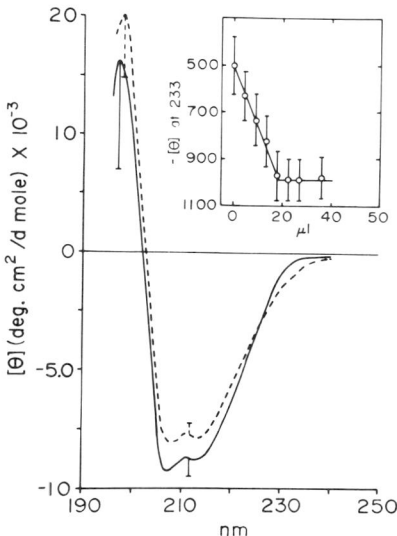

Fig. 2. Circular dichroism spectra of PBG (———) and PBG–progesterone complex (---) at pH 7.4. Progesterone-binding site concentration, 8.6×10^{-7} M. Note change of scale of ordinate. Inset: CD titration of PBG by progesterone. At the equivalence point, 1.08 moles of progesterone has been added per binding site. From Stroupe and Westphal (1975a).

more negative ellipticity between 240 and 227 nm where it becomes more positive. Both samples have minima at 213 and at 207 nm. Zero ellipticity occurs at about 203 nm; maxima are seen at 198 nm for the progesterone complex and at 197 nm for steroid-free PBG.

To demonstrate that the conformational change, indicated by the CD difference between PBG and liganded PBG, is indeed due to complex formation, a simple titration experiment was performed at 233 nm where the percentage difference between the two curves is maximal. The CD signal changes linearly with the addition of progesterone until the binding sites are saturated (Fig. 2, inset). The progesterone-binding site concentration was, thus, found to be 9.3×10^{-7} M, in agreement with the value of 8.6×10^{-7} obtained by fluorescence-quenching analysis (see below).

CD spectra of high-affinity steroid-binding proteins have not been reported previously. The spectra given in Fig. 2 are noteworthy primarily for their low ellipticity and the unusual double minima at 207 and 213 nm. Attempts to apply available methods of interpreting the PBG spectrum in terms of α-helix, β-pleated sheet, and random coil segments were unsuccessful (Stroupe and Westphal, 1975a). The reason may be the contribution to the observed ellipticity of the amide chromophores present in the carbohydrate moiety of PBG.

Conformational differences between PBG and steroid-liganded PBG were also revealed by ultraviolet difference spectra (Stroupe and Westphal, 1975a). Figure 3 shows such spectra of PBG against its complexes with progesterone and 5-pregnen-3β-ol-20-one. Both steroids induce a large positive signal at 294–295 nm, due to the perturbation of a tryptophan residue. Smaller peaks at 288 and 283 nm can be assigned to tyrosine and tryptophan, respectively. In the case of the progesterone complex, a broad and intensive negative signal appears at 268–270 nm, resulting from solvent perturbation of the Δ^4-3-keto chromophore; this is the basis of a previously published spectral method for measuring protein interactions with Δ^4-3-ketosteroids (Westphal, 1957). In accordance with this interpretation, the PBG complex with pregnenolone, a steroid lacking the Δ^4-3-keto chromophore, does not give the 268–270 nm minimum in its difference spectrum (Fig. 3).

The large positive peak at 233–234 nm in both difference spectra (Fig. 3) is assumed to result primarily from perturbation of the short wavelength transitions of aromatic amino acids (Stroupe and Westphal, 1975a); the progesterone spectrum shows, in addition to this positive contribution by the protein, the signal given by the perturbed Δ^4-3-keto grouping. This progesterone absorption accounts almost entirely for the difference between the progesterone and pregnenolone peaks at this short wavelength; the conformational change in PBG upon binding progesterone or pregnenolone is the same.

15. Steroid-Binding Serum Proteins

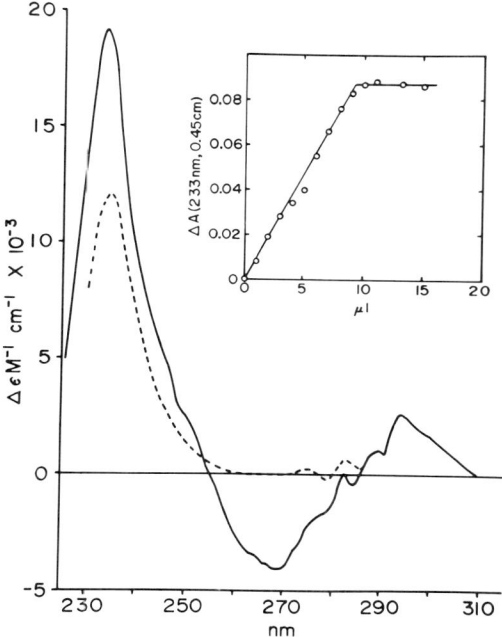

Fig. 3. Ultraviolet difference spectra of PBG complexes with progesterone (———) and 5-pregnen-3β-ol-20-one (---). Between 285 and 310 nm the difference spectra of the two complexes are identical. Inset: spectral titration of PBG with progesterone at 233 nm. At the equivalence point, 1.01 moles of progesterone have been added per binding site. From Stroupe and Westphal (1975a).

The signals at 233, 270, and 294 nm can be used to measure the concentration of binding sites. Utilizing the short wavelength signal, a titration of PBG with progesterone is given in Fig. 3, inset; similar results were obtained in titrations with both progesterone and pregnenolone following the signals at the other wavelengths. The signal changes were linear with respect to added steroid until the binding sites were saturated; no further changes were noted beyond the saturation point. This result proves that the difference spectra given by the PBG complexes of progesterone and pregnenolone result from steroid binding to a specific site on the protein and not from nonspecific solvent perturbation.

C. Fluorescence Quenching upon Interaction with Δ^4-3-Ketosteroids

The involvement of tryptophan in the steroid binding to PBG, revealed by the ultraviolet difference spectra (Fig. 3), can also be seen in fluorometric

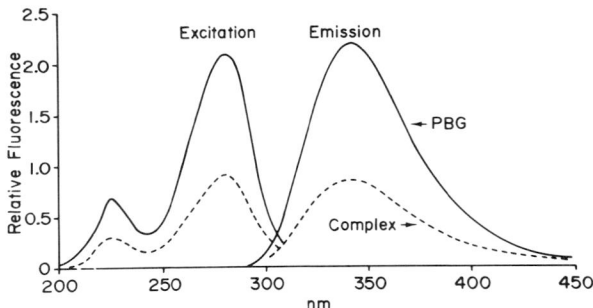

Fig. 4. Fluorescence excitation and emission spectra of PBG (solid lines) and PBG–progesterone complex (broken lines). Concentration of both PBG and the complex was 3.3×10^{-7} M. From Stroupe et al. (1975).

measurements (Stroupe et al., 1975). The intrinsic fluorescence spectrum of PBG shows an excitation maximum at 280 nm and an emission maximum at 340 nm, characteristic of polypeptides containing tryptophan (Fig. 4). Occupation of the binding site by progesterone results in strong quenching without shift of the wavelength maxima; for affinity-purified PBG, the reduction of fluorescence is over 80% (Cheng et al., 1976). This quenching phenomenon can be utilized in a simple titration method to determine the concentration of binding sites and the association constant. Addition of small aliquots of a progesterone solution to a given PBG solution results in a gradual decrease of the relative fluorescence until the binding site is saturated (Fig. 5). Further addition of progesterone does not reduce the fluorescence more, except for a small quenching contribution caused by ethanol in the steroid solution and by inner filter effects. The intersect of the extended initial linear portion and the extrapolated baseline gives the equivalence point. This determines the concentration of binding sites since the concentration of the added progesterone solution is known.

The association constant can be determined by the expression

$$K_a = \alpha/(1 - \alpha)^2 P$$

where α is the degree of association as given by the ratio of quenching at the equivalence point over total quenching, and P is the binding site concentration at the equivalence point. Drawing a smooth curve through all data points between the two linear portions (Fig. 5) makes it possible to base the value of α not on a single point, but rather on an average. The data representing the quenching curve between the linear portions can be presented as a Scatchard plot (Fig. 5, inset). As expected, the affinity constant obtained is the same as that calculated by the simple expression given above.

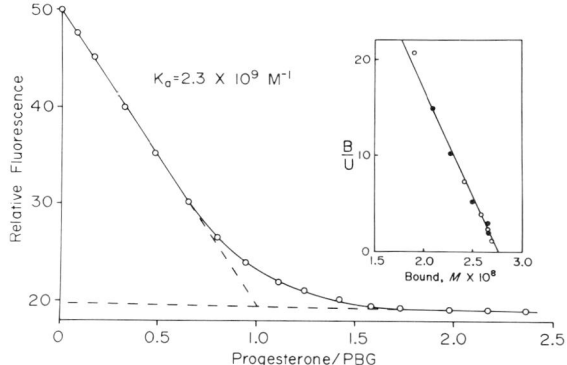

Fig. 5. Fluorescence-quenching titration of PBG with progesterone. The equivalence point gives a binding site concentration of 2.70×10^{-8} M; the solid curve yields a K_a of 2.3×10^9 M^{-1}. Inset: Scatchard plot of the data from the nonlinear region, giving a binding site concentration of 2.77×10^{-8} M and a K_a of 2.1×10^9 M^{-1}. The filled circles correspond to the actual data points, whereas the open circles are taken from the solid curve. From Stroupe *et al.* (1975).

Complex formation of AAG with steroids such as progesterone also causes a decrease of protein fluorescence, although to a lesser degree than with PBG (Fig. 6). Fluorescence-quenching titration curves may be obtained in a similar way (Fig. 7), and the concentration of binding sites and affinity constants can be determined (Stroupe *et al.*, 1975). Figure 8 shows that the fluorescence-quenching method is also sensitive to the differences in steroid binding activity that have been observed by Ganguly and Westphal (1968a) in different solvent environments. The presence of 4 M

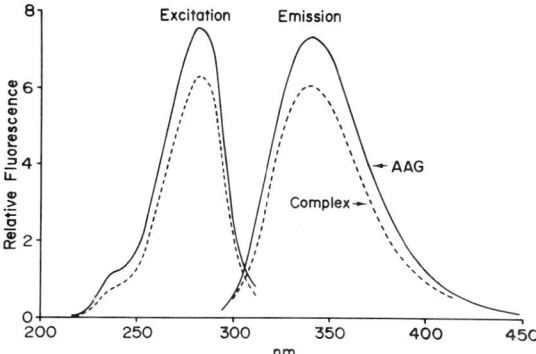

Fig. 6. Fluorescence excitation and emission spectrum of AAG (solid lines) and AAG–progesterone complex (broken lines). Concentration of both AAG and the complex was 1.3×10^{-5} M. From Stroupe *et al.* (1975).

NaCl in 50 mM phosphate buffer of pH 7.4 increases the association constant of the AAG–progesterone complex many times; accordingly, the fluorescence quenching is almost doubled (Kute, 1975). Conversely, 4 M KSCN, which drastically reduces the binding affinity, virtually eliminates the quenching phenomenon. These findings corroborate the validity of the use of fluorescence quenching as the basis for the determination of binding affinity in certain steroid–protein interactions.

The main advantages of the fluorescence quenching titration for determination of association constant and binding site concentration are (a) the small amount of binding protein required, i.e., typically 0.1 nmole or less than 10 μg of PBG per experiment; (b) the greater rapidity compared to equilibrium dialysis; and (c) the possibility to use unlabeled steroids. The binding protein must be in a purified form and the steroid must have the appropriate ultraviolet absorption. Fluorescence quenching is also a valuable method for assaying PBG activity during purification procedures without introducing radiosteroids; measurement of the fluorescence of the relevant fractions in the presence and absence of a large excess of progesterone gives a value for the progesterone-induced quenching which is proportional to PBG purity.

The fluorescence-quenching titration method has been applied in our laboratory for the determination of association constants of PBG complexes with a large number of steroids with Δ^4-3-keto and other absorbing groupings (unpublished results with A. T. Blanford, S. D. Stroupe, and

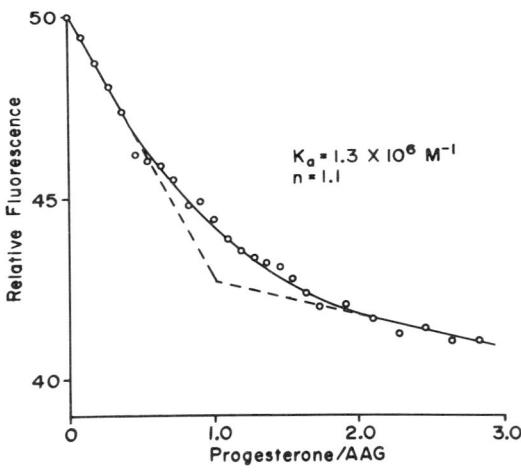

Fig. 7. Fluorescence-quenching titration of AAG with progesterone. At equivalence, the AAG concentration was 1.3×10^{-5} M. A K_a of 1×10^6 M^{-1} was calculated from the solid curve. From Stroupe *et al.* (1975).

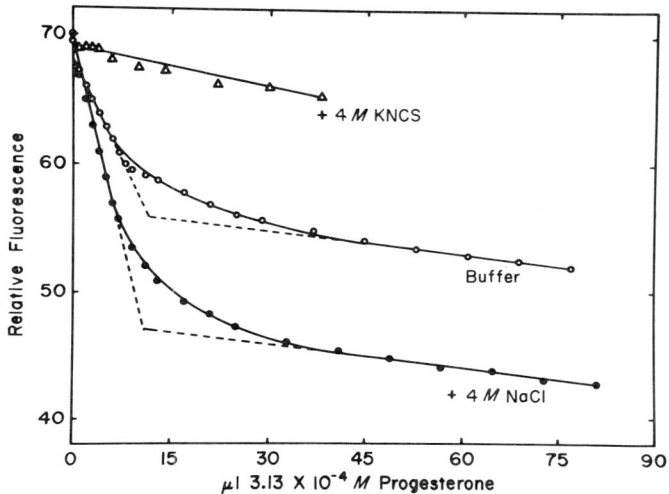

Fig. 8. Fluorescence-quenching titration of AAG with progesterone in neutral salt solutions. The AAG concentration was 2.5×10^{-6} M in all three determinations. From Kute and Westphal (1976).

W. L. Wittman). Examples of three Δ^4-3-ketosteroids more polar than progesterone are given in Fig. 9, A–C. The association constants obtained are in general agreement with those determined by a competitive equilibrium dialysis method (Lea, 1973b). Figure 9D shows the titration of two identical PBG samples with progesterone and with 5-pregnen-3β-ol-20-one. Even though pregnenolone binds to PBG over 10 times more strongly than cortisol (Lea, 1973b), quenching is only minimal, and an association constant cannot be calculated. The ultraviolet difference spectra (Fig. 3) had shown that the protein perturbation as such is virtually the same whether given by progesterone or by pregnenolone, indicating the same type of conformational change upon binding of either steroid.

If pregnenolone or any related steroid lacking the Δ^4-3-keto grouping binds to the same site in PBG as progesterone, competitive displacement of progesterone by the nonabsorbing steroid and reversal of the fluorescence quenching should be demonstrable. Figure 10 shows that this is indeed the case; addition of 5α- or 5β-pregnane-3,20-dione to a PBG solution that is maximally quenched by a stoichiometric amount of progesterone, results in restoration of the fluorescence (Stroupe *et al.*, 1975). The PBG complex formed with the saturated pregnane derivative approaches the intrinsic fluorescence of the unbound PBG as the concentration of pregnanedione is increased. The inset of Fig. 10 indicates that the fluorescence of PBG does not change even when several moles of 5β-pregnanedione are added per

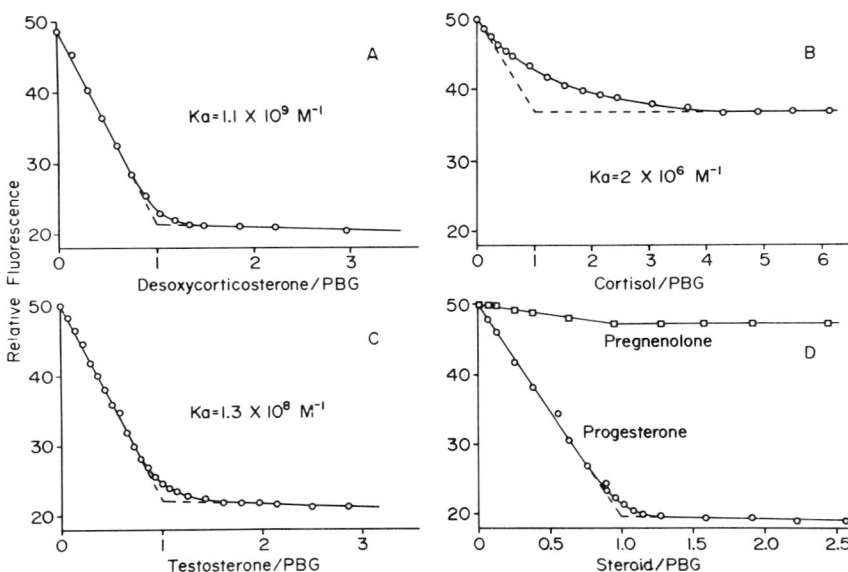

Fig. 9. Fluorescence-quenching titrations of PBG with various steroids. From Stroupe *et al.* (1975).

mole of protein. It is also evident from Fig. 10 that greater amounts of the 5β-steroid than of the 5α-isomer are needed to displace progesterone from PBG. This is explained by a lower binding affinity of the 5β-pregnanedione, in agreement with competitive equilibrium dialysis studies showing that the association constant of the PBG complex with 5α-pregnane-3,20-dione is almost 10 times higher than that of the 5β-stereoisomer (Lea, 1973b). We will see below that the change of fluorescence by competitive displacement can be utilized to measure dissociation rates of PBG–steroid complexes.

A closer analysis of the fluorescence spectrum of PBG and of the spectral properties of progesterone provided insight into the protein–steroid interaction at the molecular level (Stroupe *et al.*, 1975). Utilizing the theory of radiationless energy transfer of Förster (1948, 1959), it was calculated that the progesterone–tryptophan distance in the complex is smaller than the corresponding distance in the complex of PBG with cortisol, which has a much lower affinity. The mechanism of fluorescence quenching by energy transfer from protein fluorophores to the $n \to \pi^*$ absorption band of a conjugated carbonyl group in the steroid requires that two conditions are met. First, the contact between steroid and protein in the complex must occur very near a fluorescent group. Second, to be a suitable acceptor, the steroid must have an absorption band overlapping the fluorescence band of

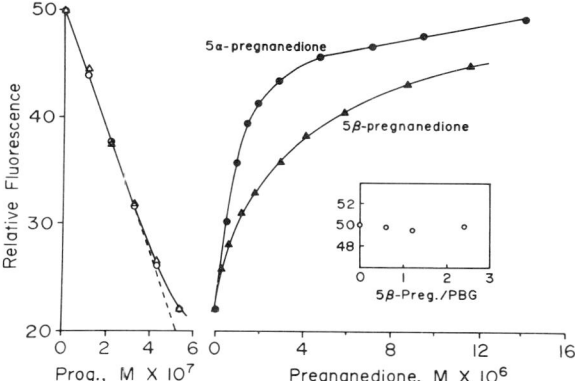

Fig. 10. Fluorescence-quenching titration of PBG with progesterone (open circles and triangles) followed by addition of an excess of 5α-pregnane-3,20-dione or 5β-pregnane-3,20-dione. Note the "unquenching" by displacement of progesterone. The inset shows that the fluorescence of PBG does not change by addition of more than 1 mole of 5β-pregnanedione per mole PBG. From Stroupe *et al.* (1975).

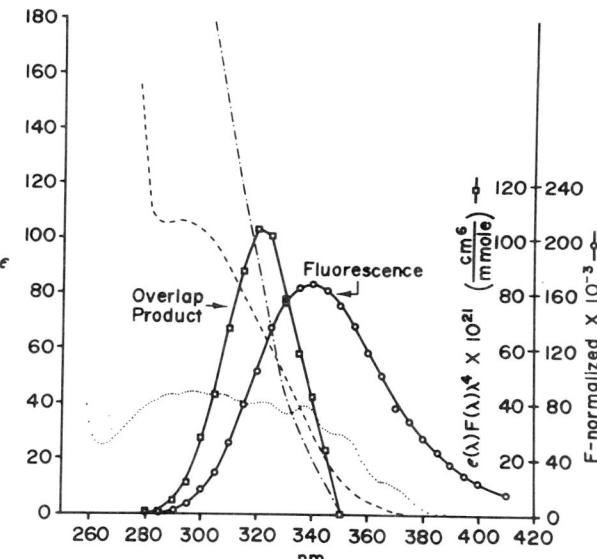

Fig. 11. Ultraviolet absorption spectra of progesterone in water containing 10% ethanol (–·–·–), in methanol (– – –), and in heptane (·····) illustrating the overlap with PBG fluorescence (–O–O–). The overlap product is given for the absorption spectrum in 10% ethanol (for details, see Stroupe *et al.*, 1975).

the protein. The magnitude of the quenching then offers information on the molecular events at the binding site. Figure 11 shows the spectral overlap of steroid absorption and fluorescence emission for progesterone and PBG; further details have been published elsewhere (Stroupe et al., 1975).

III. KINETICS OF STEROID-PROTEIN INTERACTIONS

Most of our present knowledge on interactions between steroids and proteins (Westphal, 1971) has been attained under the viewpoint of systems in equilibrium. Serum proteins with high affinity for steroid hormones have been isolated and characterized, and the strength of their association with steroids has been determined under various conditions. The emphasis has been on the end products of the reversible binding reaction, i.e., the steroid-protein complex and the unbound components formed by dissociation. For a meaningful interpretation of the interactions as they occur *in vivo* between hormones and proteins, and for an understanding of their biological significance, the association complex has to be viewed as a dynamic system; detailed information is required on the rates of association and dissociation, as well as on thermodynamic parameters. In the area of steroid-binding serum proteins, only a few quantitative kinetic studies on the interactions have been reported, as will be discussed below.

The unusual stability (Harding et al., 1974), ready availability in pure form (Cheng et al., 1976), binding affinity for a wide variety of steroids (Milgrom et al., 1973; Lea, 1973b; Tan and Murphy, 1974; Kontula et al., 1974), and suitable fluorescence properties (Stroupe et al., 1975) make PBG a very useful protein to study the rates of association and dissociation for progesterone and other steroids (Stroupe and Westphal, 1975b). Quenching of the strong fluorescence signal of PBG upon binding a Δ^4-3-ketosteroid provides a sensitive indicator for the association; the high affinity of PBG for progesterone, androgens, and other steroids permits the use of dilute reactant solutions to slow down the rapid bimolecular association reaction while still attaining complete association. Displacement of the quenching steroid from the complex by an ultraviolet-transparent steroid, such as 5α-pregnanedione or dihydrotestosterone, results in restoration of the intrinsic PBG fluorescence so that the dissociation rate of the PBG–Δ^4-3-ketosteroid complex can be measured. These unique features allow the use of stopped-flow fluorometry for the determination of association and dissociation rates of PBG–steroid complexes, thereby providing the first reported example in which a physical parameter of the binding protein is monitored to establish the time-course of steroid binding and dissociation (Stroupe and Westphal, 1975b).

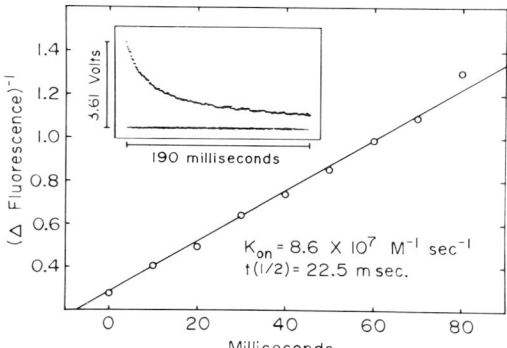

Fig. 12. Stopped-flow fluorescence measurement of association of PBG with progesterone. The decrease in photomultiplier voltage, i.e., fluorescence, was recorded as function of time and the data calculated by computer. The inset is a photograph of the oscilloscope trace of the decrease in photomultiplier voltage with time. From Stroupe and Westphal (1975b).

Figure 12 shows a representative determination of the association rate constant (k_{on}) between PBG and progesterone at pH 7.4, 20°C. A half-time of 22.5 msec was obtained at an equimolar concentration of 0.52 μM, corresponding to a rate constant of 8.6×10^7 M^{-1} s^{-1}. An average value ($\pm$ SD) of $k_{on} = 8.7 \pm 1.9 \times 10^7$ M^{-1} s^{-1} was calculated from 32 experiments, each of which was the mean of 4 runs. The association rate constant was found to be independent of concentration over a range from 33.5 nM to 1.65 μM.

To measure the dissociation rates, the PBG–Δ^4-3-ketosteroid complex was mixed at pH 7.4 with a large excess of nonquenching steroid. The inset in Fig. 13 presents the oscilloscope trace of the photomultiplier voltage, indicating the "unquenching" of fluorescence following the displacement of progesterone by 5α-pregnanedione as a function of time. The same result was obtained with dihydrotestosterone as competing steroid. In this trial, the dissociation rate constant, k_{off}, was 0.053 s^{-1} with a half-time of 13.1 seconds; the average value was $k_{off} = 0.060 \pm 0.005$ s^{-1}, with the PBG–progesterone complex concentration varying from 12.5 to 500 nM.

The rate of association of PBG and progesterone was measured over the temperature range from 5.9° to 41.2°C; the corresponding dissociation rate was determined from 20.0° to 41.4°C. An Arrhenius plot of the data obtained (Fig. 3 in Stroupe and Westphal, 1975b) shows that the temperature dependencies of the two reactions are quite different. The association reaction has a relatively low energy of activation of 10.0 kcal/mole, being constant over the entire range measured. The temperature dependency of the dissociation reaction is greater, with an activation energy rising from 17 kcal/mole at 20°C to 24 kcal/mole at 40°C.

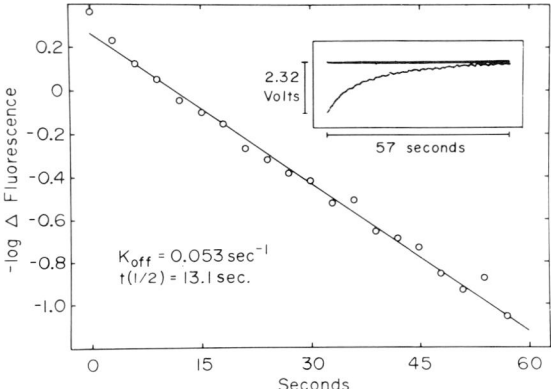

Fig. 13. Stopped-flow fluorescence measurement of dissociation of the PBG–progesterone complex. Displacement of progesterone by a ninefold molar amount of 5α-pregnane-3,20-dione produced an increase in photomultiplier voltage which was utilized to compute k_{off} and $t_{1/2}$. The inset is a photograph of the oscilloscope trace of the photomultiplier voltage as a function of time. From Stroupe and Westphal (1975b).

With the association and dissociation rate constants available over a rather wide temperature range, the general relationship $K_a = k_{on}/k_{off}$ was compared with the association constants measured by equilibrium dialysis (Stroupe and Westphal, 1975b). Table V gives the rate constants of the progesterone–PBG complex and the ratios k_{on}/k_{off} at various temperatures. The K_a values determined by the two independent procedures agree at all temperatures. The close coincidence between the kinetic and the equilibrium association constants gives assurance that the observed fluorescence changes provide a true measure for complex formation and dissociation.

TABLE V

Association Constants of PBG–Progesterone Complex from Kinetic and Equilibrium Data[a]

Temperature (°C)	k_{on} ($M^{-1}s^{-1} \times 10^{-7}$)	k_{off} (s^{-1})	k_{on}/k_{off} ($M^{-1} \times 10^{-9}$)	K_a[b] ($M^{-1} \times 10^{-9}$)
4	2.2	0.0095[c]	2.4	2.2
14	4.3	0.031	1.4	1.4
23	7.4	0.083	0.89	1.0
37	16.2	0.39	0.41	0.35
45	24.6	1.05	0.23	0.22

[a] Stroupe and Westphal (1975b).
[b] Equilibrium dialysis; unpublished results with G. B. Harding.
[c] A value of 0.011 s^{-1} was determined independently by radiosteroid displacement using gel filtration.

15. Steroid-Binding Serum Proteins

Introduction of hydroxy groups into the progesterone molecule results in a decrease of binding affinity to PBG (Lea, 1973b), in proportion to the number of hydroxy groups involved. This binding behavior is in accordance with the polarity rule (Westphal, 1971), indicating that the PBG–steroid interaction is predominantly of a hydrophobic nature. The association and dissociation rate constants, including their ratios which are equal to K_a, are given in Table VI for progesterone, deoxycorticosterone, corticosterone, and cortisol, in addition to testosterone, its acetate, and medrogestone (6,16α-dimethyl-4,6-pregnadiene-3,20-dione). For comparison, the association constants determined independently by fluorescence-quenching titration are listed. The latter values for most steroids in Table VI are somewhat higher than the association constants obtained from kinetic data, in accordance with our previous observation (Stroupe et al., 1975) that the fluorescence method slightly overestimates the affinity constants when compared with equilibrium dialysis results.

The association of PBG with the various steroids occurs at a very rapid rate, which is essentially the same for all steroids having an affinity constant of $> 10^8$ M^{-1}. Complexes of lower affinity appear to associate at a somewhat slower rate, although the values for the weakly bound corticosteroids are less certain. The rate constant for association of progesterone

TABLE VI

Association and Dissociation Rate Constants of PBG and Various Steroids at 20°C[a]

Steroid	k_{on} $M^{-1}s^{-1} \times 10^{-7}$	k_{off} s^{-1}	k_{on}/k_{off} $M^{-1} \times 10^{-8}$	K_a $M^{-1} \times 10^{-8}$
Progesterone	8.8[b]	0.060	14.5	20[c,d]
Deoxycorticosterone	8.3	0.12	6.7	10[c]
Corticosterone	~5[e]	1.4	0.4[e]	0.2[f]
Cortisol	~5[e]	90[g]	—[g]	0.02[c]
Testosterone	7.8	0.43	1.8	2.9[f]
Testosterone acetate	9.3	0.15	6.1	9.2[f]
Medrogestone[h]	8.5	0.024	35.3	45.5[f]

[a] Stroupe and Westphal (1975b).
[b] This value was determined in the experiment comparing the first four steroids.
[c] Stroupe et al. (1975).
[d] Extrapolation of equilibrium dialysis data in Table V gives $K_a = 11 \times 10^8 M^{-1}$ at 20°C.
[e] This value is less precise than the constants for the other steroids because the reaction did not go to completion under the conditions used.
[f] Determined by fluorescence quenching at 23°C. Unpublished results with A. T. Blanford and W. L. Wittman.
[g] The cortisol dissociation was biphasic with a slower reaction (1–2 s^{-1}) contributing about half of the fluorescence increase. None of the other dissociation reactions was biphasic.
[h] 6,16α-Dimethyl-4,6-pregnadiene-3,20-dione.

to PBG, $k_{on} = 8.7 \times 10^7$ M^{-1} s^{-1} at 20°C, is similar to those of a great number of protein–ligand complexes reported (Eigen and Hammes, 1963) to be in the range of 10^6 to 10^8 M^{-1} s^{-1}. The association rates of the PBG–steroid complexes are not limited by diffusion (Stroupe and Westphal, 1975b).

In contrast to the relatively invariant rates of association, the dissociation rate constants show considerable differences among the steroids studied, covering a relative range of from 1 to 3750 (Table VI). The dissociation rate thus becomes the controlling factor in steroid binding to PBG, conferring specificity to the interaction. This may be seen in several examples. Medrogestone binds to PBG with an affinity two to three times that of progesterone, yet both steroids associate at the same rate. It is the threefold slower dissociation of medrogestone which gives it the higher affinity. Similarly, testosterone acetate binds three times more tightly than testosterone and dissociates about three times more slowly. Again, the ratio between the affinity constants of progesterone and deoxycorticosterone is about 2:1, with a ratio of dissociation of 1:2. All these steroids associate with PBG at the same rate. The phenomenon of the dissociation rates controlling complex stability is similar to observations with antibody–hapten systems (Smith and Skubitz, 1975).

What is the physiological meaning of the association and dissociation rates of various steroid–protein complexes? Obviously, the dissociation rate of the serum–protein complex determines the availability of the steroid hormone to the target cell. Binding of the steroid to an intracellular receptor protein serves a different function: hormone remains attached to the receptor while conformational changes and nuclear transfer take place. It is worth examining, therefore, the proportions in which association and dissociation rates contribute to the stability of the different types of steroid–protein complexes. Table VII shows these rate constants for steroid complexes with three high-affinity binders from serum, and with several cytosol receptor proteins from chick and rat. A striking difference is evident; all serum proteins have dissociation rates that are approximately 6–400 times higher than those of the group of receptor proteins.

These differences appear to be in accordance with physiological function. At late-term pregnancy concentrations of progesterone and PBG, the half-time of association at 37°C is 0.36 msec, that of dissociation of the complex is 1.8 seconds (Stroupe and Westphal, 1975b). The corresponding half-time values for the CBG–cortisol complex at 37°C are 44 msec and 1.1 seconds. By comparison, the association rate constant of progesterone with the chick oviduct receptors, and that of dexamethasone with the rat liver binder, resemble that found for CBG. However, the half-time of dissociation for the receptor complexes is of the order of 10 hours at 0–4°C; the half-time of

TABLE VII
Association and Dissociation Rate Constants for Various Steroid Binders at 0°–4°C

Protein	Steroid[a]	k_{on} M^{-1}s^{-1} × 10^{-4}	k_{off} s^{-1} × 10^{5}	k_{on}/k_{off} M^{-1} × 10^{-8}	Reference
PBG, guinea pig	P	2200	950	24	Table V
CBG, human	C	20	41	4.9	Paterson (1973)
CBG, human	C	—	45	—	Dixon (1968)
CBG, human	C	—	230	—	Rosner et al. (1973)
CBG, rat	C	—	50	—	Koblinsky et al. (1972)
TeBG, human	T	—	90	—	Heyns and DeMoor (1971)
TeBG, human	DHT	—	15	—	Heyns and DeMoor (1971)
TeBG, rabbit	DHT	—	220	—	Hansson et al. (1974)
Chick oviduct receptor A	P	28	1.9	150	Schrader and O'Malley (1972)
Chick oviduct receptor B	P	63	2.4	260	Schrader and O'Malley (1972)
Chick oviduct receptor, purified	P	—	1.6	—	Kuhn et al. (1975)
Rat liver receptor	D	1.4	2.0	7.3	Koblinsky et al. (1972)
Rat uterus receptor	E	—	3.9[b]	—	Katzenellenbogen et al. (1973)

[a] P, progesterone; C, cortisol; T, testosterone; DHT, dihydrotestosterone; D, dexamethasone; E, estradiol.
[b] 25°C.

dissociation for the dexamethasone-binding receptor protein at 37°C is about 13 minutes.

The slow dissociation rates of the cytosol–receptor complexes are in accord with their postulated role in mediating cellular response to steroid hormones. It assures that the steroid remains bound to the cytosol–receptor protein for a sufficiently long time so that the subsequent reactions leading to nuclear hormonal effects can take place. In contrast, the requirements of a hormone transporting protein in the blood serum are different: rapid dissociation of the complex is necessary to provide immediate availability of the steroid at the target site. At the same time, the association must be fast, resulting in a high affinity so that the major portion of the circulating hormone is present in bound form, for the protection of the organism as well as of the steroid hormone.

IV. ON THE CHEMICAL NATURE OF THE BINDING SITE

A. Chemical Modification of α_1-Acid Glycoprotein

Earlier studies on the relationship of the chemical structure of AAG to its steroid binding activity have been reviewed (Westphal, 1971). It was found that the integrity of the *disulfide groups* is essential for the affinity to progesterone (Ganguly and Westphal, 1968b). Reductive cleavage of the S—S bond(s) results in decreased binding activity; this inactivation can be fully reversed by air oxidation. However, when the sulfhydryl groups formed by reduction are covalently blocked by alkylation with iodoacetic acid or its amide, the ability to bind progesterone is lost irreversibly. Although these findings might be explained as direct participation of a disulfide group in the steroid interaction at the binding site, a more likely interpretation would be that disulfide groups in the AAG molecule are essential for the particular conformation that is optimal for association with the steroid.

Modification of the ϵ-amino groups of *lysine* by acetic anhydride or ethyl thiotrifluoroacetate (Ganguly and Westphal, 1968b) results in a loss of the progesterone-binding ability of AAG. Partial removal of the modifying substituent restores part of the steroid-binding activity. Recent results (Kute and Westphal, 1976) have confirmed the significance of the lysine residue for steroid binding. Modification of AAG by phenylisocyanate decreases the nK_a value; increasing amounts of reagent per mole AAG increase the number of lysine residues modified, concomitantly with a reduction of the progesterone-binding activity. Scatchard analysis shows that the loss of binding activity, nK_a, results from a decrease of the number of binding sites, n; the association constant, K_a, for the remaining sites remains that of the native AAG. Naphthylisocyanate abolishes the progesterone-binding activity of AAG in a similar, but more specific way: whereas 9.9 lysine residues had to be modified by phenylisocyanate to reduce nK_a to 6% of its original value, only 3.2 lysine residues needed to be substituted in the naphthylisocyanate reaction to achieve the same loss of binding activity. The latter reagent appears to have a greater affinity for those lysine residues that are located in the binding site for the hydrophobic progesterone.

If the chemical modification of lysine blocks the access of progesterone to the binding site, it should in turn be possible to protect the lysine residue by complex formation with the steroid. Figure 14 shows the rate of modification of lysine in AAG by trinitrobenzenesulfonic acid (TNBS), a reagent that substitutes unprotonated amino groups (Means and Feeney, 1971). The reaction was performed in the presence and absence of 2 moles progesterone per mole AAG. No difference was seen between these two conditions for about 2 hours when more than 4 moles of lysine per mole protein had been modified. After 3 or 4 hours, the protective effect of progesterone was evident; approximately one less lysine residue was substituted in the presence of progesterone. The rate of modification then became the same up to at least 6 hrs when the temperature was raised to 70°C for 15 minutes to complete the reaction. The protection of lysine from modification by

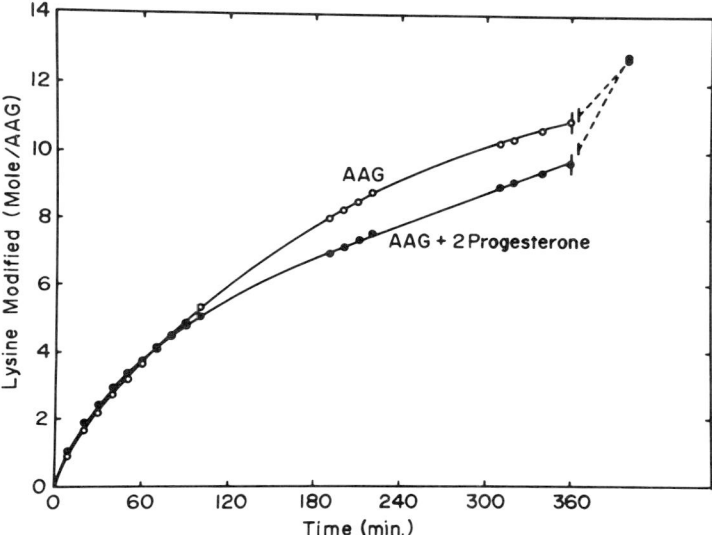

Fig. 14. Modification of AAG by trinitrobenzenesulfonic acid at 22°C in the presence and absence of 2 moles progesterone per mole AAG. At 360 minutes, the temperature was raised to 70°C for 15 minutes to complete the reaction. From Kute and Westphal (1976).

TNBS is now lost because of dissociation of progesterone from AAG at the higher temperature. A total of about 13 residues, i.e., all lysine residues of AAG, are finally modified. We conclude that a lysine residue is located in the binding site.

Introduction of a nitro group at C-3 of the phenol ring of *tyrosine* by tetranitromethane (Means and Feeney, 1971) results in a decrease of the number of active progesterone-binding sites in AAG with retention of full binding affinity at the remaining sites (Kute and Westphal, 1976). Addition of progesterone, or of a mixture of several Δ^4-3-ketosteroids to provide a higher concentration of soluble ligand, protected approximately one tyrosine residue from nitration, and left a greater fraction of n intact. This protection can be seen in Fig. 15, showing the nitration of AAG by tetranitromethane in the absence and in the presence of 2 moles of progesterone per mole AAG; the effect is evident from the first minutes of the reaction. The tetranitromethane modification of the AAG–progesterone complex is interpreted best by the presence of one tyrosyl residue in the steroid-binding site.

Fluorescence quenching of AAG upon binding of progesterone (see Section II,C) results from radiationless energy transfer from *tryptophan* to the Δ^4-3-ketosteroid. Further evidence for the involvement of tryptophan in the interaction of steroids with AAG was obtained by chemical modification studies (Kute and Westphal, 1976). Substitution of tryptophan in AAG by N-bromosuccinimide, formic acid, and 2-hydroxy-5-nitrobenzylbromide (HNBB, Koshland's reagent) decreases the binding activity. Formylation

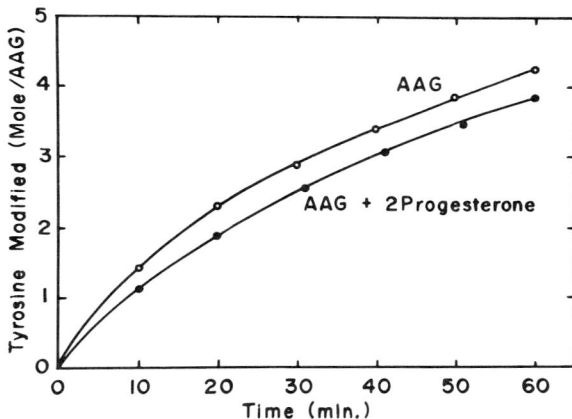

Fig. 15. Modification of AAG by tetranitromethane at 22°C in the presence and absence of 2 moles progesterone per mole AAG. From Kute and Westphal (1976).

TABLE VIII
Effect of Formylation of AAG and its Reversal on Progesterone-Binding Activity

Exp. No.	Protein	Conditions	Trp residues formylated per mole AAG	nK_a $M^{-1} \times 10^{-5}$
1	AAG	(Control)	0.00	14
	AAG	Formylation 3 minutes	0.75	3.4
	AAG	Formylation 10 minutes	1.22	2.6
	AAG	Formylation 20 minutes	1.80	1.4
2	AAG	(Control)	0.00	10.3
	AAG	Formylation	0.34	2.7
	N-Formyl-AAG	Deformylation	0.00	11.2

with formic acid in the presence of HCl gas over 20 minutes substituted almost two tryptophan residues per mole AAG, accompanied by 90% loss of binding activity. Table VIII shows that the formylation reaction and the loss of binding affinity were fully reversible; removal of the formyl group by incubation at pH 10.5 restored nK_a to its original value.

Reactions of AAG with hydroxynitrobenzylbromide reduced the number of progesterone-binding sites and did not change the association constants of the remaining sites. Attempts to protect the tryptophan residue by complex formation with progesterone did not succeed under the conditions used. This is in agreement with the absence of observable ultraviolet difference absorption signals at 281–282 nm and 291–294 nm, which would indicate binding of progesterone to a tryptophan residue as seen in PBG (Fig. 3). Whereas these results fail to support a direct binding of progesterone to tryptophan in the complex, the fluorescence quenching of AAG by progesterone (Figs. 6 and 7) clearly shows the involvement of tryptophan in the association of AAG with the steroid. Calculations of the approximate distance between progesterone and tryptophan in the complex (Kute and Westphal, 1976) are in agreement with the assumption that a tryptophan residue is located not directly in the binding site, but rather near to it.

The studies on chemical modification of AAG in relation to progesterone binding suggest that tryptophan, lysine, and tyrosine are involved in the binding site. According to Schmid *et al.* (1973), who determined the amino acid sequence of AAG, the protein consists of a chain of 181 amino acids to which five heteropolysaccharide groups are attached. The glycoprotein contains a hydrophobic amino acid sequence from residue 21 to 31 (-Ile-Thr-Gly-Lys-Trp-Phe-Tyr-Ile-Ala-Ser-Ala-) which would appear to be a possible steroid-binding site (Kute and Westphal, 1976).

B. Chemical Modification of Progesterone-Binding Globulin

The approach used to explore the significance of individual amino acids for progesterone binding to PBG was similar to that described above for AAG. The chemical reactions were performed (Kute, 1975) with PBG purified by chromatographic methods exclusive of affinity chromatography. Although the use of such PBG preparations having n values < 1 may influence some results in a quantitative manner, the basic effects of the chemical modifications on progesterone binding are not affected by it.

Substitution of *tryptophan* in PBG by reaction with hydroxynitrobenzylbromide (HNBB) resulted in a decrease of binding sites while the association constant of the remaining sites was not changed. Table IX shows the parallelism between HNBB applied per PBG molecule, number of HNB residues introduced, decline of the quenching, and decrease of n measured by fluorescence titration and by equilibrium dialysis.

In contrast to the observations with AAG, the tryptophan residues in PBG could be protected from HNB substitution by complex formation with progesterone (Table X). Whereas 90% of the binding sites are inactivated by reaction of PBG with HNBB alone, a loss of only 20% of the binding sites occurs in the presence of an excess of progesterone. Again, the K_a values of the remaining binding sites are not affected.

Modification of *lysine* in PBG by trinitrobenzenesulfonic acid (TNBS) results in decreased steroid-binding activity. Complex formation with progesterone protects the lysine residues from substitution. Figure 16 shows that this protection starts immediately, with the first residues reacting. This would indicate, in comparison with the analogous protection experiment with AAG and its latent period of more than an hour (Fig. 14), that the lysine residues most reactive to TNBS are the ones with which progesterone interacts, presumably, in the binding site.

The effect of the chemical modification of lysine on the binding activity of PBG with and without protection by progesterone was also analyzed. In

TABLE IX

Chemical Modification of PBG by HNBB at pH 7.2

HNBB/PBG	HNB/PBG	Fluorescence titration		Scatchard analysis	
		% Quench	n^a	n^a	$K_a(M^{-1} \times 10^{-9})$
0	0	56	1.00	1.00	1.1
15	0.5	47	0.61	0.70	1.7
30	1.0	39	0.54	0.46	2.5
45	1.4	33	0.39	0.41	1.9

^{a} Values adjusted relative to control $n = 1.00$.

TABLE X
Inactivation of PBG by HNBB and Protection of the Binding Site by Progesterone

Reagent per mole PBG	Trp modified per mole PBG	Equilibrium dialysis, 4°C	
		n^a	$K_a(M^{-1} \times 10^{-9})$
None	0	1.0	1.1
20 HNBB	1.2	0.1	1.1
10 Progesterone, 20 HNBB	0.7	0.8	0.8

^{a} Values adjusted relative to control $n = 1.0$.

the absence of progesterone, there was a rapid decrease of the binding activity (Fig. 17) as the number of trinitrophenyl groups incorporated into PBG increased. For example, at 2.5 minutes after addition of TNBS, 3.8 amino groups were modified, and the binding activity was reduced to 84% and 83% of the original value, as measured by multiple equilibrium dialysis

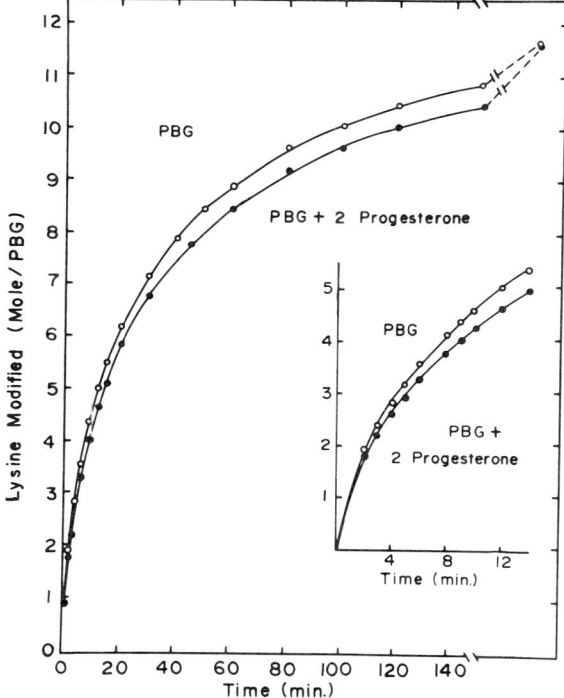

Fig. 16. Modification of PBG by trinitrobenzenesulfonic acid at 22°C in the presence and absence of 2 moles progesterone per mole PBG. At 150 minutes the temperature was raised to 70°C for 15 minutes to complete the reaction. The inset shows the lysine modification (mole/PBG) on an expanded time scale. From Kute (1975).

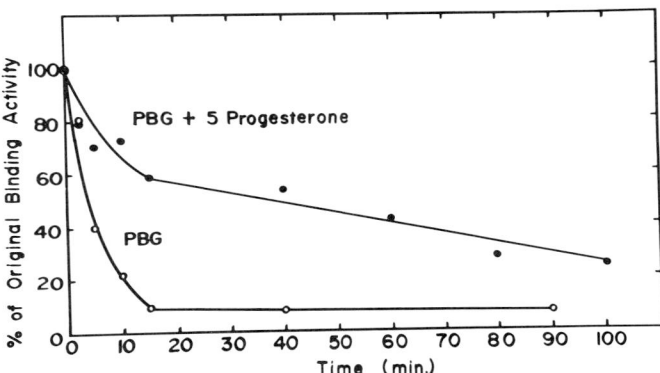

Fig. 17. Rate of inactivation of PBG and PBG–progesterone complex by trinitrobenzenesulfonic acid. The binding activity was determined by multiple equilibrium dialysis. For details, see Kute (1975).

and fluorescence quenching titration, respectively; only 63% of the original quenching was now observed. After 15 minutes of TNBS reaction, the binding activity was down to one-tenth of the original value, while the quenching was only 8% of that of the unmodified control. In contrast, the PBG that was protected by complex formation with progesterone showed a much slower loss of binding activity, as determined by multiple equilibrium dialysis (Fig. 17). After 15 minutes of reaction, 83% of the binding sites were still active, and equilibrium dialysis indicated 60% of the original binding activity. Even after 60 minutes, there was still 42% of the original binding activity present.

Reaction of PBG with tetranitromethane (TNM) reduced the number of progesterone-binding sites to 3–10% of its original value, concomitantly with introduction of nitro groups into *tyrosine* residues (Kute, 1975). The formation of nitrotyrosine was suppressed, and under the conditions applied, about two-thirds of the binding sites remained active when PBG was shielded from TNM by association with progesterone.

The results of the chemical modification studies with PBG indicate that tryptophan, lysine, and tyrosine residues are in different environments in free and progesterone-complexed PBG. The altered reactivity of these residues could result from the conformational change accompanying complex formation, or from direct interaction with progesterone at the binding site.

ACKNOWLEDGMENT

The work described from the author's laboratory has been supported by Grant AM-06369 from the National Institute of Arthritis, Metabolism, and Digestive Diseases and USPHS Research Career Award GM-K6-14,138 from the Division of General Medical Sciences.

REFERENCES

Alfsen, A. (1963). *C. R. Trav. Lab. Carlsberg, Ser. Chim.* **33**, 415–431.
Burton, R. M., Harding, G. B., Rust, N., and Westphal, U. (1971). *Steroids* **17**, 1–16.
Burton, R. M., Harding, G. B., Aboul-Hosn, W. R., MacLaughlin, D. T., and Westphal, U. (1974). *Biochemistry* **13**, 3554–3561.
Chader, G. J., and Westphal, U. (1968). *Biochemistry* **7**, 4272–4282.
Chader, G. J., Rust, N., Burton, R. M., and Westphal, U. (1972). *J. Biol. Chem.* **247**, 6581–6588.
Cheng, S. L., Stroupe, S. D., and Westphal, U. (1976). *FEBS Lett.* **64**, 380–384.
Chervenka, C. H. (1970). *Anal. Biochem.* **34**, 24–29.
Diamond, M., Rust, N., and Westphal, U. (1969). *Endocrinology* **84**, 1143–1151.
Dixon, P. F. (1968). *J. Endocrinol.* **40**, 457–465.
Eigen, M., and Hammes, G. G. (1963). *Adv. Enzymol.* **25**, 1–38.
Förster, T. (1948). *Ann. Phys. (Leipzig)* [6] **2**, 55–75.
Förster, T. (1959). *Discuss. Faraday Soc.* **27**, 7–17.
Ganguly, M., and Westphal, U. (1968a). *J. Biol. Chem.* **243**, 6130–6139.
Ganguly, M., and Westphal, U. (1968b). *Biochim. Biophys. Acta* **170**, 309–323.
Hansson, V., Ritzen, E. M., Weddington, S. C., McLean, W. S., Tindall, D. J., Nayfeh, S. N., and French, F. S. (1974). *Endocrinology* **95**, 690–700.
Harding, G. B., Burton, R. M., Stroupe, S. D., and Westphal, U. (1974). *Life Sci.* **14**, 2405–2412.
Heap, R. B. (1969). *J. Reprod. Fertil.* **18**, 546–548.
Heyns, W., and DeMoor, P. (1971). *J. Clin. Endocrinol. Metab.* **32**, 147–154.
Katzenellenbogen, J. A., Johnson, H. J., Jr., and Carlson, K. E. (1973). *Biochemistry* **12**, 4092–4099.
King, R. J. B., and Mainwaring, W. I. P. (1974). "Steroid-Cell Interactions." Univ. Park Press, Baltimore, Maryland.
Koblinsky, M., Beato, M., Kalimi, M., and Feigelson, P. (1972). *J. Biol. Chem.* **247**, 7897–7904.
Kontula, K., Jänne, O., Rajakoski, E., Tanhuanpää, E., and Vihko, R. (1974). *J. Steroid Biochem.* **5**, 39–44.
Kuhn, R. W., Schrader, W. T., Smith, R. G., and O'Malley, B. W. (1975). *J. Biol. Chem.* **250**, 4220–4228.
Kute, T. E. (1975). Ph.D. Dissertation, University of Louisville, Louisville, Kentucky.
Kute, T., and Westphal, U. (1976). *Biochim. Biophys. Acta* **420**, 195–213.
Lea, O. A. (1973a). *Biochim. Biophys. Acta* **317**, 351–363.
Lea, O. A. (1973b). *Biochim. Biophys. Acta* **322**, 68–74.
LeGaillard, F., Racadot, A., Racadot-Leroy, N., and Dautrevaux, M. (1974). *Biochimie* **56**, 99–108.
LeGaillard, F., Han, K. K., and Dautrevaux, M. (1975). *Biochimie* **57**, 559–568.
LeGaillard, F., Aubert, J. P., Dautrevaux, M., and Loucheux-LeFebvre, M. H. (1976). *FEBS Letters* **64**, 278–284.
MacLaughlin, D. T., and Westphal, U. (1974). *Biochim. Biophys. Acta* **365**, 373–388.
Means, G. E., and Feeney, R. E. (1971). "Chemical Modification of Proteins." Holden-Day, San Francisco, California.
Mickelson, K. E., and Pétra, P. H. (1975). *Biochemistry* **14**, 957–963.
Milgrom, E., Atger, M., and Baulieu, E. E. (1970). *Nature (London)* **228**, 1205–1206.
Milgrom, E., Allouch, P., Atger, M., and Baulieu, E. E. (1973). *J. Biol. Chem.* **248**, 1106–1114.
Paterson, J. Y. F. (1973). *J. Endocrinol.* **56**, 551–570.

Rosner, W., and Bradlow, H. L. (1971). *J. Clin. Endocrinol. Metab.* **33**, 193–198.
Rosner, W., and Smith, R. N. (1975). *Biochemistry* **14**, 4813–4820.
Rosner, W., Darmstadt, R., and Tauster, S. J. (1973). *J. Steroid Biochem.* **4**, 249–255.
Rosner, W., Beers, P. C., Awan, T., and Khan, M. S. (1976). *J. Clin. Endocrinol. Metab.* **42**, 1064–1073.
Ryan, M. F., and Westphal, U. (1972). *J. Biol. Chem.* **247**, 4050–4056.
Ryan, M. T. (1968). *Arch. Biochem. Biophys.* **126**, 407–417.
Ryan, M. T., and Gibbs, G. (1970). *Arch. Biochem. Biophys.* **136**, 65–72.
Schmid, K., Kaufmann, H., Isemura, S., Bauer, F., Emura, J., Motoyama, T., Ishiguro, M., and Nanno, S. (1973). *Biochemistry* **12**, 2711–2724.
Schrader, W. T., and O'Malley, B. W. (1972). *J. Biol. Chem.* **247**, 51–59.
Smith, T. W., and Skubitz, K. M. (1975). *Biochemistry* **14**, 1496–1502.
Stroupe, S. D., and Westphal, U. (1975a). *Biochemistry* **14**, 3296–3300.
Stroupe, S. D., and Westphal, U. (1975b). *J. Biol. Chem.* **250**, 8735–8739.
Stroupe, S. D., Cheng, S. L., and Westphal, U. (1975). *Arch. Biochem. Biophys.* **168**, 473–482.
Tan, S. Y., and Murphy, B. E. P. (1974). *Endocrinology* **94**, 122–127.
Westphal, U. (1957). *Arch. Biochem. Biophys.* **66**, 71–90.
Westphal, U. (1961). *In* "Mechanism of Action of Steroid Hormones" (C. A. Villee and L. L. Engel, eds.), pp. 33–89. Pergamon, Oxford.
Westphal, U. (1971). "Steroid-Protein Interactions." Springer-Verlag, New York.
Westphal, U., and Harding, G. B. (1973). *Biochim. Biophys. Acta* **310**, 518–527.

16

Progesterone-Binding Proteins in Plasma and the Reproductive Tract

E. MILGROM

I.	Progesterone-Binding Plasma Proteins	474
	A. Corticosteroid-Binding Globulin (CBG)	474
	B. Progesterone-Binding Plasma Protein (PBP)	475
II.	Progesterone Receptors	476
	A. Progesterone-Receptor Concentration Is under the Control of Estrogen and Progesterone	476
	B. Progesterone Receptors during Estrous Cycle and Pregnancy	479
III.	Female Genital Tract Secretory Proteins	485
IV.	Discussion	488
	References	489

Steroid hormones are secreted into the blood stream and carried to their target cells. In some cases, they are also excreted into the lumen of the reproductive tract ducts. At all these levels, they interact with specific binding proteins. Corticosteroid-binding globulin (CBG), sex steroid-binding protein (SBP), progesterone-binding plasma protein (PBP), and α-fetoprotein are found in the blood (Westphal, 1971); receptors (Raspé, 1971) and, perhaps, membrane carriers (Milgrom et al., 1973a) are found in the target cells, androgen-binding protein (ABP) is present in rete testis and epididymal fluid (Hansson et al., 1975), and uteroglobin (Beier, 1968) or blastokinin (Krishnan and Daniel, 1967) is found in uterine and oviductal fluid. The present discussion will be limited to those proteins which bind progesterone, and it will be centered on physiological control mechanisms, rather than on purely biochemical descriptions.

I. PROGESTERONE-BINDING PLASMA PROTEINS

A. Corticosteroid-Binding Globulin (CBG)

In most species, progesterone shares with glucocorticoids the same high-affinity binding protein: corticosteroid-binding globulin. Human CBG binds preferentially cortisol at 4°C ($K_a = 5.10^8$ M^{-1} for cortisol, $K_a = 3.10^8$ M^{-1} for progesterone), but at the physiological temperature (37°C) affinity for progesterone ($K_a = 8.10^7$ M^{-1}) is even higher than that for cortisol ($K_a = 3.10^7$ M^{-1}) (Seal and Doe, 1966; Westphal, 1971). However, plasma cortisol concentrations are one or two orders of magnitude higher than those of progesterone in pregnancy and the luteal phase, respectively. This, plus the fact that progesterone is more readily bound to albumin, explains why a higher proportion of cortisol than progesterone is bound to CBG.

Proteins similar to CBG have been found in the soluble fraction of various tissue homogenates in many species. For instances, in the rat uterine cytosol, this protein has been compared with plasma CBG by density-gradient sedimentation, paper and polyacrylamide gel electrophoresis, chromatography through Sephadex G-200, thermolability, steroid specificity and association constant, and antigenicity (Milgrom and Baulieu, 1970a). By all these criteria, no difference could be found between the plasma CBG and the uterine protein. A similar situation has been observed in the rabbit (McGuire and Bariso, 1972) and human uterus (Young and Cleary, 1974; McGuire et al., 1974) and in human mammary carcinoma (Pichon and Milgrom, 1976).

In some cases, evidence has been given that the presence of the CBG-like protein in target tissue cytosol cannot be ascribed to simple blood contamination. For instance, in the rat and rabbit uterine cytosol, its concentration is much higher than the concentrations of hemoglobin and other plasma proteins, and it cannot be washed out from uteri (Milgrom and Baulieu, 1970a), nor eliminated by perfusion (Faber et al., 1973). When uteri are incubated with radioactive progesterone and cortisol, it may be shown that the CBG-like protein is not in contact with the incubation medium and is, thus, probably intracellular (Milgrom and Baulieu, 1970b). Actually, these studies show an apparent discrepancy between cell-free and tissue experiments (Milgrom and Baulieu, 1970b). When uterine cytosol was first prepared and then incubated with [^{3}H]progesterone or [^{3}H]cortisol, both were bound to the CBG-like protein (Fig. 1, right). When uteri were incubated with the same hormones and cytosol subsequently prepared, only [^{3}H]progesterone was bound (Fig. 1, left). The explanation of this phenomenon is the preferential uptake of progesterone by the uteri and the very rapid metabolism of the low amounts of cortisol entering the cells. The

16. Progesterone-Binding Proteins

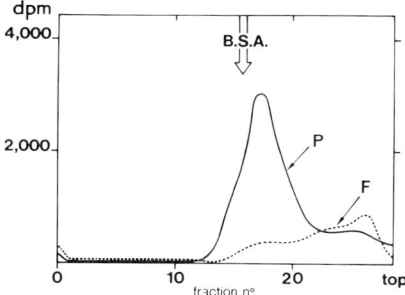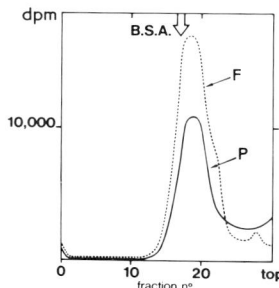

Fig. 1. [³H]progesterone (P) and [³H]cortisol (F) binding to rat uterine CBG-like protein. (Left) Sucrose gradient after incubation of uteri. Uteri were incubated 30 minutes at 37°C with 10 nM steroid. Cytosol was prepared and analyzed by sucrose-gradient ultracentrifugation. (Right) Sucrose gradient after incubation of cytosol. Cytosol was incubated with 10 nM steroid and analyzed by sucrose-gradient ultracentrifugation.

same preferential binding of progesterone was observed *in vivo*. When it is injected intravenously into the rat, [³H]progesterone is bound to the CBG-like protein in the uterus, whereas [³H]cortisol and [³H]corticosterone are not (or very weakly) bound. The role of this protein and its origin (locally synthesized or imported from the blood) are unknown.

The presence of the CBG-like protein often raises another problem; i.e., the difficulty of distinguishing progesterone binding to this high-affinity protein from its binding to the receptor. Two techniques may be used to discriminate between both proteins. One approach is to use some synthetic progestins which are bound mainly to the receptor, e.g., R5020 (17,21-dimethyl-19-norpregna-4,9-diene-3,20-dione), is frequently used (Philibert and Raynaud, 1974). Alternatively, it is possible to inhibit binding to the CBG-like protein by unlabeled cortisol. In the latter case, it may also be useful to enhance binding to receptor without modifying binding to CBG by glycerol treatment (Pichon and Milgrom, 1976).

B. Progesterone-Binding Plasma Protein (PBP)

In the guinea pig, progesterone has a relatively low affinity for CBG. In this species (Milgrom *et al.*, 1970; Burton *et al.*, 1971), and, more generally, in the hystricomorphs (Heap and Illingworth, 1974), progesterone is bound by a specific protein (progesterone-binding plasma protein, PBP) which has little affinity for glucocorticoids. PBP has been purified to homogeneity (Milgrom *et al.*, 1973b), and its physicochemical characteristics are shown in Table I. Its very high carbohydrate content and its unusually high concentration (~1 mg/ml at the end of pregnancy) are striking. The physiology of this protein is also very peculiar. It is present in blood only during pregnancy. Its distribution is restricted to the maternal circulation; no PBP can be detected in the fetal blood or in the umbilical vein or arteries. This protein cannot be induced by treatment with various estrogens, progesterone, or combinations of both (Milgrom et al., 1973b). It is possible that PBP is synthesized in the placenta.

Various hypotheses have been proposed concerning its possible role, e.g., economy of progesterone (through the reduction of the metabolic clearance rate), protection of the fetus from a high concentration of this hormone, etc. The specificity and high concentration of PBP make it an efficient tool for the assay of progesterone in human plasma (Pichon and Milgrom, 1973).

II. PROGESTERONE RECEPTORS

In target cells, progesterone is bound by specific proteins (receptors). Their biochemical characteristics and attachment to chromatin under the effect of hormone are similar to those described for other steroid hormone receptors in this book (see also review in Raspé, 1971). Very peculiar, however, is the hormonal mechanism controlling the concentration of this receptor. Two types of studies have been performed in this field: experiments in model situations (ovariectomized animals) and measurements of receptor concentrations during actual physiological events (estrous cycle and pregnancy).

A. Progesterone-Receptor Concentration Is under the Control of Estrogen and Progesterone

Guinea pigs ovariectomized at diestrus maintain, during the following weeks, a stable and low level of receptor. These animals can, thus, be used to study hormonal influences on progesterone receptor (Milgrom et al., 1973c,d).

When one single injection of estrogen was administered to these animals, an increase of receptor concentration was observed during the first day, attaining eightfold higher values. Then a slow decrease (half-life, 5 days) was observed during the following days (Fig. 2). Only binding-site concentration and sedimentation coefficient varied, the other characteristics of the receptor (affinity, specificity, sensitivity to SH-blocking agents) were unchanged.

The effect of estradiol could be abolished by a simultaneous injection of RNA or protein synthesis inhibitors (Fig. 3). This suggests that the receptor is synthesized under the effect of estrogen. However, an alternative possi-

TABLE I

Physicochemical Properties of Progesterone-Binding Plasma Protein (PBP)

Parameter	Value
Molecular weight	77,500
$s^°_{20,w}$	4.5
E^1_1 cm/mg/ml at 280 nm	0.49
pHi	3.6
f/f_0	1.685
Carbohydrate content	48.7%
Binding sites/molecule	1
K_a progesterone (at 4°C)	$9 \cdot 10^8$ M^{-1}
K_a testosterone (at 4°C)	$1.6 \; 10^7$ M^{-1}
Stokes radius	47 Å

bility is that the receptor may be in an inactive form (not binding the hormone) and that an hypothetical activator of receptor is synthesized under the effect of estradiol. There is no evidence in favor of the latter hypothesis. When RNA or protein synthesis inhibitors are injected 1 day or later after estradiol, there is no decrease of receptor concentration. This probably means that receptor synthesis has become negligible at this period of time. Thus, the decrease of receptor concentration, which starts 1 day after estradiol injection, probably reflects its turnover. According to these data, the progesterone receptor is a fairly stable molecule (half-life, 5 days). A similar half-life has been found by Sarff and Gorski (1971) for the estrogen receptor.

In this respect, receptors should not be considered regulatory proteins, that usually turn over rapidly, but as markers of cellular differentiation. The latter proteins are usually quite stable (Kafatos, 1972).

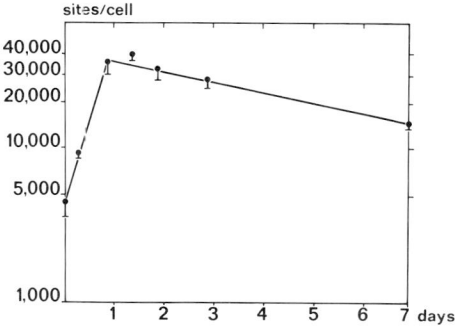

Fig. 2. Effect of estrogen administration on progesterone–receptor concentrations in castrated guinea pigs. Estradiol (10 μg/100 g) was administered to guinea pigs at time 0.

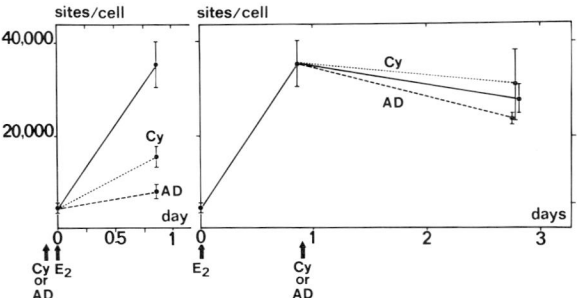

Fig. 3. RNA and protein synthesis inhibitors and estrogen effect on progesterone receptor. (Left) Inhibitor administered 15 minutes before estradiol. (Right) Inhibitor administered 20.5 hours after estradiol. Cy, cycloheximide; AD, actinomycin D; E, estradiol.

Uterine progesterone receptor is also controlled by its own physiological ligand. An important decrease in progesterone receptor is observed if progesterone is administered to guinea pigs when the concentration of estrogen-stimulated receptor is at its highest level (Fig. 4). In these experiments, receptor was measured 1, 2, and 6 days after progesterone injection, and it was verified that the decrease of receptor could not be attributed to masking by endogenous hormone or to transfer of receptor into the nuclei. This effect of progesterone could not be due to a decrease of receptor rate of synthesis, since the latter has been shown to be negligible at this period of time. Therefore, progesterone probably exerts its effect through an enhancement of receptor inactivation rate. The molecular mechanism of this inactivation is unknown; the receptor molecule may be proteolyzed or it may simply lose its ability to bind the hormone. Protein synthesis inhibitors did not abolish the effect of progesterone, showing that this hormone did not induce the appearance of a receptor-inactivating enzyme. It is possible that the inactivation of the receptor is linked in some way to its attachment to

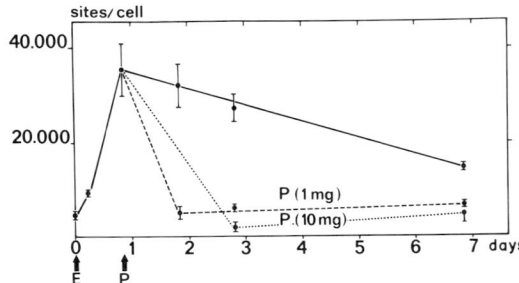

Fig. 4. Progesterone effect on uterine progesterone-receptor concentrations in estrogen-treated guinea pigs. E, estradiol injection; P, progesterone injection.

the nucleus, as shown in the following experiment. [³H]progesterone was injected into guinea pigs, and uterine cytosol and nuclei prepared. Both were then heated at 25°C and stability of [³H]progesterone–receptor complexes measured. It was observed that, whereas the concentration of cytosol complexes did not change after 1 hour exposure at 25°C, nuclear complexes decreased with a half-life of 20 minutes. Various inhibitors of proteases had no effect on this decrease. These experiments are perhaps not relevant to the situation existing *in vivo*, since it is well known that homogenization of uterine tissues releases proteolytic enzymes. However, it may be considered, at least as a working hypothesis, that progesterone receptor (stable when not attached to the chromatin) is translocated into the nuclei under the effect of the hormone, modifies gene transcription, and, thereafter (or simultaneously), is inactivated. There seems to be an autolimitation of progesterone action, i.e., while exerting its biologic effect, the hormone decreases the concentration of its receptor, thus diminishing its further effects.

B. Progesterone Receptors during Estrous Cycle and Pregnancy

The previous experiments performed in model situations have shown that progesterone receptor concentration is under a dual hormonal control; i.e., increased by estrogen, decreased by progesterone. How these hormones modify receptor concentration in actual physiological situations remained to be established.

1. Estrous Cycle

a. In the Guinea Pig (Milgrom et al., 1972). An exchange method was used to measure the total concentration (hormone-bound and free) of cytosol receptor in guinea pig uteri.

It was observed that the affinity constant of receptor for progesterone did not change during the estrous cycle, but there were marked variations of binding-site concentration (Fig. 5). Receptor peaked at proestrus ($\sim 40,000$ binding sites/cell) and decreased rapidly during estrus and postestrus, reaching 16-fold lower values at diestrus. Variations in the sedimentation coefficient of the radioactive hormone–receptor complexes were also observed.

In proestrus, a 6.7 S peak was observed with a shoulder in the 4.5 S region (Fig. 6). In the presence of *p*-hydroxymercuribenzoate (PHMB), the 6.7 peak disappeared, and some radioactivity had shifted to the 4.5 S region. It is known that treatment with SH-blocking reagents inhibits binding of progesterone to its receptor. In estrus, the sucrose gradient showed two peaks of about equal height, one in the 4.5 S region and another one at

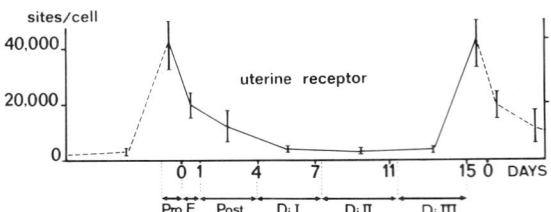

Fig. 5. Progesterone–receptor concentrations in the uterine cytosol of guinea pigs during estrous cycle. Pro, proestrus; E, estrus; Post, postestrus; Di, diestrus.

6.7 S. The latter was completely destroyed by *p*-hydroxymercuribenzoate, whereas only a part of the former disappeared. In postestrus, only a shoulder was seen in the 6.7 S region. In diestrus, the heavier binding had nearly completely disappeared, and the only observed binder had a sedimentation coefficient of about 4.5 S.

Thus, there appeared to be a progressive decay of the 6.7 S binder from proestrus to diestrus. The heavier (6.7 S) binding seems to be composed only of receptor protein sensitive to *p*-hydroxymercuribenzoate, is found only in target organs and specifically binds progestagens. In the 4.5 S region of the cytosol ultracentrifugation pattern, there seems to be a mixture of receptor that adheres to the above-mentioned criteria and of other uncharacterized binding macromolecules which do not. It was verified that the variations of the sedimentation coefficient did not reflect an aggregation–dissociation equilibrium due to concentration variations or an artifact due to partial proteolysis. Their function and meaning are not understood. For most steroid receptors, 6–10 S and 3–5 S forms have been described, but no specific functions could be attributed to these apparently different molecular entities.

b. In the Rat (Vu Hai *et al.*, 1977). In the guinea pig, for technical reasons, only cytosol receptors were measured. Even though various experiments (castration of animals, subcellular distribution of radioactive hormone after injection at different periods of the cycle) indicated that the total cellular content of receptor varied in a similar manner, there was no direct evidence for this.

To solve this problem we developed "exchange assays" to measure total receptor (hormone-bound and free) in rat uterine cytosol and nuclei. These assays are based on the use of R5020, a synthetic progestin having a high affinity for the progesterone receptor and a very low affinity for CBG (Philibert and Raynaud, 1974). Advantage has also been taken of the fast dissociation rate of progesterone–receptor complexes in the rat, allowing exchange reactions to be performed at 0°C. Briefly, endogenous hormone

16. Progesterone-Binding Proteins

was removed from the cytosol by dextran-coated charcoal under conditions which have been shown not to harm the receptor. [^{3}H]R5020 was then added to the cytosol and receptor–[^{3}H]R5020 complexes were measured. In the nuclei, a 6-hour incubation at 0°C allowed complete exchange of endogenous progesterone with added [^{3}H]R5020, and, thus, it was possible to measure progesterone–receptor complexes present in the nuclei. Figure 7 shows the variations of nuclear and cytosol receptors in the rat uterus during the estrous

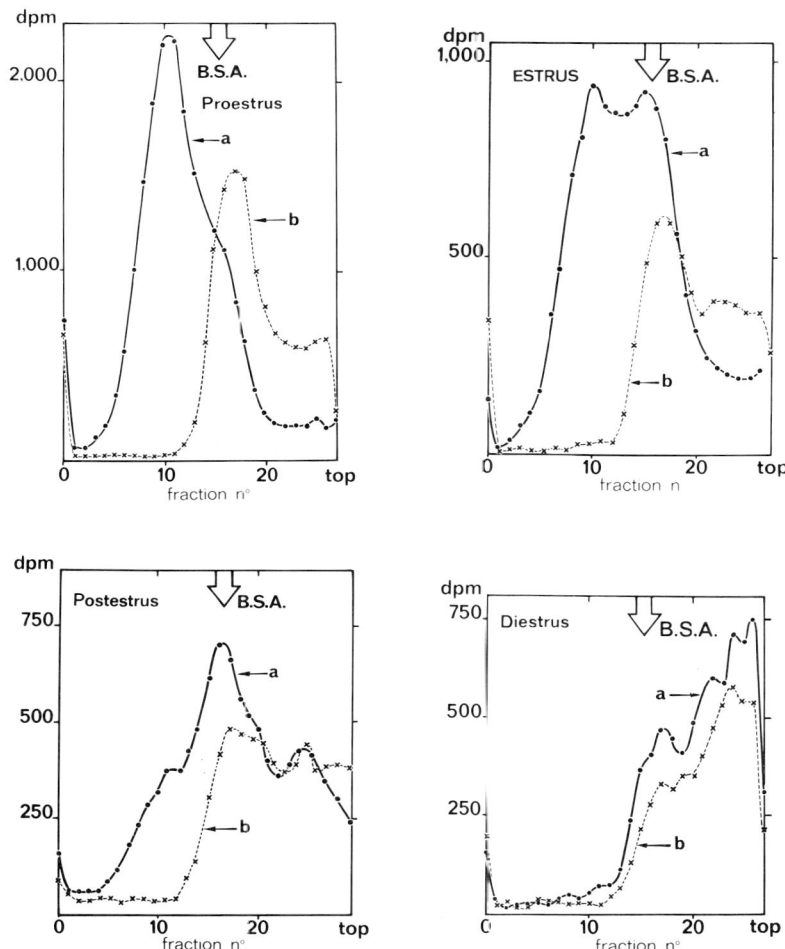

Fig. 6. Sucrose-gradient ultracentrifugation of [^{3}H]progesterone guinea pig uterine cytosol incubate at various periods of the estrous cycle. a, incubation in the absence of *p*-hydroxymercuribenzoate; b, incubation in the presence of *p*-hydroxymercuribenzoate.

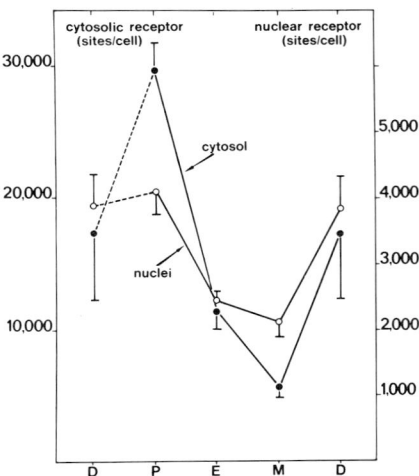

Fig. 7. Cytosol and nuclear progesterone receptor during the estrous cycle in the rat uterus. Total receptor (hormone bound and free) was measured in the cytosol and nuclei.

cycle. Cytosol receptors show the same pattern as in guinea pigs; i.e., a peak at proestrus (~30,000 binding sites per cell) followed by a decrease at estrus and metestrus (~5000 sites per cell) and a beginning increase at diestrus. In the nuclei, maximal concentrations were observed at proestrus and diestrus (~4000 sites per cell). Low concentrations were present at estrus and metestrus. The highest ratio of nuclear receptor to cytosol receptor was seen at metestrus. This ratio was very low in the rat in all physiological situations, including pregnancy. This phenomenon is perhaps related to the strikingly low affinity of receptor for its physiological ligand (K_d for progesterone 10 nM) when compared to other receptors in other target organs. The concentration of nuclear receptor depends, as expected, on both the concentration of cytosol receptor and plasma progesterone. A correlation coefficient of $r = 0.78$ was obtained when comparing nuclear-receptor concentration with the product of cytosol-receptor concentration times the plasma progesterone concentration.

c. Autoradiographic Studies. All the experiments reported above measured the concentration of receptor in total uteri. However since this organ contains many different cell types, one could ask if the observed receptor variations were due to molecular changes in individual cells or to cell population variations. We have isolated endometrial and myometrial parts of the guinea pig uterus and shown that, although some differences could be observed, the overall mechanisms controlling receptor concentration were identical (Luu Thi et al., 1975). However, since these tissues are still very heterogeneous, autoradiographic studies were undertaken to obtain a clear answer. Guinea pigs were injected with [^{3}H]progesterone at various periods of the estrous cycle and autoradiographs of uterine horns, cervix, and vagina performed. Previous studies (Warembourg, 1974) have shown that the labeling, which is observed, has the characteristics of hormone interaction with receptor, i.e., saturability (abolished by excess unlabeled progesterone), hormone specificity (not inhibited by excess unlabeled cortisol), tissue specificity (absence in nontarget organs), and nuclear localization.

A very heavy labeling was observed in uterine horns, cervix, and vagina at proestrus and estrus. It decreased at postestrus, and only a few silver grains were observed at diestrus. In all cell types of these three target organs, the same pattern was observed during the cycle (Warembourg and Milgrom, 1976).

Since it could be argued that the decrease in labeling observed at diestrus was due to occupation of receptor sites by endogenous hormone, the following experiment was undertaken. The guinea pigs were ovariectomized at diestrus and [^{3}H]progesterone was injected 24 hours after castration. This did not change the observed pattern, showing that the decreased labeling was probably due to a low concentration of intracellular binding sites.

These experiments suggest that similar mechanisms probably regulate progesterone receptor concentration in the various cell types of uterine horns, cervix, and vagina.

2. *Pregnancy*

Although high concentrations of progesterone are necessary for maintaining pregnancy, the mechanisms by which the hormone exerts this regulation are still unknown. The events leading to blastocyst implantation and to parturition have been especially discussed with emphasis on the timing of progesterone action and its interplay with other hormones. However, only plasma concentrations of hormone were taken into account. In this respect, the evaluation of receptor variations could give new insights into the mechanism of control of pregnancy. Few such studies have been previously performed. Davies *et al.* (Davies and Ryan, 1973; Davies *et al.*, 1974) have measured the binding of progesterone to rat and rabbit myometrial cytosol, but under experimental conditions where the contribution to the total binding of the CBG-like protein known to be present in rat and rabbit uterine cytosol was not precisely known. We have previously reported receptor concentrations in guinea pig uterine cytosol, but only at the very beginning of pregnancy (Milgrom *et al.*, 1972) [later the very high concentrations of plasma progesterone-binding protein (PBP) interfered with the assay].

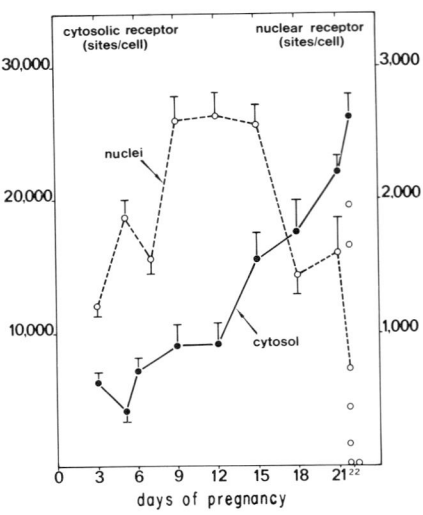

Fig. 8. Cytosol and nuclear progesterone receptor in the rat uterus during pregnancy.

As shown in Fig. 8, the concentration of cytosol receptor is very low at the beginning of pregnancy. A temporary decrease is observed on day 5 (with a parallel increase in the nuclei, suggesting that there is a transfer of complexes into the nuclei under the influence of increased plasma progesterone). Then the cytosol receptor starts to increase slowly from days 6 to 12 and very rapidly from days 15 to 22. A sixfold increase is observed between days 3 and 22. It may, however, be noticed that there is a parallel variation in the total protein content of the uterus and that receptor concentration per milligram of protein showed a smaller increase. The pattern was very different in the nuclei. The concentration of nuclear receptor was low on day 3 of pregnancy, increased abruptly on day 5 (reflecting the decrease of cytosol receptor), and then decreased on day 6. The highest concentrations were attained during a "plateau" period extending from days 9–15 (~2600 binding sites/cell). Then the concentration of nuclear receptor started to fall. On day 22, the mean concentration was very low (~700 binding sites per cell); however, the measurements in individual animals were very scattered with some of them, probably on the verge of parturition, having no detectable receptor in the nuclei.

As already observed in guinea pigs, the concentration of receptor was low at implantation in both nuclei and cytosol. The concentration of nuclear receptor fell shortly before parturition. Since nuclear receptor–steroid complexes are supposed to be obligatory intermediates in hormone action this suggests that progesterone effect is markedly diminished or even abolished shortly before parturition. This fall in the concentration of nuclear complexes is not explained by a decrease of receptor (since the latter is very high in the cytosol), but by a decrease in plasma hormone levels. In this respect, it is possible that the increase of receptor in cytosol during the second half of pregnancy prevents a premature onset of parturition which could be provoked by the decreasing hormonal concentrations. It still remains possible that in other species (in humans, for instance) the "progesterone block" is removed, not by a fall in circulating progesterone concentrations, but by a decrease of its receptor.

III. FEMALE GENITAL TRACT SECRETORY PROTEINS

Only in the rabbit have there been extensive studies of progesterone-binding proteins in female genital tract secretions.

Uteroglobin (Beier, 1968) or blastokinin (Krishnan and Daniel, 1967) is a protein found in the uterine fluid during pregnancy (days 3-12 with a maximal concentration at day 5) and pseudopregnancy. It can be induced in the nonpregnant animal by a treatment with progesterone. The same protein has been found in various other organs (Feigelson, 1977), but studies on steroid binding have been restricted only to the uterine fluid. There had been considerable controversy on whether uteroglobin does (Arthur et al., 1972; Urzua et al., 1970; Garcea et al., 1974; Beato and Baier, 1975) or does not (Goswami and Feigelson, 1974; Rahman et al., 1975) bind progesterone and estradiol.

These discrepancies were probably due to the fact that lyophilization, which has been extensively used in these studies, decreases steroid binding by uteroglobin. This binding is, on the contrary, increased by production of SH groups (Beato and Baier, 1975; Fridlansky and Milgrom, 1976). Non-controlled oxidation of SH groups, thus, probably led to a diminished interaction between progesterone and uteroglobin. As shown in Fig. 9, dithiothreitol (Cleland's reagent) was, among the tested SH-reducing agents, the most powerful compound. A maximal effect was observed at a concentration of 20 mM. Dithioerythritol had about 60% of the efficiency of dithiothreitol at comparative concentrations. β-Mercaptoethanol was also effective but only at very high concentrations (10-100 mM). SH-blocking agents (iodoacetate, iodoacetamide, p-hydroxymercuribenzoate, dithiobisnitrobenzoic acid) are inhibitors of progesterone binding to uteroglobin. Affinity for progesterone was very similar in the presence ($K_d = 4.1 \; 10^{-7} \; M$ at 0°C) and in the absence ($K_d = 8.8 \; 10^{-7} \; M$ at 0°C) of SH-reducing agents (Fig. 10). The small difference can probably be ascribed to differences in the technique which had to be used to measure bound hormone. In the absence of SH reducing agents, one in every 500

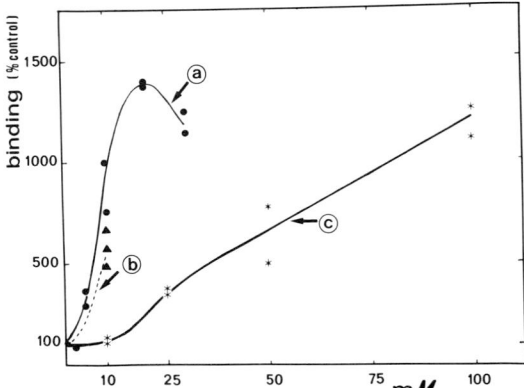

Fig. 9. Effect of SH reducing agents on progesterone binding to uteroglobin. Binding of [³H]progesterone to purified uteroglobin was measured by equilibrium dialysis in the presence of increasing concentrations of dithiothreitol (a), dithioerythritol (b), and β-mercaptoethanol (c), 100 = binding in the absence of SH reducing agent.

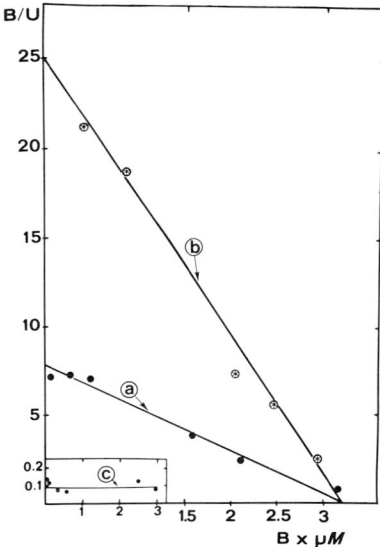

Fig. 10. Binding of [³H]progesterone (a), [³H]5α-pregnane-3,20-dione (b), and [³H]estradiol (c) to purified uteroglobin. Binding was studied by equilibrium dialysis at 4°C.

TABLE II

Compared Steroid Specificity of Uteroglobin and Progesterone Receptor from Rabbit Uterus[a]

Steroid	Uteroglobin	Receptor
Progesterone	100	100
5α-Pregnane-3,20-dione	317	108
R5020	10	158
Norethisterone	2.5	141
Chlormadinone acetate	1.8	127
17-Hydroxyprogesterone	6.8	3
Testosterone	0	1.5
5α-Dihydrotestosterone	2.1	—
Cortisol	0	—
Estradiol	0.8	2.5
Estriol	0	—
Estrone	1	—
Diethylstilbestrol	15	0

[a] For both uteroglobin and progesterone receptor, the concentrations of unlabeled steroid giving a 50% inhibition of binding were determined. They were compared to that of progesterone taken as a reference (= 100).

molecules of uteroglobin bound progesterone; in 20 mM dithiothreitol, one in every two molecules had this property.

5α-Pregnanedione (K_d = 1.3 10^{-7} M at 0°C) is bound by uteroglobin with a higher affinity than is progesterone (Fig. 10). Estradiol is bound in a nonspecific, nonsaturable way (at concentrations up to 50 μM).

Steroid-binding specificity of uteroglobin was compared with that of rabbit uterine progesterone receptor (Table II). Especially striking in this respect was the high affinity of receptor for synthetic progestins (norethisterone, chlormadinone acetate, R5020). These compounds had only a low affinity for the secretory protein.

The equilibrium dissociation constant of uteroglobin–progesterone complexes was at the lower limit of the values observed for Michaelis constant of enzymes. Thus, the possibility that uteroglobin was actually a progesterone-metabolizing protein had to be examined. Uteroglobin was incubated with [³H]progesterone under various experimental conditions (presence or absence of cofactors, presence or absence of SH reducing agents). No metabolism of progesterone was observed.

IV. DISCUSSION

The physiological role of the three types of specific progesterone-binding proteins described to date is not clearly understood.

The receptor is supposed to be an obligatory intracellular intermediate in steroid hormone action. In this respect, receptor concentration variations, as well as plasma hormone variations, might regulate the importance of the biologic response to the hormone. However, it is still unknown if there is a limited number of nuclear acceptor sites (Milgrom and Atger, 1975). If this were the case, some of the above described regulating mechanisms might lead to the appearance of "spare receptor sites" without physiological significance. It is also unknown if, for a given concentration of steroid-receptor complexes, a constant concentration of nuclear complexes will be obtained; regulatory mechanisms may also exist at the level of receptor-steroid complex activation (Bailly et al., 1977).

The existence of precise variations of progesterone receptor concentration during the cycle and pregnancy suggests that a very strict timing may be necessary for successful implantation and maintenance of pregnancy. This suggests the possibility of either suppressing fertility by pharmacologic manipulations or of restoring it in cases where pathological conditions interfere with the physiological pattern of receptor variations.

Steroid-binding plasma proteins have been supposed to play a role of "reservoir" for rapidly available free active hormone. This might be an oversimplification, especially if one considers the occurrence of the CBG-like protein in the target cells. The appearance of such proteins (PBP) or the increase of their concentration (CBG) during pregnancy is also very remarkable. This suggests the possibility of a specific role in pregnancy.

The problem of uterine secretory proteins is even less clearly understood. In the case of uteroglobin it is not known if there is any significant binding of progesterone in *in vivo* conditions. The extent of the binding depends on the presence of SH groups and the oxidoreduction conditions prevailing *in vivo* in the uterine lumen are ignored. The relatively low affinity of uteroglobin for progesterone is not a real problem, since the concentration of uteroglobin is extremely high (40–60% of the secretory proteins at day 5 of pregnancy). The threefold higher affinity for 5α-pregnane-3,20-dione, when compared to progesterone, suggests that this steroid might have a physiological role. It has been suggested that uteroglobin (bastokinin) has a stimulatory effect on blastocyst; however, this is still controvertial and the possibility that the steroid-binding property of uteroglobin may be related to this hypothetical effect on the blastocyst has been ignored. The occurrence of uteroglobin in other species and especially in women, is still discussed and it is unknown if this (or a similar protein of the uterine fluid) binds progesterone in humans.

ACKNOWLEDGMENT

Studies reported in this paper were performed with the help of my collegues: P. Allouch, M. Atger, F. Fridlansky, F. Logeat, M. Perrot, and M. T. Vu Hai. Support was obtained from the INSERM, the CNRS, and the UER Kremlin-Bicêtre.

REFERENCES

Arthur, A. T., Cowan, B. O., and Daniel, J. C. (1972). *Fertil. Steril.* **23**, 85–92.
Bailly, A., Sallas, N., and Milgrom, E. (1977). *J. Biol. Chem.* **252**, 858–863.
Beato, M., and Baier, R. (1975). *Biochim. Biophys. Acta* **392**, 346–356.
Beier, H. M. (1968). *Biochim. Biophys. Acta* **160**, 289–291.
Burton, R. M., Harding, G. B., Rust, N., and Westphal, U. (1971). *Steroids* **17**, 1–16.
Davies, I. J., and Ryan, K. J. (1973). *Endocrinology* **92**, 394–401.
Davies, I. J., Challis, J. R. G., and Ryan, K. J. (1974). *Endocrinology* **95**, 165–173.
Faber, L. E., Sandmann, M. L., and Stavely, H. E. (1973). *Endocrinology* **93**, 74–80.
Feigelson, M., Noske, I. G., Goswami, A. K., and Kay, E. (1977). *Ann. N.Y. Acad. Sci.* **286**, 273–286.
Fridlansky, F., and Milgrom, E. (1976). *Endocrinology* **99**, 1244–1251.
Garcea, N., Campo, S., Caruso, A., Milano, L., and Bompiani, A. (1974). *Int. J. Fertil.* **19**, 197–201.
Goswami, A., and Feigelson, M. (1974). *Endocrinology* **95**, 669–675.
Hansson, V., Ritzen, M. E., French, F. S., Weddington, S. C., and Nayfeh, S. N. (1975). *Mol. Cell. Endocrinol.* **3**, 1–20.
Heap, R. B., and Illingworth, D. V. (1974). *In* "The Biology of Hystricomorph Rodents" (I. W. Rowlands and B. J. Weir, eds.) pp. 385–416. Academic Press, New York.
Kafatos, F. C. (1972). *Gene Transcription Reprod. Tissue, Trans. Karolinska Symp. Res. Methods Reprod. Endocrinol., 5th, 1972* pp. 319–345.
Krishnan, R. S., and Daniel, J. C. (1967). *Science* **158**, 490–492.
Luu Thi, M., Baulieu, E. E., and Milgrom, E. (1975). *J. Endocrinol.* **66**, 349–356.
McGuire, W. L., and Bariso, C. D. (1972). *Endocrinology* **90**, 496–506.
McGuire, W. L., Bariso, C. D., and Fuller, B. S. (1974). *Acta Endocrinol. (Copenhagen)* **75**, 579–583.
Milgrom, E., and Atger, M. (1975). *J. Steroid Biochem.* **6**, 487–492.
Milgrom, E., and Baulieu, E. E. (1970a). *Endocrinology* **87**, 276–287.
Milgrom, E., and Baulieu, E. E. (1970b). *Biochem. Biophys. Res. Commun.* **40**, 723–730.
Milgrom, E., Atger, M., and Baulieu, E. E. (1970). *Nature (London)* **228**, 1205–1206.
Milgrom, E., Atger, M., Perrot, M., and Baulieu, E. E. (1972). *Endocrinology* **90**, 1071–1078.
Milgrom, E., Atger, M., and Baulieu, E. E. (1973a). *Biochim. Biophys. Acta* **320**, 267–283.
Milgrom, E., Allouch, P., Atger, M., and Baulieu, E. E. (1973b). *J. Biol. Chem.* **248**, 1106–1114.
Milgrom, E., Luu Thi, M., Atger, M., and Baulieu, E. E. (1973c). *J. Biol. Chem.* **248**, 6366–6374.

Milgrom, E., Luu Thi, M., and Baulieu, E. E. (1973d). *Acta Endocrinol. (Copenhagen), Suppl.* **180,** 380–403.
Philibert, D., and Raynaud, J. P. (1974). *Endocrinology* **94,** 627–632.
Pichon, M. F., and Milgrom, E. (1973). *Steroids* **21,** 335–346.
Pichon, M. F., and Milgrom, E. (1977). *Cancer Res.* **37,** 464–471.
Rahman, S. S., Velayo, N., Domres, P., and Billiar, R. B. (1975). *Fertil. Steril.* **26,** 991–995.
Raspé, G. (1971). *Adv. Biosci.,* **7,** 1–417.
Sarff, M., and Gorski, J. (1971). *Biochemistry* **10,** 2557–2565.
Seal, U. S., and Doe, R. P. (1966). *Steroid Dyn., Proc. Symp., 1965* p. 63.
Urzua, M., Stambaugh, R., Flickingor, G., and Mastroianni, L. (1970). *Fertil. Steril.* **21,** 860–865.
Vu Hai, M. T., Logeat, F., Warembourg, M., and Milgrom, E. (1977). *Ann. N.Y. Acad. Sci.* **286,** 199–209.
Warembourg, M. (1974). *Endocrinology* **94,** 665–670.
Warembourg, M., and Milgrom, E. (1977). *Endocrinology* **100,** 175–181.
Westphal, U. (1971). "Steroid-Protein Interactions." Springer-Verlag, Berlin and New York.
Young, P. C. M., and Cleary, R. C. (1974). *J. Clin. Endocrinol. Metab.* **39,** 425–439.

17

Androgen-Binding Proteins of the Male Rat Reproductive Tract

ELIZABETH M. WILSON, OSCAR A. LEA, AND FRANK S. FRENCH

I.	Introduction	492
II.	Androgen-Binding Protein (ABP)	492
	A. Distinguishing ABP from Other Androgen-Binding Proteins	493
	B. Quantitation of ABP by Steady-State Polyacrylamide Gel Electrophoresis	493
	C. Physical and Chemical Properties of ABP	495
	D. Steroid Specificity of ABP	496
	E. Control of ABP Concentration by FSH and Androgens in the Sertoli Cell	497
III.	9 S Androgen- and Progesterone-Binding Protein	501
	A. Chemical Properties	504
	B. Steroid-Binding Properties	505
IV.	Androgen Receptor	507
	A. Stabilization of the *in Vitro* Receptor–Androgen Interaction	509
	B. Procedures for Quantitation of Androgen Receptor	511
	C. Steroid Specificity of the Androgen Receptor	519
	D. Kinetics of Receptor–Androgen Interaction	520
	E. Thermodynamics of Receptor–Testosterone Interaction	522
	F. Influence of Androgen Metabolism on Receptor Binding	523
	G. Significance of Testosterone Versus Dihydrotestosterone Binding	525
V.	Concluding Remarks	525
	References	528

I. INTRODUCTION

Androgens are essential for the development and function of the male reproductive tract. Thus far, three types of androgen-binding proteins have been identified in androgen-dependent organs of the male rat. Each of the three proteins exhibits a degree of specificity for biologically active androgens.

The tubular fluid of testis and epididymis of the male rat contains an androgen-binding protein referred to as ABP. ABP is thought to have a carrier function, perhaps influencing the accumulation and distribution of androgens in the testis germinal epithelium, as well as the transport of androgens from testis to epididymis. In addition to its apparent role in androgen action, the identification of ABP as a secretory product of the Sertoli cell has provided an effective new way to study the hormonal control of Sertoli cell function. In this chapter, we will review earlier studies on the physical and chemical properties of ABP and some more recent results on the hormonal control of ABP production.

A second protein with properties distinct from ABP has recently been identified in tissues of the reproductive tract of the male rat. This protein, which is characterized by its high binding capacity for progesterone and androgens and a sedimentation coefficient of 9 S, is referred to as the 9 S binding protein. Although studies are as yet preliminary, the properties of this protein suggest that it may have an intracellular storage function.

A third protein is the intracellular androgen receptor. When bound with androgen, it is this protein which is believed to move into nuclei where it alters the transcriptional specificity of the DNA in chromatin. Despite the efforts of many laboratories, numerous discrepancies remain in the literature concerning its physical properties and androgen-binding specificity. A difficulty in studying the receptor is its low concentration relative to nonspecific steroid-binding proteins and other androgen-binding proteins. We will present in this chapter some data on the binding properties of the partially purified androgen receptor.

II. ANDROGEN-BINDING PROTEIN (ABP)

Testes of several mammalian species produce a specific androgen-binding protein, ABP, which has a high affinity for both dihydrotestosterone ($K_a = 1.25 \times 10^9 \, M^{-1}$) and testosterone ($K_a = 0.5 \times 10^9 \, M^{-1}$) (French and Ritzén, 1973a,b; Hansson et al., 1973a, 1975a; Ritzén et al., 1973; Ritzén and French, 1974; Sanborn et al., 1974; Vernon et al., 1974). ABP is secreted by Sertoli cells of the germinal epithelium. Sertoli cell cytoplasm extends from the wall of the seminiferous tubule to its lumen and surrounds the developing germ cells. As it leaves the Sertoli cell, ABP enters the seminiferous tubular fluid and passes into the lumen of the epididymis. Production of ABP by the Sertoli cell is regulated by pituitary gonadotropins and androgens. Although the precise function of ABP remains to be clarified, most available data indicate that ABP enhances the accumulation of androgen within seminiferous tubules and facilitates transport of androgen from testis to epididymis via the testicular fluid through the efferent ducts. Within the lumen of caput epididymis, ABP becomes concentrated as testicular fluid is absorbed, and it binds androgen diffusing into the epididymis from blood as well. Below follows a description of some of the most pertinent experimental results which have contributed to our understanding of this protein.

A. Distinguishing ABP from Other Androgen-Binding Proteins

ABP was first identified in the rat, which lacks the serum testosterone-binding globulin (French and Ritzén, 1973a,b; Ritzén *et al.*, 1973). In the rabbit, ABP and testosterone-binding globulin have remarkably similar properties (Ritzén and French, 1974; Hansson *et al.*, 1975b; Weddington *et al.*, 1975b), and are immunologically indistinct. They can be separated, however, on the basis of charge properties using isoelectric focusing (Hansson *et al.*, 1975b). Experiments described herein were carried out in the rat.

ABP can be distinguished from intracellular androgen receptors on the basis of electrophoretic mobility and other physicochemical properties. ABP is a smaller molecule, more acidic, and less susceptible to degradation on heating. Its steroid specificity is like that of the androgen receptor; however, the kinetics of ligand binding are very different. Rapid androgen association and dissociation to ABP contrast sharply with the slower rates of receptor binding and dissociation. Like the androgen receptor, ABP is a low-capacity binder which enables it to be readily distinguished from the 9 S binding protein described in a later section.

B. Quantitation of ABP by Steady-State Polyacrylamide Gel Electrophoresis

ABP can be quantitated precisely in polyacrylamide gels containing tritiated androgens, a technique referred to as steady-state polyacrylamide gel electrophoresis (Ritzén *et al.*, 1974). This method combines the advantages of high resolution with those of steady-state conditions. It is applicable only to binding proteins with rapid rates of ligand association

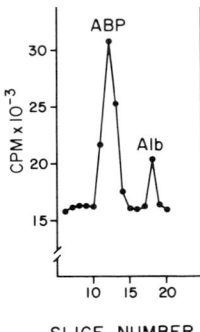

Fig. 1. Steady-state polyacrylamide gel electrophoresis of rat ABP labeled with [³H]dihydrotestosterone. Testes (decapsulated) were homogenized in 3 volumes of 50 mM Tris, pH 7.4 containing 1.5 mM EDTA, 0.5 mM 2-mercaptoethanol, and 10% glycerol and centrifuged at 105,000 g for 1 hour. Samples of testis supernatant were treated overnight at 0°C with dextran-coated charcoal (1 mg Norit A/mg protein) to remove endogenous steroid. Charcoal was removed by centrifugation twice at 10,000 g. The sample (0.4 ml, 2.2 mg protein) was layered onto a 6½% acrylamide gel (10 × 70 mm) containing 10% glycerol, to which 2nM [³H]dihydrotestosterone had been added before polymerization. Electrophoresis was run at 0°C for 5 hours at 5 mAmp/gel. Following electrophoresis, the gel was sliced into 2.3-mm segments and placed directly into counting vials with toluene scintillation fluid. After standing overnight at room temperature, more than 98% of the radioactivity is extracted into toluene. Steady state between bound and free [³H]DHT is obtained when the level of radioactivity in front of the ABP peak is identical to that behind the peak (French et al., 1974).

and dissociation, such as ABP, which has a half-time of dissociation of the [³H]dihydrotestosterone–ABP complex at 0°C of approximately 6 minutes (McLean et al., 1976; Tindall et al., 1975) and 3 minutes for [³H]testosterone (Sanborn et al., 1974). For measurement of ABP in rat testis and epididymis, samples containing 0.4–0.5 mg total protein are applied to 5 × 50-mm gels. Stacking gels are made to contain 10 nM [³H]dihydrotestosterone to ensure that steady state is reached within the separating gel, which contains 2 nM [³H]dihydrotestosterone. As ABP moves through the gel, it binds an increasing amount of [³H]dihydrotestosterone until a steady state between association and dissociation is reached. Gels are then sliced, and radioactivity in gel slices is measured after extracting into toluene scintillation mixture (Fig. 1). Removal of endogenous unlabeled androgen by charcoal adsorption is not required, since dissociation and replacement by [³H]dihydrotestosterone occurs during electrophoresis.

In order to calculate the total number of ABP binding sites in a preparation, the law of mass action can be applied (Ritzén et al., 1974):

$$K_d [S_b] = [\text{ABP}_u] [S_u] \tag{1}$$

17. Androgen-Binding Proteins

where K_d = apparent equilibrium dissociation constant, $[S_b]$ = concentration of [³H]androgen bound to ABP, $[ABP_u]$ = concentration of unoccupied ABP binding sites and $[S_u]$ = concentration of unbound [³H]androgen. Since $[ABP_u] = [ABP_{tot}] - [S_b]$, where $[ABP_{tot}]$ = concentration of total binding sites, it follows from Eq. (1) that

$$[ABP_{tot}] = [S_b](K_d/[S_u] + 1) \tag{2}$$

Since ABP_{tot} and S_b are distributed in essentially identical volumes in the gel, the absolute amount of ABP_{tot} may be obtained from S_b, the amount of [³H]androgen bound to ABP as follows:

$$ABP_{tot} = S_b(K_d/[S_u] + 1) \tag{3}$$

S_b and S_u can be calculated from the total radioactivity recovered from the peak minus background. Arrangement of S_b and S_u in the form of a Scatchard plot allows one to estimate K_d and $[ABP_{tot}]$. Once the K_d has been determined for a particular gel system, it is sufficient to run gels at one [³H]dihydrotestosterone concentration to determine $[ABP_{tot}]$.

C. Physical and Chemical Properties of ABP

ABP has been demonstrated and characterized in 105,000 g supernatant fractions from rat testis and epididymal homogenates (French and Ritzén, 1973b; Hansson et al., 1973a; Ritzén et al., 1973) or in rete testis fluid (French and Ritzén, 1973a) using a variety of techniques. ABP is absent in other organs of the rat male reproductive tract. ABP is an acidic protein with an isoelectric pH of 4.6 (Hansson, 1972). On electrophoresis in 6.5% polyacrylamide gels using glycine buffer, pH 8.6, the relative mobility is 0.5 when compared to bromophenol blue (Ritzén et al., 1973). Using sucrose-gradient centrifugation, ABP sediments at 4.5 S in buffers of low or high ionic strength. A Stokes radius of 47 Å has been estimated by gel filtration chromatography on Sephadex G-200. ABP elutes between human immunoglobulin G and bovine serum albumin. The molecular weight (MW) and frictional ratio (f/f_o) of rat ABP have been determined from gel filtration and gradient centrifugation according to Siegel and Monty (1966), Hansson (1972) and Hansson et al., (1973a):

$$MW = 6\eta\pi Nas/(1 - \bar{v}d)$$

$$f/f_o = a/(3\bar{v}MW/4\pi N)^{1/3}$$

where ν = viscosity of the buffer, N = Avogadro's number, a = Stokes radius (47 Å), s = sedimentation coefficient (4.5 S), $\bar{v}$ = partial specific volume and d = density of the medium. Assuming $\bar{v} = 0.74$ cm³/g, the MW is 90,000, and the frictional ratio is 1.6. Molecular weight has also been determined from the "mean molecular radius" as measured by polyacrylamide gel electrophoresis in gels of different pore size (Ritzén et al., 1973). Retardation coefficients (K_R) have been calculated from the relative mobilities (R) of hemoglobin, testosterone-binding globulin, and ABP in 5% and 8% acrylamide gels in relation to the mobility of bovine serum albumin as follows:

$$\log R = \log R_o - K_R G$$

where R_0 = free electrophoretic mobility and G = gel concentration. From the linear relationship between K_R and mean molecular radius, the molecular radius of ABP could be estimated using standard radii for testosterone-binding globulin (2.95 nm), hemoglobin (2.66 nm), and bovine serum albumin (2.69 nm) (Corvol et al., 1971; Rodbard and Chrambach, 1970, 1971; Mahoudeau and Corvol, 1973). Assuming a spherical molecule, the molecular weight is calculated: MW = $\bar{R}^3 \, 4N/3\bar{v}$ where $\bar{R}$ = mean molecular radius and N = Avogadro's number. Assuming a partial specific volume $\bar{v}$ of 0.74, the MW of rat ABP is 90,000.

The binding of dihydrotestosterone to ABP is sensitive to pH, heat, and certain sulfhydryl reagents. A pH between 7 and 9 is required for optimal binding (Hansson et al., 1973a; Ritzén et al., 1973). [³H]Dihydrotestosterone–ABP complexes in epididymis 105,000 g supernatant are stable to heating at 50°C for 30 minutes, but are destroyed at 60°C (Hansson et al., 1973a). ABP binding is unaffected by the sulfhydryl reagent, p-chloromercuriphenylsulfonate (1 mM), but is inhibited by similar concentrations of other sulfhydryl reagents including Ellman's reagent [5,5′-dithiobis(2-nitrobenzoic acid)] and N-ethylmaleimide. N-Ethylmaleimide (10 mM) inhibited binding to 20% of control. Disulfide reducing agents, 2-mercaptoethanol and dithiothreitol (10 mM) caused a similar reduction in binding, indicating that disulfide groups are essential for maintaining the active binding site (Hansson et al., 1973a; Ritzén et al., 1973).

D. Steroid Specificity of ABP

The binding of various ³H-steroids to ABP has been examined by direct binding and by competitive inhibition of [³H]dihydrotestosterone binding by unlabeled steroids. Analysis of *in vitro* labeled 105,000 g supernatants by electrophoresis on unlabeled gels showed that the amount of [³H]testosterone binding was 50% that of [³H]dihydrotestosterone. Binding of [³H]progesterone, [³H]17β-estradiol, [³H]androstenedione, or [³H]5α-androstanediol was low or undetectable. Competitive binding studies with [³H]dihydrotestosterone and unlabeled steroids using polyacrylamide gel electrophoresis indicated relative affinities as follows: dihydrotestosterone (100), testosterone (50), 17β-estradiol (10–15), progesterone (2–6), and hydrocortisone (0) (Hansson *et al.*, 1973a; Ritzén *et al.*, 1971, 1973). Cyproterone acetate did not compete with [³H]dihydrotestosterone for binding to ABP *in vitro* in a concentration 200 times greater than [³H]dihydrotestosterone (Tindall *et al.*, 1974b). Similarly cyproterone acetate did not inhibit [³H]androgen binding to ABP when 1 mg was injected intravenously 5 minutes prior to [³H]testosterone (60 μCi), but caused 80% inhibition of binding to receptor (Smith *et al.*, 1975a; Tindall *et al.*, 1975). The steroid specificity of ABP otherwise closely resembles that of androgen receptors. Similarities in steroid specificity between ABP and receptor might be expected if the function of ABP is to transport biologically active androgens to intracellular receptors.

E. Control of ABP Concentration by FSH and Androgens in the Sertoli Cell

Production of ABP in the testis and secretion into seminiferous tubular fluid was demonstrated by ligation of the efferent ducts. It was found that ABP accumulated in the testis and disappeared from epididymis (French and Ritzén, 1973a). The concentration of ABP in rete testis fluid collected 18 hours following efferent duct ligation approached 100 nM (Fig. 2), which was similar to the concentration of testosterone (French and Ritzén, 1973b; Ritzén *et al.*, 1977). In rete testis fluid of rabbits, Guerrero *et al.* (1975) have also shown that the concentration of dihydrotestosterone correlates with the concentration of ABP. Since primary seminiferous tubular fluid becomes diluted before reaching the rete testis (Tuck *et al.*, 1970), the concentration of ABP surrounding the germinal epithelium is probably higher than that of efferent duct fluid. Within the lumen of the caput epididymis, the ABP concentration may become extraordinarily high due to absorption of water from the testicular fluid as it passes through the efferent ducts and the first portion of the caput epididymis (Crabo, 1965).

An abundance of evidence now indicates that ABP is produced by the Sertoli cell under the hormonal control of pituitary gonadotropins. Moreover, the observation that FSH stimulates production of ABP supports the concept that Sertoli cells are target cells for FSH. ABP disappears from testis and epididymis after prolonged hypophysectomy and reappears after treatment with FSH (Hansson *et al.*, 1973c, 1974a, 1975c; Fritz *et al.*, 1974; Sanborn *et al.*, 1974). When hypophysectomized rats are injected with FSH, the accumulation of ABP in epididymis is dose dependent (Hansson *et al.*, 1974a). Several FSH preparations have been shown to have similar relative potencies with respect to stimulation of ABP production and

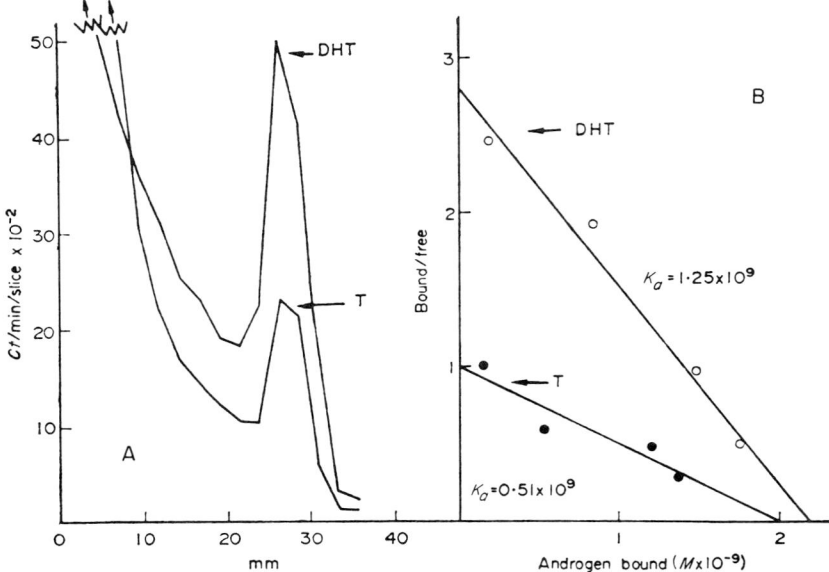

Fig. 2. ABP binding of [³H]testosterone and [³H]dihydrotestosterone. (A) Polyacrylamide gel electrophoresis of ABP in efferent duct fluid after equilibration with [³H]testosterone or [³H]dihydrotestosterone (40 Ci/mmole). Testicular efferent ducts were ligated close to the epididymis. After 3 days, fluid was collected and centrifuged to remove spermatozoa. Fluid was diluted 1:4.5 with buffer containing 1.5 mM EDTA, 2 mM 2-mercaptoethanol, 10% glycerol, and 0.5% bovine serum albumin. Endogenous free androgen was reduced by incubation with charcoal (1 mg/mg albumin) for 12 hours at 0°C. Aliquots (0.5 ml) were labeled with saturating concentrations of [³H]dihydrotestosterone ([³H]DHT) or [³H]testosterone ([³H]T) (35 or 72 nM) for 2 hours at 0°C and separated on 6.5% acrylamide gels as previously described (Ritzén et al., 1971). (B) Scatchard plots of [³H]DHT and [³H]T binding to ABP in testicular fluid as determined by Sephadex gel equilibration. Samples were prepared as in (A), except they were diluted 1:7 with the same buffer. Aliquots (0.25 ml) were further diluted to 1 ml and labeled with 0.8 nM [³H]T or [³H]DHT plus 0, 3.3, 10, 20, or 40 nM unlabeled T and DHT, respectively. The Sephadex gel equilibration assay was as previously described (Pearlman and Crèpy, 1967). Sephadex G-25 (200 mg), swelled in 1 ml of the above buffer for 18 hours at 25°C, was incubated with samples by shaking at 0°C for 1 hour. Radioactivity in the clear supernatant was measured, and the bound radioactivity was calculated (French and Ritzén, 1973a).

increase in ovarian weight in the Steelman–Pohley assay (Hansson et al., 1975c). Studies by Means and Tindall (1975) have demonstrated that ABP formation can be stimulated rapidly. Testicular ABP increases within 1 hour after administration of FSH or 8-bromo-cyclic AMP to prenatally X-irradiated rats. X-irradiation of prenatal rats produces testes which are essentially free of germ cells (Sertoli cell-enriched testis). The effect of a single intravenous injection is short-lived, and turnover of ABP in the testis is rapid, since ABP concentrations return to control levels within 4–6 hours. The rapid effect of FSH on ABP in the immature rat testis has been confirmed by Kotite et al. (1976) using ovine FSH (NIH-FSH-S10) as well as highly purified human FSH (LER 1577 and LER 1563). Finally, FSH stimulation of ABP production *in vitro* has been demonstrated both in organ (Ritzén et al., 1975) and cell cultures (Fritz et al., 1974; Steinberger et al., 1975).

Androgens are involved in regulating the sensitivity of the Sertoli cell to FSH in an as yet little understood way. Sertoli cell response to FSH, as measured by ABP concentration, decreases dramatically after hypophysectomy, but can be maintained by pretreatment with high doses of testosterone propionate. When hypophysectomized immature rats are treated with 2 mg testosterone daily beginning at day 1 after hypophysectomy, Sertoli cell sensitivity to FSH is increased compared to that seen in 2-day hypophysectomized controls which received no testosterone (Hansson et al., 1975a). Testosterone augmentation of Sertoli cell responsiveness has also been demonstrated in 15-day-old intact rats. Prior treatment with testosterone propionate causes testicular levels of ABP to rise higher in response to FSH (Fig. 3). Treatment with testosterone in very high doses maintains

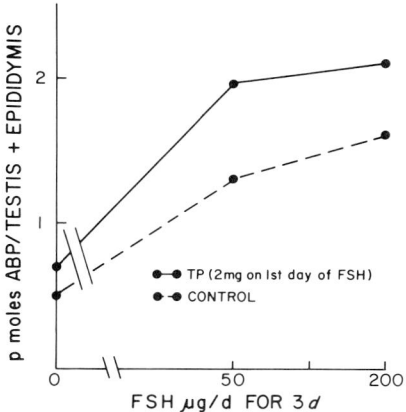

Fig. 3. Testosterone augmentation of ABP response to FSH in immature intact rats. Fifteen-day-old rats in groups of five were injected twice daily for 3 days with different doses of NIH-FSH-S10 (●--------●) (control). At each dosage, a parallel group received 2 mg testosterone propionate intramuscularly in 0.1 ml sesame oil on the first day of treatment (●———●). Twelve hours following the last injection, testes were removed and homogenized in 8 volumes 50 mM Tris buffer containing 1 mM EDTA and 10% glycerol, pH 7.4 at 25°C; 105,000 g supernatants were analyzed by steady-state polyacrylamide gel electrophoresis (Ritzén et al., 1974). Stacking gels contained 10 nM and running gels 2 nM [1,2-^{3}H]dihydrotestosterone (Kotite et al., 1976).

ABP production if started immediately following hypophysectomy (Hansson et al., 1975d).

Administration of testosterone in various doses to intact rats results in a biphasic effect on ABP production (Fig. 4). Low doses of testosterone suppress ABP secondary to suppression of pituitary gonadotropins. High doses, sufficient to raise the intratesticular concentration of testosterone to normal levels, stimulate ABP production even though blood levels of gonadotropins remain suppressed (Weddington et al., 1976). LH and testosterone are both effective in stimulating a rapid increase in the intratesticular concentration of ABP in immature intact rats (Kotite et al., 1976), suggesting that the response to LH is mediated by testosterone. Tindall and Means (1976) have recently suggested that the binding activity of ABP in the testis may be regulated acutely by testosterone, rather than by a direct effect of FSH on Sertoli cells. However, if the testis has undergone regression for several days following hypophysectomy, testosterone administration is less effective than FSH in initiating production and secretion of ABP (Hansson et al., 1975d; Weddington et al., 1975a). It seems that FSH is a specific requirement for initiation of the secretion process as measured by ABP in the epididymis. The secretion of ABP and its stimulation by testosterone are blocked by inhibitors of protein synthesis (Means et al., 1976; Tindall et al., 1976).

Although these *in vivo* studies point to the Sertoli cell as a target cell for androgens, the possibility remained that hormones injected *in vivo* might exert their effects indirectly through other organs. Ritzén et al. (1975) have

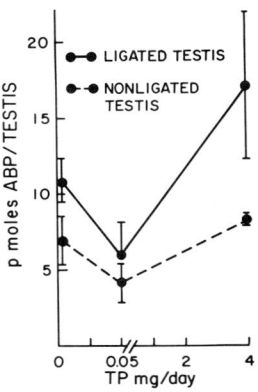

Fig. 4. Androgen suppression and stimulation of ABP production in immature intact rats. Twenty-one-day-old rats in groups of four were injected daily for 8 days with 0.05 or 4 mg testosterone propionate in 0.1 ml sesame oil i.m. On the eighth day, testicular efferent ducts on one side were ligated. Rats were sacrificed 24 hours later and ABP was measured in the ligated (●———●) and nonligated (●--------●) testes as described in Fig. 1. The difference in total ABP of ligated and nonligated testes gives an estimate of production during the 24-hour period of ligation (Weddington et al., 1976).

demonstrated in testis organ culture that ABP synthesis can be stimulated by testosterone. Testosterone acts, therefore, directly on the testis to stimulate Sertoli cell production of ABP.

Although testosterone alone is capable of stimulating ABP production, studies with Stanley–Gumbreck androgen-insensitive (Tfm) rats, which are characterized by a deficiency of androgen receptors, indicate that ABP production may not have an absolute dependence on receptor-bound androgen. ABP is present in near normal levels in testes of these androgen-insensitive rats (French and Ritzén, 1973b). Furthermore, Ritzén has demonstrated *in vitro* production of ABP by the androgen-insensitive rat testis, although the rate of production is only 30% of normal control littermates (Hansson *et al.*, 1976). Altogether, androgens and FSH seem to act independently in stimulating ABP production by mechanisms that are synergistic.

Although the role of ABP in androgen action in the testis and epididymis remains to be established, it appears that ABP may provide these organs with a means to accumulate androgen from its site of production within Leydig cells. It has been shown recently that testosterone and dihydrotestosterone enter testicular fluid more readily than other steroids, which are not bound by ABP (Cooper and Waites, 1975). In rete testis fluid of the ram, testosterone concentrations were increased more by administration of FSH and LH than by LH alone, although plasma concentrations were similar (Bartke *et al.*, 1975). These studies suggest that ABP may facilitate the accumulation of androgen within seminiferous tubular fluid. In addition, ABP may serve to channel testosterone and dihydrotestosterone to androgen receptors within the cytoplasm of the Sertoli cell itself or in adjacent germ cells.

FSH stimulation of ABP production may enhance the transport of androgen from the testis to epididymis by way of the testicular efferent duct fluid. Within the lumen of the caput epididymis where ABP becomes concentrated and binds the androgen diffusing into the epididymis from blood, a very high concentration of androgen is maintained in close proximity to spermatozoa and to androgen-dependent cells of the epithelium. Thus, it would appear that ABP may have a role in the accumulation, transport and storage of androgen in testis and epididymis.

III. 9 S ANDROGEN- AND PROGESTERONE-BINDING PROTEIN

Early studies on androgen uptake *in vivo* following injection of [^{3}H]testosterone demonstrated that radioactivity is retained by androgen-dependent organs at higher levels than in blood or nondependent organs

(Bruchovsky and Wilson, 1968a; Fang et al., 1969; Tveter et al., 1975). A major portion of the retained radioactivity is [^{3}H]testosterone and [^{3}H]dihydrotestosterone (Bruchovsky and Wilson, 1968a; Fang et al., 1969; Tveter and Aakvaag, 1970; Tveter et al., 1975). The accumulation and retention of tracer amounts of these biologically active androgens is highest in cells with a high receptor concentration and may be, thus, explained in part by binding to receptor and subsequent nuclear translocation. For at least two reasons, however, it is suspected that androgen-binding components other than the receptor are involved in retention of androgens and other steroids. The total accumulation of tracer amounts of testosterone in target tissues is not appreciably reduced by simultaneous injection of 60–250-fold excess amounts of unlabeled testosterone (Smith et al., 1975a), even though under these conditions, binding of labeled testosterone to the receptor is inhibited completely (Rennie and Bruchovsky, 1973; Smith et al., 1975b). Furthermore, recent measurements of endogenous testosterone and dihydrotestosterone in androgen-dependent organs indicate that the concentrations of these androgens are much greater than can be expected by binding to receptor proteins alone (Robel et al., 1973; Vreeburg, 1975; Vreeburg et al., 1976). For example, rat prostate and seminal vesicle contain 5 ng testosterone plus dihydrotestosterone per gram tissue (approximately 15–20 nM), which is twice the concentration in peripheral plasma and 100 times the receptor concentration (0.1–0.5 nM, assuming one binding site per receptor molecule). Much higher levels of testosterone are present in testis (150 ng/g tissue or about 500 nM). In epididymis, the dihydrotestosterone concentration is 40 ng/g tissue or about 130 nM in caput and 3 ng/g tissue or about 10 nM in cauda (Vreeburg et al., 1976). In testis and epididymis, ABP may contribute substantially to androgen accumulation; however, high tissue androgen levels may also result from the presence of an active uptake mechanism or steroid-binding protein serving a storage function. Recent studies carried out in our laboratory have demonstrated a high molecular weight protein that binds large amounts of androgen and progesterone (Wilson et al., 1977).

It is well known that a variety of proteins bind androgens. However, with exception of the receptor, most of the steroid-binding proteins, including ABP and serum albumin, sediment exclusively in the 4 S region on sucrose gradients. The androgen-binding macromolecule described in this section has a sedimentation coefficient of approximately 9 S, corresponding to an MW of approximately 200,000. The 9 S binding protein has been identified in 105,000 g supernatants from rat testis, epididymis, prostate, seminal vesicle, and lung, but was not detected in spleen, liver, and serum. In contrast to ABP, the 9 S binding protein remains in testis and epididymis

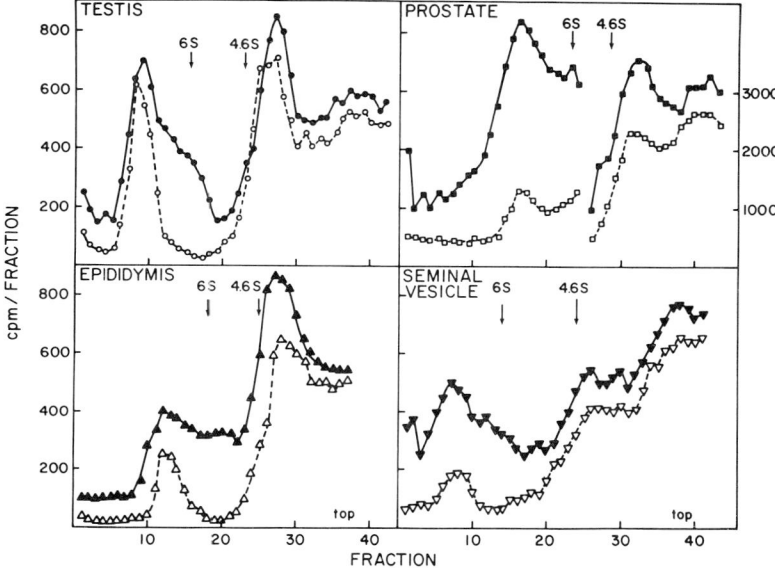

Fig. 5. Sucrose density-gradient centrifugation of 105,000 g supernatants from rat testis, epididymis, prostate, and seminal vesicle labeled with [³H]testosterone; 105,000 g supernatants were prepared from tissues removed 24 hours after castration or 30 days following hypophysectomy. Minced tissues were homogenized in 4 volumes of 50 mM Tris, pH 7.5, containing 1 mM EDTA and 10% glycerol using an Ultra Turrax at 4°C and centrifuged for 75 minutes. Supernatants were incubated with [³H]testosterone (15 nM) in the presence (open symbols) or absence (solid symbols) of a 100-fold excess unlabeled testosterone for 20 hours at 0°C. Samples were run in parallel on 5–20% (w/v) sucrose gradients containing 1 mM EDTA, 10% glycerol, and 50 mM Tris, pH 7.5, by centrifuging in a Beckman SW50.1 rotor for 18–22 hours at 2°C. Gradients were fractionated from the bottom by collecting 8–10-drop fractions and counted in Aquasol–toluene (1:1).

following hypophysectomy and in epididymis for a prolonged period following castration. A characteristic property of the 9 S protein is that binding of [³H]androgen or [³H]progesterone is not abolished by addition of 50- to 100-fold excess of unlabeled androgen. It can, thus, be clearly distinguished from the androgen receptor by gradient centrifugation of supernatants labeled in the presence and absence of a 100-fold excess of unlabeled androgen (Fig. 5). Since the receptor and ABP are saturable at low steroid concentrations, [³H]androgen binding is negligible in the presence of a large excess of unlabeled androgen. The 9 S binding protein is also different from "complex I" in rat ventral prostate, which is a 3–3.5 S androgen-binding protein described by Fang and Liao (1971).

A. Chemical Properties

The 9 S binding protein was found to be easily separable from the androgen receptor by $(NH_4)_2SO_4$ fractionation. Only a small amount of the 9 S binding activity ($\simeq 10\%$) precipitated at 0–40% saturation where the androgen receptor is found. About 80% of the 9 S binding activity of the 105,000 g supernatant from rat testis precipitated at 40–70% saturation with $(NH_4)_2SO_4$. The 9 S protein has a low charge at neutral pH and is, therefore, not adsorbed by either anion or cation exchangers in media of low ionic strength (Fig. 6). DEAE–Sephadex or DEAE–cellulose column chromatography in 50 mM Tris buffer, pH 8.0, thus, provides a way of

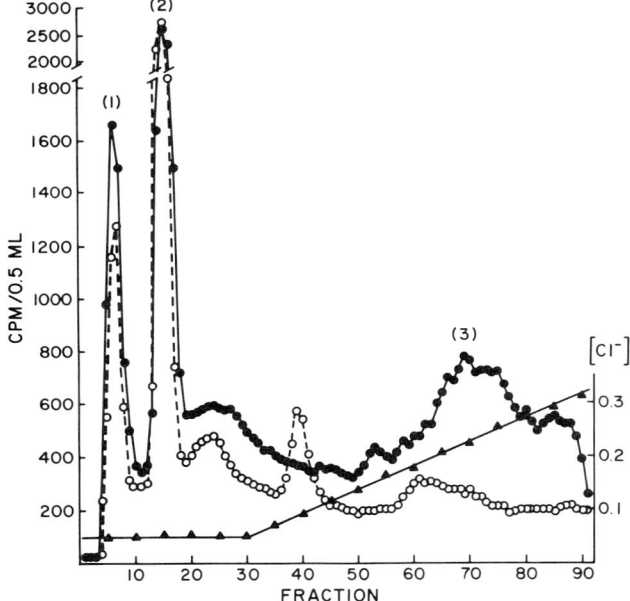

Fig. 6. DEAE–Sephadex chromatography of epididymis 105,000 g supernatant labeled with [³H]dihydrotestosterone. Ten milliliters of epididymis 105,000 g supernatant, prepared as described in Fig. 5, was incubated with 10 nM [³H]dihydrotestosterone (³H-DHT) (●———●) or 10 nM ³H-DHT plus 100-fold excess unlabeled DHT (○---------○) for 20 hours at 0°C. Radioactivity bound by ABP was displaced 3 hours before chromatography by making the sample 10 μM with unlabeled DHT. Free steroid was reduced by incubating with 2% charcoal for 10 minutes at 0°C. Charcoal was removed by centrifugation. Samples were applied to a 1.6 × 25-cm DEAE–Sephadex A-50 column equilibrated with 50 mM Tris, pH 7.4, at 4°C. Adsorbed proteins were eluted with 300 ml of 0–0.4 M linear KCl gradient in 50 mM Tris, pH 7.4, at a flow rate of 25 ml/hr; (▲———▲) represents chloride ion concentration. (Peak 1 contains the 9 S binding protein, peak 2 is mainly free [³H]dihydrotestosterone, and peak 3 represents binding to androgen receptor. ABP would elute at approximately 0.2 M KCl.)

separating this protein from ABP and androgen receptor, both of which are adsorbed to the column under these conditions. The gel filtration effect of Sephadex A-50 facilitates a separation of the 9 S binding protein from free steroid and from the bulk of $3\alpha/\beta$-hydroxysteroid oxidoreductase activity.

The possibility that the 9S binding protein might be composed of subunits was tested by sucrose gradient centrifugation in the presence of 0.4 M KCl. No shift in sedimentation occurred in the high salt concentration, suggesting that subunits, if present, were not associated through weak ionic bonds. The presence of 4 M urea resulted in loss of about 70% of binding activity, with no apparent change in sedimentation, suggesting further than the 9 S protein may be a single polypeptide. It is somewhat more sensitive to heat inactivation than ABP but less sensitive than the androgen receptor. Approximately 40% of binding activity was destroyed by heating at 37°C for 30 minutes, while 85% was lost at 50°C. The binding of [^{3}H]progesterone or [^{3}H]dihydrotestosterone to the 9 S protein was enhanced by 10 mM 2-mercaptoethanol and partially inhibited to 1 mM p-chlorohydroxyphenylsulfonate, indicating that sulfhydryl groups may be important for maintenance of the active binding site. At a concentration of 100 mM 2-mercaptoethanol, binding was decreased by about 40%, suggesting that disulfide bonds may also be a structural requirement (Wilson *et al.*, 1977).

B. Steroid-Binding Properties

Studies on the specificity of the 9 S binding protein for labeled steroids using continuous or tritiated steroid-containing discontinuous sucrose gradient centrifugation (Fig. 7) and equilibrium dialysis, indicate a selectively for [^{3}H]progesterone and [^{3}H]dihydrotestosterone. Detection of binding on unlabeled sucrose gradients required labeling of the protein at concentrations of 10–15 nM. Binding was not detectable at steroid concentrations of 2 nM unless labeled steroid was distributed throughout the gradient prior to centrifugation. The amount of radioactivity bound in sucrose gradients following incubation with 20–40 nM [^{3}H]progesterone or [^{3}H]dihydrotestosterone plus a 100-fold excess of unlabeled progesterone or dihydrotestosterone was either the same or even greater than the amount bound after incubation with [^{3}H]steroid alone; however, equilibrium dialysis showed 30% to 70% inhibition of binding by a 1000-fold excess unlabeled steroid. Relatively little binding was observed with [^{3}H]testosterone and [^{3}H]17β-estradiol, and there was lower binding of [^{3}H]5α-androstanediol or [^{3}H]androstenedione. A 100-fold excess unlabeled cyproterone acetate did not inhibit [^{3}H]progesterone or [^{3}H]dihydrotestosterone binding. The specificity of the 9 S binding protein for progesterone and dihydrotestosterone

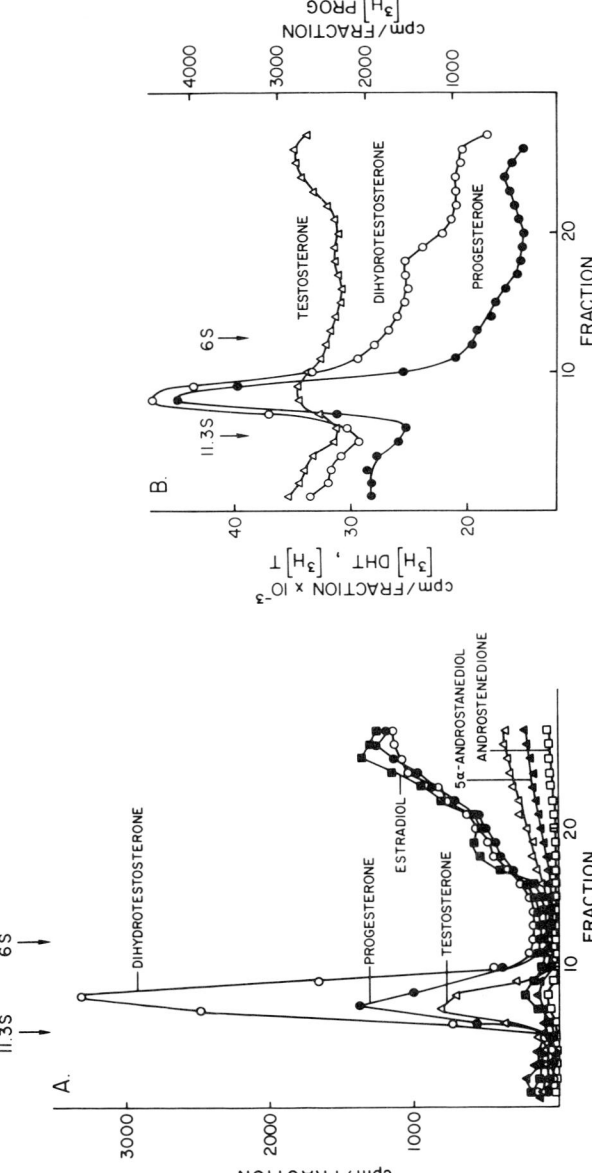

Fig. 7. Steroid specificity of 9 S binding protein from epididymis on sucrose gradients. The 9 S protein fraction was partially purified by DEAE Sephadex chromatography (cf. Fig. 6) from the 105,000 g supernatant of epididymis from rats castrated for 24 hours. (A) Aliquots (0.7 ml) from the pooled fractions of peak I were incubated at 0°C for 2 hours with 40 nM [³H]dihydrotestosterone (O), [³H]testosterone (△), [³H]progesterone (●), [³H]17β-estradiol (■), [³H]5α-androstanediol (▲), or [³H]androstenedione (□). Free radioactive steroids were extracted for 2 minutes with charcoal and aliquots of 0.5 ml were analyzed by linear 5–20% (w/v) sucrose gradient centrifugation as described in Fig. 5. Marker proteins are indicated for bovine γ-globulin (6 S) and bovine liver catalase (11.3 S). The same relative binding was observed when samples were not extracted with charcoal. (B) Partially purified 9 S binding protein from the DEAE-Sephadex flowthrough fraction was incubated with 2 nM [³H]steroid for 2 hours at 0°C. Aliquots (0.5 ml) were applied to discontinuous gradients of 1.2 ml each of 20, 15, 10, and 5% (w/v) sucrose in the same buffer, but containing 2 nM [³H]steroid. Recovery of [³H]testosterone and [³H]dihydrotestosterone was above 80%, while there was considerable loss of [³H]progesterone (~75% of total radioactivity) probably due to sticking to cellulose nitrate tubes (Wilson et al., 1977).

differs from the androgen receptor and ABP. Both the androgen receptor and ABP have high affinities for dihydrotestosterone and testosterone and little affinity for progesterone. All three proteins have low but detectable affinities for 5α-androstanediol. The selective binding of progesterone and dihydrotestosterone suggests that this 9 S binding protein may serve to maintain high intracellular concentrations of androgen or progesterone in target tissues. A summary of the properties of the 9 S protein is given in Table III.

In the testis, progesterone is a precursor in the biosynthesis of testosterone; however, it is uncertain whether progesterone has any hormonal function in androgen-dependent organs. A high-affinity binding protein for progesterone has been reported in rat testis (Galena et al., 1974) and prostate (Karsznia et al., 1969), and synandrogenic actions of progestins and testosterone have been described in other organs (Mowszowicz et al., 1974). The low concentration of progesterone relative to androgens, especially in epididymis, makes uncertain the physiological importance of progesterone binding to the 9 S protein.

IV. ANDROGEN RECEPTOR

Intracellular receptor proteins for testosterone and dihydrotestosterone have been demonstrated in nearly all reproductive organs of the male rat, including prostate (Baulieu and Jung, 1970; Bruchovsky and Wilson, 1968b; Fang et al., 1969; Mainwaring, 1969; Rennie and Bruchovsky, 1972; Unhjem et al., 1969; Ritzén et al., 1971) epididymis (Blaquier, 1971; Blaquier and Calandra, 1973; Hansson et al., 1973b; Tindall et al., 1972, 1974a, 1975), seminal vesicle (Stern and Eisenfeld, 1969), bulbocavernosus and levator ani muscles (Jung and Baulieu, 1972; Krieg et al., 1974), and testis (Hansson et al., 1974b; McLean et al., 1976; Mulder et al., 1975; Sanborn et al., 1975; Sar et al., 1975; Smith et al., 1975b; Wilson and Smith, 1975). In this section, we will deal primarily with an examination of the binding kinetics and the *in vitro* steroid specificities of androgen receptors from rat testis, epididymis, prostate, and seminal vesicle. Remarkable similarities in the *in vitro* binding properties of androgen receptors in different target organs contrast *in vivo* differences in apparent binding specificity. These differences observed *in vivo* seem to result from the extent of metabolism of [^{3}H]testosterone and [^{3}H]dihydrotestosterone.

[^{3}H]Testosterone is converted rapidly to dihydrotestosterone in most androgen responsive cells (Fig. 8). It has not been clear, however, whether this conversion of testosterone is an absolute requirement for androgen action. Reports that [^{3}H]dihydrotestosterone is exclusively associated with

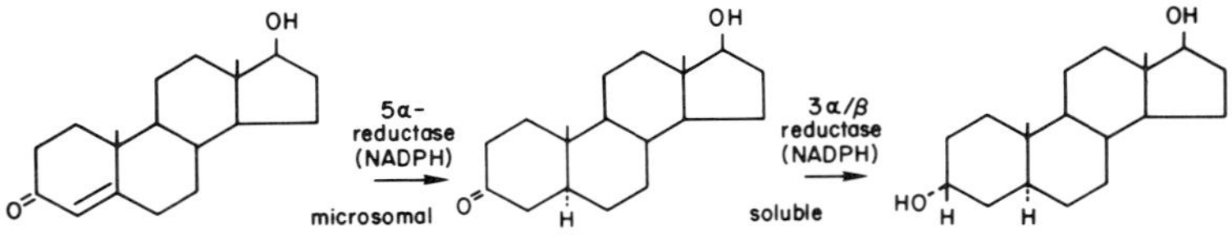

Fig. 8. Metabolism of testosterone.

the cytoplasmic receptor protein and retained in nuclei after labeling with [^{3}H]testosterone *in vivo* have indicated that dihydrotestosterone is in fact an active intracellular form of androgen. Differences in the apparent *in vivo* binding specificity of androgen receptors in various androgen-responsive tissues prompted our *in vitro* studies on steroid affinity and specificity of the androgen receptor. For instance, receptors in prostate and epididymis have been observed to bind only dihydrotestosterone (Mainwaring and Mangan, 1973; Liao *et al.*, 1973), while receptors in testis bind both testosterone and dihydrotestosterone (Hansson *et al.*, 1974d; Smith *et al.*, 1975b) or predominantly testosterone (Mulder *et al.*, 1975), and receptors in levator ani bind only testosterone (Jung and Baulieu, 1972).

Nuclear accumulation of androgen seems to be receptor dependent (Bruchovsky *et al.*, 1975). Accordingly, the cytoplasmic receptor-binding specificity for androgen *in vivo* was paralleled in nuclei. In prostate of castrate rats (Bruchovsky and Wilson, 1968b; King and Mainwaring, 1974; Liao and Fang, 1969; Tveter *et al.*, 1974) and epididymis of castrated or hypophysectomized rats (Tindall *et al.*, 1972, 1974a), predominantly [^{3}H]5α-dihydrotestosterone accumulates in nuclei following *in vivo* injection of [^{3}H]testosterone. In testis of hypophysectomized rats, however, nuclei accumulate [^{3}H]testosterone and [^{3}H]dihydrotestosterone (Smith *et al.*, 1975a) or [^{3}H]testosterone alone (Mulder *et al.*, 1975). Recent data on prostate indicates that, under conditions favoring high concentrations of [^{3}H]testosterone relative to [^{3}H]dihydrotestosterone, substantial amounts of [^{3}H]testosterone accumulate in prostate nuclei as well (Gustafsson and Pousette, 1975; Rennie and Bruchovsky, 1973). The apparent differences in receptor binding of testosterone and dihydrotestosterone *in vivo* suggested the possibility that receptor proteins in target organs might have different binding properties, even though their other physical and chemical properties are remarkably similar (Bardin *et al.*, 1975; Mainwaring and Irving, 1973; Mainwaring *et al.*, 1973; McLean *et al.*, 1976; Smith *et al.*, 1975b). Our *in vitro* binding studies, however, indicate that receptor proteins from different androgen target organs have similar, if not identical, binding properties. Organ differences in binding of testosterone or dihydrotestosterone *in vivo* appear, then, to be determined not by receptor affinity, but rather, by the intracellular availability of these androgens for binding to receptor.

A. Stabilization of the *in Vitro* Receptor–Androgen Interaction

Analysis of receptor binding *in vitro* makes it possible to compare the binding properties of receptors from different organs under relatively similar conditions. Stabilization of the *in vitro* binding reaction involves both the elimination of factors that promote androgen metabolism as well as the establishment of conditions that maintain receptor stability. These requirements were satisfied using a charcoal adsorption assay and a receptor–protein preparation partially purified by $(NH_4)_2SO_4$ fractionation.

1. Androgen Stability

Enzymes that convert testosterone to active and inactive metabolites have been identified in subcellular fractions of most androgen responsive tissues (Fig. 8). Δ^4-3-Ketosteroid-5α-oxidoreductase, which converts testosterone to dihydrotestosterone, is present largely in the microsomal fraction. Accordingly, this enzyme activity was not detected in 105,000 g supernatants since [^{3}H]testosterone was stable both at 0°C and 23°C for periods up to 24 hours. On the other hand, $3\alpha/\beta$-hydroxysteroid oxidoreductase, which converts dihydrotestosterone to 5α-androstanediol, is present in the soluble fraction of some tissue homogenates. [^{3}H]Dihydrotestosterone metabolism in crude supernatant preparations was negligible in epididymis and seminal vesicle at 0°C with or without added NADPH, low in prostate (10% in 24 hours at 0° or 23°C) and high in testis (95% within 24 hours at 0°C or 1 hour at 23°C) (Fig. 9A). This metabolic activity was found to be dependent on the cofactor NADPH. $(NH_4)_2SO_4$ precipitation of receptor eliminated this enzyme activity (Fig. 9B) and permitted incubations with [^{3}H]dihydrotestosterone for prolonged periods under stable conditions. Since addition of an NADPH-generating system restored $3\alpha/\beta$-reductase activity, it is likely that treatment with $(NH_4)_2SO_4$ either removed or inactivated the cofactor required for reductase activity.

Androgen bound to proteins may be protected from steroid-metabolizing enzymes. For example, ABP may promote a lower free testosterone and dihydrotestosterone concentration available to the reductase by binding these androgens within the Sertoli cell and protecting them for later secretion into the seminiferous tubular fluid (see Section II). Moreover, the 9 S binding protein (see Section III) may sequester the biologically active androgens in intracellular regions apart from metabolizing enzymes. Our *in vitro* studies indicate that binding to the receptor protects dihydrotestosterone from enzymatic conversion to 5α-androstanediol. Under conditions where all free [^{3}H]dihydrotestosterone was metabolized (Fig. 10), [^{3}H]dihydrotestosterone bound to receptor remained unchanged. Analysis of the dissociation rate (in presence of 1000-fold excess unlabeled testosterone) showed little change in rate after addition of $3\alpha/\beta$-hydroxysteroid oxidoreductase. Metabolism of free [³H]dihydrotestosterone in the control yielded 5α-androstanediol and androsterone, as determined by thin-layer chromatography on silica gel in methylene chloride:ether 9:1.

2. Receptor Stability

Stability of the androgen receptor *in vitro* was found to be sensitive to pH, temperature, and the presence of [³H]testosterone or [³H]dihydrotestosterone. Optimal receptor-binding activity was observed between pH 7 and 8.6. The presence of [³H]androgen stabilizes the receptor. As shown in Fig. 11, [³H]testosterone rendered the receptor completely stable at 0°C. In the absence of [³H]testosterone, receptor is inactivated with a rate which tends to vary with the preparation, the $t_{1/2}$ in the range of 6–40 hours. Higher

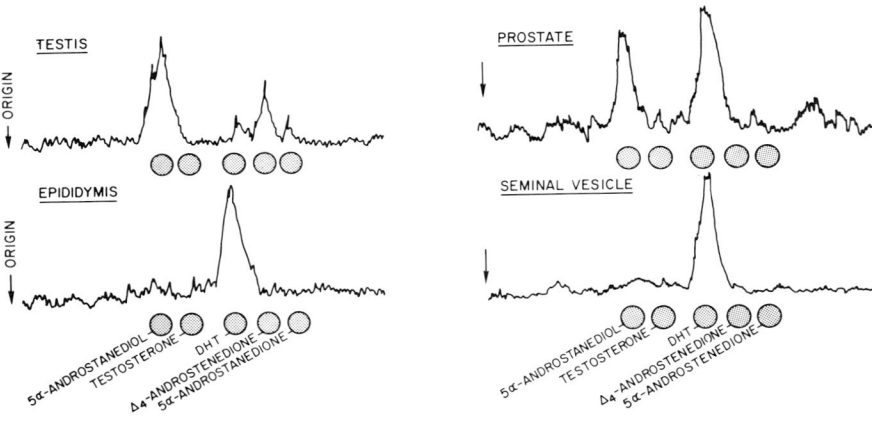

A

Fig. 9. Metabolism of [³H]dihydrotestosterone in 105,000 g supernatants and $(NH_4)_2SO_4$ fractions; 105,000 g supernatants were prepared (see Fig. 5) from testis, epididymis, prostate, and seminal vesicle from either hypophysectomized or castrated rats. The 0–32% and 0–40% saturated $(NH_4)_2SO_4$ fractions from testis and prostate 105,000 g supernatants, respectively, were redissolved in 10% glycerol, 1 mM EDTA, 50 mM Tris, pH 7.5. Aliquots (0.5 ml) labeled with [³H]dihydrotestosterone (10–20 nM) for 24 hours at 0°C were combined with unlabeled carrier steroids (100 μg each in 0.1 ml ethanol of 5α-androstanediol, testosterone, dihydrotestosterone, androsterone, androstenedione, and 5α-androstanedione) and extracted three times with 10 volumes methylene chloride. Extracts were dried at 37°C under N_2 and dissolved in ethanol. Steroids were separated on precoated silica gel sheets (0.2 mm No. 60 F-254 E Merck, Darmstadt, Germany) by developing twice with methylene chloride:ether (4:1) and scanned using a Packard radiochromatogram scanner. Represented are thin-layer chromatograms of extracted radioactivity following incubation with [³H]dihydrotestosterone in 105,000 g supernatants in the four tissues (A) and in $(NH_4)_2SO_4$ fractions of testis and epididymis (B).

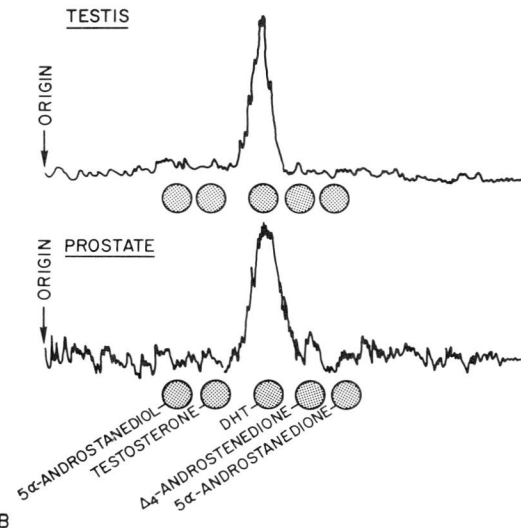

Fig. 9. (Continued)

temperature was observed to increase the rate of receptor inactivation. At 23°C, rapid inactivation of the free receptor occurred. This rate was considerably slowed, however, by the presence of [^{3}H]testosterone. These results suggest that the [^{3}H]androgen–receptor complex is less susceptible to degradation caused by proteolytic breakdown or thermal inactivation than the unbound receptor. A conformational change upon binding of androgen may increase the stability of the complex. The instability of the free receptor complicated determination of binding constants, as discussed later.

B. Procedures for Quantitation of Androgen Receptor

The low concentration of androgen receptors in target tissues has provoked the development of a variety of techniques which can be used to assess receptor-binding activity. Quantitation of receptor in crude 105,000 g supernatant preparations is complicated by its low concentration and by the presence of other proteins that display both low or high affinity binding for androgens. For an analytical method to be effective, it must distinguish between the various binding components. In addition to the charcoal adsorption assay, some limitations and advantages of several other techniques, including sucrose gradient centrifugation, DEAE–cellulose filter assay, ion-exchange chromatography, and polyacrylamide gel electrophoresis are mentioned below.

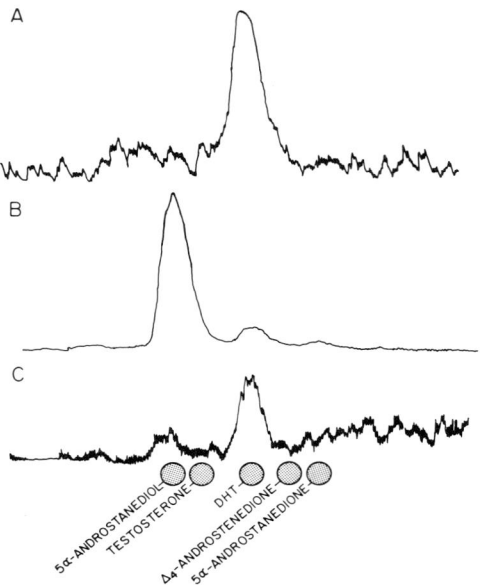

Fig. 10. Influence of $3\alpha/\beta$-hydroxysteroid oxidoreductase activity on free and receptor bound [^{3}H]dihydrotestosterone. The androgen receptor present in the (NH$_4$)$_2$SO$_4$ fraction (0–40% saturated) from prostate of rats castrated for 24 hours was incubated with 10 nM [^{3}H]dihydrotestosterone for 18 hours at 0°C. $3\alpha/\beta$-Hydroxysteroid oxidoreductase activity was obtained from submaxillary gland 105,000 g supernatant, which was preincubated with 20 nM unlabeled dihydrotestosterone for 18 hours at 0°C to bind the androgen receptor. Free steroid was removed from both prostate and submaxillary supernatants by suspending charcoal to make 1% suspensions for 15 minutes at 0°C. Charcoal was removed by centrifugation and prostate supernatant containing receptor-[^{3}H]DHT incubated with 1 mM NADPH and $\frac{1}{2}$ volume submaxillary gland supernatant. (A) Thin-layer chromatogram of radioactivity extracted from (NH$_4$)$_2$SO$_4$ fraction of prostate supernatant after incubation with 10 nM [^{3}H]dihydrotestosterone for 24 hours at 0°C showing absence of metabolism. (B) Chromatogram of radioactivity extracted from submaxillary gland supernatant after 1 hour incubation at 0°C with 10 nM [^{3}H]dihydrotestosterone plus 1 mM NADPH showing nearly complete metabolism to androstanediol. (C) Radioactivity extracted from prostate supernatant containing [^{3}H]dihydrotestosterone–receptor complexes incubated with submaxillary gland supernatant at 0°C for 24 hours. The small conversion to [^{3}H]androstanediol is consistent with the amount of [^{3}H]dihydrotestosterone dissociating from the receptor during the 24-hour incubation.

Quantitation of the receptor appears to reflect methodology, since the absolute amount of receptor measured depends on the assay. Of the methods investigated, polyacrylamide gel electrophoresis yielded the lowest quantity of receptor-binding activity. This method utilizes 3.25% acrylamide gels containing 0.5% agarose as previously described (McLean et al., 1976;

Tindall et al., 1975). Some loss of receptor may result from failure to enter the gel, dissociation of the [³H]androgen–receptor complex during electrophoresis, or partial inactivation caused by high pH (pH 8.9). An advantage is a negligible level of nonspecific binding. Receptors from several tissues exhibited a mobility of 0.4–0.5 relative to bromophenol blue in 3.25% acrylamide gels containing 0.5% agarose using a glycine buffer at pH 8.9 (Hansson et al., 1974d; Smith et al., 1975b; Tindall et al., 1975). Androgen

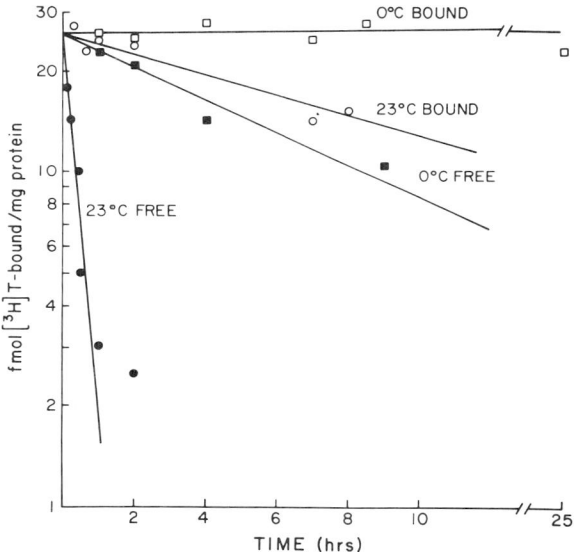

Fig. 11. Stability of bound and free androgen receptor. The 105,000 g testis supernatant (see Fig. 5) from rats hypophysectomized for 30 days was incubated at 0° or 23°C in the presence and absence of 10 nM [³H]testosterone ([³H]T). For determination of bound receptor inactivation rates, receptors were saturated with [³H]T at 0°C for 18 hours and then placed at 0° or 23°C. Total specific binding remaining at time intervals between 0 and 9 hours was determined using the charcoal adsorption assay as follows: Charcoal (Norit A) is washed in 0.1 N HCl, H₂O, 0.1 N NaOH, and then H₂O, and dried with ethanol and ether rinses. Aliquots (0.6 ml) taken from a stirring stock solution containing 1% charcoal, 0.1% Dextran-80, 0.1% gelatin (purified from calf skin), 1 mM EDTA, and 10 mM Tris, pH 7.5, are added to receptor samples (0.1–0.3 ml in 10% glycerol, 1 mM EDTA, 50 mM Tris, pH 7.5; 2–10 mg protein/ml) which were labeled with [³H]androgen in the presence and absence of 100-fold excess unlabeled androgen. Incubation is for 20 minutes at 0°C with frequent shaking, followed by centrifugation at 2000 g for 15 minutes. An aliquot (0.5 ml) is counted in Aquasol : toluene (1 : 1) (5 ml) in plastic minivials. The difference in radioactivity in presence and absence of excess unlabeled steroid gives a measure of receptor-binding activity. Free receptor inactivation rates were obtained by incubating receptor preparations at 0 or 23°C in the absence of [³H]T. Aliquots (0.2 ml) taken at various times were labeled for 18 hours at 0°C in the presence of 10 nM [³H]T. Shown is the amount of specific binding remaining for [³H]T-bound receptor at 0°C (□) and 23°C (○) and the free receptor at 0°C (■) and 23°C (●) (Wilson and French, 1976).

receptors in prostate, seminal vesicle, bulbocavernosus–levator ani (Krieg et al., 1974), and testis (Mulder et al., 1975) have previously been shown also to have similar mobilities by agar gel electrophoresis at pH 8.5.

Charcoal adsorption and sucrose-gradient assays measured similar concentrations of receptor, which were approximately twice the amount detected by polyacrylamide gel electrophoresis. Both of these methods are discussed in more detail below. A DEAE–cellulose filter assay (Whatman DE 81) (Baxter et al., 1975) indicated equivalent or higher binding activity than that detected by the charcoal assay. This method depends on the binding of androgen receptors to positively charged diethylaminoethyl groups (anion exchanger) at low ionic strength to which free [^{3}H]androgens bind minimally (about 0.7% of total radioactivity). Regardless of the type of assay, saturation of receptor-binding sites occurs between 10 and 25 nM [^{3}H]testosterone or [^{3}H]dihydrotestosterone, depending on the tissue being studied. Androgen-binding activity detected by ion exchange chromatography is usually lower than that detected by other assay methods due to poor recoveries and dissociation of the [^{3}H]androgen–receptor complex.

1. Sucrose-Gradient Centrifugation—Determination of Sedimentation Coefficients

Sucrose density-gradient centrifugation has been used to demonstrate that androgen receptors vary in size, depending on the method of preparation and the ionic strength. Generally, 5–20% sucrose gradients buffered to pH 7.5–8 with or without glycerol, thioglycerol, or KCl are used. Simultaneous centrifugation of standard marker proteins allows estimation of receptor sedimentation coefficients. When analyzing receptor activity, parallel gradients containing samples labeled with ^{3}H-steroid in the presence of 100-fold excess unlabeled steroid are required to account for nonspecific binding.

Though discrepancies in androgen–receptor sedimentation exist in the literature, many have reported that there are two forms in cytosol, sedimenting at approximately 8 S and 4 S. In rat ventral prostate, both 8 S and 4 S forms have been reported (Baulieu and Jung, 1970; Ritzén et al., 1971; Unhjem et al., 1969) although others have sometimes found only the 8 S (Mainwaring, 1969; Davies and Griffiths, 1975) or 3.5–4 S form (Fang et al., 1969). Similarly in rat epididymis, either both forms (Blaquier, 1971) or only the 3.5–4 S or 7–8 S forms have been detected (McLean et al., 1976; Tindall et al., 1974a). In testes of immature hypophysectomized rats labeled in vivo with [^{3}H]testosterone, the 6–8 S receptor was the predominant form recovered (McLean et al., 1976). Different forms of the androgen receptor at low ionic strength may result largely from aggregation. Nuclear androgen–receptor complexes have been extracted in 3 to 3.5 S forms (Fang et al., 1969; Baulieu et al., 1971; Tindall et al., 1974a; Bruchovsky et al., 1975; Baker et al., 1977).

Receptor sedimentation can be markedly influenced by ionic strength. In the presence of 0.4 M KCl or higher salt concentrations, receptors tend to disperse from the 8–12 S form to a 3–4 S form (Hansson et al., 1973b; Mainwaring and Irving, 1973). Precipitation of receptor in 105,000 g supernatants, 30% saturated with $(NH_4)_2SO_4$, has been reported to yield the 8 S form, and incubation of the $(NH_4)_2SO_4$-treated receptor at 30°C for 20 minutes converts the 8 S form to 4 S (Mainwaring and Irving, 1973). The conversion of the receptor from 8 S to 4 S in the presence of salt or heat may represent separation into subunits. No biologic significance can yet be attributed to the propensity of androgen-receptor molecules to aggregate with themselves or with other proteins. Dimerization of the estrogen receptor is believed to be a prerequisite for nuclear translocation (Notides et al., 1975).

We have found that receptors from rat testis, epididymis, prostate and seminal vesicle display similar sedimentation patterns when crude 105,000 g supernatants are analyzed on linear sucrose gradients (Fig. 5). In agreement with previous reports, receptor binding determined as displaceable radioactivity in the presence of 100-fold excess unlabeled steroid, was found to be approximately 4 S and 5–8 S. A crude supernatant fraction from testes of rats injected with [^{3}H]testosterone showed predominantly a 6–8 S peak (Fig. 12). Also apparent on the gradients in Fig. 5 is nondisplaced bound radioactivity in the 9 S region of the gradient. This binding activity represents a 9 S androgen binding protein which is distinct from the receptor, as described in Section III. It is possible that previous failure to account for so-called nonspecific binding may have caused errors in assessing receptor sedimentation properties.

Partial purification of androgen receptors using $(NH_4)_2SO_4$ revealed differences in the sedimentation patterns of receptors from various tissues. As shown in Fig. 13, single broad peaks of displaceable radioactivity from testis were 5–8 S, epididymis 4–5 S, and prostate 3–4 S. Exposure to 0.4 M KCl shortly prior to and during centrifugation caused a shift in the testis peak from 5–8 S to 4–5 S, but had little effect on receptors from epididymis or prostate. Essentially one form of the receptor was present, and each sedimented in a different region of the gradient, indicating differences in size.

2. Ion-Exchange Chromatography

Androgen receptors exhibit dipolar charge characteristics. A pI of 5.8 has been reported for androgen receptors in prostate (Mainwaring and Irving,

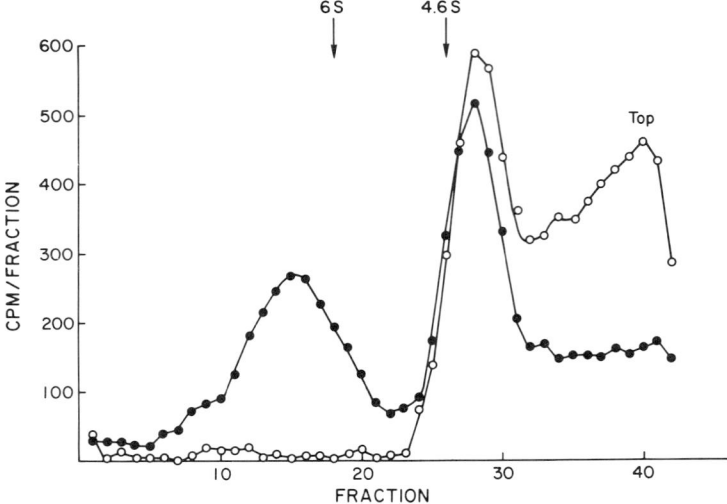

Fig. 12. Sucrose density-gradient centrifugation of *in vivo* labeled testis supernatant. Eighty-day-old rats hypophysectomized 30 days earlier were injected in the femoral artery with 100 μCi [³H]testosterone in 15% ethanol–saline. Rats were sacrificed 1 hour later, and 105,000 g testis supernatant was prepared as described in the legend to Fig. 5. Aliquots (0.46 ml) were kept at 0°C (●) or heated at 37°C for 5 hours in the presence of 0.2 μM unlabeled testosterone (○). Samples were centrifuged on linear 5–20% (w/v) sucrose gradients as described in the legend to Fig. 5 with the marker proteins bovine serum albumin (4.6 S) and bovine gamma globulin (6 S). The peak between 5–8 S represents binding to androgen receptor. Note that the 9 S binding protein is not detected, due to the low concentration of [³H]androgen in the supernatant, about 2 nM.

1973), epididymis (Tindall, *et al.*, 1975), and testis (McLean *et al.*, 1976), as determined by isoelectric focusing, and indicates a net negative charge at neutral pH. Accordingly, receptors are adsorbed to anion exchange media like DEAE-cellulose (Sullivan and Strott, 1973) and DEAE-Sephadex at low ionic strength (Fig. 6). Receptors are eluted in a disperse pattern between 0.1 and 0.3 M KCl at pH 7.4. An area of high positive charge density also is present since androgen receptors interact strongly with the cation exchanger, phosphocellulose (Rennie and Bruchovsky, 1972; Norris and Kohler, 1976) (Fig. 14).

3. *Charcoal Assay for Androgen-Receptor Binding*

The use of charcoal as a rapid means to remove free steroid as applied to estrogens by Korenman (1968) and others (Katzenellenbogen *et al.*, 1973) is also useful in the study of steroid binding to androgen receptors (for procedure, see legend of Fig. 11) (Wilson and French, 1976). The technique is simple and rapid to perform but has the disadvantage that specific high-affinity binding must be measured over a rather high background of low-affinity binding. Dilution of [^{3}H]androgens with 50- to 100-fold excess unlabeled androgen is a reliable way to eliminate binding to receptor. Total

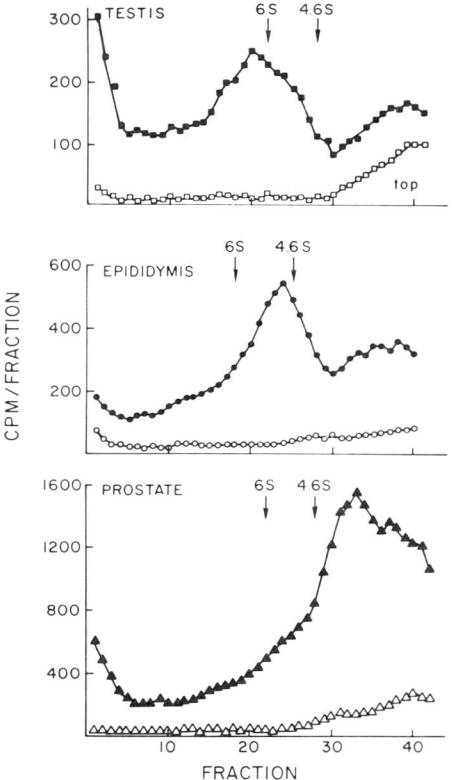

Fig. 13. Sucrose density-gradient centrifugation of $(NH_4)_2SO_4$ fractions from testis, epididymis, and prostate 105,000 g supernatants; 105,000 g supernatants of tissues from rats castrated for 24 hours or hypophysectomized for 30 days were incubated at 0°C for 20 hours with 15 nM [^{3}H]testosterone in the presence (open symbols) or absence (solid symbols) of a 100-fold excess unlabeled testosterone. Supernatants were then partially purified by precipitating the 0–32% saturated $(NH_4)_2SO_4$ fraction from testis and the 0–40% fraction from epididymis and prostate and redissolving in 10% glycerol, 1 mM EDTA, 50 mM Tris, pH 7.5. Samples (0.3–0.5 ml) and marker proteins (bovine serum albumin, 4.6 S and bovine gamma globulin, 6 S) were centrifuged in 5–20% (w/v) sucrose gradients as described in the legend of Fig. 5. Gradient scans are shown for testis (■), epididymis (●) and prostate (▲) (Wilson and French, 1976).

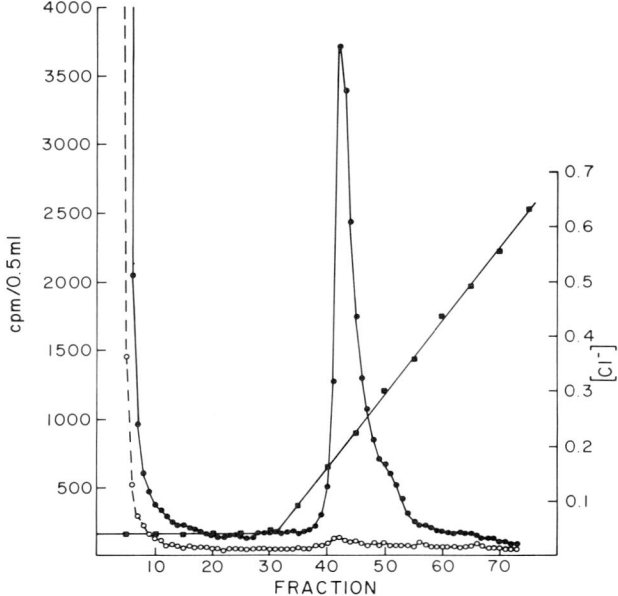

Fig. 14. Phosphocellulose chromatography of androgen receptors from rat epididymis. The 105,000 g supernatant of epididymis from rats castrated for 24 hours was incubated with 15 nM [³H]dihydrotestosterone (³H-DHT) for 20 hours at 0°C in the absence (●──────●) and presence of 1.5 μM unlabeled dihydrotestosterone (○---------○). Samples (5 ml) were applied to 0.9 cm × 3-cm phosphocellulose columns (Whatman P-11, potassium form) which were equilibrated with 50 mM Tris, pH 7.4. A linear 0–0.7 M KCl gradient in 100 ml was applied to elute adsorbed material at a flow rate of 18 ml/hr. Fractions 1–21 were 4.5 ml, and then 1.8 ml. Chloride ion concentration (■──────■) of the effluent fractions was monitored with an ion-specific electrode. ABP and the 9 S binding protein are not retained on phosphocellulose (Lea et al., 1977).

receptor binding can then be determined as a difference in counts in the presence and absence of excess unlabeled steroid. At low concentrations of androgens (below 6 nM), receptor binding represents 50% or more of total androgen binding. At concentrations between 6 and 20 nM, which are frequently required to saturate receptor, nonspecific binding increases rapidly (see Section III) so that receptor binding measurements are less precise. Nonspecific binding usually ranges between 0.1–3% of total free [³H]androgen. Part of this activity is due to free [³H]androgen not removed by charcoal (0.3% for [³H]testosterone and 0.7% for [³H]dihydrotestosterone). Despite these limitations, the charcoal assay could be used to assess factors which influence receptor stability, the steroid specificity of the receptor as well as the kinetics of androgen–receptor interaction, as described in the remaining sections.

C. Steroid Specificity of the Androgen Receptor

Hormone receptors must be capable of distinguishing between various chemically distinct steroids which circulate in the blood stream. The cytoplasmic androgen receptor from rat testis, epididymis, prostate, and seminal vesicle distinguishes testosterone and dihydrotestosterone from other steroids and binds them with much higher affinity. Figure 15 shows that a

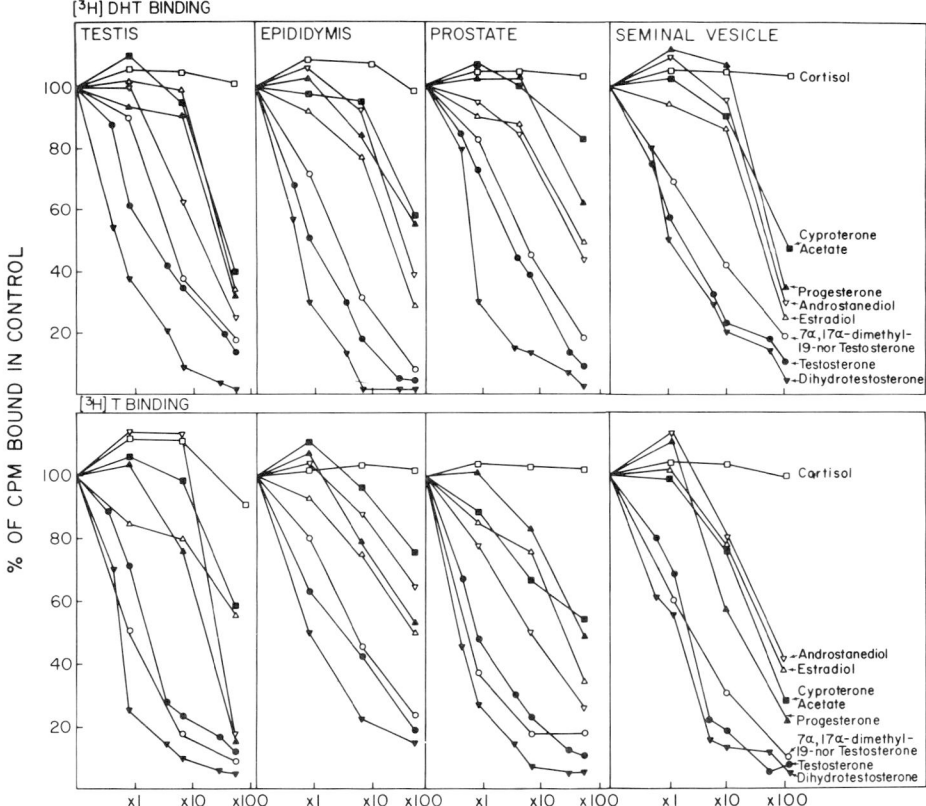

Fig. 15. Inhibition of [³H]dihydrotestosterone or [³H]testosterone binding to androgen receptors by unlabeled steroids in testis, epididymis, prostate, and seminal vesicle; 0.15–0.25-ml aliquots of $(NH_4)_2SO_4$ fractions (testis, epididymis, prostate) or 105,000 g supernatants (seminal vesicle) were incubated with saturating concentrations of [³H]dihydrotestosterone ([³H]DHT) or [³H]testosterone ([³H]T) (15–20 nM) and various unlabeled steroids (15–2000 nM) for 18–24 hours at 0°C. Binding reactions were quantitated by the charcoal adsorption assay (see Fig. 11). Data represent the binding of [³H]DHT (top) and [³H]T (bottom) in the presence of unlabeled dihydrotestosterone (▼), testosterone (●), 7α, 17α-dimethyl-19-nortestosterone (○), 17β-estradiol (△), 5α-androstanediol (▽), progesterone (▲), cyproterone acetate (■) and cortisol (□).

50- to 100-fold molar excess of unlabeled estrogen, progesterone, or 5α-androstanediol was required to inhibit *in vitro* receptor binding of [³H]testosterone or [³H]dihydrotestosterone. The synthetic androgen 7α, 17α-dimethyl-19-nortestosterone has a biologic activity several times higher than testosterone or dihydrotestosterone (Segaloff, 1963; Liao *et al.*, 1973). However, its ability to inhibit *in vitro* binding of [³H]testosterone or [³H]dihydrotestosterone was similar to testosterone and dihydrotestosterone. Thus, the greater biologic activity of 7α, 17α-dimethyl-19-nortestosterone is not due to a higher affinity for receptor as previously reported (Liao *et al.*, 1973), but results very likely from its slower rate of catabolism.

The antiandrogen, cyproterone acetate, has been found previously to inhibit receptor binding to androgens *in vivo* (Krieg *et al.*, 1974; Tindall *et al.*, 1975) and to block nuclear accumulation of radioactive androgens (Fang and Liao, 1969; Smith *et al.*, 1975a). High concentrations (50- to 100-fold excess) of cyproterone acetate also inhibit binding of [³H]testosterone or [³H]dihydrotestosterone *in vitro*. Low concentrations of cyproterone acetate, as well as other steroids, like 5α-androstanediol, hydrocortisone, or progesterone, enhance receptor binding of [³H]testosterone or [³H]dihydrotestosterone *in vitro*. This potentiation of receptor binding at low steroid concentrations was variable, and its significance is not clear. It may be that interaction of these steroids with receptor stabilizes the receptor against inactivation. An alternative explanation is that they promote an allosteric change in the receptor, which increases its affinity for [³H]testosterone and [³H]dihydrotestosterone.

All of the organs studied, including rat prostate, epididymis, testis, and seminal vesicle, contain androgen receptors which have nearly identical relative affinities for the various steroids. Highest affinities are for dihydrotestosterone, testosterone, and 7α, 17α-dimethyl-19-nortestosterone. Hydrocortisone did not inhibit receptor binding of [³H]testosterone or [³H]dihydrotestosterone, indicating a low receptor affinity. Similarities in receptor steroid specificity support the concept that androgen binding sites on receptor proteins in these tissues are identical.

D. Kinetics of Receptor–Androgen Interaction

One of the problems inherent in kinetic analysis of the receptor protein is its low concentration within the cell (about 0.05–0.5 nM). This difficulty is partly overcome through the use of ³H-androgens with high specific activities (60–100 Ci/mmole). The low concentration of the receptor also complicates its purification in sufficient quantities to perform kinetic studies on the isolated protein. In all of our studies, the receptor has,

17. Androgen-Binding Proteins

teins, some of which might lower free-steroid concentration by interacting nonspecifically with androgen.

Table I summarizes the binding and release rates of [³H]testosterone and [³H]dihydrotestosterone–receptor complexes from rat testis, epididymis, prostate, and seminal vesicle. In all cases, [³H]dihydrotestosterone dissociated and associated more slowly than [³H]testosterone, resulting in similar equilibrium dissociation constants for the two androgens as determined from the ratio of the rate constants. A comparison of the therefore, necessarily been examined in the presence of other soluble pro-

TABLE I
Rate and Equilibrium Constants of Androgen–Receptor Binding at 0°C[a]

Tissue	[³H]Androgen	Rate of association (k_a) $(M^{-1}hr^{-1})$	Rate of dissociation $t_{1/2}$ (hr)	k_d (hr^{-1})	Equilibrium dissociation constant $\left(K_d = \dfrac{k_d}{k_a}\right)$ (M)
Testis	Testosterone	1.6×10^8	15	0.046	2.9×10^{-10}
	Dihydrotestosterone	4.5×10^7	45	0.015	3.3×10^{-10}
Epididymis	Testosterone	1.7×10^8	16	0.043	2.5×10^{-10}
	Dihydrotestosterone	8.0×10^7	37	0.019	2.4×10^{-10}
Prostate	Testosterone	1.4×10^8	10	0.069	4.9×10^{-10}
	Dihydrotestosterone	5.3×10^7	38	0.018	3.4×10^{-10}
Seminal vesicle	Testosterone	1.8×10^8	14	0.050	2.8×10^{-10}
	Dihydrotestosterone	1.4×10^8	38	0.018	1.3×10^{-10}

[a] Constants were determined at 0°C using 105,000 g supernatant fractions (seminal vesicle) or fractions partially purified with $(NH_4)_2SO_4$ (testis, epididymis, prostate). Association rate constants were determined by measuring androgen–receptor complex formation using the charcoal adsorption assay at short time intervals in the presence of 1.5–3 nM [³H]androgen and correcting data for inactivation of free receptor, using the following equation:

$$1 - \frac{RS(k_a[S] + k_1)}{R_t k_a[S]} = e^{-(k_a[S] + k_1)t}$$

where RS is receptor–androgen complex, k_a is association rate constant, S is [³H]androgen concentration, k_1 is inactivation rate constant of unbound receptor, R_t is total receptor, and t is time. Inactivation rate constants of unbound receptor were determined as described in Fig. 11. At 0°C, the inactivation rate constant k_1 ranged between 0.02 and 0.11 hr^{-1}, depending on the preparation, so that the standard error of association rate constants was ±50% for [³H]testosterone and [³H]dihydrotestosterone. The half-time of receptor dissociation, $t_{1/2}$, and the dissociation rate constants ($k_d = 0.6933/t_{1/2}$) were determined for receptors as described in Fig. 15. The range of variation of $t_{1/2}$ was ±2 and ±10 hours for T and DHT, respectively. Equilibrium dissociation constants were determined as the ratio of dissociation and association rate constants ($K_d = k_d/k_a$).

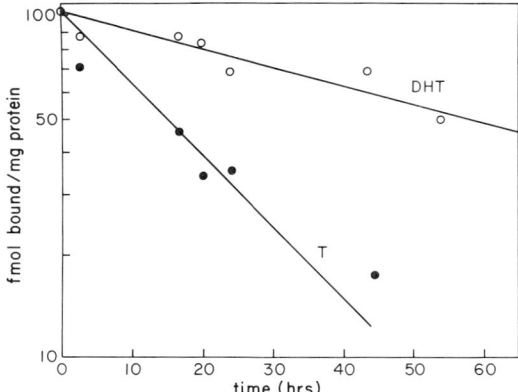

Fig. 16. Dissociation of [³H]testosterone or [³H]dihydrotestosterone from epididymis androgen receptor. The 105,000 g supernatant prepared from epididymis from rats 4 days after castration was incubated with 15 nM [³H]testosterone ([³H]T) or [³H]dihydrotestosterone ([³H]-DHT) for 24 hours at 0°C. A 1000-fold excess of unlabeled testosterone or dihydrotestosterone, respectively, was added to half of the labeled supernatant to measure dissociation of the [³H]T-receptor complex. The other half served as control. At various times, specific binding to receptor was analyzed using the charcoal adsorption assay (see Fig. 11). No significant decrease in binding was detected in the control over the time periods indicated. Dissociation of [³H]T (●) and [³H]DHT (○) from epididymis receptor is shown with respect to time. The $t_{1/2}$ for receptor complexed with [³H]T and [³H]DHT is 15 hours and 55 hours, respectively (Wilson and French, 1976).

dissociation rates for the epididymis receptor at 0°C is shown in Fig. 16, where the $t_{1/2}$ is 15 hours for [³H]testosterone and about 40 hours for [³H]]dihydrotestosterone. The remarkable similarities in rate constants indicate similarities in the binding-site properties for the androgen receptor in these tissues.

These slow rates of association and dissociation for the interaction of androgen with the receptor contrast with those of other androgen binding proteins, although equilibrium constants are similar (K_d of 10^{-9} to 10^{-10} M) (French and Ritzén, 1973a; Hansson et al., 1975b; King and Mainwaring, 1974). For example, the ABP-[³H]dihydrotestosterone complex dissociates very fast ($t_{1/2}$ of about 6 minutes at 0°C, see Section II). The plasma-binding protein, testosterone-binding globulin, interacts with androgens at intermediate rates (Heyns and DeMoor, 1971). In contrast, receptors for estrogen (Katzenellenbogen et al., 1973; Mester and Robertson, 1971), progesterone (Schrader and O'Malley, 1972), and androgen exhibit slower rates which may reflect a property necessary for the accumulation of receptor-steroid complexes within nuclei.

E. Thermodynamics of Receptor–Testosterone Interaction

Measurement of the effect of temperature on the binding and release rates of androgens from the receptor gives an indication of the thermodynamic properties of the interaction. When receptor inactivation was corrected as described in the legend of Table I, association and dissociation rates increased proportionally with temperature (Table II) (Wilson and French, 1976) in a manner similar to the progesterone receptor (Hansen et al., 1976). Activation energies calculated using the Arrhenius equation (Table II) were similar for the binding and release reaction, indicating that a small net change in enthalpy occurs as a result of androgen–receptor interaction.

The influence of temperature on binding allowed estimation of several thermodynamic constants. The apparent free energy, ΔG, at 0°C was approximately -12 kcal/mole for androgen receptors from testis, epididymis, and prostate, when calculated using the Gibbs–Helmholtz equation, $\Delta G_{0°C} = -RT \ln K_a$, where K_a is the equilibrium binding constant. The apparent enthalpy, ΔH can be computed using the van't Hoff equation, $\Delta H = -R \ln K_a/(1/T_1 - 1/T_2)$ where T is temperature in degrees Kelvin. In agreement with the activation energy data, the apparent enthalpy ΔH was approximately -2 kcal/mole for androgen receptors from testis and epididymis. The apparent entropy was estimated to be $+35$ cal mole^{-1}K^{-1} [$\Delta S = (-\Delta G - \Delta H)/T$]. The entropy change contributes strongly to the free energy (ΔG), suggesting that hydrophobic interactions are involved.

F. Influence of Androgen Metabolism on Receptor Binding

Studies on androgen–receptor binding in different organs following injection of [^{3}H]testosterone *in vivo* have led to the contention that the steroid specificity and, thus, the receptor proteins themselves, are different in various tissues. In prostate and epididymis, the receptor binds [^{3}H]dihydrotestosterone almost exclusively, while in other tissues, like kidney and testis, more [^{3}H]testosterone is bound. A cursory look at androgen metabolism in the various tissues suggests that it is the metabolism of [^{3}H]testosterone and [^{3}H]dihydrotestosterone that determines the relative amounts bound to the receptor. The microsomal enzyme Δ^4-3-ketosteroid-5α-oxidoreductase is high in most organs of the male reproductive tract (King and Mainwaring, 1974; McLean et al., 1976; Smith et al., 1975a; Tindall et al., 1975; Wilson, 1975). Soluble $3\alpha/\beta$-hydroxysteroid oxidoreductase activity, however, appears relatively low in epididymis and prostate supernatants at 0°C *in vitro*, even in the presence of NADPH. Low $3\alpha/\beta$-reductase activity would enable [^{3}H]dihydrotestosterone to accumulate while high activity would cause it to be converted rapidly to 5α-

TABLE II
Kinetics of Androgen Receptor–[³H]T Binding at Different Temperatures[a]

Tissue	Temperature (°C)	Inactivation rate (k_1) (hr^{-1})	Association			Dissociation		Equilibrium dissociation constant (K_d) (M)
			Rate k_a (M^{-1}hr^{-1})	Activation energy ΔH_a (kcal/mole)		Rate (k_d) (hr^{-1})	Activation energy (ΔH_d) (kcal/mole)	
Testis	0	0.03–0.11	1.6×10^8			0.046		2.9×10^{-10}
	15	0.10	7.0×10^8	14.4		0.126	13.2	1.8×10^{-10}
	23	2.8	2.0×10^9			0.277		1.4×10^{-10}
Epididymis	0	0.03–0.09	1.7×10^8			0.043		2.5×10^{-10}
	15	0.35	6.5×10^8	15.5		0.100	12.4	1.5×10^{-10}
	23	1.8	1.5×10^9			0.231		1.5×10^{-10}
Prostate	0	0.02–0.05	1.4×10^8			0.069		4.9×10^{-10}
	15	0.17	—	—		0.416	17.0	—
	23	0.46	—			0.578		—
Seminal vesicle	0	0.05	1.8×10^8			0.055		3.0×10^{-10}
	15	0.92	3.3×10^8	8.7		0.266	16.1	8.0×10^{-10}
	23	2.8	5.1×10^8			0.515		1.0×10^{-9}

[a] Constants were determined using 105,000 g supernatants (seminal vesicle) or partially purified receptor fractions (testis, epididymis, or prostate). Association and dissociation rate constants at 0°, 15°, and 23°C were calculated as described in Table I. The [³H]androgen–receptor complex from prostate and seminal vesicle was susceptible to inactivation at 15° and 23°C. Therefore, the k_d was estimated as the difference between the apparent k_d and the inactivation constant, k_1. Activation energy was estimated by plotting the corrected association (see Table I) or dissociation rate constant versus the reciprocal of temperature (in degrees Kelvin) and using the slope in the following Arrhenius equation: $\Delta H = -\text{slope } (1.987)(2.303)$.

androstanediol. Accumulation of [^{3}H]dihydrotestosterone in prostate and epididymis would make it more available for binding by the receptor. In testis, submaxillary gland, and kidney, where [^{3}H]dihydrotestosterone conversion to 5α-androstanediol is high, androgen receptors bind [^{3}H]testosterone to the same or greater extent as [^{3}H]dihydrotestosterone *in vivo*. Thus, a correlation exists between metabolism and the apparent binding specificity of androgen receptors *in vivo*. The binding kinetics and androgen specificity of receptors *in vitro* indicate that receptors in prostate, testis, epididymis, and seminal vesicle have similar capabilities to bind testosterone and dihydrotestosterone. It appears then that the receptor binding of [^{3}H]testosterone relative to [^{3}H]dihydrotestosterone *in vivo* is determined by the intracellular concentrations of the androgens, which are controlled largely by the activities of the 5α- and 3α-reductases.

G. Significance of Testosterone Versus Dihydrotestosterone Binding

It remains to be established whether a distinction exists in the nuclear response to receptor-bound testosterone or dihydrotestosterone. It is conceivable that receptor–androgen complexes could activate the same genes, or the two androgens could induce different conformational forms of receptor, causing interaction at different sites on chromatin or with polymerases. Another possibility is that the nuclear retention time of testosterone and dihydrotestosterone receptor complexes may differ in a way analogous to estriol and estradiol–receptor complexes in nuclei of rat uterus (Anderson *et al.*, 1975). The more rapid dissociation of testosterone–receptor complexes relative to those with dihydrotestosterone could result in faster turnover of receptor in the nucleus, thereby effecting differential gene activation.

V. CONCLUDING REMARKS

We have described the properties of three unique proteins which appear to function in the action of androgens on cells within the male rat reproductive tract. While two appear to have extracellular carrier or intracellular storage functions, i.e., ABP and the 9 S binding protein, respectively, the receptor probably acts in the nucleus to promote alterations in gene transcription. Table III summarizes the properties of the three androgen-binding proteins.

ABP in the rat is a protein unique to the testis and epididymis. Its discovery more than 4 years ago has led to further studies on its chemical properties and the control of its secretion by pituitary gonadotropins. Many

TABLE III
Properties of Three Androgen-Binding Proteins

	ABP	9 S Binding Protein	Androgen receptor
Androgen specificity	DHT > T	Progesterone > DHT > T	DHT ≤ T
Equilibrium binding constant (M^{-1})	1×10^9	10^5–10^6	5×10^{9} [a]
Dissociation rate ($t_{1/2}$) at 0°C	≃ 3 minutes T	~7 minutes[a] T and DHT	15 hours—T[a]
	≃ 6 minutes DHT		40 hours—DHT
Response to 100-fold excess unlabeled androgen	Saturated	Unsaturated	Saturated
Precipitation with $(NH_4)_2SO_4$ (% saturation)	50%	40–70%	40%
Sedimentation coefficient	4.6 S	9 S	3–8 S
+0.4 M KCl	4.6 S	9 S	3–5 S
Mobility on polyacrylamide gels (R_f)	0.75	0.1	0.45
Isoelectric pH	4.6	7.0	5.8
Molecular weight	~90,000	≤200,000	60,000–200,000
Stokes radius	47 Å	56 Å	53 Å
DEAE–Sephadex	Eluted at 0.2 M KCl	Unretarded	Eluted at 0.1–0.3 M KCl
Heat stability of binding (50°C for 30 min)	Stable	Destroyed	Destroyed
Sulfhydryl sensitivity of binding (1 mM PCMB)	Stable	Reduced	Destroyed

[a] Values were estimated using the charcoal assay.

of the studies carried out on ABP have been facilitated by the development of the steady-state polyacrylamide gel electrophoresis system worked out by Ritzén et al. (1974). The chemical properties of ABP are not unusual—it is an acidic protein of medium size, an MW of about 90,000, and like most proteins, is moderately sensitive to alterations in its environment, including pH and heat. Like other androgen-binding proteins, including the androgen receptor, ABP has a preference for dihydrotestosterone and testosterone over other steroids. Cyproterone acetate, a well-known inhibitor of androgen binding to receptors, does not interact with ABP. ABP's home is the Sertoli cell of the testis where it may serve to enhance the accumulation of androgens. Its synthesis is dependent on FSH and androgen, whose actions are independent yet synergistic. ABP is secreted into the tubular fluid and leaves the testis to perform its predestined function of carrying androgens to the epididymis. With the help of ABP, therefore, the testis shares its abundant androgen with its neighbor, the epididymis, whose need is great for the maturation of spermatozoa. Here it becomes concentrated in the lumen of the caput and can bind androgens diffusing into the epididymis via the circulating blood. Once performing these functions, its life cycle is complete. As it passes through the epididymis, ABP loses its binding activity and is probably put to rest by degradative enzymes.

The story of the 9 S binding protein is much less clear and far from complete. It can be distinguished from both ABP and the androgen receptor by its size, its low charge causing it not to stick to anion exchangers, and its high binding capacity. The steroid affinity appears greatest for progesterone, followed by dihydrotestoterone and testosterone. High concentrations are detected in testis, epididymis, and lung. Based on its apparent high capacity for binding progesterone and androgens and its apparent absence from serum and other tissues, this large 9 S binding protein may play a role in the intracellular retention of androgens.

The androgen receptor from all types of cells has been battered and bruised in laboratories for many years in an attempt to decipher its properties. Yet, uncertainties about its steroid specificity and size remained despite modern technology. We offer here data which leads us to believe that the androgen-binding kinetics of receptors from different tissues are quite similar. Testosterone is bound and released faster than dihydrotestosterone; however, equilibrium constants for the androgens are similar. Although $(NH_4)_2SO_4$ purification of androgen receptors caused differences in their sedimentation coefficients, it did not alter their binding properties. The extent of androgen metabolism *in vivo* may explain differences in the apparent *in vivo* receptor specificity for testosterone and dihydrotestosterone. Our results indicate that organs in which the receptor binds [^{3}H]testosterone, as well as [^{3}H]dihydrotestosterone after [^{3}H]testosterone injection *in vivo*, are those containing high $3\alpha/\beta$-hydroxysteroid oxidoreductase activity or low 5α-reductase activity.

ACKNOWLEDGMENT

This work was supported by USPHS Research Grant HD04466, USPHS Training Grants AM05330 and CA09156, World Health Organization Grant H9/181/83, and American Cancer Society Grant IN-15Q.

REFERENCES

Anderson, J. N., Peck, E. J., and Clark, J. H. (1975). *Endocrinology* **96**, 160–167.
Baker, H. W. G., Bailey, D. J., Feil, P. D., Jefferson, L. S., Santen, R. J., and Bardin, C. W. (1977). *Endocrinology* **100**, 709–721.
Bardin, C. W., Jänne, O., Bullock, L. P., and Jacob, S. T. (1975). *In* "Hormonal Regulation of Spermatogenesis" (F. S. French *et al.*, eds.), pp. 237–255. Plenum, New York.
Bartke, A., Harris, M. E., and Voglmayr, J. K. (1975). *In* "Hormonal Regulation of Spermatogenesis" (F. S. French *et al.*, eds.), pp. 197–212. Plenum Press, New York.
Baulieu, E. E., and Jung, I. (1970). *Biochem. Biophys. Res. Commun.* **38**, 599–606.
Baulieu, E. E., Jung, I., Blondeau, J. P., and Robel, P. (1971). *In* "Advances in Biosciences," (G. Raspé, ed.), Vol. 7, p. 179. Pergamon, Oxford.
Baxter, J. D., Santi, D. V., and Rousseau, G. G. (1975). *In* "Methods in Enzymology" (B. W. O'Malley and J. G. Hardman, eds.), Vol. 36, pp. 234–239. Academic Press, New York.
Blaquier, J. A. (1971). *Biochem. Biophys. Res. Commun.* **45**, 1076–1082.
Blaquier, J. A., and Calandra, R. S. (1973). *Endocrinology* **93**, 51–60.
Bruchovsky, N., and Wilson, J. D. (1968a). *J. Biol. Chem.* **243**, 2012–2021.
Bruchovsky, N., and Wilson, J. D. (1968b). *J. Biol. Chem.* **243**, 5953–5960.
Bruchovsky, N., Rennie, P. S., Lesser, B., and Sutherland, D. J. A. (1975). *J. Steroid Biochem.* **6**, 551–560.
Cooper, T. G., and Waites, G. M. H. (1975). *J. Endocrinol.* **65**, 195–205.
Corvol, P. L., Chrambach, A., Rodbard, D., and Bardin, C. W. (1971). *J. Biol. Chem.* **246**, 3435–3443.
Carbo, B. (1965). *Acta Vet. Scand., Suppl.* **6**, 5.
Davies, P., and Griffiths, K. (1975). *Mol. Cell. Endocrinol.* **3**, 143–164.
Fang, S., and Liao, S. (1969). *Mol. Pharmacol.* **5**, 428–431.
Fang, S., and Liao, S. (1971). *J. Biol. Chem.* **246**, 16–24.
Fang, S., Anderson, K. M., and Liao, S. (1969), *J. Biol. Chem.* **244**, 6584–6595.
French, F. S., and Ritzén, E. M. (1973a). *J. Reprod. Fertil.* **32**, 479–483.
French, F. S., and Ritzén, E. M. (1973b). *Endocrinology* **93**, 88–95.
Fritz, I. B., Kopec, B., Lam, K., and Vernon, R. G. (1974). *In* "Hormone Binding and Target Cell Activation in the Testis" (M. L. Dufau and A. R. Means, eds.), pp. 311–327. Plenum, New York.
Galena, H. J., Pillai, A. K. and Terner, C. (1974). *J. Endocrinol.* **63**, 223–237.
Guerrero, R., Ritzén, E. M., Purvis, K., Hansson, V., and French, F. S. (1975). *In* "Hormonal Regulation of Spermatogenesis" (F. S. French, *et al.*, eds.), pp. 213–221. Plenum, New York.

Gustafsson, J. A., and Pousette, A. (1975). *Biochemistry* **14**, 3094–3101.
Hansen, P. E., Johnson, A., Schrader, W. T., and O'Malley, B. W. (1976). *J. Steroid Biochem.* **7**, 723–732.
Hansson, V. (1972). *Steroids* **20**, 575–596.
Hansson, V., Djoseland, O., Reusch, E., Attramadal, A., and Torgersen, O. (1973a). *Steroids* **21**, 457–474.
Hansson, V., Djoseland, O., Reusch, E., Attramadal, A., and Torgersen, O. (1973b). *Steroids* **22**, 19–33.
Hansson, V., Reusch, E., Trygstad, O., Torgersen, O., Ritzén, E. M., and French, F. S. (1973c). *Nature (London), New Biol.* **246**, 56–59.
Hansson, V., Trygstad, O., French, F. S., McLean, W. S., Smith, A. A., Tindall, D. J., Weddington, S. C., Petrusz, P., Nayfeh, S. N., and Ritzén, E. M. (1974a). *Nature (London)* **250**, 387–391.
Hansson, V., McLean, W. S., Smith, A. A., Tindall, D. J., Weddington, S. C., Nayfeh, S. N., French, F. S., and Ritzén, E. M. (1974b). *Steroids* **23**, 823–832.
Hansson, V., Ritzén, E. M., French, F. S., and Nayfeh, S. N. (1975a). *Handb. Physiol., Sect. 7: Endocrinol.* **5**, 173–201.
Hansson, V., Ritzén, E. M., French, F. S., Weddington, S. C., and Nayfeh, S. N. (1975b). *Mol. Cell. Endocrinol.* **3**, 1–20.
Hansson, V., Weddington, S. C., Petrusz, P., Ritzén, E. M., Nayfeh, S. N., and French, F. S. (1975c). *Endocrinology* **97**, 469–473.
Hansson, V., Weddington, S. C., Naess, O., Attramadal, A., French, F. S., Kotite, N., Nayfeh, S. N., Ritzén, E. M., and Hagenas, L. (1975d). *In* "Hormonal Regulation of Spermatogenesis" (F. S. French, *et al.*, eds.), pp. 323–336. Plenum, New York.
Hansson, V., Calandra, R., Purvis, K., Ritzén, E. M., and French, F. S. (1976). *Vitam. Horm. (N.Y.)* **34**, 187–214.
Heyns, W., and DeMoor, P. (1971). *J. Clin. Endocrinol. Metab.* **32**, 147–154.
Jung, I., and Baulieu, E. E. (1972). *Nature (London), New Biol.* **237**, 24–26.
Karsznia, R., Wyss, R. H., Heinrichs, W. L. and Herrman, W. L. (1969). *Endocrinology* **84**, 1238–1246.
Katzenellenbogen, J. A., Johnson, H. J., and Carlson, K. E. (1973). *Biochemistry* **12**, 4092–4099.
King, R. J. B., and Mainwaring, W. I. P. (1974). "Steroid-Cell Interactions," pp. 41–101. Butterworth, London.
Korenman, S. G. (1968). *J. Clin. Endocrinol. Metab.* **28**, 127–130.
Kotite, N. J., Morris, M. A., Petrusz, P., Nayfeh, S. N., and French, F. S. (1976). *Program 58th Annu. Meet. Am. Endocr. Soc., San Francisco* p. 237.
Krieg, M., Szalay, R., and Voigt, K. D. (1974). *J. Steroid Biochem.* **5**, 453–459.
Lea, O. A., Wilson, E. M., Smith, A. A., and French, F. S. (1977). In preparation.
Liao, S., and Fang, S. (1969). *Vitam. Horm.* **27**, 17–91.
Liao, S., Liang, T., Fang, S., Castañeda, E., and Shao, T. C. (1973). *J. Biol. Chem.* **248**, 6154–6162.
McLean, W. S., Smith, A. A., Hansson, V., Naess, O., Nayfeh, S. N., and French, F. S. (1976). *Mol. Cell. Endocrinol.* **4**, 239–255.
Mahoudeau, J. A., and Corvol, P. (1973). *Endocrinology* **92**, 1113–1119.
Mainwaring, W. I. P. (1969). *J. Endocrinol.* **45**, 531–541.
Mainwaring, W. I. P., and Irving, R. (1973). *Biochem. J.* **134**, 113–127.
Mainwaring, W. I. P., and Mangan, F. R. (1973). *J. Endocrinol.* **59**, 121–139.
Mainwaring, W. I. P., Mangan, F. R., Wilce, P. A., and Milroy, E. G. P. (1973). *In* "Recep-

tors for Reproductive Hormones" (B. W. O'Malley and A. R. Means, eds.), pp. 197–231. Plenum, New York.
Means, A. R., and Tindall, D. J. (1975). *In* "Hormonal Regulation of Spermatogenesis" (F. S. French *et al.*, eds.), pp. 383–398. Plenum, New York.
Means, A. R., Fakunding, J. L., Huckins, C., Tindall, D. J., and Vitale, R. (1976). *Recent Prog. Horm. Res.* **32**, 477–527.
Měster, J., and Robertson, D. M. (1971). *Biochim. Biophys. Acta* **230**, 543–549.
Mowszowicz, I., Bieber, D. E., Chung, K. W., Bullock, L. P., and Bardin, C. W. (1974). *Endocrinology* **95**, 1589–1599.
Mulder, E., Peters, M. J., de Vries, J., and Van der Molen, H. J. (1975). *Mol. Cell. Endocrinol.* **2**, 171–182.
Norris, J. S., and Kohler, P. O. (1976). *Science* **192**, 898–900.
Notides, A. C., Hamilton, D. E., and Auer, H. E. (1975). *J. Biol. Chem.* **250**, 3945–3950.
Pearlman, W. H., and Crèpy, O. (1967). *J. Biol. Chem.* **242**, 182–189.
Rennie, P., and Bruchovsky, N. (1972). *J. Biol. Chem.* **247**, 1546–1554.
Rennie, P., and Bruchovsky, N. (1973). *J. Biol. Chem.* **248**, 3288–3297.
Ritzén, E. M., and French, F. S. (1974). *J. Steroid Biochem.* **5**, 151–154.
Ritzén, E. M., Nayfeh, S. N., French, F. S., and Dobbins, M. C. (1971). *Endocrinology* **89**, 143–151.
Ritzén, E. M., Dobbins, M. C., Tindall, D. J., French, F. S., and Nayfeh, S. N. (1973). *Steroids* **21**, 593–607.
Ritzén, E. M., French, F. S., Weddington, S. C., Nayfeh, S. N., and Hansson, V. (1974). *J. Biol. Chem.* **249**, 6597–6604.
Ritzén, E. M., Hagenäs, L., Hansson, V., and French, F. S. (1975). *In* "Hormonal Regulation of Spermatogenesis" (F. S. French *et al.*, eds.), pp. 353–366. Plenum, New York.
Ritzén, E. M., Hagenäs, L., Purvis, K., Guerrero, R., Johnsonbaugh, R. E., Dym, M., French, F. S., and Hansson, V. (1977). *In* "Maldescensus Testis" (J. R. Bierich, K. Rager, and M. B. Ranke, eds.) pp. 79–87. Urban and Schwarzenberg, Baltimore, Maryland.
Robel, P., Corpéchot, C., and Baulieu, E. E. (1973). *FEBS Lett.* **33**, 218–220.
Rodbard, D., and Chrambach, A. (1970). *Proc. Natl. Acad. Sci. U.S.A.* **65**, 970–977.
Rodbard, D., and Chrambach, A. (1971). *Anal. Biochem.* **40**, 95–134.
Sanborn, B. M., Elkington, J. S. H., and Steinberger, E. (1974). *In* "Hormone Binding and Target Cell Activation in the Testis" (M. L. Dufau and A. R. Means, eds.), pp. 291–310. Plenum, New York.
Sanborn, B. M., Elkington, J. S. H., Steinberger, A., and Steinberger, E. (1975). *In* "Hormonal Regulation of Spermatogenesis" (F. S. French *et al.*, eds.), pp. 293–309. Plenum, New York.
Sar, M., Stumpf, W. E., McLean, W. S., Smith, A. A., Hansson, V., Nayfeh, S. N., and French, F. S. (1975). *In* "Hormonal Regulation of Spermatogenesis" (F. S. French *et al.*, eds.), pp. 311–319. Plenum, New York.
Schrader, W. T., and O'Malley, B. W. (1972). *J. Biol. Chem.* **247**, 51–57.
Segaloff, A. (1963). *Steroids* **1**, 299–315.
Siegel, L. M., and Monty, K. J. (1966). *Biochim. Biophys. Acta* **112**, 346–362.
Smith, A. A., McLean, W. S., Hansson, V., Nayfeh, S. N., and French, F. S. (1975a). *Steroids* **25**, 569–586.
Smith, A. A., McLean, W. S., Nayfeh, S. N., French, F. S., Hansson, V., and Ritzén, E. M. (1975b). *In* "Hormonal Regulation of Spermatogenesis" (F. S. French *et al.*, eds.), pp. 257–280. Plenum, New York.
Steinberger, A., Elkington, J. S. H., Sanborn, B. M., Steinberger, E., Heindel, J. J., and

Lindsey, J. N. (1975). *In* "Hormonal Regulation of Spermatogenesis" (F. S. French *et al.*, eds.), pp. 399–411. Plenum, New York.
Stern, J. M., and Eisenfeld, A. J. (1969). *Science* **166**, 233–235.
Sullivan, J. N., and Strott, C. A. (1973). *J. Biol. Chem.* **248**, 3202–3208.
Tindall, D. J., and Means, A. R. (1976). *Endocrinology* **99**, 809–818.
Tindall, D. J., French, F. S., and Nayfeh, S. N. (1972). *Biochem. Biophys. Res. Commun.* **49**, 1391–1397.
Tindall, D. J., Hansson, V., Sar, M., Stumpf, W. E., French, F. S., and Nayfeh, S. N. (1974a). *Endocrinology* **95**, 1119–1128.
Tindall, D. J., French, F. S., and Nayfeh, S. N. (1974b). *J. Steroid Biochem.* **5**, (Abst. 162), 334.
Tindall, D. J., Hansson, V., McLean, W. S., Ritzén, E. M., Nayfeh, S. N., and French, F. S. (1975). *Mol. Cell. Endocrinol.* **3**, 83–101.
Tindall, D. J., Cunningham, G. R., and Means, A. R. (1976). *Program 58th Annu. Meet. Am. Endocr. Soc., San Francisco* p. 204.
Tuck, R. R., Setchell, B. P., Waites, G. M. H., and Young, J. A. (1970). *Pfluegers Arch.* **318**, 225–243.
Tveter, K. J., and Aakvaag, A. (1970). *Acta Endocrinol. (Copenhagen)* **65**, 723–730.
Tveter, K. J., Hansson, V., and Unhjem, O. (1975). *In* "Advances in Sex Steroid Research" (J. A. Thomas and R. L. Singhal, eds.), pp. 17–76. Univ. Park Press, Baltimore, Maryland.
Unhjem, O., Tveter, K. J., and Aakvaag, A. (1969). *Acta Endocrinol.* **62**, 153–164.
Vernon, R. G., Kopec, B., and Fritz, I. B. (1974). *Mol. Cell. Endocrinol.* **1**, 167–187.
Vreeberg, J. T. M. (1975). *J. Endocrinol.* **67**, 203–210.
Vreeberg, J. T. M., Bielska, M., and Ooms, M. (1976). *Endocrinology* **99**, 824–830.
Weddington, S. C., Hansson, V., Ritzén, E. M., Hagenas, L., French, F. S., and Nayfeh, S. N. (1975a). *Nature (London)* **254**, 145–146.
Weddington, S. C., Brandsaag, P., Hansson, V., French, F. S., Petrusz, P., and Ritzén, E. M. (1975b). *Nature (London)* **258**, 257–259.
Weddington, S. C., Hansson, V., Purvis, K., Varaas, T., Verjans, H. L., Eik-Nes, K. B., Ryan, W. H., French, F. S., and Ritzén, E. M. (1976). *Mol. Cell. Endocrinol.* **5**, 137–145.
Wilson, E. M., and French, F. S. (1976). *J. Biol. Chem.* **251**, 5620–5629.
Wilson, E. M., and Smith, A. A. (1975). *In* "Hormonal Regulation of Spermatogenesis" (F. S. French *et al.*, eds.), pp. 281–286. Plenum, New York.
Wilson, E. M., Lea, O. A., and French, F. S. (1977). *Proc. Natl. Acad. Sci. U.S.A.* **74** 1960–1964.
Wilson, J. D. (1975). *Handb. Physiol., Sect. 7: Endocrinol.* **5**, 491–508.

18

Vitamin D Receptors and Biologic Responses

ANTHONY W. NORMAN AND
WAYNE R. WECKSLER

I.	Introduction	533
	A. Background	533
	B. Chemical Structure of Vitamin D	535
	C. Vitamin D as a Steroid Hormone	537
II.	Receptors for Vitamin D	541
	A. General Comments	541
	B. Purification and Physical Properties of Vitamin D Plasma-Binding Protein	543
III.	Receptors for 25-(OH)D	545
	A. General Comments	545
	B. Purification and Physical Properties of 25-(OH)D Plasma-Binding Protein	548
IV.	Receptors for 1,25-(OH)$_2$D$_3$	553
	A. Interactions with Receptors under *in Vivo* Conditions	553
	B. Interactions with Receptors under *in Vitro* Conditions	558
V.	Summary	567
	References	568

I. INTRODUCTION

A. Background

The primary homeostatic regulator involved in the mediation of calcium absorption is the fat-soluble vitamin D or calciferol. Physicians and scientists have known since the 1600's of the correlation between incidence of rickets and lack of sunshine (Whistler, 1645; Hess, 1929). These intuitive observations ultimately led to the report of Melanby (1919) who provided the first experimental production of rickets. This was followed very shortly in 1922 by the report of Hess and Gutman (1922) and McCollum et al. (1922) who identified "vitamin D" as the antirachitic factor. Shortly thereafter, Goldblatt and Soames (1923) as well as Steenbock and Black (1924) demonstrated the critical role of ultraviolet light in producing vitamin D. Once the connection between antirachitic activity, ultraviolet light, and Δ^7 unsaturated sterols, such as 7-dehydrocholesterol or ergosterol was appreciated, then it was possible for Askew et al. (1932) and Windaus et al. (1932) to carry out a formal chemical characterization of vitamin D. The surprising observation was that chemically vitamin D was in reality a steroid; cholecalciferol, the natural form of vitamin D, is termed 9,10-secocholesta-5,7,10(19)-trien-3β-ol. Thus vitamin D is officially a secosteroid.*

Vitamin D, along with the peptide hormones, parathyroid hormone (PTH) and calcitonin (CT), are three of the most important regulators of calcium and phosphorus metabolism. Together these substances work to affect an efficient homeostasis of these important minerals. The major pathways of calcium and phosphorus metabolism are intake and absorption by the intestinal mucosal tissue, transport within the body by the blood to various sites, deposition and resorption from bone and other calcified structures, and excretion in the urine and feces. The concentration of calcium in the blood is maintained at a remarkably constant 2.5 mM, considering the fluxes that occur between these various bodily compartments.

It is also important to recognize that the constant plasma level of calcium is maintained in spite of wide fluctuations in the dietary availability of calcium. Thus, a challenging problem to the organism is to adapt its intestinal absorption mechanism to reflect both the needs dictated by his physiological system and the availability of calcium present in his diet. It has long been known that both animals and man have a capacity to alter their efficiency of intestinal calcium absorption (Nicolaysen, 1943; Malm, 1953; Adams and Norman, 1970).

The primary homeostatic regulator involved in mediation of calcium absorption is vitamin D (Norman, 1968; Omdahl and DeLuca, 1973; Norman and Henry, 1974a). The last decade has seen a steady increase in our understanding of the biochemical mechanism of action of vitamin D. While 10 years ago little was known considering either the absorption, tissue localization, or proposed mode of action of this nutritionally

---

* Secosteroids are those in which one of the rings has undergone fission by breakage of a carbon–carbon bond. In the instance of vitamin D, this is ring B and is indicated by the inclusion 9,10-seco in the official nomenclature.

important steroid, there has emerged in the intervening period of time a new model for the mechanism of action of vitamin D. The model is based on the concept that, in terms of its structure and mode of action, vitamin D is similar to the classical steroid hormones estradiol, testosterone, hydrocortisone, aldosterone, and ecdysone. It now seems virtually certain that there is, in reality, an endocrine system for processing the parent vitamin D into its hormonally active form 1,25-dihydroxyvitamin D. This substance then carries out its biologic functions in a manner similar to that for other steroid hormones. It is the purpose of this review article to present some of the recent data which support the existence of this new endocrine and steroid hormone system.

B. Chemical Structure of Vitamin D

Shown in Fig. 1 is a summary of the development of our understanding of the structure of vitamin D. Structure **1** in Fig. 1 depicts the initial formulation of the steroidal structure put forth by Askew and Windaus in the early 1930's. It is apparent that when a structure of vitamin D is depicted in this

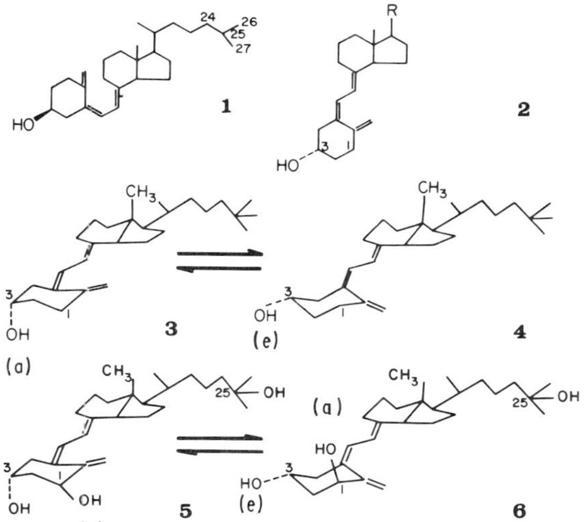

Fig. 1. Evolution of conformational representations of vitamin D. The structure for vitamin D_3 represented in **1** resulted from the original structure determination. The extended structure depicted in **2** was deduced from X-ray crystallographic analysis. Structures **3** and **4** illustrate the rapid equilibrium between the two A-ring chair conformations, while structures **5** and **6** show the same relationship for 1,25-$(OH)_2D_3$. The (*e*) and (*a*) refer, respectively, to the equatorial and axial orientations of the indicated hydroxyl group (i.e., either the 3β- or 1α-hydroxyl).

manner that there are many similarities to that of other classical steroid hormones; the only difference being the absence of the 9,10 carbon–carbon bond. This bond is broken or cleaved by the photochemical reaction which converts the provitamin, either 7-dehydrocholesterol or ergosterol, into vitamin D_3 or D_2, respectively.

It also should be apparent that structure **1** of Fig. 1 does not adequately describe the stereochemistry of this molecule. This was only accomplished by Crowfoot and Dunitz (1948) and Hodgkin *et al.* (1963). Their results established that the diene system extending from carbons 5–8 is coplanar and transoid, as opposed to the cisoid configuration given in the representation in structure **2** of Fig. 1. The primary characteristic feature of structure **2** is the emphasis on the "opened-up" B ring with a concomitant extension of the molecule in the A ring region. While such a representation tends to some extent to deemphasize the structural similarity between vitamin D and other steroids, this is only a superficial effect and would not necessarily dictate a change in the biologic mode of action for this substance.

The X-ray crystallographic data of Hodgkin also indicated that the A ring is in a single chair conformation. This feature, however, is rarely incorporated into the planar structure, either in that given in panel 1 or panel 2. More recently, Knobler *et al.* (1972) reported X-ray crystallographic determination of another vitamin D analogue that indicated the presence of an opposite chair conformation to that reported by Hodgkin's group. This difference resulted from the fact that the A ring could be frozen in either of two chair conformations which was dependent upon the nature of these analogues as they existed in their crystal lattice state. The existence of these two different A-ring conformations is a direct consequence of the open ring structure of vitamin D.

More recently dramatic new advances have been made in our understanding of the shape of vitamin D secosteroids. It is now apparent from the work carried out in our own laboratory (Wing *et al.*, 1974, 1975) as well as that of Lamar and Budd (1974) that, in solution, vitamin D secosteroids have a high degree of conformational mobility. The consequences of this mobility, as illustrated in structures **3** and **4** of Fig. 1 are that secosteroids exist in solution as a pair of dynamically equilibrating chair conformers. Through the use of high resolution PMR spectroscopy, it was possible to demonstrate the rapid interconversion of these two A-ring chair–chair conformers. It had long been known that cyclohexane itself existed in solution as a pair of rapidly equilibrating chair conformers. Thus, it is not completely unexpected that the conformationally mobile A ring of vitamin D should also be capable of exhibiting similar physical properties. It is now quite apparent that the molecular shape or conformation of vitamin D has certain unique properties not shared by other classical steroid hormones.

One of the important consequences of the rapid chair–chair conformational inversion equilibrium is that, for each conformational inversion, every equatorial position becomes axial and every axial position becomes equatorial. Further, it is known from other chemical studies (Eliel *et al.*, 1967) that the equilibrium constant between the two chair forms depends upon the nature and localization of the substituent groups on the conformationally mobile ring. For example, as shown in structures **5** and **6** (Fig. 1) the 1α-hydroxyl of 1,25-dihydroxy vitamin D_3 [1,25-$(OH)_2D_3$], depending upon the chair conformer, will be either equatorial or axial. In fact, experimental analysis of the conformational ratio of 1,25-$(OH)_2D_3$ indicates an equatorial-to-axial ratio (e/a ratio) of 55/45 (Wing *et al.*, 1974, 1975). That is to say in a population of 1,25-$(OH)_2D_3$ molecules in solution, 45% will have their 1α-hydroxyl oriented in the axial direction, while the other 55% of the molecules will have their 1α-hydroxyl oriented in the equatorial configuration. Distribution or partitioning is governed by a dynamic equilibrium between the two chair forms so that the A ring of any one molecule may flip from one chair conformation to the other some million times per second.

A challenging problem, then, is to identify the consequences of this unique chemical "fact of life" concerning the dynamic structure of vitamin D and its metabolites and derivatives in biologic systems and to relate it to any proposed mechanism of action. A particularly interesting aspect of this problem is the challenge offered to the synthetic organic chemist. As indicated above, the equilibrium ratio between the two A-ring conformers is determined by the nature and distribution of the chemical substituents on the A ring. It is possible to conceive of chemically synthesized analogues in which the equilibrium ratio of the two A ring conformers is drastically different from that of the hormonally active form of vitamin D, 1,25$(OH)_2D_3$. For a detailed discussion of these matters, the reader is referred to Norman *et al.* (1976) and Procsal *et al.* (1976).

C. Vitamin D as a Steroid Hormone

The most notable advance in our understanding of the mechanism of action of vitamin D has been the elucidation of a complex metabolic pathway of production of the biologically active form. These relationships are summarized in Fig. 2. It is now generally agreed (Norman, 1971; Lewin, 1973; Avioli and Haddad, 1973; Kodicek, 1974; DeLuca, 1976) that the biologically active form of vitamin D is the steroid 1,25-dihydroxyvitamin D_3 [1,25-$(OH)_2D_3$].

To date, four and possibly five naturally occurring, biologically active metabolites of vitamin D_3 have been identified. The first was 25-hydroxy-

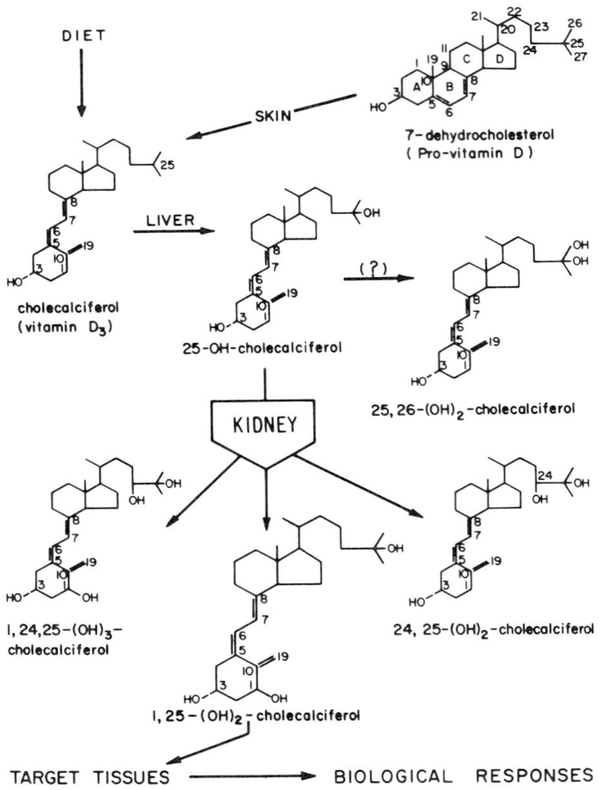

Fig. 2. Metabolic pathway for the production of the hormonally active form of vitamin D, 1,25-dihydroxycholecalciferol [1,25-$(OH)_2D_3$].

vitamin D_3 [25-$(OH)D_3$] (Blunt *et al.*, 1968). This steroid was found to be 1.4 times more active than vitamin D in stimulating intestinal calcium transport and bone calcium mobilization *in vivo*. Soon thereafter, Blunt and DeLuca (1969) achieved the chemical synthesis of 25-$(OH)D_3$ and proposed that this steroid was the biologically active form of vitamin D (DeLuca, 1969). However, Norman's laboratory had already reported the existence of a more polar metabolite (Haussler *et al.*, 1968) which was then subsequently shown to have much greater biologic activity than 25-$(OH)D_3$ (Myrtle and Norman, 1971; Haussler and Rasmussen, 1972). Ultimately, this more polar metabolite was isolated and chemically characterized by three laboratories (Norman *et al.*, 1971; Lawson *et al.*, 1971; Holick *et al.*, 1971).

Also two other dihydroxy metabolites of vitamin D have been chemically characterized; these are 24,25-dihydroxyvitamin D_3 [24,25-$(OH)_2D_3$] (Holick et al., 1972) and 25,26-dihydroxyvitamin D_3 [25,26-$(OH)_2D_3$] (Suda et al., 1970). A trihydroxy metabolite of vitamin D has also been detected under *in vitro* conditions; this is the steroid 1,24,25-trihydroxyvitamin D_3 [1,24,25-$(OH)_3D_3$] (Holick et al., 1973). However, on the basis of the results of Friedlander and Norman (1975), it is not yet certain whether this metabolite actually circulates *in vivo* in the animal.

As diagrammed in Fig. 2, vitamin D, which may be either ingested dietarily or produced in the skin by a photochemical reaction, is first transported to the liver where it is hydroxylated at the 25-position to yield 25-$(OH)D_3$. This steroid is then transported systemically to the kidney where it further undergoes metabolism to produce 1,25-$(OH)_2D_3$. Evidence will be presented in this article which supports the thesis that 1,25-$(OH)_2D_3$ is a steroid hormone produced by the endocrine organ, the kidney, and which in a variety of other target organs elicits the characteristic responses formally attributed to vitamin D. The kidney also has the capability of metabolizing 25-$(OH)D_3$ to 24,25-$(OH)_2D_3$. At the present time, no known function for this steroid has been yet identified with certainty. Some preliminary evidence has been presented by Henry et al. (1977) implicating this steroid along with 1,25-$(OH)_2D_3$ in modulating parathyroid gland function. At the present time, no information is available identifying the site of synthesis of 25,26-$(OH)_2D_3$ or as to whether 1,24,25-$(OH)_2D_3$ actually exists *in vivo*.

It is now generally accepted that the kidney, in addition to carrying on its normal renal functions, also functions as an endocrine organ for the metabolism of 25-$(OH)D_3$ into principally 1,25-$(OH)_2D_3$ and also 24,25-$(OH)_2D_3$ (see Fig. 2). A hormone is classically defined as being a systemic-acting substance produced by a specialized cell in response to a specific set of physiological stimuli or signals; very small amounts of the substance then are released into the circulation and transported to distal target organs where it interacts to elicit a set of specific physiological responses. It is the lack of these responses that usually generates indirectly the signal that results in the secretion of the hormone.

The classical method of demonstrating that an organ has an endocrine role in the economy of the organism is to create a deficit of its hormone by surgical removal or chemical inactivation of the organ in question. With reference to vitamin D and its renal product, 1,25-$(OH)_2D_3$, this criterion was first satisfied by the observations of Fraser and Kodicek (1970) who found that a nephrectomized rat could not produce 1,25-$(OH)_2D_3$. Furthermore, Wong et al. (1970) clearly demonstrated that a vitamin D-deficient nephrectomized rat was unable to generate a biologic response to moderate doses of either cholecalciferol or 25-(OH)D$_3$. In marked contrast, these same vitamin D-deficient, nephrectomized animals gave a completely normal spectrum of biologic responses when administered 1,25-(OH)$_2$D$_3$. These observations demonstrate that a deficit of the biologically active (hormonally active) form of vitamin D could be created by surgical removal of the kidney and that this deficit could be overcome by administration of the hormone, 1,25-(OH)$_2$D$_3$. Thus, these results collectively support the concept that the kidney is, indeed, an endocrine organ for the production of the biologically/hormonally active form of vitamin D, 1,25-(OH)$_2$D$_3$.

In other biochemical studies by Henry and Norman (1974), Henry et al. (1974), Tanaka and DeLuca (1973), Boyle et al. (1971), and Larkins et al. (1974), it has been clearly shown that the production of 1,25-(OH)$_2$D$_3$ by the kidney is subject to regulation. The present hypothesis is that the production of 1,25-(OH)$_2$D$_3$ is stimulated by hypocalcemic conditions and current data support the view that the parathyroid hormone functions as a tropic factor to stimulate the rate of biosynthesis of the 1-hydroxylase.

More recently, our laboratory (Henry and Norman, 1975a; Wecksler et al., 1977), as well as Haussler and associates (Brumbaugh et al., 1975), have presented evidence that 1,25-(OH)$_2$D$_3$ may localize in the parathyroid gland; presumably, this is some kind of "feedback" designed to perhaps regulate the synthesis or secretion of the tropic factor, parathyroid hormone. Shown in Fig. 3, then, is a summary of the proposed endocrine system for vitamin D action.

It is quite apparent that vitamin D undergoes a multiple series of

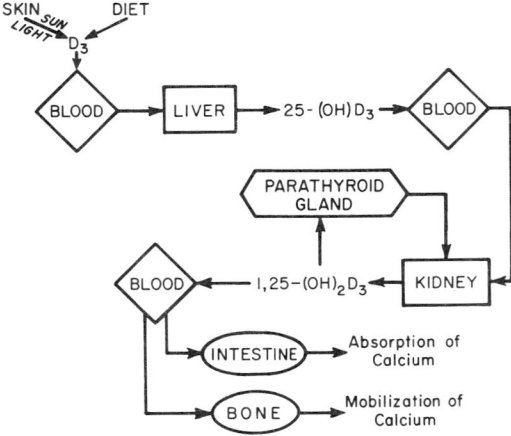

Fig. 3. Endocrine system of vitamin D action. For a detailed discussion of these relationships, see Norman and Henry (1974b).

transformations and multisite interactions in the organism from the time of ingestion of the vitamin or production photochemically, until it generates its biologic response in either the target intestine or bone. This multifaceted system offers many opportunities to carry out a study of how the detailed structure of the relevant vitamin D metabolite, including its pair of dynamically equilibrating conformers, is related to its particular interaction at any one site. Of necessity, this interaction implies a ligand–receptor interaction. Ultimately, a detailed molecular description of the mode of action of the steroid vitamin D will necessitate an understanding of how the structure and conformation of vitamin D is related to its specific receptor interactions and which, in turn, generate various specific biologic responses. In the remainder of this article, we wish to review efforts by a number of investigators to characterize, in broad terms, the structural requirements for interaction of vitamin D steroids and analogues at several selected receptor sites within the total chain of interactions related to the endocrine system of action (see Fig. 3) that are required to produce a vitamin D-related biologic response.

II. RECEPTORS FOR VITAMIN D

A. General Comments

In view of our current understanding of the complex metabolic pathway concerned with the conversion of vitamin D to its hormonally active form(s), it is not unreasonable to anticipate the existence of plasma-binding proteins for the parent vitamin, as well as its daughter metabolites. They would be essential to the orderly translocation of these hydrophobic steroids through the aqueous internal milieu. The general water insolubility of these secosteroids would also dictate the existence of specific binding proteins for the steroids in their various target tissues, e.g., liver [vitamin D and 25-$(OH)D_3$]; kidney [25-$(OH)D_3$, 1,25-$(OH)_2D_3$, and 24,25-$(OH)_2D_3$]; plasma [vitamin D, 25-$(OH)D_3$, 1,25-$(OH)_2D_3$, and 24,25-$(OH)_2D_3$]; intestine [1,25-$(OH)_2D_3$]; and bone [as yet unspecified metabolites].

Over the years, many workers have studied the binding of vitamin D to not only plasma-binding proteins but to proteins present in other tissues. Prior to the advent of the understanding of the metabolic pathway for vitamin D, these studies were carried out in the expectation that a receptor for vitamin D could be identified which would be involved in initiating the biological responses characteristic of the vitamin. As is apparent from evaluation of Table I, there is a widespread generalized distribution of vitamin D-binding or vitamin D receptors in a variety of different tissues.

Using vitamin D_2, Bukin and Areshkina (1958) first showed that vitamin

TABLE I
Compilation of Vitamin D Binding to Different Tissues[a]

Tissues	Species	References
Serum	Human	Bukin and Areshkina (1958); Morgan et al. (1958); Thomas et al. (1959); DeCrousaz et al. (1965); Peterson (1971); Smith and Goodman (1971); Nilsson et al. (1972); Daiger et al. (1975)
	Chick	Rikkers and DeLuca (1967); Edelstein et al. (1973, 1974); Belsey et al. (1974); Daiger (1975)
	Rat	Rikkers and DeLuca (1967); Chalk and Kodicek (1961); Oku et al. (1972); Daiger (1975)
	Dog	Chen and Lane (1965)
	Baboon	Rosenstreich et al. (1971)
	Rabbit	Daiger (1975)
	Mice	Daiger (1975)
	Cow	Daiger (1975)
	Monkey	Edelstein et al. (1973); Daiger (1975)
Lymph	Rat	Schachter et al. (1964)
Liver	Human	Rojanasathit and Haddad (1976)
Kidney	Human	Greenberg et al. (1974)
Urine	Human	Peterson (1971)
Cerebrospinal fluid	Human	Peterson (1971)
Intestine	Rat	Hosoya et al. (1970)

[a] The criteria for binding were any of the following techniques: charcoal—dextran assay, electrophoresis, or autoradiography.

D was associated with the protein fraction of plasma both after the administration of physiological quantities, as well as after pharmacologic doses (10,000–50,000 IU*) which induced a state of hypervitaminosis D. Subsequently, Morgan et al. (1958), Thomas et al. (1959), as well as DeCrousaz et al. (1965), separated the serum proteins from patients given large doses of vitamin D_2 by electrophoresis on starch and agar gels. The protein fractions on the gels were evaluated for antirachitic activity (a measure of biologic activity) via the rat line test (U. S. Pharmacopeia, 1947) and it was noted that the activity migrated with the α_2-globulins and albumins. In later studies the fate of vitamin D in terms of its plasma binding was followed by using either ^{14}C- or ^{3}H-labeled molecules. [^{14}C]vitamin D_2 was added to rat serum and the protein subsequently fractionated by starch-block electrophoresis; Chalk and Kodicek (1961) reported that the radioactivity was associated with the albumin and α_2-globulin fraction. In other studies,

* One international unit (IU) of vitamin D_3 is equivalent to 0.025 µg or 65 pmoles. The minimum daily requirement of vitamin D_3 for the rat or chick is equivalent to approximately 650 picomoles while for man is equivalent to 400 IU/day.

[³H]vitamin D_3 when given to dogs and the serum sample subsequently analyzed by an ultracentrifugal flotation technique, indicated that, whereas 80% of the radioactivity in the serum was sedimentable, the remaining 20% floated and was associated with the lipoprotein fractions (Chen and Lane, 1965).

The existence of specific vitamin D-binding proteins in other tissues has also been reported by a variety of investigators (see Table I). However, little information is currently available regarding the biochemical properties or functional significance of these putative tissue receptors for the present vitamin.

B. Purification and Physical Properties of Vitamin D Plasma-Binding Protein

Several rigorous biochemical studies have been carried out to isolate and purify serum-binding proteins for vitamin D. In reviewing this work, it should be appreciated that there is a difference in species responses to vitamin D_2 and vitamin D_3. Vitamin D_3 (the naturally occurring form) is produced from 7-dehydrocholesterol and is the most biologically active form of the vitamin in both mammals and birds. Vitamin D_2 (produced from the provitamin ergosterol) is fully active in mammals, but is only approximately one-tenth as active in birds, particularly the chick (Hibberd and Norman, 1969).*

Shown in Table II is a compilation of the physical properties of purified serum-binding proteins for vitamin D. Peterson and co-workers (Peterson, 1971; Nilsson et al., 1972) have thoroughly evaluated the properties of the purified vitamin D-binding protein obtained from human plasma, whereas Edelstein et al. (1972, 1973, 1974) have evaluated the biochemical properties of the plasma-binding protein for vitamin D obtained from the chick.

Peterson (1971) has carried out a rigorous purification of the vitamin D binding protein present in human plasma via the sequential steps of ammonium sulfate precipitation, followed by chromatography on columns of Sephadex G-200, DEAE-Sephadex, sulfoethyl–Sephadex, and finally Sephadex G-100. The protein was characterized by its high association constant $K_a = 2.8 \times 10^8$ M^{-1} for vitamin D_3 as determined under completely specified conditions. The reported molecular weight (MW) is approximately 53,000 daltons; the electrophoretic mobility is that of an α_1-globulin; and the sedimentation coefficient is 3.8 S. The studies of Peterson (1971) indicated that the concentration of the vitamin D-binding protein in normal human serum is of the order of 5 μg/ml or 9.4×10^{-8} M.

---

* Vitamin D_2 has the same chemical structure as D_3, except for the presence of a 22,23 double bond and an additional methyl group at C-24 of the side chain.

TABLE II

Compilation of Physical Properties of Serum-Binding Protein for Vitamin D

Properties	Human[a]	Chick[b]
Molecular weight	53,000	60,000
Sedimentation coefficient (S)	3.8	3.5
Electrophoretic mobility	α_1	β
Association constant (K_a)		
Vitamin D_3 (M^{-1})	2.8×10^8	—
Vitamin D_2 (M^{-1})	1.25×10^8	—
Hydrated density (g/cm^3)	1.21	—
Frictional ratio (f/f_o)	1.22	—
Stokes molecular radius (Å)	31	—
Subunits	No	—

[a] References: Peterson (1971) and Nilsson et al. (1972).
[b] Edelstein, et al. (1972, 1973).

Nilsson et al. (1972) carried out a detailed quantitative evaluation of the comparative association constants (K_a) for the binding of vitamin D_3 and D_2 to their preparation of highly purified vitamin D-binding protein by the technique of fluorescence spectroscopy. The K_a for vitamin D_3 and vitamin D_2 were reported to be 2.8 and 1.3×10^8 M^{-1}, respectively. This is the first evidence that vitamins D_2 and D_3 may be bound to the same vitamin D-binding protein. These same workers further noted that the binding of 2-p-toluidinylnaphthalene-6-sulfonate (TNS) to human vitamin D serum-binding protein is associated with a strong increase of fluorescence intensity. Concomitant with this finding was noted a shift in the wavelength of maximum emission. Interestingly, neither vitamin D_2 or D_3 was found to quench the TNS fluorescence. The observed binding was felt to satisfy a mechanism of noncompetitive interaction and suggested, accordingly, that TNS and vitamin D do not bind to identical sites. Nilsson et al. (1972) further suggested that the binding of vitamin D to a plasma carrier protein results in a conformational change in the environment of the receptor site, which is responsible for the enhancement of the fluorescence.

Chick serum contains two vitamin D_3-binding proteins, one of which binds chiefly vitamin D_3 and the other which binds both vitamin D_3 and 25-(OH)D_3 (Edelstein et al., 1972, 1973, 1974). These proteins have been partially purified by means of Cohn fractionation (Cohn et al., 1950) followed by ammonium sulfate precipitation, gel filtration on Sephadex G-200, ion exchange chromatography on DEAE–Sephadex, and an additional gel filtration step on Sephadex G-100. Some of the physical properties of this vitamin D_3-binding protein have been determined and its properties are listed in Table II. The MW was found to be approximately 60,000 daltons.

The protein possessed β-globulin mobility upon analytical polyacrylamide disc gel electrophoresis and a sedimentation coefficient of 3.5 S. The association constant for vitamin D was not determined.

Recently Daiger *et al.* (1975) have reported that the human plasma binding protein for vitamin D is identical with previously described human group-specific component (Gc) protein.* This conclusion was based on their identical electrophoretic mobilities, as well as immunologic cross-reactivity with monospecific antisera to human Gc.

III. RECEPTORS FOR 25-(OH)D

A. General Comments

With the unveiling of the metabolic pathway for conversion of vitamin D to its hormonally active forms, much effort and interest has focused on understanding the interaction of the first metabolite with not only plasma-binding proteins but various putative receptors claimed to be present in a wide variety of tissues. Under normal circumstances, 25-(OH)D circulates in the plasma of both man and all experimental animals studied to date at a concentration of approximately 15–30 ng/ml of plasma or $3.7–7.4 \times 10^{-8}$ M. Further, it should be appreciated that 25-(OH)D occupies a pivotal position in the overall endocrine system of action of vitamin D; clearly it is necessary to have receptors present in the liver for 25-(OH)D, where it is enzymatically produced from vitamin D, as well as in the kidney, where it is further metabolized to other active vitamin D-related steroids. An intriguing question, though, pertains to whether or not 25-(OH)D has any unique biologic activity of its own. That is to say, in various vitamin D-related target tissues, wherever they may be, are certain of the actions of vitamin D mediated exclusively through the association of 25(OH)D with these tissues? If, so, then, of necessity, there are specific tissue receptors for 25-(OH)D. A summary of work supporting the existence of widespread, specific, high-affinity receptors for 25-(OH)D is given in Table III. These results were mostly obtained by the technique of sucrose-gradient ultracentrifugation of 100,000 *g* supernatant fractions or Scatchard analysis. It can be noted, for example, in the rat that the K_a for 25-(OH)D in a wide variety of tissues varies from $1–4 \times 10^9$ M^{-1}.

To date, there is no definitive evidence which specifically resolves the question of whether 25-(OH)D has biologically significant interactions with

---

* Group-specific component (Gc) proteins are a group of immunologically identifiable serum proteins that exist in all human populations (Lay and Nussenzweig, 1968). They exist as two alleles, Gc[1] and Gc[2], and have not previously been assigned a physiological role.

TABLE III

Compilation of 25-OH-D Binding (K_a, M^{-1}) to Different Tissues[a]

Tissue	Chick	Rat[b]
Bone	$+$[c]	4.0×10^{9}[d]
Brain	—	$+$[e]
Cartilage	—	$+$[e]
Heart	—	$+$[e]
Intestinal mucosa	—	2.0×10^{9}[d]
Kidney	3.6×10^{8}[c]	1.1×10^{9}[d]
Liver	—	$+$[e]
Lung	—	$+$[e]
Skeletal muscle	—	1.7×10^{9}[d]
Skin	—	1.0×10^{9}[d]
Testis	—	$+$[e]
Serum	3.0×10^{8}[f]	1.8×10^{9}[d]
	1.9×10^{8}[d]	
Erythrocytes	—	No[d]

[a] The symbol + indicates that a saturable binding of 25-OHD$_3$ was reported.
[b] Haddad and Birge (1975).
[c] Greenberg et al. (1974); Osborn (1976).
[d] Edelstein et al. (1974); Hosoya and Oku (1971).
[e] Oku et al. (1972).
[f] Edelstein et al. (1973).

receptor systems. It should be appreciated that this is an unusually difficult point to firmly establish because all the metabolites of vitamin D are chemical analogues of one another. That is to say, 25-(OH)D can function as an analogue for 1,25-(OH)$_2$D$_3$ in receptors that are normally receptive to the latter metabolite (see later section) and, conversely, 1,25-(OH)$_2$D$_3$ could theoretically function as an analogue of 25-(OH)D in a receptor designed for this circulating metabolite. An inherent assumption present in such studies is that one can identify a receptor as being either a "25-(OH)D-receptor" or "1,25-(OH)$_2$D-receptor," on the basis of which ligand exhibits the highest K_a, i.e., has the tightest binding with its receptor.

Shown in Fig. 4 are representative data obtained in this laboratory indicating the presence of high-affinity receptors for 25-(OH)D in a variety of tissues from chicken and rat. Analysis of cytoplasm for 25(OH)D$_3$ receptors on 5–20% sucrose gradients shows the presence of 5–6 S binding components in mucosa (Figs. 4A,F), parathyroid glands (Figs. 4E), kidney (Figs. 4B,G), and liver (Figs. 4C,H). The presence of a 3.7–4.1 S serum-binding protein is shown in Figs. 4D, 4I. The sedimentation property (3.7–4.1 S) of the highly purified chick serum binding protein (Osborn, 1976) is shown in Fig. 4J. The serum-binding protein differs in sedimentation properties on sucrose gradients from tissue cytoplasmic receptors. This is clearly shown in the gradients of kidney (Fig. 4C) and liver (Fig. 4D), where serum contamination in these highly vascularized tissues results in the appearance of the 3.7–4.1 S-binding peak. These results are in good agreement with those of Haddad and Birge (1975) and Haussler and associates (Brumbaugh and Haussler, 1975).

Hay and Watson (1976a,b) carried out a remarkably thorough study of the phylogenetic distribution of plasma transport proteins for 25(OH)D in 22 species of fish, 12 species of amphibians, 5 species of reptiles, 19 species of birds, as well as 72 species from 14 separate orders of mammals. They found that fish with a cartilage skeleton and amphibia use lipoproteins for the transport of 25-(OH)D and that bony fish and reptiles choose to carry this steroid in the plasma bound to an α-globulin. Twelve species of birds,

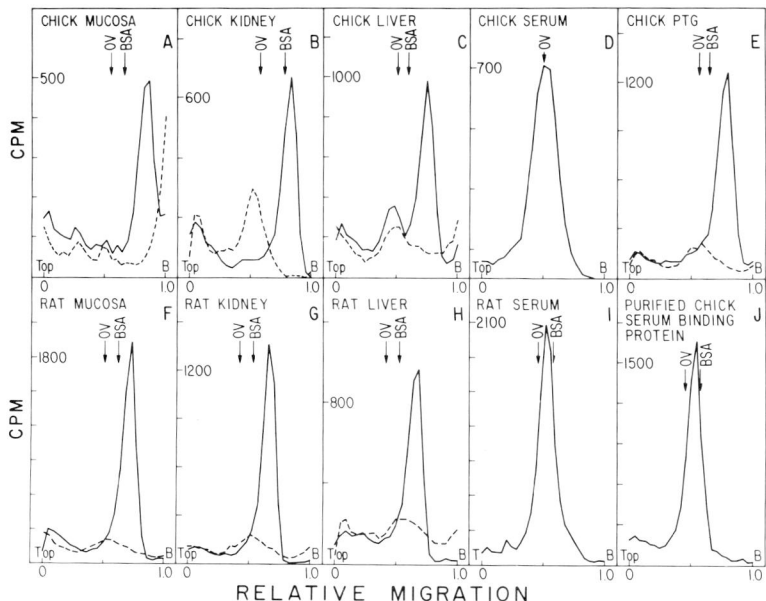

Fig. 4. Sucrose gradient analysis of binding proteins for 25-(OH)D_3. Cytosol from the indicated tissues or serum was incubated with 6.8 nM ^{3}H-25-(OH)D_3 in the presence (------) or absence (———) of 3.4 μM competing, nonradioactive 25-(OH)D_3 for 90–120 minutes at 0°C; 0.15 ml of incubation mix was layered on a 4.2 ml 5–20% sucrose gradient containing 10 mM Tris, 1mM EDTA, and 0.3 M KCl, pH 7.4 and the samples were centrifuged for 20 or 21 hours at 50,000 rpm in a Beckman Model L5-50 ultracentrifuge (SW 56 or SW 60 rotor); 5–6 S receptors are present in all tissue cytosols from chick and rat that were examined. Serum contains a 3.7–4.1 S binding component. The partially purified chick serum binding protein (J) also migrated as a 3.7–4.1 S compound. Sedimentation values were calculated using [^{14}C] ovalbumin (3.7 S) and [^{14}C] bovine serum albumin (4.4 S) as standards.

however, employed β-globulin transport proteins, while four species of birds were noted to use albumin and three species used an α-globulin. Of the 72 species of mammals studied, 65 employed an α-globulin transport protein, while a few chose to use albumin as their transport protein for 25-(OH)D. This remarkable series of studies is strongly complementary to the earlier evaluation by Henry and Norman (1975b) of the species distribution of the kidney 25-(OH)D-1-hydroxylase; they reported the presence of this key enzyme system in 17 separate classes of animals. Thus, from the combined results of these two studies, it is apparent that transport proteins for the intermediate form of vitamin D, 25-(OH)D, as well as enzymes to convert this steroid into the hormonally active form of 1,25-$(OH)_2D_3$, are widely distributed in the various classes and orders of higher animals. Clearly, vitamin D plays an integral role in normal calcium and phosphorus metabolism in a wide variety of differing species.

B. Purification of Physical Properties of 25-(OH)D Plasma-Binding Protein

Shown in Table IV is a compilation of the physical properties of plasma-binding proteins for 25(OH)D. Haddad and Chyu (1971) labeled human plasma-binding proteins, both under *in vivo* and *in vitro* conditions, with tritiated 25(OH)D_3 and observed that the bulk of the radioactivity was associated with a protein of α-globulin mobility as determined by disc gel electrophoresis. They suggested that the protein had an MW of 40,000–

TABLE IV

Compilation of Physical Properties of Plasma-Binding Proteins for 25(OH)D

Properties	Human	Rat	Chick[a]	Chick[b]
No. of binding proteins	1	1	1	2–3
Molecular weight (approx.)	50,000–60,000[c] 40,000–50,000[d]	?	54,000	60,000
Sedimentation coefficient (S)	3.1[d]	6.8[e], 4.1[f]	3.5	3.7–4.1[f]
Association constant (M^{-1})	?	1.8×10^9	3.0×10^8 0.9×10^{8b}	6×10^6 1×10^8
Electrophoretic mobility	α	α	β	β
Hydrated density (g/cm³)	1.21[c]	?	?	?
pH Optimum	8–9[d]	8.6[c]	?	>10.2

[a] Edelstein *et al.* (1972, 1973, 1974).
[b] Osborn (1976).
[c] Smith and Goodman (1971).
[d] Haddad and Chyu (1971).
[e] Oku *et al.* (1972).
[f] See Fig. 4.

50,000 daltons and a sedimentation coefficient of 3.1 S. These results are consistent with the report of Smith and Goodman (1971), as well as the more recent report of Kida and Goodman (1976), who reported a mobility for the human plasma-binding protein for 25-(OH)D, which was slightly greater than that of plasma albumin, as well as having an MW of 50,000–60,000 daltons.

Edelstein et al. (1973) reported that serum obtained from rat, pig, monkey, and human all contained a single binding protein that was responsible for the transport of vitamin D as well as 25-(OH)D. Thus, the characterization by Peterson (1971) of a plasma-binding protein for vitamin D described in the preceding section, must also give the physical properties of a 25-(OH)D binding protein (see Table II). In the rat, one protein is known to transport both metabolites, but few physical properties are yet known. The more recent purification studies of Osborn (1976) indicate that, in the chick, there may be several "iso-binders" present in the plasma for 25-(OH)D, all of which have relatively high association constants for this steroid. In these studies, the predominant plasma-binding protein for 25-(OH)D was purified some 470-fold starting from Cohn fraction IV via sequential chromatography steps of DEAE-Sephadex, SP-Sephadex (2x), Sephadex G-100, DEAE-Sephadex, and Sephadex G-75. It was estimated on the basis of isoelectric focusing that a further 10-fold purification would be necessary to isolate the binding protein to homogeneity. We have used this highly purified preparation of chick plasma-binding protein for 25-(OH)D to evaluate certain biochemical properties of this plasma "receptor."

Shown in Fig. 5 is a summary of the effects of pH and urea on the interaction of 25(OH)D with this protein. As shown in Fig. 5A, there is apparently no optimal pH for interaction of the ligand 25-(OH)D with its purified binding protein. As the pH range was extended from 4.5 to 10, there was a virtually linear increase in the amount of 25-(OH)D bound to the binding protein (under saturating conditions), irrespective of the buffer employed. As shown in Fig. 5B, when the urea concentration was increased from 0 to 8.5 M three distinctive levels of 25-(OH)D binding were noted. We have also examined our purified preparations to determine if they were glycoproteins. After isoelectric focusing of our most highly purified preparations, when the gels were stained with periodic acid fuchsin sulfite, a negative result for glycoproteins was obtained.

We have also utilized our preparation of purified chick plasma-binding protein for 25-(OH)D to carry out a detailed study of the interaction of various structural analogues of this ligand with the binding protein. Studies of this nature were particularly important to us in light of our previously described observation that vitamin D secosteroids exist in solution as a pair of rapidly equilibrating conformers. Shown in Fig. 6 is a summary of the

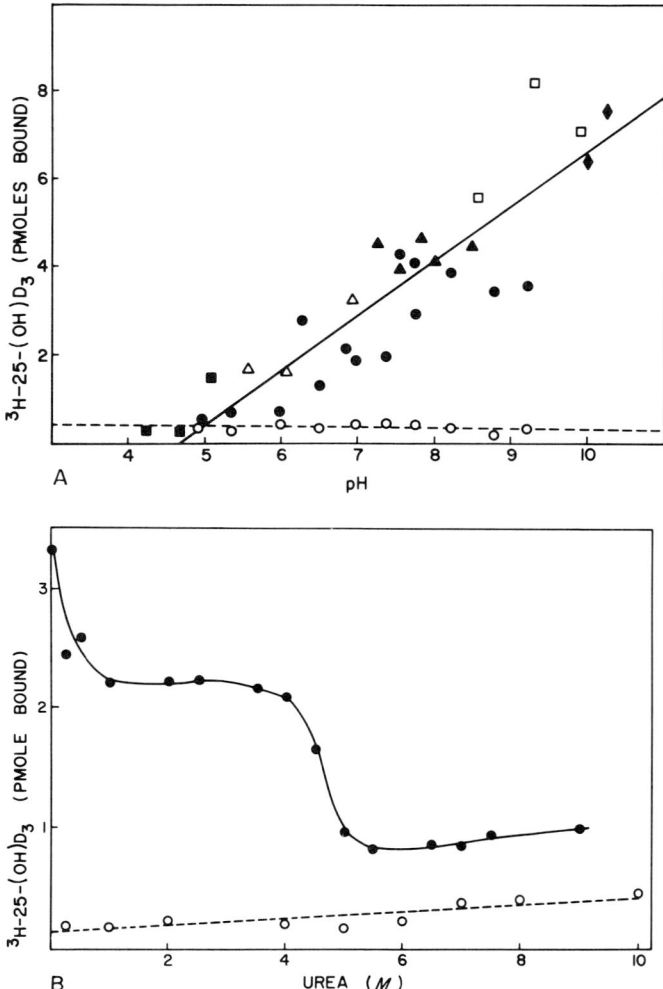

Fig. 5. Effects of pH (A) and urea (B) on the binding of 25-(OH)D_3 to its purified chick serum-binding protein. The general binding assay procedure was that of Osborn (1977). (A) The protein solutions were made with the corresponding 0.09 M buffers and pH. The different buffers are denoted: acetate; carbonate; glycine–sodium hydroxide; cacodylate; phosphate; Tris–HCl. The linear coefficient for the picomoles bound of 25-(OH)D_3 versus pH from 5–10 was 0.88. (B) The protein solutions for the general binding assay procedure (Osborn 1977) were made with a corresponding urea concentration prior to incubation with ^{3}H-25-(OH)D_3, at 25°C.

A. D₃ AND METABOLITES

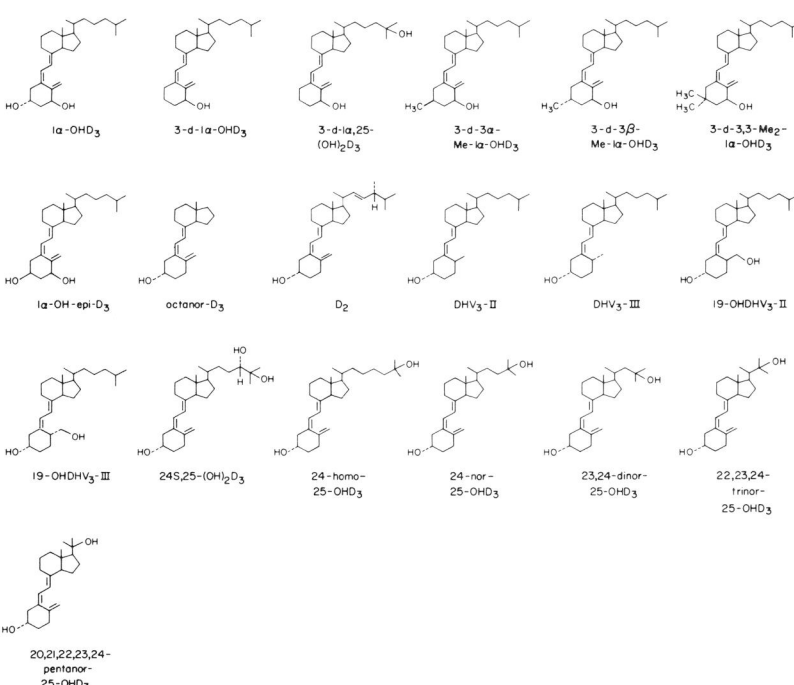

B. 5Z (5,6-cis) ANALOGUES

C. 5E (5,6-trans) ANALOGUES

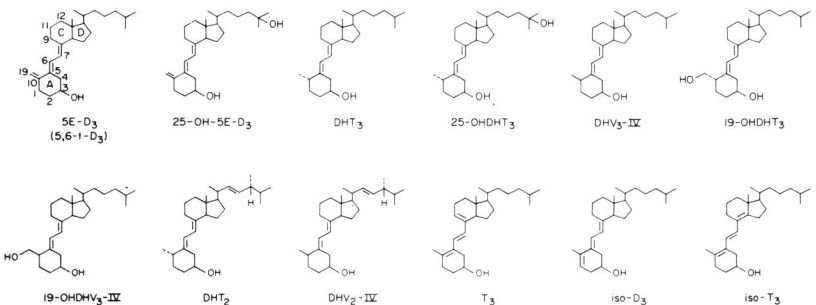

Fig. 6. Structure of vitamin D₃, its metabolites, and analogues.

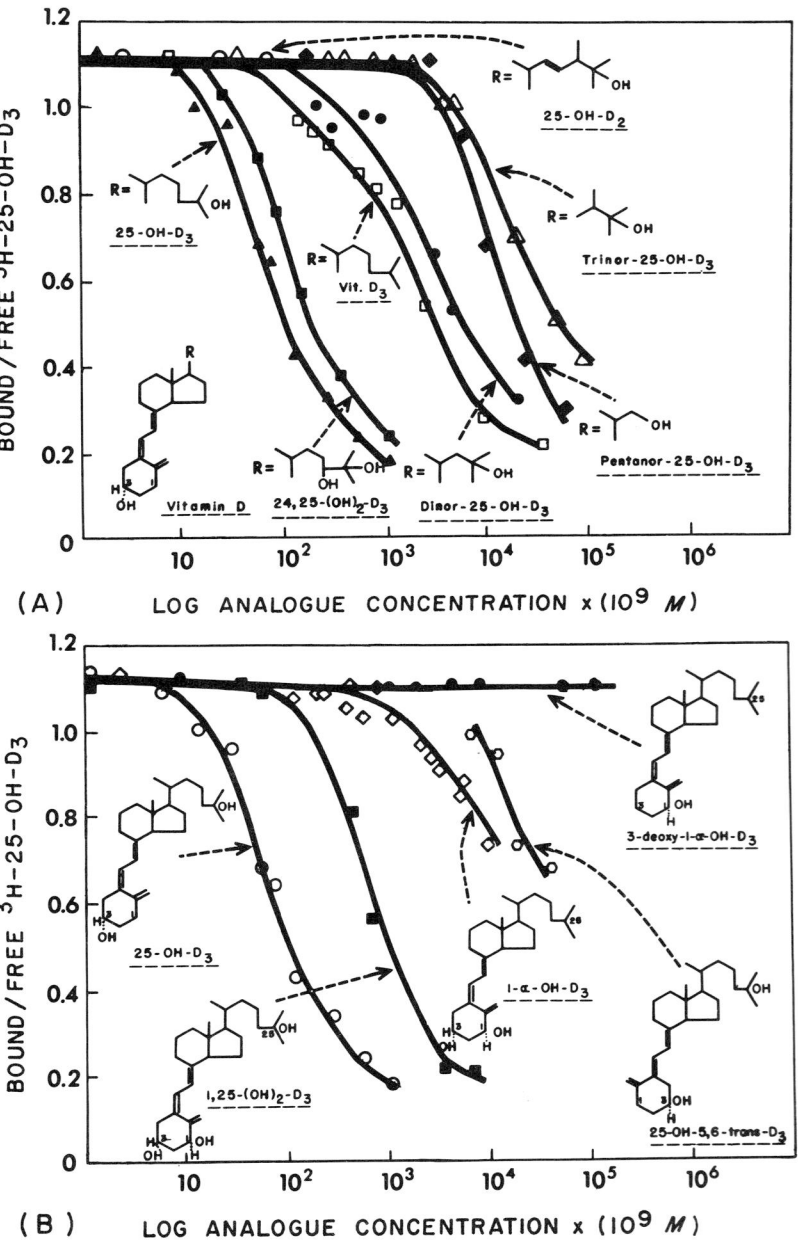

Fig. 7. Competition of vitamin D side-chain analogues (A) and vitamin D–A-ring analogues (B) with 25-(OH)D for its chick serum-binding protein. The general binding assay procedure was that of Osborn (1977). The structure of the various analogues employed are listed in Fig. 6.

structure of many of the various vitamin D metabolites and analogues to which we have access.

Our efforts have focused on two aspects of the 25-(OH)D molecule; the side chain and the A ring. Shown in Fig. 7A are results of experiments with analogues of 25-(OH)D which varied in their length of the side chain (Johnson et al., 1975). These series of analogues maintained the tertiary hydroxyl moiety characteristic of 25-(OH)D, but varied the length of the side chain, so that it was either one carbon longer or one to four carbons shorter than the native 25-(OH)D. Shown in Fig. 7B is a parallel series of studies where analogues of 25-(OH)D were employed which had alterations in the A ring. In both of these studies, a classical steroid competition assay was developed where increasing concentrations of analogue were incubated with a standardized amount of radioactive 25-(OH)D. After incubation at 0°C for 30 minutes, then the bound steroids were separated from the free steroids by the addition of charcoal–dextran. In terms of the structural features of the ligand 25-(OH)D, we noted that optimum interaction with its plasma receptor occurs in those analogues which have an open B ring and which have both a 3β-OH and a 25-hydroxyl group, with the 3β-OH being relatively more important. Inhibition of ligand binding occurred when the side chain was either lengthened or shortened, and when the A ring was present in the 5,6-trans configuration, as opposed to the 5,6-cis configuration, or when there was a 1αOH present. This later observation concerning the inhibitory contribution of a 1α-hydroxyl group is particularly intriguing in light of the fact that, to date, no investigator has isolated a specific plasma receptor or binding protein for $1,25$-$(OH)_2D_3$. In fact most investigators are of the opinion that both $1,25$-$(OH)_2D_3$ and 25-$(OH)D_3$, as well as possibly $24,25$-$(OH)_2D_3$, are all carried by the same plasma-binding protein.

IV. RECEPTORS FOR $1,25$-$(OH)_2D_3$

A. Interaction with Receptors under *in Vivo* Conditions

The primary focus of interest with regard to $1,25$-$(OH)_2D_3$ has been in evaluation of its interaction with the target intestinal mucosa. The primary biologic response of vitamin D is to stimulate the intestinal absorption of calcium. It has long been known that one of the puzzling aspects of this action of vitamin D has been the marked time lag which occurs after its administration before any stimulation of intestinal calcium absorption may be documented. The existence of this time lag was first commented on by Irving (1944). Since then the time lag has been documented by virtually every investigator concerned with the action of vitamin D in the intestine. When a physiological dose of vitamin D_3 (10–50 IU; 0.65–1.3 nmoles) is administered, there is a lag of 24–48 hours before the maximum stimulation of intestinal calcium absorption occurs. This lag can be shortened somewhat by administration of the intermediate metabolite 25-(OH)D_3 (20–24 hours duration) and shortened even further by the administration of 1,25-(OH)$_2D_3$ (see Fig. 8D). However, even when large doses of 1,25-(OH)$_2D_3$

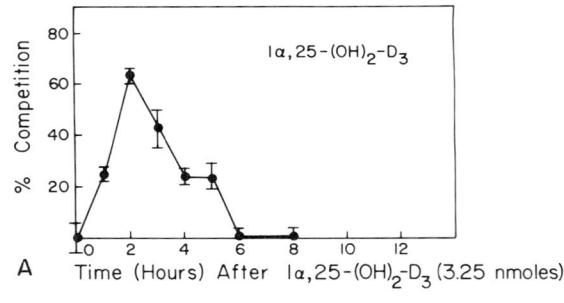

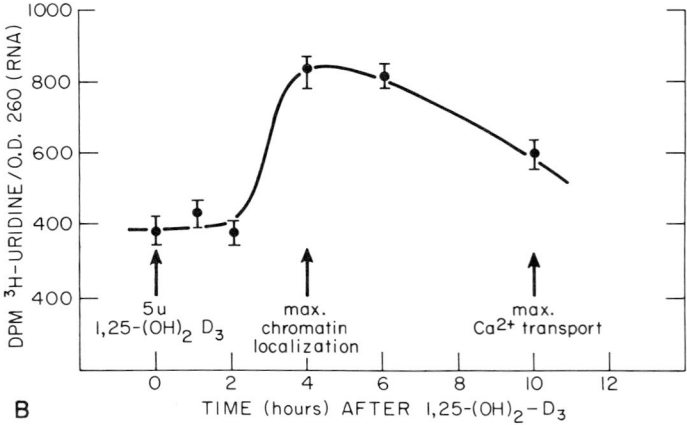

Fig. 8. Time course of several intestinal response after administration of 1,25-(OH)$_2D_3$ to a rachitic chick. (A) A time course of localization of 1,25-(OH)$_2D_3$ in the chick intestinal mucosa chromatin fraction. Nonradioactive 1,25-(OH)$_2D_3$, 3.25 nmoles, was administered orally; at varying time intervals the saturation of the intestinal chromatin receptor was assessed *in vitro* (Procsal *et al.* 1975). (B) Effect of 1,25(OH)$_2D_3$ on incorporation *in vivo* of [^{3}H]uridine into intestinal mucosal RNA. Groups of rachitic chicks were given doses of 325 pmoles of 1,25-(OH)$_2D_3$ intracardially. At varying time periods after administration of the steroid, 5 μCi of [^{3}H]uridine were administered intracardially, and 20 minutes later the birds were killed, the total RNA of the intestinal mucosa was isolated, and its radioactivity content was determined. (C) Appearance of calcium-binding protein (CaBP) after intracardial administration of 1,25-(OH)$_2D_3$ to vitamin D-deficient chicks. (D) Increase in intestinal Ca^{2+} transport measured *in vivo* (Myrtle and Norman, 1971).

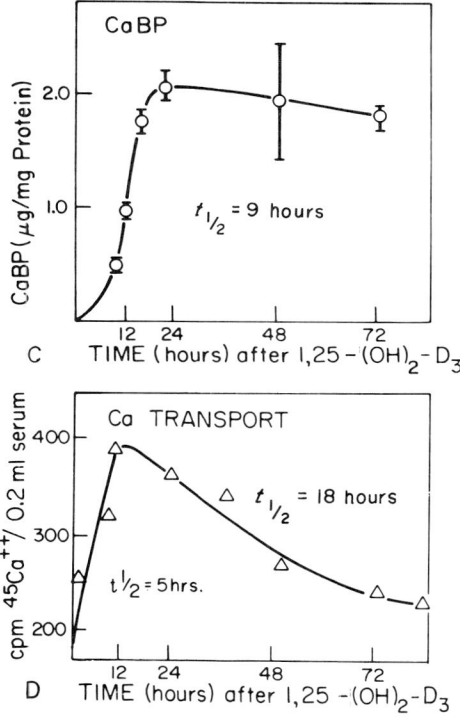

Fig. 8. (Continued)

are given, it is still an irreconcilable fact that there is a finite duration to the time lag before the initiation of intestinal calcium absorption begins. In principle, there are several possible explanations for this time lag. There could be a necessity for (a) a slow transport of the unaltered vitamin to the target organ; (b) a metabolism of the vitamin to a biologically active metabolite(s); or (c) mediation of its activity by an inductive mechanism, perhaps requiring new RNA and/or protein synthesis.

Figure 8 summarizes our current understanding of various steps of the action of $1,25\text{-}(OH)_2D_3$ in initiating intestinal calcium transport. The basic effect of the steroid is to promote the intestinal movement of calcium from the lumen to the blood; however, a lag period of 9–12 hours is required for a maximal biologic effect (See Fig. 8D). Wasserman and Taylor (1968) were the first to describe the production of a specific protein in response to the administration of vitamin D; this was identified as being a calcium-binding protein (CaBP). While the precise subcellular localization of this protein is not known with certainty, it is now known that it is produced specifically in response to the presence of 1,25-$(OH)_2D_3$, and that it binds specifically calcium, strontium, or barium in preference to other divalent or monovalent cations. We have shown, in collaboration with Wasserman and Taylor (Norman and Henry, 1974b), that the kinetics of the appearance of the CaBP after administration of 1,25$(OH)_2D_3$ are chronologically consistent with the hormone-mediated stimulation of intestinal calcium transport (see Fig. 8C). However, recently Spenser et al. (1976) have claimed that there is a 1–3-hour inconsistency between the onset of calcium absorption and the delayed initiation of biosynthesis of CaBP.

Also, a number of workers have found that vitamin D or 1,25-$(OH)_2D_3$ administration results in an increase in intestinal mucosal levels of alkaline phosphatase (Norman et al., 1970; Holdsworth, 1970). There is a time delay of 36–40 hours after administration of 1,25-$(OH)_2D_3$ before the increase in this enzyme activity is maximum.

One additional potential contribution to the time delay may be the process of turnover and renewal of the intestinal columnar epithelial cells. It is known that these cells undergo progressive maturation or differentiation as they proceed up to the intestinal villus. Originally, there was some concern (Spielvogel et al., 1972) that a portion of the lag in response to vitamin D might be due to some complex time-dependent requirement for differentiation of the columnar epithelial cells to a state where they would be "receptive" to the presence of vitamin D or its metabolites. It is now known that the $t_{1/2}$ for appearance or decay of all the known intestinal vitamin D-related responses is shorter than the 90–100 hours necessary for the complete turnover of the intestinal cells (Spielvogel et al., 1972).

Figure 8A shows a time course of localization of 1,25-$(OH)_2D_3$ in the intestinal mucosa, and more particularly its nuclear or chromatin fraction. The original approach pioneered in this laboratory towards developing a biochemical description of the action of vitamin D was to administer small physiological doses of radioactive vitamin D and to trace the appearance of the radioactive label in the target tissue and ascertain its subcellular localization. In the course of these studies (Haussler and Norman, 1967, 1969; Hausser et al., 1968; Myrtle et al., 1970), it became apparent not only that there was a specialized localization of radioactivity within the target intestinal nuclear and chromatin fraction, but also that this radioactivity was not chemically identical to the parent vitamin D. Further extensive studies eventually resulted in the unequivocal demonstration that this substance, which selectively localized in the target intestine and its nuclear fraction, was chemically distinct from both vitamin D and the intermediate 25-$(OH)D_3$ (Myrtle et al., 1970). With the concomitant demonstration that this polar metabolite was highly biologically active in terms of stimulating the intestinal transport of calcium (Haussler et al., 1968; Myrtle and Norman, 1971), the extensive effort necessary to chemically characterize this substance was undertaken. This resulted in simultaneous, yet independent reports from three laboratories that the chemical structure of this vitamin D metabolite was 1,25-$(OH)_2D_3$ (Norman et al., 1971; Lawson et al., 1971; Holick et al., 1971). As shown in Fig. 8A, when the physiological dose of 5 U or 325 pmoles of 1,25-$(OH)_2D_3$ are given, maximum localization occurs in the chromatin within 4 hours.

Also in results not described here, it has been shown by a variety of workers (Norman, 1965; Zull et al., 1966; Tsai et al., 1973) that actinomycin D, an inhibitor of DNA-directed RNA synthesis, was capable of blocking the biologic responses of intestinal calcium absorption which was produced by both vitamin D and 1,25-$(OH)_2D_3$. As reported in detail by Tsai et al. (1973), this inhibition was not due to a blockage by actinomycin D of the localization of 1,25-$(OH)_2D_3$ in the intestine. It could be unequivocally demonstrated that there were normal quantities of this steroid present in the intestine after dosing the animals with the antibiotic.

The logical extension of the results described in panels A, C, and D of Fig. 8 is that a significant contribution to the time lag and action of 1,25-$(OH)_2D_3$ may be due to the "activation" or utilization of information in the genome which is necessary for the expression of the biologic response. As shown in Fig. 8B, this was tested directly by measuring the effects of administration of small amounts of 1,25-$(OH)_2D_3$ on the subsequent synthesis of RNA. The administration incardially to vitamin D-deficient chicks of as little as 325 pmoles of 1,25-$(OH)_2D_3$ resulted in a 100-150% stimulation of the incorporation of [^{3}H]uridine into the RNA isolated from the whole intestinal mucosa (Fig. 8B). As can be noted by comparison with the time course in the other panels of Fig. 8, the kinetics of the stimulatory effect on RNA synthesis correlated well with the time-course for maximal localization of this steroid in the intestine (3-4 hours) and the maximal appearance of the intestinal CaBP which occurs 9-12 hours after administration of this steroid, as well as with the maximal stimulation of intestinal calcium absorption (which occurs at 9-12 hours). At the present time, it is not known what class of RNA is being synthesized in response to the presence of the steroid. In separate studies, Emtage et al. (1973) have isolated a messenger RNA present in the intestinal mucosa associated with polysomes, which is capable of synthesizing a protein which cross-reacts immunologically with the antibody for calcium binding protein.

Thus, it appears that there is almost complete confirmation of the genome-activation theory for the mechanism of action of 1,25-$(OH)_2D_3$, at least with regard to the synthesis of calcium-binding protein. What is not confirmed at this time is whether the complete action of vitamin D and its mediator, 1,25-$(OH)_2D_3$ in the intestinal mucosa is dependent upon gene activation.

Shown in Table V is a compilation of the relative amounts of steroids accumulated by their target organs. In the case of 1,25-$(OH)_2D_3$ and its target receptor organ, the intestinal mucosa, it can be calculated that there are approximately 2400 molecules of metabolite per intestinal mucosal cell, which is comparable to a metabolite concentration of approximately 9.0×10^{-9} M in the entire intestinal mucosa. Also it is apparent from Table V that the amount of the steroid hormone 1,25$(OH)_2D_3$ present in its target intestinal mucosa is quite comparable to that previously reported for other classic steroid hormones.

B. Interactions with Receptors under *In Vitro* Conditions

The specificity with which steroid hormones are able to initiate their characteristic physiological response apparently is dependent upon the presence of specific receptor proteins in their target tissue(s). Studies on the mechanism of action of such hormones as estradiol, progesterone, testosterone, aldosterone, and glucocorticoids have established that these steroids participate in a two-step mechanism prior to the initiation of nuclear events required for manifestation of their biologic activity. The steroids first must bind to a specific extranuclear receptor protein to form steroid hormone–receptor complexes; these then undergo an obligatory "activation" process,

TABLE V

Compilation of Amounts of Steroids Accumulated by Target Organs

Steroid hormone	Target organ	Estimated molecules per cell	Reference
1,25-$(OH)_2D_3$	Rachitic chick intestine chromatin	2,300	Procsal et al. (1975)
Aldosterone	Rat kidney chromatin	600	Swaneck et al. (1970)
Estrogens	Rat uterus (immature) nuclei	7,700	Higgins et al. (1973)
Progesterone	Chick oviduct nuclei	9,000	Buller et al. (1975)
	Chick oviduct chromatin	3,400	Buller and O'Malley (1976)
Glucocorticoids	Rat liver nuclei	10,000	Kalimi et al. (1973)
	HTC cell nuclei	15,500	Higgins et al. (1973)
Androgens	Rat ventral prostate	2,000	Fang and Liao (1971)
	Rat ventral prostate nuclei	6,000	Mainwaring and Peterken (1971)

prior to entry of the complexes into the nucleus, where they become selectively associated with the chromatin fraction. Following this sequence of events, it is proposed that an enhancement of genetic expression ensues, ultimately leading to an increase synthesis of key proteins responsible for the development of the characteristic physiological response.

Studies performed in this laboratory (Haussler et al., 1968; Haussler and Norman, 1969; Tsai et al., 1972; Tsai and Norman, 1973) and others (Lawson et al., 1969; Lawson and Wilson, 1974; Chen and DeLuca, 1973; Brumbaugh and Haussler, 1974a,b) have established a similar mode of action for the biologically active form of vitamin D, 1,25-$(OH)_2D_3$, in its target tissue, the intestine. In previous reports from our laboratory, a specific macromolecular receptor, judged to be a protein on the basis of its sensitivity to pronase, but not RNase or DNase, has been identified in the cytosol fraction of the chick intestine (Tsai and Norman, 1973). Evidence has also been presented for the mandatory binding of 1,25-$(OH)_2D_3$ to the cytoplasmic receptor protein prior to the association of the steroid with the intestinal chromatin fraction (Tsai and Norman, 1973; Brumbaugh and Haussler, 1974a). Finally, a 167-fold purified chromasomal receptor for 1,25-$(OH)_2D_3$ has been isolated from chick intestinal mucosa (Haussler and Norman, 1969). Thus, a strong causal relationship between the two-step association of 1,25-$(OH)_2D_3$ with a specific receptor system in the intestine and the development of the physiological response has been established to an extent comparable to that for other classical steroid hormones.

Shown in Fig. 9 are the results of an experiment demonstrating the temperature dependence of the saturable binding of 1,25-$(OH)_2D_3$ to its intestinal cytosol plus chromatin receptor under *in vitro* conditions. These data demonstrate that maximal binding of 1,25-$(OH)_2D_3$ at a level of about 21–24 pmoles per chick intestinal chromatin (15 mg of DNA) occurs at a concentration of 2.0×10^{-8} M 1,25-$(OH)_2D_3$ at 25°C. When rigorous efforts are made to maintain all incubation components at 0°C, only a much reduced amount of 1,25-$(OH)_2D_3$ localizes in the reisolated chromatin pellet. This result is consistent with a temperature-dependent "activation" process of the cytosol receptor, which is required for optimum transfer of the steroid to the chromatin. This value of 21–24 pmoles is approximately two times higher than that which occurs *in vivo* when radioactive vitamin D is administered. However, the renal metabolism of 25-$(OH)D_3$ to 1,25-$(OH)_2D_3$ is known to be stringently regulated (Henry et al., 1974). This may account for the lower value observed *in vivo* when vitamin D is administered. When radioactive 1,25-$(OH)_2D_3$ is given *in vivo* to rachitic chicks, within 2–4 hours, 20–24 pmoles of hormone per chick intestinal chromatin are maximally localized (see Fig. 8A and Table V), which compares favorably with the value reported here.

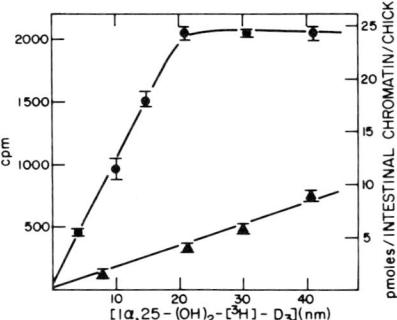

Fig. 9. Temperature dependence of the satural binding of $1\alpha,25\text{-}(OH)_2D_3$ to chick intestinal mucosal chromatin. Increasing amounts of steroid were incubated with a standardized amount of reconstituted cytosol–chromatin receptor system.

The time-course for the binding of $1,25\text{-}(OH)_2D_3$ to the intestinal chromatin under *in vitro* conditions is shown in Fig. 10; we have observed that saturation occurs 30 minutes after incubation of the components at 25°C and can remain at this level for at least 30 minutes longer. These results define a concentration of steroid (2.0×10^{-8} M), temperature (25°C), and time (45 minutes) required for maximal binding of $1,25\text{-}(OH)_2D_3$ to chick intestinal chromatin under the *in vitro* conditions described here.

Shown in Fig. 11 are the results of sucrose-gradient centrifugation of the intestinal cytosol receptor (Fig. 11A) and a KCl-extracted protein fraction obtained from intestinal chromatin (Fig. 11B). Both the cytosol receptor (presumably unactivated), as well as the receptor retrieved from the intestinal chromatin (which has been "activated") have identical sedimentation values of 3.5–3.7 S. On the basis of experiments of this type, it can be tentatively concluded that "activation" of the intestinal cytosol receptor for 1,25-

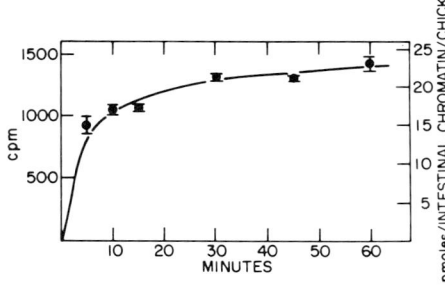

Fig. 10. Time-course for the saturation of chick intestinal mucosa chromatin-binding sites with $1\alpha,25(OH)_2D_3$.

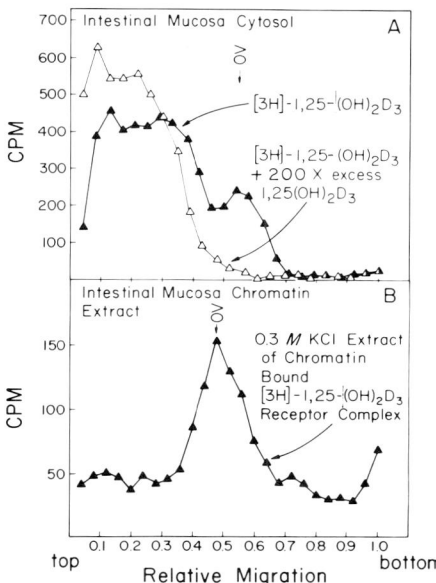

Fig. 11. Sucrose gradient analysis of intestinal cytosol and KCl-extracted intestinal mucosal chromatin after incubation with 1,25-$(OH)_2D_3$. (A) Intestinal cytosol was incubated with 11 nM ^{3}H-1,25-$(OH)_2D_3$ in the presence (△———△) or absence (▲———▲) of 200-fold excess nonradioactive 1,25$(OH)_2D_3$ and run on 4.2 ml 5–20% sucrose gradients at 50,000 rpm for 20 hours. (B) Reconstituted chromatin and cytosol from a 40% intestinal mucosa homogenate were incubated with 14 nM ^{3}H-1,25-$(OH)_2D_3$, the chromatin fraction was isolated, extracted with a 0.3 M KCl buffer, and run on 5–20% sucrose gradients as above. [^{14}C]ovalbumin was run on a parallel gradient. All gradients contained 0.3 M KCl.

$(OH)_2D_3$ does not involve major modification in either the size or shape of the receptor protein. This seems to be a somewhat simpler situation than that observed in other steroid hormone-receptor systems, where many different-sized receptors may be isolated dependent on salt concentration, temperature, or other factors. As discussed previously, an unresolved question concerns the significance and possible function of an intestinal cytosol receptor protein for 25-$(OH)D_3$ (see Fig. 4A–D). Since the 25-$(OH)D$ receptor protein has a quite significantly different S value, it is not identical with that under discussion for 1,25-$(OH)_2D_3$.

In the course of conducting the experiments described above, it became apparent that another possible target tissue for 1,25-$(OH)_2D_3$ was the parathyroid gland. Besides its effects on bone calcium mobilization and renal phosphate excretion, parathyroid hormone (PTH) is believed to be a tropic factor, which is capable of stimulating the production of 1,25-

$(OH)_2D_3$ by the kidney (Henry et al., 1974; Fraser and Kodicek, 1970). It is then possible to postulate that a "feedback loop" might exist between production of $1,25\text{-}(OH)_2D_3$ and the diminution of secretion of PTH. Henry and Norman (1975a) observed that, when tritiated $1,25\text{-}(OH)_2D_3$ of high specific activity was administered to rachitic chicks, a specific concentration of this steroid occurred within 2 hours in the parathyroid glands. The concentration gradient of $1,25\text{-}(OH)_2D_3$ between the plasma and the parathyroid gland tissue was comparable to that observed for the known target organ, the intestine. In follow-up studies, Henry et al. (1977) demonstrated a striking effect of $1,25\text{-}(OH)_2D_3$ alone and in conjunction with $24,25\text{-}(OH)_2D_3$ in reduction of parathyroid gland size in vitamin D-deficient chicks. This was felt to be a manifestation of the return of the hypertrophied gland of vitamin D-deficient chicks (40–50 mg) to a size

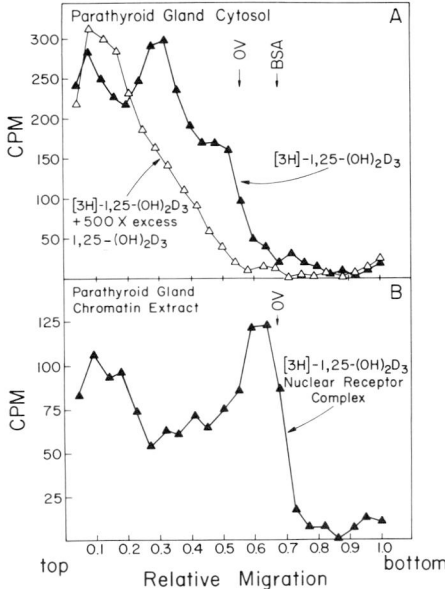

Fig. 12. Sucrose gradient analysis of cytosol and KCl-extracted chromatin fractions obtained from chick parathyroid glands after incubation with $1,25\text{-}(OH)_2D_3$. (A) Parathyroid gland cytosol was incubated with 5.5 nM ^{3}H-$1,25\text{-}(OH)_2D_3$ in the presence (△————△) or absence (▲————▲) of 500-fold excess nonradioactive $1,25\text{-}(OH)_2D_3$; 0.15-ml aliquots were layered on 5–20% sucrose gradients and run for 20 hours at 50,000 rpm. (B) Reconstituted chromatin and cytosol from a 20% parathyroid gland homogenate were incubated with 14 nM ^{3}H-$1,25\text{-}(OH)_2D_3$; chromatin was isolated and extracted with 0.3 M KCl, and 0.15 ml of this KCl extract was applied to a 5–20% sucrose gradient and centrifuged as above. [^{14}C]ovalbumin (3.7 S) was included as a sedimentation marker on a parallel gradient. All gradients contained 0.3 M KCl.

TABLE VI
Reconstituted Chromatin and Cytosol Studies

Cytosol source	Chromatin source	pmoles [^{3}H]-1,25(OH)$_2$D$_3$ specifically bound to chromatin
Mucosa	Mucosa	0.72
Mucosa	Parathyroids	0.033
Mucosa	Kidney	0.12
Mucosa	Liver	0.13
Parathyroids	Parathyroids	0.23
Parathyroids	Mucosa	0.11
Kidney	Kidney	0.020
Kidney	Mucosa	0.11
Liver	Liver	0.006
Liver	Mucosa	0.012
BSA[a]	Mucosa	0.018
50 mM Tris (pH 7.5)	Mucosa	0.028

[a] 20 mg/ml bovine serum albumin in 50 mM Tris (pH 7.5).

more comparable to that of a vitamin D-replete chick's parathyroid gland (15–20 mg), which could be consistent with the reduction of secretion of parathyroid hormone that might occur upon conversion from a D-deficient state to a D-replete state. Unfortunately, there are no radioimmunoassay techniques available for measuring avian PTH.

In parallel studies, Wecksler et al. (1977) carried out a detailed study of the subcellular localization of tritiated 1,25-(OH)$_2$D$_3$ in parathyroid glands obtained from vitamin D-deficient chicks. We have shown that parathyroid glands appear to specifically localize 1,25-(OH)$_2$D$_3$ under both *in vivo* and *in vitro* conditions in the chromatin fraction. As shown in Fig. 12, both the parathyroid cytosol and nuclear receptors for 1,25-(OH)$_2$D$_3$ have identical S values of 3.1–3.5 S. Once again, it is evident that no major change in sedimentation properties occurs as a consequence of a possible activation process during the translocation of the steroid from the cytosol to the chromatin fraction.

It is further interesting to note that the sedimentation rate for the parathyroid tissue (3.1–3.5 S) is somewhat different than that reported in Fig. 12 for the intestinal cytosol receptor (3.5–3.7 S). This suggests that these 1,25-(OH)$_2$D$_3$ receptor proteins are not identical. One way of pursuing this possibility was to carry out "crossover experiments" in which the relative ability of the parathyroid gland cytosol and the intestinal cytosol were compared with regard to their ability to translocate 1,25-(OH)$_2$D$_3$ to chromatin fractions. Shown in Table VI are the results of such experiments. It is

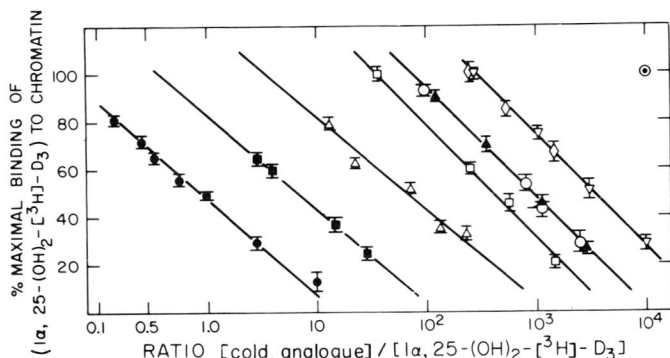

Fig. 13. Competition of structural analogues of 1,25-(OH)$_2$D$_3$ for its chick intestinal receptor system. Analogues denoted as follows: ●———●, 1α,25-(OH)$_2$D$_3$; ■———■, 3-D-1α,25-(OH)$_2$D$_3$; △———△, 25-OH-DHT$_3$; □———□, 25-OH-5,6-trans-D$_3$; ○———○, 25-OH-D$_3$; ▲———▲, 1α-OH-D$_3$; ▼———▼, 24,25-(OH)$_2$D$_3$; ◊———◊, 3-D-1α)OH)D$_3$; ◉, D$_3$.

apparent that intestinal mucosal chromatin has a greater capacity to bind 1,25-(OH)$_2$D$_3$ than all other tissues evaluated; however, parathyroid gland chromatin is clearly a superior concentrator of 1,25-(OH)$_2$D$_3$ than the liver or kidney tissues.

On the basis of the preceding studies employing chick intestinal mucosa chromatin and cytosol, it has been possible to devise a competitive binding assay for 1,25-(OH)$_2$D$_3$. As shown in Fig. 13, a linear standard curve is obtained when increasing amounts of nonradioactive 1,25-(OH)$_2$D$_3$ are added to the radioactive 1,25-(OH)$_2$D$_3$ that is employed in the assay. The decreased radioactive steroid bound is due to a dilution of the pool of 1,25-(OH)$_2$D$_3$ such that, at a ratio of nonradioactive steroid and radioactive steroid equal to 1.0, 50% of the maximal radioactivity bound is measured. One important use of this assay has been to assess the structural requirements of the ligand steroid, 1,25-(OH)$_2$D$_3$ for its cytosol chromatin receptor.* Tabulated in Table VII are the relative concentrations of steroids required to produce half-maximal competition under these assay conditions.

Several interesting relationships may be deduced by evaluation of the data in Fig. 13 and Table VII. A basic requirement is that any analogue must be a 9,10-secosteroid. This conclusion is supported by the observation that 1,25-(OH)$_2$-cholesterol did not compete, even at a concentration 10,000 times greater than that of 1,25-(OH)$_2$D$_3$. The dramatically decreased ability

---

* These studies were only possible as a result of the determined efforts of Professor William H. Okamura and associates, Department of Chemistry, University of California, Riverside (Okamura *et al.*, 1974a,b; Mitra *et al.*, 1974; Johnson *et al.*, 1975, 1977).

of either 25-(OH)D or 1α-OH-D to compete with 1,25-$(OH)_2D_3$ emphasizes the great importance that must be attributed to the presence of both the 25- and 1α-hydroxyl groups in order for a compound to obtain biologic activity. The 100 times greater ability of 3-deoxy-1,25-$(OH)_2D_3$ to compete than either 1-$(OH)D_3$ or 25-$(OH)D_3$ argues strongly that the requirement for the 3β-OH group is relatively less stringent than for either the 25-(OH)D or 1α-OH functional groups. The relatively greater importance of the 1α-hydroxyl over that of the 3β-OH is further emphasized by the observation that vitamin D_3, which lacks both a 25-OH and 1α-hydroxyl but possesses a 3β-

TABLE VII

Relative Effectiveness of Structural Analogues of Vitamin D in the 1α,25-$(OH)_2D_3$ Chick Intestinal Receptor Assay

Compound	Relative concentration of steroid required for 50% competition[a]
1α,25-$(OH)_2D_3$	1
5,6-cis (Z) series	
3-deoxy-1α,25-$(OH)_2D_3$	8
1α-OH-D_3	900
25-$(OH)D_3$	900
3-deoxy-1α-OH-D_3	5,000
24R,25-$(OH)_2D_3$	5,000
24S,25-$(OH)_2D_3$	5,000
D_3	>10,000
19-OH-DHV_3-II	>10,000
10-OH-DHV_3-III	>10,000
5,6-trans (E) series	
25-OH-DHT_3	90
25-OH-5,6-trans-D_3 (25-OH-5E-D_3)	600
5,6-trans-D_3 (5E-D_3)	>10,000
DHT_3	>10,000
DHV_3-IV	>10,000
19-OH-DHT_3	>10,000
19-OH-DHV_3-IV	>10,000
Other	
1α,25-dihydroxycholesterol	>10,000

[a] The data shown are the concentrations of analog required to reduce the binding of ^{3}H-1α,25-$(OH)_2D_3$ to its intestinal cytosol–chromatin receptor system by 50%. The assay was conducted as described by Procsal et al. (1975).

hydroxyl, is an ineffective competitor, whereas 3-deoxy-1-OH-D_3, which lacks 25 and 3β-hydroxyls but does have a 1α-hydroxyl, will compete.

The consequence of a 180° rotation of the A ring about the 5,6 double bond to produce analogues of the 5,6-trans series has also been evaluated. A primary consequence of the cis-trans isomerization is the change in the orientation of the C-19 methylene group. Although isomerization also moves the 3β-hydroxyl to a position sterically equivalent to the 1α-hydroxyl of steroids of the 5,6-*cis* series, this is apparently not sufficient to permit either 25-OH-5,6-*trans*-D_3 or 5,6-*trans*-D_3 to compete as effectively as their 5,6-*cis* counterparts, 3-D-1α, 25(OH)$_2$$D_3$, and 3-D-1$\alpha$-OH-$D_3$, respectively. Presumably, this difference is the consequence of the change in orientation of the C-19 methylene group. Our laboratory has recently succeeded (Norman *et al.*, 1975a), in introducing a hydroxyl into the 19-position of the 5,6-*cis* analogues to give 19-OH-DHV$_3$-II and 19-OH-DHV$_3$-III (see Fig. 6 for structures). It was reasoned that the presence of a hydroxyl group at the 19-position might, to some limited degree, satisfy the requirements for a pseudo-1α-OH group in the 5,6-trans series, or the 1-OH in the 5,6-cis series. However, no significant competition was observed for any of these compounds in our competitive binding assay. It may be that these compounds will first have to be hydroxylated in the 25-position before their relative ability to bind to the receptor can be evaluated.

The insertion of a hydroxyl group into the 24-position of 25-(OH)D_3 to give either the *R* or *S* epimer of 24,25-(OH)$_2$$D_3$ significantly reduced the ability of a compound to compete with 1,25-(OH)$_2$$D_3$. Under these assay conditions, it was not possible to discern any significant difference between the two epimers. The naturally occurring epimer of 24,25-(OH)$_2$$D_3$ has been shown to have its 24-hydroxyl in the *R* configuration (Tanaka *et al.*, 1975).

In general, there is a remarkable correlation between the relative binding of analogues in the chick intestinal receptor system, and their relative ability to stimulate intestinal calcium absorption. The following conclusions may, therefore, be drawn with respect to the structural features required for vitamin D-like biologic activity in the intestinal cell:

(a) All biologically active compounds must have a 1α-hydroxyl or its geometric equivalent and a 25-hydroxyl group.

(b) The presence of a hydroxyl group at a geometrically equivalent position to the 3β-hydroxyl of 1α,25-(OH)$_2$$D_3$ is not an absolute requirement.

(c) 5,6-cis geometry of the A ring is preferred to 5,6-trans geometry. A comparison of the biologic and binding activities of 25(OH)DHT$_3$ with those of 25(OH)-5,6-*trans*-D_3 suggest that in compounds of the 5,6-trans series a C-19 methyl is preferred over a C-19 methylene group.

(d) Altering the length or modifying the side chain, including the insertion of a hydroxyl group as in 24,25-$(OH)_2D_3$ or 25,26-$(OH)_2D_3$ significantly decreases the activity of the compound.

A further refinement of the requirement for biological activity has recently been proposed by Okamura et al., (1974b). Our model takes into account the chairlike nature of the A ring (illustrated in Fig. 1) and proposes that the chain conformer in which the 1α-OH is equatorial is the preferred biologically active form. The evidence to support this model is largely derived by a comparison of the significant biologic activity of DHT_3 (e/a ratio of 91/2) with the inactivity of its structural congener, DHV_3-IV (e/a ratio of 50/50) (Knobler et al., 1972; Okamura et al., 1974a; Wing et al., 1974, 1975).

The structure–function studies described here have made it possible to design and construct a number of analogues for clinical use. Compounds, such as 1,25-$(OH)_2D_3$ and 1α-OH-D_3, are already being used clinically to treat patients who suffer from several vitamin D-related diseases, principally renal osteodystrophy (Brickman et al., 1974, 1975). As our understanding of the structural basis for biologic activity increases, it may be possible to synthesize analogues with predetermined activities or that can act as antivitamins (Johnson et al., 1975). The availability of such compounds will undoubtedly serve as a further stimulus for this rapidly expanding area of research.

V. SUMMARY

The metabolism of vitamin D to its hormonally active form, 1,25-$(OH)_2D_3$, and its subsequent mode of action requires the presence of specific proteins for the vascular transport and intracellular handling of these steroids. Serum-binding globulins are involved in the circulation in the blood stream of all the metabolites. There exist 25-$(OH)D_3$ binding proteins or receptors in a variety of tissues, but their function is not known with certainty. The target tissues for 1,25-$(OH)_2D_3$ that have been extensively studied (intestinal mucosa and parathyroid gland) contain both cytoplasmic and chromatin-extractible receptors for this steroid. This receptor system is involved in the chromatin localization of the steroid where it is believed to exert its effects on transcriptional events. Figure 14 is a summary of the two-stage mode of action of 1,25-$(OH)_2D_3$. Also included in this figure are other steroid hormones and their target tissues in which this type of receptor system appears to be a common feature. The general mode of action of all steroid hormones seems to be a highly conserved mechanism, the details

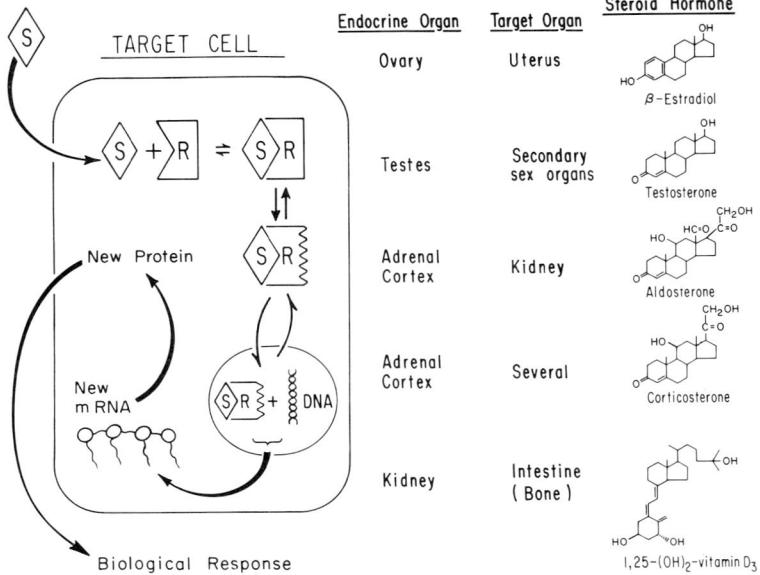

Fig. 14. Summary of two-step steroid hormone mechanism of action of 1,25-$(OH)_2D_3$ and other steroid hormones.

of which appear to be only slightly modified in the different steroid hormone systems.

REFERENCES

Adams, T. H., and Norman, A. W. (1970). *J. Biol. Chem.* **245**, 4421.
Askew, F. A., Bourdillon, R. B., Bruce, H. M., Callow, R. K. St. L., Philpot, J., and Webster, T. A. (1932). *Proc. R. Soc. London, Ser. B* **109**, 488.
Avioli, L. V., and Haddad, J. G. (1973). *Metab. Clin. Exp.* **22**, 507.
Belsey, R. E., DeLuca, H. F., and Potts, J. T. (1974). *Nature (London)* **247**, 208.
Blunt, J. W., and DeLuca, H. F. (1969). *Biochemistry* **8**, 671.
Blunt, J. W., DeLuca, H. F., and Schnoes, H. K. (1968). *Biochemistry* **7**, 3317.
Boyle, I. T., Gray, R. W., and DeLuca, H. F. (1971). *Proc. Natl. Acad. Sci. U.S.A.* **68**, 2131.
Brickman, A. S., Coburn, J. W., Massry, S. G., and Norman, A. W. (1974). *Ann. Intern. Med.* **80**, 161.
Brickman, A. S., Coburn, J. W., Friedman, G. R., Okamura, W. H., Massry, S. G., and Norman, A. W. (1975). *J. Clin. Invest.* **57**, 1540.
Brumbaugh, P. F., and Haussler, M. R. (1974a). *J. Biol. Chem.* **249**, 1251.
Brumbaugh, P. F., and Haussler, M. R. (1974b). *J. Biol. Chem.* **249**, 1258.
Brumbaugh, P. F., and Haussler, M. R. (1975). *Life Sci.* **16**, 353.

Brumbaugh, P. F., Hughes, M. R. and Haussler, M. R. (1975). *Proc. Nat. Acad. Sci. U.S.A.* **72**, 4871.
Bukin, U. N., and Areshkina, Y. L. (1958). *Proc. Int. Symp. Enzyme Chem., 1958* p. 475.
Buller, R. E., and O'Malley, B. W. (1976). *Biochem. Pharmacol.* **25**, 1.
Buller, R. E., Schrader, W. T., and O'Malley, B. W. (1975). *J. Biol. Chem.* **250**, 809.
Chalk, K. J. J., and Kodicek, E. (1961). *Biochem. J.* **79**, 1.
Chen, P. S., Jr., and Lane, K. (1965). *Arch. Biochem. Biophys.* **112**, 70.
Chen, T. C., and DeLuca, H. F. (1973). *J. Biol. Chem.* **248**, 4890.
Cohn, E. J., Gurd, F., Surgenor, D., Barnes, B., Brown, R., Derouaux, G., Gillespie, J., Kahnt, F., Lever, W., Liu, C., Mittelman, D., Mouton, R., Schmid, K., and Uroma, E. (1950). *J. Am. Chem. Soc.* **72**, 465.
Crowfoot, D., and Dunitz, J. D. (1948). *Nature (London)* **162**, 608.
Daiger, S. P. (1975). Ph. D. Dissertation, Stanford University, Stanford, California.
Daiger, S. P., Schoenfield, M. S., and Cavalli-Sforza, L. L. (1975). *Proc. Natl. Acad. Sci. U.S.A.* **72**, 2076.
DeCrousaz, P., Blanc, B., and Antener, I. (1965). *Helv. Odontol. Acta* **9**, 151.
DeLuca, H. F. (1969). *Am. J. Clin. Nutr.* **22**, 412.
DeLuca, H. F. (1976). *Clin. Endocrinol. (Oxford)* **5**, 97s.
Edelstein, S., Lawson, D. E. M., and Kodicek, E. (1972). *Biochim. Biophys. Acta* **270**, 570.
Edelstein, S., Lawson, D. E. M., and Kodicek, E. (1973). *Biochem. J.* **135**, 417.
Edelstein, S., Charman, M., Lawson, D. E. M., and Kodicek, E. (1974). *Clin. Sci. Mol. Med.* **46**, 231.
Eliel, E. N., Allinger, N. L., Angyal, N. L., and Morrison, G. A. (1967). "Conformational Analysis," Chap. 2. Wiley (Interscience), New York.
Emtage, J. S., Lawson, D. E. M., and Kodicek, E. (1973). *Nature (London), New Biol.* **246**, 100.
Fang, S., and Liao, S. (1971). *J. Biol. Chem.* **246**, 16.
Fraser, D. R., and Kodicek, E. (1970). *Nature (London)* **228**, 764.
Friedlander, E. J., and Norman, A. W. (1975). *Arch. Biochem. Biophys.* **170**, 731.
Goldblatt, H., and Soames, K. M. (1923). *Biochem. J.* **17**, 294.
Greenberg, P. B., Hillyard, C. J., Galante, L. S., Colston, K. W., Evans, I. M. A., and MacIntyre, I. (1974). *Clin. Sci. Mol. Med.* **46**, 143
Haddad, J. G., and Birge, S. F. (1975). *J. Biol. Chem.* **250**, 299.
Haddad, J. G., and Chyu, K. (1971). *Biochim. Biophys. Acta* **248**, 471.
Haussler, M. R., and Norman, A. W. (1967). *Arch. Biochem. Biophys.* **118**, 145.
Haussler, M. R., and Norman, A. W. (1969). *Proc. Natl. Acad. Sci. U.S.A.* **62**, 155.
Haussler, M. R., and Rasmussen, H. (1972). *J. Biol. Chem.* **247**, 2328.
Haussler, M. R., Myrtle, J. F., and Norman, A. W. (1968). *J. Biol. Chem.* **243**, 4055.
Hay, A. W. M., and Watson, G. (1976a). *Comp. Biochem. Physiol. B* **53**, 163.
Hay, A. W. M., and Watson, G. (1976b). *Comp. Biochem. Physiol. B* **53**, 167.
Henry, H. L., and Norman, A. W. (1974). *J. Biol. Chem.* **249**, 7529.
Henry, H. L., and Norman, A. W. (1975a). *Biochem. Biophys. Res. Commun.* **62**, 781.
Henry, H. L., and Norman, A. W. (1975b). *Comp. Biochem. Physiol. B* **50**, 431.
Henry, H. L., Midgett, R. J., and Norman, A. W. (1974). *J. Biol. Chem.* **249**, 7584.
Henry, H. L., Taylor, A., and Norman, A. W. (1977). *J. Clin. Nutrit.* **107**, 1918.
Hess, A. F. (1929). "Rickets Including Osteomalacea and Tetany." Lea & Febiger, Philadelphia.
Hess, A. F., and Gutman, M. G. (1922). *J. Am. Med. Assoc.* **78**, 29.
Hibberd, K. A., and Norman, A. W. (1969). *Biochem. Pharmacol.* **18**, 2347.

Higgins, S. J., Rousseau, G. G., Baxter, J. D., and Tompkins, G. M. (1973). *J. Biol. Chem.* **248,** 5873.
Hodgkin, D. C., Rimmer, B. M., Dunitz, J. D., and Trueblood, K. N. (1963). *J. Chem. Soc.* p. 4945.
Holdsworth, E. A. (1970). *J. Membr. Biol.* **3,** 43.
Holick, M. F., Schnoes, H. K., DeLuca, H. F., Suda, T., and Cousins, R. J. (1971). *Biochemistry* **10,** 2799.
Holick, M. F., Schnoes, H. K., DeLuca, H. F., Gray, R. W., Boyle, I. T., and Suda, T. (1972). *Biochemistry* **11,** 4251.
Holick, M. F., Kleiner-Bossaller, A., Schnoes, H. K., Kasten, P. M., Boyle, I. T., and DeLuca, H. F. (1973). *J. Biol. Chem.* **248,** 6691.
Hosoya, N., and Oku, T. (1971). J. of Vitaminology **17,** 119.
Hosoya, N., Oku, T., and Moriuchi, S. (1970). *Vitamins* **41,** 325.
Irving, J. T. (1944). *J. Physiol. (London)* **103,** 9.
Johnson, R. L., Okamura, W. H., and Norman, A. W. (1975). *Biochem. Biophys. Res. Commun.* **67,** 797.
Johnson, R. L., Carey, S. C., Norman, A. W., and Okamura, W. H. (1977). *J. Med. Chem.* **20,** 5.
Kalimi, M., Beato, M., and Feigelson, P. (1973). *Biochemistry* **12,** 3365.
Kida, K., and Goodman, D. S. (1976). *J. Lipid Res.* **17,** 485.
Knobler, C., Romero, C., Braun, P. B., and Hornstra, J. (1972). *Acta Crystallogr., Sect. B* **28,** 2097.
Kodicek, E. (1974). *Lancet* **1,** 325.
Lamar, G. D., and Budd, D. L. (1974). *J. Am. Chem. Soc.* **96,** 7317.
Larkins, R. G., MacAuley, S. J., Rapoport, A., Martin, T. J., Tulloch, B. R., Byfield, P. G. H., Matthews, E. W., and MacIntyre, I. (1974). *Clin. Sci. Mol. Med.* **46,** 569.
Lawson, D. E. M., and Wilson, P. W. (1974). *Biochem. J.* **144,** 573.
Lawson, D. E. M., Wilson, P. W., and Kodicek, E. (1969). *Nature (London)* **222,** 171.
Lawson, D. E. M., Fraser, D. M., Kodicek, E., Morris, H. R., and Williams, D. H. (1971). *Nature (London)* **230,** 228.
Lay, W. H., and Nussenzweig, V. (1968). *J. Exp. Med.* **128,** 991.
Lewin, R. (1973). *New Sci.* **57,** 371.
McCollum, E. V., Simmonds, N., Becker, J. E., and Shipley, P. G. (1922). *J. Biol. Chem.* **53,** 293.
Mainwaring, W. I. P., and Peterken, B. M. (1971). *Biochem. J.* **125,** 285.
Malm, O. J. (1953). *Scand. J. Clin. Lab. Invest.* **5,** 75.
Melanby, E. (1919). *Lancet* **2,** 407.
Mitra, M. N., Norman, A. W., and Okamura, W. H. (1974). *J. Org. Chem.* **39,** 2931.
Morgan, H. G., Thomas, W. C., Haddock, L., and Eager, J. (1958). *Trans. Assoc. Am. Physicians* **71,** 93.
Myrtle, J. F., and Norman, A. W. (1971). *Science* **171,** 79.
Myrtle, J. F., Haussler, M. R., and Norman, A. W. (1970). *J. Biol. Chem.* **245,** 1190.
Nicolaysen, R. (1943). *Acta Physiol. Scand.* **5,** 201.
Nilsson, S. F., Ostberg, L., and Peterson, P. A. (1972). *Biochem. Biophys. Res. Commun.* **46,** 1380.
Norman, A. W. (1965). *Science* **149,** 184.
Norman, A. W. (1968). *Biol. Rev. Cambridge Philos. Soc.* **43,** 97.
Norman, A. W. (1971). *Am. J. Clin. Nutr.* **24,** 1346.
Norman, A. W., and Henry, H. (1974a). *Clin. Orthop. Relat. Res.* **98,** 258.
Norman, A. W., and Henry, H. (1974b). *Recent Prog. Horm. Res.* **30,** 431.

Norman, A. W., Mircheff, A. K., Adams, T. H., and Spielvogel, A. (1970). *Biochim. Biophys. Acta* **215**, 348.
Norman, A. W., Myrtle, J. F., Midgett, R. J., Nowicki, H. G., Williams, V., and Popjak, G. (1971). *Science* **173**, 51.
Norman, A. W., Johnson, R. L., Osborn, T. W., Procsal, D. A., Carey, S. C., Hammond, M. L., Mitra, M. N., Pirio, M. R., Rego, A., Wing, R. M., and Okamura, W. H. (1976). *Clin. Endocrinol. (Oxford)* **5**, 121.
Norman, A. W., Mitra, M. N., Okamura, W. H., and Wing, R. M. (1975). *Science* **188**, 1013.
Okamura, W. H., Mitra, M. W., Wing, R. M., and Norman, A. W. (1974a). *Biochem. Biophys. Res. Commun.* **60**, 179.
Okamura, W. H., Norman, A. W., and Wing, R. M. (1974b). *Proc. Natl. Acad. Sci. U.S.A.* **71**, 4194.
Oku, T., Matsura, J., and Hosoya, N. (1972). *Vitamins* **45**, 90.
Omdahl, J. L., and DeLuca, H. F. (1973). *Phys. Rev.* **53**, 327.
Osborn, T. W. (1976). Ph.D. Dissertation, University of California, Riverside.
Peterson, P. A. (1971). *J. Biol. Chem.* **246**, 7748.
Procsal, D. A., Okamura, W. H., and Norman, A. W. (1975). *J. Biol. Chem.* **250**, 8382.
Procsal, D. A., Okamura. W. H., and Norman, A. W. (1976). *Am. J. Clin. Nutr.* **29**, 1271.
Rikkers, H., and DeLuca, H. F. (1967). *J. Physiol. (London)* **213**, 380.
Rojanasathit, S., and Haddad, J. G. (1976). *Biochim. Biophys. Acta* **421**, 12.
Rosenstreich, S. J., Volwiler, W., and Rich, C. (1971). *Am. J. Clin. Nutr.* **24**, 897.
Schachter, D., Finkelstein, J. D., and Kowarski, S. (1964). *J. Clin. Invest.* **43**, 787.
Smith, J. E., and Goodman, D. S. (1971). *J. Clin. Invest.* **50**, 2159.
Spenser, R., Charman, M., Wilson, P., and Lawson, E. (1976). *Nature (London)* **263**, 161.
Spielvogel, A. M., Farley, R. D., and Norman, A. W. (1972). *Exp. Cell Res.* **74**, 359.
Steenbock, H., and Black, A. (1924). *J. Biol. Chem.* **61**, 405.
Suda, T., DeLuca, H. F., Schnoes, H. K., Tanaka, Y., and Holick, M. F. (1970). *Biochemistry* **9**, 4776.
Swancek, G. E., Chu, L. L. H., and Edelman, I. S. (1970). *J. Biol. Chem.* **245**, 5382.
Tanaka, Y., and DeLuca, H. F. (1973). *Arch. Biochem. Biophys.* **154**, 566.
Tanaka, Y., DeLuca, H. F., Ikekawa, N., Masuo, M., and Koizumi, N. (1975). *Arch. Biochem. Biophys.* **170**, 620.
Thomas, W. C., Morgan. H. G., Connor, T. B., Haddock, L., Bills, C. E., and Howard, J. E. (1959). *J. Clin. Invest.* **38**, 1078.
Tsai, H. C., and Norman. A. W. (1973). *J. Biol. Chem.* **248**, 5967.
Tsai, H. C., Wong, R. G., and Norman, A. W. (1972). *J. Biol. Chem.* **247**, 5511.
Tsai, H. C., Midgett, R. J., and Norman, A. W. (1973). *Arch. Biochem. Biophys.* **157**, 339.
U.S. Pharmacopoeia. (1947). 13th revision. p. 718.
Wasserman, R. H., and Taylor, A. N. (1968). *J. Biol. Chem.* **243**, 3987.
Wecksler, W. R., Henry, H., and Norman, A. W. (1977). *Arch. Biochem. Biophys.* **183**, 168.
Whistler, D. (1645). Ph.D Dissertation, University of Leiden.
Windaus, A., Linsert, O., Lüttringhaus, A., and Weidlich, A. (1932). *Justus Liebigs Ann. Chem.* **492**, 226.
Wing, R. M., Okamura, W. H., Pirio, M. R., Sine, S. M., and Norman, A. W. (1974). *Science* **186**, 939.
Wing, R. M., Okamura, W. H., Rego, A., Pirio, M. R., and Norman, A. W. (1975). *J. Am. Chem. Soc.* **97**, 4980.
Wong, R. G., Norman, A. W., Reddy, C. R., and Coburn, J. W. (1970). *J. Clin. Invest.* **51**, 1287.
Zull, J. E., Misztal, C., and DeLuca, H. F. (1966). *Proc. Natl. Acad. Sci. U.S.A.* **55**, 177.

19

Cellular-Binding Proteins for Compounds with Vitamin A Activity

FRANK CHYTIL AND DAVID E. ONG

I.	Introduction	573
II.	The Vitamin A-Deficient Animal	574
III.	Vitamin A Acid (Retinoic Acid)	576
IV.	Fate of Vitamin A-Active Compounds *in Vivo*	577
V.	Vitamin A and Cellular Differentiation	578
VI.	Cellular Retinol-Binding Protein (CRBP)	579
VII.	Cellular Retinoic Acid-Binding Protein (CRABP)	580
VIII.	Properties of the Cellular-Binding Proteins	581
IX.	Other Vitamin A-Binding Proteins	587
X.	Cellular Binding Proteins and Cancer	587
	A. Vitamin A and Cancer	587
	B. Binding Proteins in Experimental Tumors	587
	C. Binding Proteins in Human Tumors	589
XI.	Conclusions	589
	References	590

I. INTRODUCTION

The dietary component "fat-soluble factor A", now vitamin A, was discovered to be a growth factor in 1915 (McCollum and Davis, 1915). The structure of its most active form, all-*trans*-retinol (Fig. 1) has been known for 40 years (Karrer *et al.*, 1931). In spite of numerous investigations, understanding of its essential role in growth and development still eludes us. This is in contrast to the role of vitamin A in vision where substantial

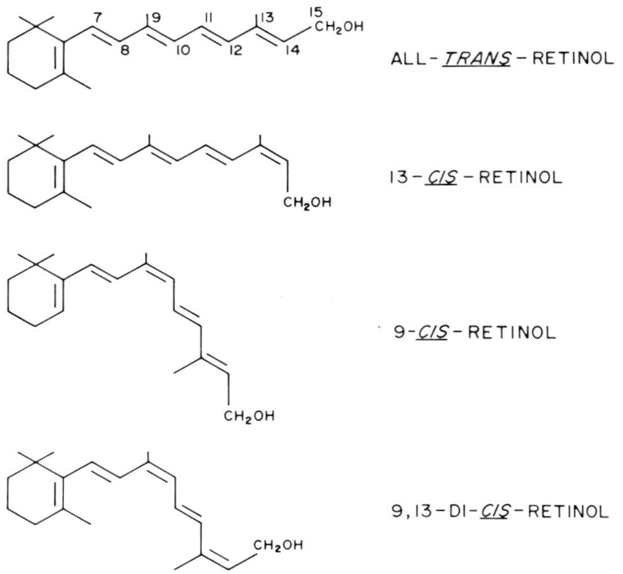

Fig. 1. Structure of all-*trans*-retinol and *cis* isomers.

progress has been made due to the brilliant work of Wald and others (Wald, 1968). But the visual role of vitamin A is clearly separable from its role in growth and development. This chapter describes recent work on two intracellular binding proteins for vitamin A-active compounds. The first is called cellular retinol-binding protein, CRBP. The second is the cellular retinoic acid-binding protein or CRABP. This nomenclature has been suggested to avoid confusion with another retinol-binding protein discovered in serum and abbreviated RBP (Kanai *et al.*, 1968; Peterson, 1971). Serum RBP has been studied intensively and is responsible for the transport of retinol from the liver to the target organs (for recent reviews, see Glover *et al.*, 1974; Goodman, 1974; Peterson *et al.*, 1974).

The intracellular-binding proteins discussed here may play an essential role in mediating vitamin A action in processes other than vision.

II. THE VITAMIN A-DEFICIENT ANIMAL

Investigation of the lesions in animals restricted to vitamin A-deficient diets have been essential for identifying processes and tissues requiring this nutritional factor (Moore, 1967). The animals deficient in the vitamin cease to grow and eventually die. As 11-*cis*-retinal, derived from all-*trans*-retinol, is the chromophore that combines with opsin (protein of MW 28,000) to form the visual pigment rhodopsin, vision is impaired and blindness may result (Wald, 1968). However, failure of vision takes place relatively late in the progression of the deficient state. One of the earliest observable lesions is found in many epithelial tissues (Wolbach and Howe, 1925). Normal columnar epithelial cells are replaced by squamous cells, frequently keratinized. The proliferation of these cells is frequently rapid leading to stratified epithelium of an epidermoid type. In advanced cases, the proliferation can be invasive. Among the first sites affected are the respiratory, genitourinary, and alimentary tracts. The lesions are fully reversible, as refeeding retinol promotes replacement by the normal epithelial cell type (Wolbach and Howe, 1933). Vitamin A is also required for normal reproductive function. A severely deficient female will not conceive; uterine and vaginal epithelium show keratinization (Moore, 1967). A less severe deficiency may allow conception, but the fetuses are aborted or malformed neonates are delivered. The male reproductive system is also affected; in the testes, the germinal epithelium fails to produce sperm, and the epididymal epithelium may undergo metaplasia to a keratinized state (Moore, 1967).

Although the morphological effects of vitamin A deficiency have been clearly defined, it is unclear which biochemical systems are involved, so there is no clear path to the mechanism of vitamin A action. By investigating the deficient animal, regulation of many metabolic and enzymatic functions have been attributed to this vitamin (Moore, 1967; Sundaresan, 1972), but evaluation of the degree of vitamin A deficiency is difficult, and similar effects can be observed in food-restricted animals (pair-fed). Moreover, effects of vitamin A deficiency, such as decreased food intake, infection, or other secondary effects complicate the interpretation of the results. It was long believed that adrenal function required vitamin A; in particular, lower levels of 3β-hydroxysteroid dehydrogenase have been observed in retinol-depleted rats (Johnson and Wolf, 1960). Recently it was reported, however, that this lesion in steroidogenesis may be caused by ascorbic acid depletion (Gruber *et al.*, 1976), as vitamin A deficiency causes a reduction in the biosynthesis of ascorbic acid by rat liver (Malathi and Ganguly, 1964; Ghosh *et al.*, 1965).

Large, nonphysiological doses of vitamin A-active compounds cause labilization of lysozomal membranes (Roels, 1967), but there appears to be no unequivocal defect in the deficient state. It seems most likely now that the changes observed with high doses of vitamin A are due to nonspecific surface-active properties of the vitamin, as discussed recently (Smith and Goodman, 1976).

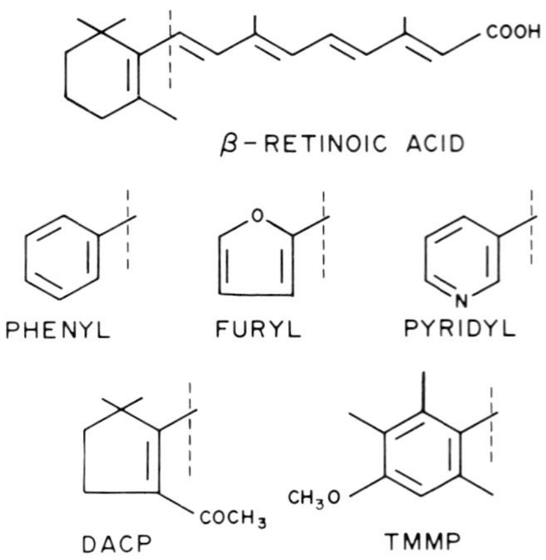

Fig. 2. Structure of β-retinoic acid and analogues with ring modifications.

The deficient animal appears to have altered glycoprotein synthesis (DeLuca et al., 1970a), and a possible role for retinol as carrier of sugars in such syntheses has been investigated with suggestive results (DeLuca et al., 1970b). A carrier role for the polyisoprenols–dolichols, which have some structural similarities to retinol, has been described (Behrens et al., 1971).

III. VITAMIN A ACID (RETINOIC ACID)

Much later after the discovery of retinol, retinoic acid (Fig. 2) was synthesized and found to promote growth in the retinol-deprived animal (Ahrens and Van Dorp, 1946). Closer investigation revealed that, although epithelial tissues seemed to be normal in the retinoic acid-fed animal, vision failed (Dowling and Wald, 1960), spermatogenesis stopped, and pregnancies were not carried to term, with fetuses being resorbed (Thomson et al., 1964). The failure of vision has suggested retinoic acid cannot be reduced to retinal *in vivo*. More recently it was shown that a small quantity of retinoic acid is formed *in vivo* from radioactive retinol administered in physiological doses (Emerick et al., 1967), and later it was suggested that retinoic acid is a normal intermediate in the metabolism of retinol (Ito et al., 1974). The exact sites of formation of retinoic acid as well as its functions are still obscure. It has been suggested (Thompson, 1969) that, in some tissues, retinol was oxidized to retinoic acid, but acted unchanged in others (e.g., testis). Our working hypothesis has been that the modes of action of the two compounds are not necessarily identical.

IV. FATE OF VITAMIN A-ACTIVE COMPOUNDS *IN VIVO*

Vitamin A is obtained in the diet as esters of retinol or carotenes (Fig. 3). The esters are hydrolyzed to free retinol by specific pancreatic esterases or intestinal brush border hydrolases before absorption (Sundaresan, 1972; Mathur *et al.*, 1974). β-Carotene is oxidatively cleaved to two molecules of retinal then reduced to retinol in the mucosa (Goodman and Huang, 1965). Free retinol is esterified with long-chain fatty acids and transported mainly by the lymph to the liver, the storage organ for retinol in the form of esters (Huang and Goodman, 1965). As has been shown by Goodman and Peterson and their co-workers (Kanai *et al.*, 1968; Peterson, 1971), the liver synthesizes a specific serum transport protein called retinol-binding protein (MW about 20,000). This transport protein is stored in the liver parenchymal cells in the form of particles (Poole *et al.*, 1975). It is released to the blood only after complexing with free retinol. The retinol–RBP complex binds with serum prealbumin to form the circulating complex, retinol–RBP–prealbumin. Generalizing from a recent report (Heller, 1975), target cells appear to have specific plasma membrane receptors for the complex. Retinol enters the cell, but RBP does not (Peterson *et al.*, 1974). After

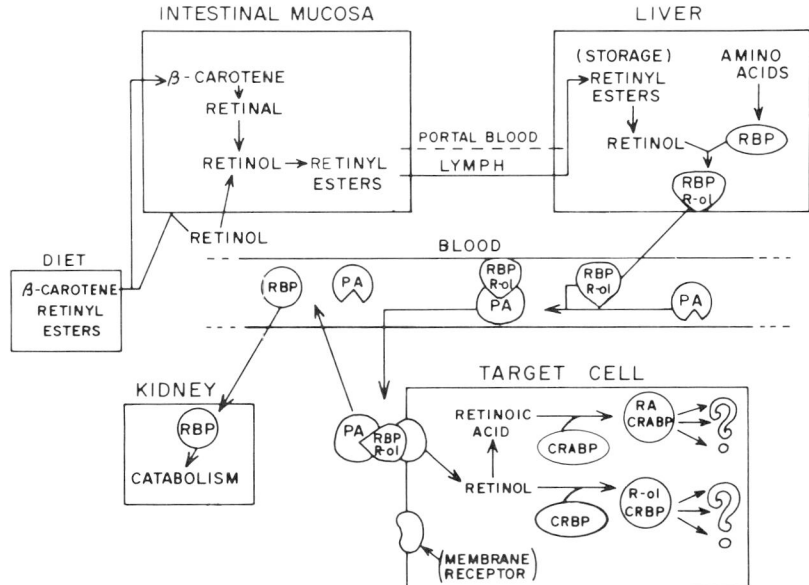

Fig. 3. Metabolic fate of vitamin A.

delivery of retinol, serum RBP appears to lose the ability to bind to prealbumin and is degraded in the kidney. Several forms of retinol-binding proteins have been described in the urine (Peterson et al., 1974; Glover et al., 1974; Clark et al., 1975).

This elaborate transport system apparently delivers only all-*trans*-retinol to the target cell. Retinol is the only vitamin A-active compound found bound to serum RBP *in vivo*, although RBP is able to bind retinal and retinoic acid *in vitro*. Administered [^{14}C]retinoic acid is transported by serum albumin (Smith et al., 1973). In addition to the lack of a specific transport system for retinoic acid, there is also no storage capability for the administered compound, and it is metabolized rapidly and excreted. It is doubtful that it is obtained in the diet. Evidence for a physiological role has been only circumstantial.

V. VITAMIN A AND CELLULAR DIFFERENTIATION

Although the mechanism of vitamin A action remains obscure, it seems reasonable that any proposed mechanism should take into account the apparent ability of vitamin A to affect cellular differentiation. It is now generally accepted that the process of cellular differentiation involves changes in nuclear transcription, whether it occurs during time-dependent perinatal development (Church and McCarthy, 1967) or after induction by steroid hormones (O'Malley and Means, 1974). Formation of new specific proteins, changes in RNA metabolism, alterations in nuclear enzymes, and changes in the characteristics of chromatin have been described in steroid hormone-induced differentiation (Spelsberg et al., 1973), as well as in perinatal development (Chytil et al., 1974).

Unlike steroid hormones, where the source of the hormone can be surgically removed, the experimental control of availability of vitamin A to the target cell is complicated by its liver storage. The liver can apparently contain sufficient retinol for the lifetime of the small animal. In addition, no specific "marker" protein has been discovered as being induced by vitamin A. However, it has been shown that changes in incorporation of radioactive precursors into nuclear RNA of various tissues occur in retinol deficiency or under the influence of administered retinol (Zachman, 1967; Johnson et al., 1969; Zile and DeLuca, 1970; DeLuca et al., 1971; Tryfiates and Krause, 1971). In addition, the spectrum of nuclear RNA extracted from tracheal epithelium of the vitamin A-deficient animal differs from that of the normal animal when analyzed by gel electrophoresis (Kaufman et al., 1972). Synthesis of protein, RNA, and DNA is elevated when organ cultures of newborn mouse skin are exposed to vitamin A-active compounds

(Sporn et al., 1975). These biologic changes, when considered with the described morphological alterations, suggest that vitamin A influences cellular differentiation. Since the differentiation process induced by steroid hormones is known to be mediated by specific intracellular binding protein receptors, impetus was provided for the search for intracellular binding proteins for vitamin A compounds by this laboratory as well as others.

VI. CELLULAR RETINOL-BINDING PROTEIN (CRBP)

Using the working hypothesis that vitamin A works by a mechanism similar to that of the steroid hormones, Mark Bashor, in this laboratory, investigated the possibility that target cells for vitamin A would contain an intracellular binding protein for retinol. Applying the technique of sucrose-gradient centrifugation as adapted by Toft and Gorski (1966) for detection of steroid hormone receptors, cytosols of various organs were layered on linear 5–20% sucrose gradients after prior incubation with [15-^{3}H]retinol. After centrifugation the profile of radioactivity showed a peak in the 2 S region, suggesting binding of retinol to a macromolecule (Fig. 4). The bind-

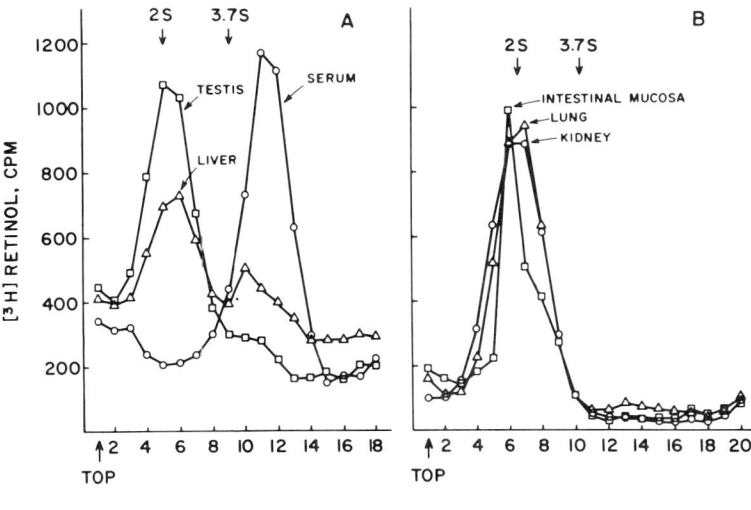

Fig. 4. Sucrose-gradient centrifugation of serum (diluted 1:6) and liver and testis cytosols (A) and kidney, lung, and intestinal mucosal cytosols (B) after incubation with [^{3}H]retinol. Myoglobin (2 S) and ovalbumin (3.7 S) on separate gradients were used as markers. Centrifugation was for 18 hours at 189,000 g. (A) Serum (○); liver cytosol (△); testis cytosol (□). (B) Kidney cytosol (○); lung cytosol (△); intestinal mucosal cytosol (□). (Reproduced from Bashor et al., 1973).

ing component was shown to be a protein, and saturable, as nonradioactive retinol reduced binding. The binding was specific, as retinal and retinoic acid in 200-fold molar excess over [^{3}H]retinol did not reduce binding (Bashor et al., 1973). This binding was not observed in serum, where retinol was found associated with serum albumin in the 4.6 S region of the gradient (Bashor and Chytil, 1975). The binding protein was widely distributed; only serum and muscle were negative. This is consistent with the fact that vitamin A appears to be required by most tissue; skeletal muscle is perhaps the most prominent exception. Subsequently, a similar binding protein for retinol has been also detected in retina of chick embryo (Wiggert and Chader, 1975).

It should be stressed that ability to detect a binding protein is limited by the specific activity of the ligand used. Currently retinol is available at 1–2 Ci/mmole, fully 10–100 times less than commercially available for steroid hormones.

VII. CELLULAR RETINOIC ACID-BINDING PROTEIN (CRABP)

As mentioned previously, retinoic acid was also a candidate for an active form of vitamin A. As retinoic acid did not compete for binding of retinol by CRBP, it appeared unlikely its action was mediated by the binding protein. However, we soon discovered that some tissues appeared to have a second binding protein, this one specific for retinoic acid (Ong and Chytil, 1975a). Cytosols were incubated with [^{3}H]retinoic acid and submitted to sucrose-gradient centrifugation. In cytosols from some organs, a peak of radioactivity in the 2 S region was again observed (Fig. 5). Nonspecific binding to albumin (4.6 S) was also noted. The binding was saturable and specific as retinal and retinol did not compete for binding of [^{3}H]retinoic acid, but unlabeled retinoic acid did. The organ distribution of this binding activity was different than that observed for CRBP (Table I). Consequently, it appeared some tissues contained two binding proteins, one specific for retinol (CRBP) and one specific for retinoic acid (CRABP).

That there were indeed two separate proteins was confirmed by separation of the two binding activities by column chromatography (Fig. 6). The step illustrated is the last step in purification attempts for the two binding proteins from rat testis. Both of the proteins at this stage have been purified approximately 1000-fold; however, it appears that about 20–30-fold more will be required for homogeneity. Using a detection procedure very similar to that described here, a binding protein for retinoic acid has also been

19. Cellular Binding Proteins for Vitamin A Compounds 581

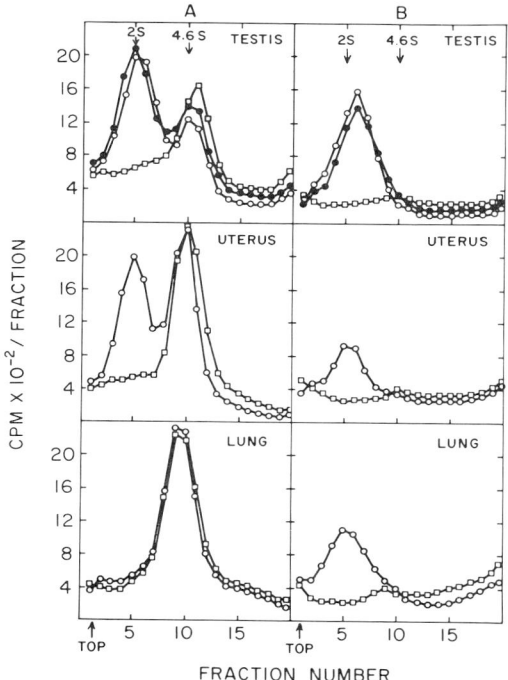

Fig. 5. Detection of CRABP and CRBP in rat testis, uterus, and lung by sucrose-gradient centrifugation. Cytosols were incubated with [³H]retinoic acid (○) and with addition of unlabeled retinoic acid (□) or retinol (●) (A) or were incubated with [³H]retinol (○) and with addition of unlabeled retinoic acid (●) or retinol (□) (B) (Ong and Chytil, 1975a).

demonstrated in crude cytosol from chick embryonic skin (Sani and Hill, 1974, 1976).

VIII. PROPERTIES OF THE CELLULAR-BINDING PROTEINS

Most of the characteristics of these proteins have been obtained by using partially purified preparations. As determined by gel filtration, the apparent MW are 14,000 for CRBP and 14,500 for CRABP. Steroid-receptor proteins are considerably larger.

During purification we noted that CRBP had fluorescent properties (excitation max. 350 nm emission max. 480 nm), suggesting it carried retinol *in vivo* (Fig. 7). The endogenous fluorescence was abolished by exposure to UV

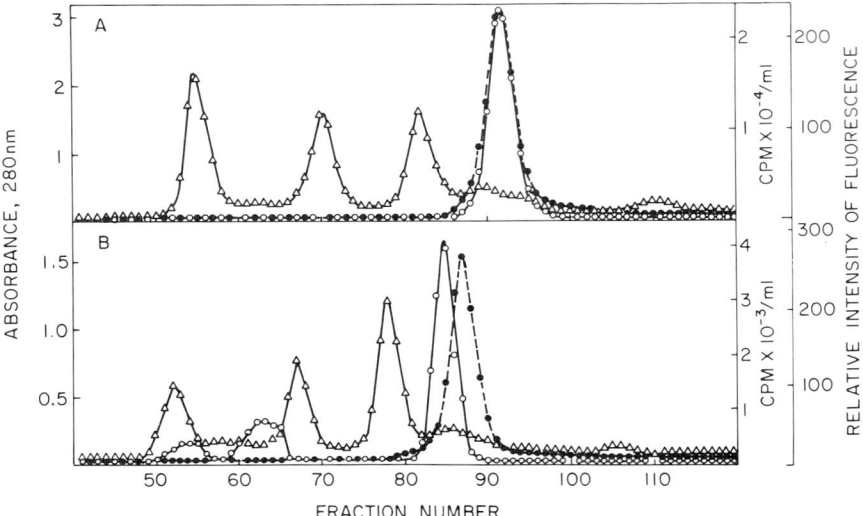

Fig. 6. Separation of CRBP from CRABP by chromatography on DEAE–cellulose. Extracts prepared from rat testis were labeled with [^{3}H]retinol or with [^{3}H]retinoic acid prior to Sephadex G-75 chromatography. The radioactive fractions from the Sephadex chromatography were then applied to columns of DEAE–cellulose and eluted with a linear gradient of NaCl from 0 to 0.2 M. Protein was measured by absorbance at 280 nm (△). Retinol binding was determined by measurement (○) of radioactivity (A) and by measurement of fluorescence (●) at 480 nm with excitation at 350 nm (A and B). Retinoic acid binding (○) was determined by measurement of radioactivity (Panel B) (reproduced from Ong and Chytil, 1975a).

light, known to degrade retinol. After extraction of a preparation of CRBP with cyclohexane, the extract had fluorescence excitation and emission spectrum identical to all-*trans*-retinol. Addition of all-*trans*-retinol to CRBP previously exposed to UV light generated fluorescence spectra identical to the spectra of CRBP with the endogenous ligand. Finally, CRBP from testes of retinol-depleted rats does not show these characteristic fluorescent properties, indicating the absence of bound retinol. In the pair-fed animal, approximately 40% of the CRBP is occupied by retinol, as estimated by fluorescence (Ong *et al.*, 1976).

Table II summarizes some of the basic properties of CRBP from rat testes, contrasted with the properties of rat serum RBP, the transport protein for retinol. The differences in size, fluorescence spectra, and antigenicity indicate the two proteins are distinctly different.

The binding specificity of CRBP was investigated by determining the ability of various vitamin A-active compounds to compete for binding of [^{3}H]retinol. Structures of some of the compounds are shown in Fig. 1

TABLE I
Detectability of CRBP and CRABP in Adult Organ Extracts[a]

Organ	CRBP	CRABP	Reference[b]
Brain	+	+	3
Eye	+	+	3
Gastrocnemius	−	−	3,6
Heart	−	−	3,6
Intestinal mucosa	+	−	1,3
Kidney	+	−	1,3
Liver	+	−	1,3
Lung	+	−	1,3; Human, 1,5; Rabbit, 2
Ovary	+	+	3,6
Serum	−	−	1,3
Skin	+	+	Mouse, 7
Spleen	+	−	1,3
Testis	+	+	1,3
Trachea	N.D.[c]	+	Hamster, 7
Uterus	+	+	3; Human, 4,6

[a] Rat, unless otherwise indicated.
[b] Key to references: (1) Bashor et al., 1973; (2) Ong and Chytil, 1974; (3) Ong and Chytil, 1975a; (4) Chytil et al., 1975; (5) Ong et al., 1975; (6) Bashor and Chytil, 1975; (7) Chytil and Ong, 1976.
[c] N.D., not done.

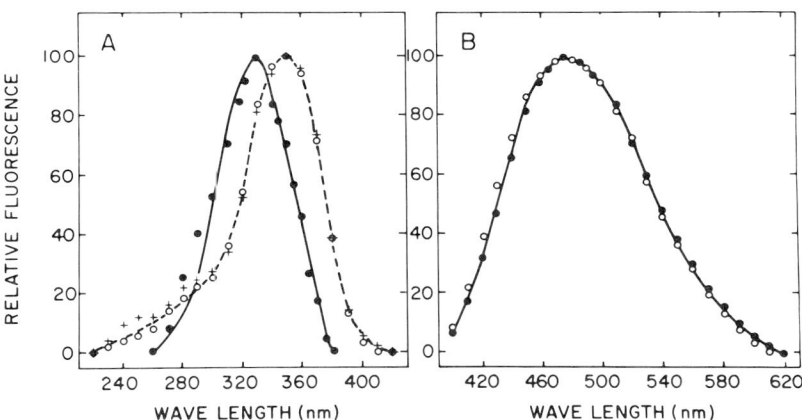

Fig. 7. Fluorescence excitation and emission spectra of free or protein-bound ligand and all-trans-retinol. (A) Fluorescence excitation spectra of partially purified cellular retinol-binding protein with endogenous ligand (+) or reconstituted with all-trans-retinol (O), and of hexane extract of endogenous ligand (●) or all-trans-retinol in hexane (———). Emission was measured at 480 nm. (B) Fluorescence emission spectra of partially purified retinol-binding protein with endogenous ligand (O), excitation at 350 nm; of hexane extract of endogenous ligand (●); and of all-trans-retinol in hexane (———), excitation at 330 nm. Spectra are expressed in arbitrary units from 0 to 100 (Ong et al., 1976).

TABLE II

Characteristics of Rat Serum Retinol-Binding Protein (RBP) and Cellular Retinol-Binding Protein (CRBP) from Rat Testis

Characteristic	RBP	CRBP
Molecular weight	20,000[a]	14,000[b]
Binding of retinoic acid or retinal	Yes[c]	No[d,e]
Fluorescence excitation spectrum (maximum, nm)	334[a]	350[b]
Antigenic toward anti-RBP serum	Yes[f]	No[g]
Level in testis in vitamin A deficiency	Depressed[f]	No change[h]

[a] Muto and Goodman (1972).
[b] Ong and Chytil (1975a).
[c] Glover *et al.* (1974).
[d] Bashor *et al.* (1973).
[e] Ong and Chytil (1975b).
[f] Muto *et al.* (1972).
[g] Bashor and Chytil (1975).
[h] Ong *et al.* (1976).

and 8. The results of the competition experiments are shown in Table III, column 1.

Of the cis isomers tested, 13-*cis*-retinol showed the greatest ability to compete, although less than all-*trans*-retinol, while 9-*cis* and 9,13-di-*cis* competed less well for binding of [^{3}H]retinol. It is significant that the ability of these compounds to promote growth in the vitamin A-deficient rat shows the same pattern. 13-*cis*-Retinol is the most effective, while 9-*cis* and 9,13-di-*cis* had lower and approximately equal activities, compared to all-*trans*-retinol (Table III, column 2). This is suggestive evidence that CRBP is mediating the action of these compounds *in vivo*.

In apparent contrast, α-retinol and 3-dehydroretinol are effective competitors but have *in vivo* activities of only 2% and 40%, respectively. However, the low *in vivo* activity of α-retinol is due to the fact that, although stored efficiently, it cannot enter the normal blood transport

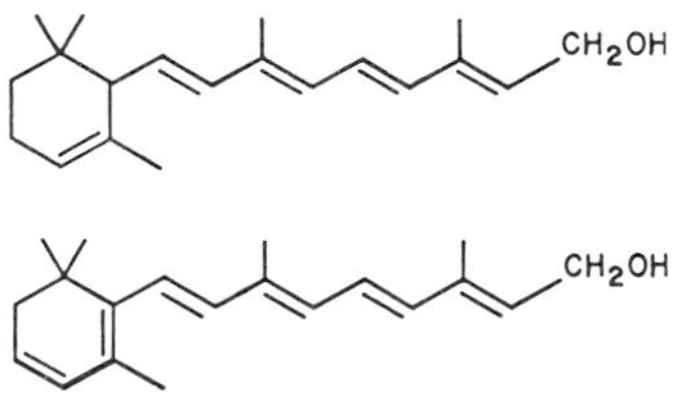

α — RETINOL

3 – DEHYDRORETINOL
(VITAMIN A_2)

Fig. 8. Structure of α-retinol and vitamin A_2.

TABLE III

Percentage Inhibition of Binding of All-*trans*-[³H]Retinol to Proteins by Vitamin A-Active Compounds[a]

Compound	CRBP (%)	*in vivo* activity in rat (%)
All-*trans*-retinol	100	100
Cis isomers		
13-*cis*-retinol	95	75
9-*cis*-retinol	51	22
9,13-di-*cis*-retinol	64	24
Ring isomers		
α-retinol	100	2
3-dehydroretinol (vitamin A$_2$)	100	40
C-15 modifications		
Retinal	0	91
Retinoic acid	0	100
Retinyl acetate	0	100
Retinyl palmitate	0	100

[a] Adapted from Ong and Chytil (1975b).

system and so is essentially trapped in the liver (Goodman *et al.*, 1974). In organ culture, α-retinol appears to be as active as all-*trans*-retinol (Clamon *et al.*, 1974) consistent with its ability to interact with CRBP. It may be that 3-dehydroretinol also does not enter the normal transport system as efficiently, giving it a lower *in vivo* activity.

CRBP shows a stringent requirement for the alcohol function at C15, as the aldehyde, acid, and esters of retinol apparently do not bind. Except for retinoic acid (discussed later), the growth-promoting ability of these compounds is almost certainly due to their conversion to all-*trans*-retinol.

In a similar manner, the binding specificity of CRABP was investigated for a series of analogues of retinoic acid (Fig. 2). As shown in Table IV, the DACP and TMMP analogues are effective competitors of binding of [³H]retinoic acid. The phenyl, furyl, and pyridyl analogues were less effective, in the order listed, with presumably decreasing affinities for CRABP. It is of interest that these results correlate fully with the ability of these compounds to promote growth in epidermal cell cultures derived from mouse skin and with their ability to reverse the metaplasia of hamster tracheas explanted from vitamin A-deficient hamsters to organ culture. As described by Sporn *et al.* (1975), retinoic acid and the DACP and TMMP analogue had marked activity in these systems, while the phenyl analogue had minimal activity, and the furyl and pyridyl analogues showed no activity. As both mouse skin and hamster trachea contain CRABP, this

TABLE IV

Percentage Inhibition of Binding of All-*trans* [³H]Retinoic Acid to Cellular Retinoic Acid-Binding Protein by Analogues of Retinoic Acid[a]

Compound	Rat testis-binding protein (%)	Mouse papilloma-binding protein (%)	Human breast tumor-binding protein (%)
All-*trans*-retinoic acid	100	100	100
DACP analogue	100	100	100
TMMP analogue	100	100	100
Phenyl analogue	42	36	36
Furyl analogue	34	16	24
Pyridyl analogue	22	0	0

[a] Reproduced from Chytil and Ong (1976).

striking correlation provides strong, suggestive evidence that the binding protein is mediating the action of these compounds in growth promotion and control of differentiation.

Table I shows the distribution of the two binding proteins in adult organs. Interestingly in all fetal organs examined so far, including lung, liver, kidney, and heart, both CRBP and CRABP are clearly present. It is obvious that alterations in levels of CRBP and CRABP must be occurring in some organs during perinatal development. In particular, CRABP (and, consequently, retinoic acid) seems to be more involved in fetal organs than adult. Factors controlling this developmental change are under investigation in this laboratory.

The organ distribution of CRBP and CRABP in the adult would appear to be at variance with what would be expected from observations reported on retinol-deprived animals fed retinoic acid. As mentioned previously in this review, such animals do not show the characteristic lesions in epithelial tissues of organs, such as lung and kidney, leading to the assumption that retinoic acid is maintaining the tissue. However, only CRBP, but not CRABP, is detectable in lung and kidney, apparently in contradiction to the postulate that the binding proteins are mediating the action of their respective ligands. It is possible, of course, that the level of CRABP in such organs is too low to detect by the procedures employed here.

We would suggest the possibility that the apparent ability of retinoic acid to replace retinol may in fact be due to a sparing effect on the animals' stores of retinol followed by conservation of retinol when stores become low. Evidence for conservation has been presented (Clausen, 1969), as well as evidence for sparing of retinol by administered retinoic acid (Krishnamurphy *et al.*, 1963; Nelson *et al.*, 1964). The failure of retinoic acid-fed animals to maintain pregnancy or spermatogenesis, as well as vision, may indicate differential depletion or utilization of retinol by different organs when availability of retinol is limited.

IX. OTHER VITAMIN A-BINDING PROTEINS

In a preliminary report (Gambhir and Ahluwalia, 1974), a protein was described to be present in seminiferous tubules of rat testis showing an MW of 4800. This binding component was detected by incubating the seminiferous tubules with tritiated retinyl acetate with subsequent gel filtration. No data showing specificity of the binding has been reported yet.

By fractionation of urine of rats injected with ^{15}C-tritiated retinol, two labeled proteins were detected, one of an MW of more than 100,000 and the second of 4600 (Clark et al., 1975).

X. CELLULAR-BINDING PROTEINS AND CANCER

A. Vitamin A and Cancer

A possible role for compounds with vitamin A activity in malignant growth has been investigated since the discovery of retinol as a growth factor (for reviews, see Burk and Winzler, 1944; Bollag, 1970; Sporn et al., 1976; Ong and Chytil, 1976). In summary, it has been established that dietary deficiency of vitamin A can lead to increased incidence of spontaneous or carcinogen- or virus-induced epithelial metaplasias and tumors in experimental animals and possibly in man (Bjelke, 1975). High doses of retinol esters, retinoic acid and particularly some of its analogues, developed by the Hoffman-LaRoche Company, have proved to be effective in reducing incidence of carcinogen-induced malignant growth in experimental animals. Furthermore, it appears that these compounds cause regression of preneoplastic lesions in experimental animals and man. Transplantable tumors in rodents generally do not appear to be inhibited by administration of vitamin A-like compounds (for review, see Ong and Chytil, 1976), although exceptions have been reported recently (Felix et al., 1975; Heilman and Swarm, 1975).

B. Binding Proteins in Experimental Tumors

As vitamin A appears to have a therapeutic effect on some tumors, we were encouraged to investigate whether experimental tumors contained either CRBP or CRABP. Earlier screening had shown that Novikoff hepatoma, ascites hepatoma AS-30, mouse Ehrlich ascites tumor, and mouse pituitary cell line At-20 did not contain CRBP (Bashor and Chytil, 1975). After the discovery of CRABP, the survey was expanded to included the second binding protein and more tumors. The results are presented in Table V, along with an indication of sensitivity of the tumor to treatment with vitamin A analogues. As can be seen, there is some correlation between presence of CRABP and responsiveness to vitamin A treatment. That is, of the tumors examined, all tumors that respond contain CRABP; no tumors that do not contain CRABP respond; some tumors contain CRABP but do not respond.

That CRABP mediates not only the action of retinoic acid in the normal cell, but also the anti-tumor effects observed, is suggested by its binding specificity (Chytil and Ong, 1976) (Table IV). The mouse skin papillomas, which are induced by topical application of dimethylbenzanthracene, are richly supplied with CRABP. The papillomas are also very sensitive to treatment by retinoic acid and the TMMP analogue of retinoic acid (Bollag, 1972, 1974). As shown, the TMMP analogue binds well to CRABP of mouse papilloma. In general, the binding specificity of CRABP from the papillomas is the same as shown for CRABP from rat testis.

In addition, 13-*cis* retinoic acid is an effective competitor for binding of [^{3}H]retinoic acid by CRABP (unpublished observation) and also inhibits the growth of chondrosarcomas (Heilman and Swarm, 1975). Finally, the DACP analogue of retinoic acid is reported to block the ability of 3-methylcholanthrene to induce hyper- and metaplasia of mouse prostate epithelium (Lasnitzki and Goodman, 1974).

TABLE V
Presence of CRBP and CRABP in Extracts of Experimental Tumors

Tumor	CRBP	CRABP	Sensitivity to vit. A
Mouse skin papilloma	++	++++	+[a]
Human adenocarcinoma HAD-1	+	+	N.R.
Dunning leukemia	+	+	N.R.
Walker 256 carcinoma	+	+	−[a]
Chondrosarcoma	0	+	+[b]
Sarcoma 180	0	+	−[a]
Ehrlich carcinoma	0	0	−[a]
L 1210 leukemia	0	0	−[a]
Novikoff hepatoma	0	0	N.R.
Ascites hepatoma AS-30	0	0	N.R.

[a] Bollag (1971).
[b] Heilman and Swarm (1975).
N.R., not reported.

The observations have led to the suggestion that presence of CRABP may be a required, although not necessarily sufficient condition for a tumor to be sensitive to treatment with retinoic acid and its analogues. Furthermore, evaluating analogues of retinol and retinoic acid for their ability to bind to CRBP and CRABP may be a useful preliminary screening step to identify those with anti-tumor activity. As a further extension, screening tumors for the presence of the binding proteins may indicate possible responsiveness of the tumors to treatment by such compounds (Ong et al., 1975; Chytil and Ong, 1976; Ong and Chytil, 1976).

C. Binding Proteins in Human Tumors

Alterations in the levels of CRBP and CRABP have been observed when limited numbers of human breast and lung carcinomas have been screened for the presence of these proteins. Whereas CRBP was not detectable in the malignant portion of the tissue, CRABP was clearly present but was not detectable in adjacent normal tissue (Ong et al., 1975). Investigation of the binding specificity of CRABP from human breast tumor revealed no significant difference from that found for CRABP from mouse skin papillomas or rat testis (Table IV).

XI. CONCLUSIONS

The discovery of two separate intracellular binding proteins, one for retinol, the second for retinoic acid, poses the crucial question as to whether and how these proteins might mediate vitamin A activity. Though much more work is necessary in this direction, we believe that the evidence presented here indicates these proteins are involved in the action of their respective ligands. The fact that distinct binding proteins for retinol and retinoic acid do exist suggests that these compounds are not interchangeable in function in molecular events of cell differentiation. Furthermore, the appearance of the cellular retinoic acid protein in some cancerous tissue adds to our knowledge of alterations occurring during malignant transformation.

ACKNOWLEDGMENT

The experimental work discussed in this article was supported by USPHS Research Grants HD-05384 and HD-09195 from the National Institute of Child Health and Human Development, by Grants HL-14214 and HL-15341 from the National Heart and Lung Institute. We thank Hoffman-LaRoche Company for support.

We are indebted to Dr. Patrick W. Trown for supplying us with some experimental tumors and to Mrs. I. Chrastil and Mrs. L. Chytil for excellent technical assistance.

REFERENCES

Ahrens, J. F., and Van Dorp, D. A. (1946). *Nature (London)* **157**, 190.
Bashor, M. M., and Chytil, F. (1975). *Biochim. Biophys. Acta* **411**, 87.
Bashor, M. M., Toft, D. O., and Chytil, F. (1973). *Proc. Natl. Acad. Sci. U.S.A.* **70**, 3483.
Behrens, N. H., Parodi, A. F., and Leloir, L. F. (1971). *Proc. Natl. Acad. Sci. U.S.A.* **68**, 2857.
Bjelke, E. (1975). *Int. J. Cancer* **15**, 561.
Bollag, W. (1970). *Int. J. Vitam. Res.* **40**, 299.
Bollag, W. (1971). *Schweiz. Med. Wochenschr.* **101**, 11.
Bollag, W. (1972). *Eur. J. Cancer* **8**, 689.
Bollag, W. (1974). *Eur. J. Cancer* **10**, 731.
Burk, D., and Winzler, R. J. (1944). *Vitam. Horm. (N.Y.)* **2**, 305.
Church, R. B., and McCarthy, B. J. (1967). *J. Mol. Biol.* **23**, 477.
Chytil, F., and Ong, D. E. (1976). *Nature (London)* **260**, 49.
Chytil, F., Glasser, S. R., and Spelsberg, T. S. (1974). *Dev. Biol.* **37**, 295.
Chytil, F., Page, D. L., and Ong, D. E. (1975). *Int. J. Vitam. Nutr. Res.* **45**, 293.
Clamon, G. H., Sporn, M. B., Smith, J. M., and Saffiotti, V. (1974). *Nature (London)* **250**, 64.
Clark, J. N., Nathaniel, R. S., Kleinman, M. K., and Wolfe, G. (1975). *Biochem. Biophys. Res. Commun.* **62**, 233.
Clausen, J. (1969). *Eur. J. Biochem.* **7**, 575.
DeLuca, L., Schumacher, M., and Wolf, G. (1970a). *J. Biol. Chem.* **245**, 4551.
DeLuca, L., Rosso, G., and Wolf, G. (1970b). *Biochem. Biophys. Res. Commun.* **41**, 615.
DeLuca, L., Kleinman, M. K., Little, E. P., and Wolf, G. (1971). *Arch. Biochem. Biophys.* **145**, 332.
Dowling, J. E., and Wald, G. (1960). *Proc. Natl. Acad. Sci. U.S.A.* **46**, 587.
Emerick, R. J., Zile, M., and DeLuca, M. F. (1967). *Biochem. J.* **102**, 606.
Felix, E. L., Loyd, B., and Cohen, M. H. (1975). *Science* **189**, 886.
Gambhir, K. K., and Ahluwalia, B. S. (1974). *Biochem. Biophys. Res. Commun.* **61**, 501.
Ghosh, N. C., Chaterjee, I., and Chaterjee, G. C. (1965). *Biochem. J.* **92**, 521.
Glover, J., Jay, C., and White, G. M. (1974). *Vitam. Horm. (N.Y.)* **32**, 215.
Goodman, D. S. (1974). *Vitam. Horm. (N.Y.)* **32**, 167.
Goodman, D. S., and Huang, H. S. (1965). *Science* **149**, 879.
Goodman, D. S., Smith, J. E., Hembry, R. M., and Dingle, J. T. (1974). *J. Lipid Res.* **15**, 406.
Gruber, K. A., O'Brien, L. V., and Gerstner, R. (1976). *Science* **191**, 472.
Heilman, C., and Swarm, R. L. (1975). *Fed. Proc., Fed. Am. Soc. Exp. Biol.* **34**, 822.
Heller, J. (1975). *J. Biol. Chem.* **250**, 3613.
Huang, H. S., and Goodman, D. S. (1965). *J. Biol. Chem.* **240**, 2839.
Ito, Y., Zile, M., DeLuca, H. F., and Ahrens, H. M. (1974). *Biochim. Biophys. Acta* **369**, 338.
Johnson, B. C., and Wolf, G. (1960). *Vitam. Horm. (N.Y.)* **18**, 457.
Johnson, B. C., Kennedy, M., and Chiba, N. (1969). *Am. J. Clin. Nutr.* **22**, 1048.
Kanai, M., Raz, A., and Goodman, D. S. (1968). *J. Clin. Invest.* **47**, 2025.
Karrer, P. A., Morf, R., and Schöpp, K. (1931). *Helv. Chim. Acta* **14**, 1036.
Kaufman, D. G., Baker, M. S., Smith, J. M., Henderson, W. R., Harris, C. C., Sporn, M. B., and Saffiotti, U. (1972). *Science* **177**, 1105.

Krishnamurphy, S., Bieri, J. G., and Andrews, E. L. (1963). *J. Nutr.* **79**, 503.
Lasnitzki, I., and Goodman, D. S. (1974). *Cancer Res.* **34**, 1564.
McCollum, E. V., and Davis, M. (1915). *J. Biol. Chem.* **23**, 181.
Malathi, P., and Ganguly, J. (1964). *Biochem. J.* **92**, 521.
Mathur, S. N., Joshi, P. S., Murthy, S. K., and Ganguly, J. (1974). *Indian J. Biochem. & Biophys.* **11**, 105.
Moore, T. (1967). *In* "The Vitamins" (W. H. Sebrell, Jr. and R. S. Harris, eds.), Vol. 1, pp. 245–266. Academic Press, New York.
Muto, Y., and Goodman, D. S. (1972). *J. Biol. Chem.* **247**, 2533.
Muto, Y., Smith, J. E., Milch, P. O., and Goodman, D. S. (1972). *J. Biol. Chem.* **247**, 2542.
Nelson, E. C., Dehority, B. A., Teague, H. S., Grifo, A. P., and Sangel, V. L. (1964). *J. Nutr.* **82**, 263.
O'Malley, B. W., and Means, A. R. (1974). *Science* **183**, 610.
Ong, D. E., and Chytil, F. (1974). *Biochem. Biophys. Res. Commun.* **59**, 221.
Ong, D. E., and Chytil, F. (1975a). *J. Biol. Chem.* **250**, 6113.
Ong, D. E., and Chytil, F. (1975b). *Nature (London)* **255**, 74.
Ong, D. E., and Chytil, F. (1976). *Cancer Lett.* **2**, 25.
Ong, D. E., Page, D. L., and Chytil, F. (1975). *Science* **190**, 60.
Ong, D. E., Tsai, C. H., and Chytil, F. (1976). *J. Nutr.* **105**, 204.
Peterson, P. A. (1971). *J. Biol. Chem.* **246**, 34.
Peterson, P. A., Nilsson, S. F., Ostberg, L., Rask, L., and Vahlquist, A. (1974). *Vitam. Horm. (N.Y.)* **32**, 181.
Poole, A. R., Dingle, J. T., Mallia, A. K., and Goodman, D. S. (1975). *J. Cell Sci.* **19**, 379.
Roels, O. (1967). *In* "The Vitamins" (W. H. Sebrell, Jr. and R. S. Marriss, eds.), Vol. 1, pp. 167–245. Academic Press, New York.
Sani, B. P., and Hill, D. L. (1974). *Biochem. Biophys. Res. Commun.* **61**, 1276.
Sani, B. P., and Hill, D. L. (1976). *Cancer Res.* **36**, 409.
Smith, F. R., and Goodman, D. S. (1976). *N. Engl. J. Med.* **294**, 805.
Smith, J. E., Milch, P. O., Muto, Y., and Goodman, D. S. (1973). *Biochem. J.* **132**, 821.
Spelsberg, T. C., Mitchell, W. M., Chytil, F., Wilson, E. M., and O'Malley, B. W. (1973). *Biochim. Biophys. Acta* **312**, 765.
Sporn, M. B., Dunlop, N. M., and Yuspa, S. H. (1975). *Nature (London)* **253**, 47.
Sporn, M. B., Dunlop, N. M., Newton, L., and Smith, S. M. (1976). *Fed. Proc., Fed. Am. Soc. Exp. Biol.* **35**, 1332.
Sundaresan, P. R. (1972). *J. Sci. Ind. Res.* **31**, 581.
Thompson, J. N. (1969). *In* "The Fat Soluble Vitamins" (M. F. DeLuca and J. W. Suttie, eds.), p. 267. Univ. of Wisconsin Press, Madison.
Thompson, J. N., Howell, J. McC., and Pitt, G. A. (1964). *Proc. R. Soc. London, Ser. B* **159**, 510.
Toft, D., and Gorski, J. (1966). *Proc. Natl. Acad. Sci. U.S.A.* **70**, 3483.
Tryfiates, G. P., and Krause, R. F. (1971). *Life Sci.* **10**, 1097.
Wald, G. (1968). *Science* **162**, 230.
Wiggert, B. O., and Chader, G. J. (1975). *Exp. Eye Res.* **21**, 143.
Wolbach, S. B., and Howe, P. R. (1925). *J. Exp. Med.* **42**, 753.
Wolbach, S. B., and Howe, P. R. (1933). *J. Exp. Med.* **57**, 511.
Zachman, R. D. (1967). *Life Sci.* **6**, 2207.
Zile, M., and DeLuca, H. F. (1970). *Arch. Biochem. Biophys.* **140**, 210.

Index

A

Acceptors (nuclear) for steroid-receptor complexes
  abundance
    in cell, 272-273
    in cell-free nuclei, 273-274
    of high-affinity sites, 278-279, 299
  characterization as proteins
    by affinity chromatography, 142-143
    in chromatin by sequential deproteinization, 142
    by recombination with DNA, 139-142
  DNA complexes with nonhistone chromatin proteins as, 215, 219-220
  relation to histones, 140, 143-144
  release of receptor from complexes bound by, 144, 270-271
α_1-Acid glycoprotein (AAG)
  amino acid sequence, 467
  binding ability after chemical modification
    of disulfide linkage, 464
    of lysine amino group, 464-466
    of tryptophan residue, 466-467
    of tyrosine residue, 466
  progesterone binding by, 444
Actinomycin D, as inhibitor of DNA and protein synthesis, 9, 67-68, 72, 185, 238, 286, 304, 383, 478
Adrenalectomy, for revealing progesterone receptors, 383
Affinity chromatography
  of hormone-receptor complexes, 111-112
  of progesterone-binding globulin, 446
Aldosterone
  distribution and effects: Na^+ reabsorption and K^+ excretion, 323-329
  genetic differences in binding, 347-349
Aldosterone receptor
  binding of nonmineralocorticoids, 344-347
  in cytosol
    affinity constants, 331
    binding properties, 329-339
    competitive binding of steroids, 329, 333-337
    purification problems, 328, 338-339
    time course of reaction, 342-344
    types, 330, 332-339
  evidence for, 326-329
  nuclear
    competitive binding of steroids, 339-341
    isolation and properties, 340-341
Androgens (*see also* Androgen receptors; Steroid hormones; Testosterone)
  anabolic action, 83-101
    assay, 84, 111
    model for: evidence for and against, 106-110
    in protein synthesis, 151-152
  antagonists, 109, 148-149, 428; *see also* Cyproterone
  characterization
    with anti-steroid antibody, 126-129
    by other methods, 129-130
  complexes with receptors
    formation in cytoplasm, 136-137
    function, 106-108, 116-117
    nuclear acceptor for, 138-144
    possible techniques for purification, 111-113
    sedimentation, 126-127
    translocation to and retention in nucleus:

temperature effects, 137–138
in mammary tumor therapy, 428–430
metabolism
  to improve binding, 134–135
  in mouse kidney, 85–87
potentiation by prolactin, 109–110
relative activities: variation with structure, 132–134
specificity of tissues for uptake, 122–123
stimulation
  of enzymes in mouse kidney, 97–100
  of female sexual receptivity, 378
Androgen-binding protein (ABP)
assay by gel electrophoresis, 493–495
binding of steroids
  after modification, 496
  specificity, 496–497
control in the Sertoli cell
  by FSH, 497–501
  by testosterone, 499–501
differentiation from other similar proteins, 493
general characteristics, 492–493
physical properties, 495–496, 525–527
Androgen-binding protein 9 S
evidence for, 501–503
chemical properties, 504–505, 525–527
specificity of steroid binding, 505–507
Androgen receptor
binding of androgens
  assay by charcoal removal of free androgen, 516–518
  envelopment in, 136
  equilibria and thermodynamic parameters in, 521–524
  influence of androgen metabolism on, 523, 525
  kinetics (and release-reaction kinetics), 520–522, 524
  specificity, 373–374, 508, 519–521
binding of progestins, 94–96
interaction
  with divalent cations and mononucleotides, 144–146
  with polynucleotides and ribonucleoproteins, 146–148
  with progesterone, 423
isolation
  by ion-exchange chromatography, 515–516, 518

by sucrose-gradient centrifugation: sedimentation coefficients, 514–517
lack in Tfm mice, 90–91
M sites in, 134–135
measurements on, 511–522
occurrence
  in mouse kidney, 87–89
  in rat prostate, 89
  in various tissues, 108, 110, 125–126, 130–131, 507
properties, 87, 89, 124–126, 372–374, 525–527
relationship to mammary tumors, 429
stability, 510–513
types, 124–126, 514–515
5α-Androstane-3α (and 3β),17β-diol, as metabolite of testosterone, 85–86, 106, 374, 376, 427
Androstenedione
as metabolite of testosterone, 86, 376
conversion to estrogens, 377–378, 384
Antiandrogens (see also Cyproterone), 148–149, 428
Antibiotics (see also Actinomycin D; Rifampicin), 68, 184–185, 238, 303, 332, 364, 383, 478
Antiestrogens (see also Nafoxidine)
blocking receptors of estrogens, 361, 364, 386–387, 390
as estrogen agonists-antagonists, 18–21, 365
for mammary tumor therapy, 414–416
relative binding affinity for uterine estrogen receptor, 178–181
Aromatization (conversion of androgens to estrogens), 384, 389–390, 429

B

Brain, role of gonadal steroids in sexual differentiation, 384–385, 389–391

C

Cations
interaction with androgen receptors and mononucleotides, 144–146
transport mediated by mineralocorticoids, 324–325, 342, 346, 348

Index 595

Chromatin transcription
  assay of RNA initiation sites in
    by incorporation of $\gamma[^{32}P]GTP$, 214
    by titration with receptor complexes, 211–212
  of ovalbumin mRNA *in vitro*, 215–216
  stimulation
    differential, by receptor subunits, 216–218
    by receptor-hormone complex, 212–214
    by testosterone, 92–94
    in various chromatins, 214–215
Circular dichroism, 449–450
Corticosteroid-binding globulin (CBG)
  human
    binding affinities, 474
    conformational change caused by steroids, 449
    kinetics of association and dissociation of cortisol complex, 463
  -like protein of uterus, 161, 163–164, 166–168, 170–171, 176, 474–475, 483
  of liver
    binding properties, 228–230
    physical properties, 228–229
  of rat, 463
Corticosteroid hormones, *see* Aldosterone; Corticosterone; Cortisol
Corticosterone, 382–383, 461, 475
Cortisol, 263–264, 461, 463, 474–475
Cyclic AMP (cAMP), comparison with glucocorticoids as bioregulator, 288–290
Cyproterone, as inhibitor of steroid-receptor complexing, 87, 148–149, 152, 370, 373–374, 428–429, 497, 520

D

Deoxycorticosterone
  for purification of receptors, 338
  receptors, 329, 334, 347
Dexamethasone
  as ACTH inhibitor, 416
  competition with aldosterone, 328, 331, 333–337
  induction of mammary tumor virus RNA
    kinetics, 304–305
    in rat hepatoma cells, 307–311
    study via pulse labeling with [³H]uridine, 305–306

Dihydroprogesterone (DHP), 159, 181–182
5α-Dihydrotestosterone (DHT) (*see also* Steroid hormones)
  as competitor of aldosterone, 336
  binding in various tissues
    compared to estradiol, 357
    compared to testosterone, 374–376, 523, 525
  complexes with receptors, 125–129
  distribution in tissues, 376–377
  effect
    on brain sexual differentiation, 389–390
    on sexual behavior, 379
  formation from testosterone, 85, 90, 106–107, 130, 158, 376–377, 427, 508
  levels as evidence for androgen-binding protein 9 S, 502–503
  metabolism to other steroids, 85–86, 106–107, 374, 427, 508–510
  receptor, *see* Androgen receptor
  retention by nucleus, 371–372, 508
  uptake by tissue, 370
1,25-Dihydroxyvitamin D_3
  formation
    discovery, 538, 557
    from hydroxyvitamin D_3 in kidney, 538–540
  interaction with parathyroid hormone, 540, 562–563
  localization in intestinal chromatin, 556–558
  as mediator of calcium absorption
    via production of calcium-binding protein, 555–556, 558
    time lag in effect, 553–558
  receptor *in vitro*, 560–566
    competitive binding of structural analogs: necessity for hydroxyl groups, 564–566
    intestinal vs. parathyroid, 564
    sedimentation, 561–562
    temperature effect, 560–561
DNA (Deoxyribonucleic acid)
  binding of glucocorticoid-receptor complex, 232–237, 271–279
    agonists vs. antagonists, 266–268
    comparison with binding of cAMP, 289
    evidence for participation, 274–279
  complementary, use in assays of mRNA, 210, 283–284, 302–303, 305–306, 310

effect of successive doses of estrogen
  in chick oviduct (stimulation), 74, 78
  in mouse and rat uterus (inhibition), 73–78
mammary tumor virus
  integrated into rat hepatoma genome, 308–309, 311
  unintegrated: assay, size, and distribution, 311–315
  as part of acceptor system for androgen-receptor complex, 139–144, 147
  synthesis stimulated by estrogens, 63–79
DNA polymerases
  inhibition by repeated doses of estrogen, 76
  stimulation by estrogens, 70–73
  types and molecular weights, 70
DNase I, for studying acceptors of hormone-receptor complex, 247–248, 276–277, 344
DNase II, for studying acceptors of hormone-receptor complex, 277

E

Enzymes, kidney, increase in activities or levels by androgens, 97–100; *see also* DNA synthetase; DNase I; DNase II; Glucuronidase; Glutamine synthetase; RNA polymerases I and II; Tryptophan oxygenase; Tyrosine aminotransferase
Estradiol (*see also* Estrogen; Steroid hormones)
  agonist-antagonist effects
    of estriol on, 11–17
    of nafoxidine on, 18–24
  binding, *see* Estradiol receptors
  competition
    with aldosterone, 336, 339
    with testosterone, 374, 384
  effects
    blocking by drugs, 364–365
    on DNA synthesis in rat uterus, 68–69, 75–78
    on enzyme synthesis, 365–366
    on neural activity and hormone levels, 362–363, 367–368
    time lag in, 363–364
  as estrogen, 2–9, 178–179

formation from androgens, 377–378
retention in nucleus, 371–372, 385–387
stimulation of prolactin and rat mammary tumors, 403
Estradiol receptors
  binding capacity
    in cytosol, 357–358, 444
    in nucleus, 358, 361
  complexes, translocation to nucleus, 360–361
  distribution, 369–370
    in brain, 355–360, 382, 384–385
    between sexes, 361–362
  nuclear
    distribution in neonatal rat brain, 385–388
    production and nature, 359–360
Estriol
  agonist-antagonist action
    competition for retention sites in, 11, 14
    in relation to estradiol, 11–18
    effect on DNA synthesis in rat uterus, 68–69, 75–76
  function, 15–16
  possible antitumor action, 415–416
  transient estrogenic action from single dose, 2–9
Estrogens (*see also* Estradiol; Steroid hormones)
  antimitotic effects, 78
  binding
    by fetoneonatal protein, 388–389
    by mammary tumors, 410
  effect on formation of progesterone receptor, 176–180, 476–478
  interrelationship with other steroid hormones, 422–423, 429
  of neonatal brain
    binding intensity for various hormones, 387–388
  binding sites, 384–388
  promotion of male sexual behavior, 378, 390
  short-acting vs. long-acting, 16–17
  stimulation of DNA synthesis
    via activation of DNA polymerases, 70–73
    dependence on RNA and protein synthesis, 67–69

Index

involvement of the prereplicative (G_1) phase, 66–67
by shortening of cell cycle, 64–66
suppression and use in mammary tumor therapy, 416–418
Estrogen receptors
activated forms
4S form, 55–57
5S form, 57–59
binding, 1–29, 181
competition with antiestrogens, 18–21
relation to uterine growth, 2–5, 10–15, 18
complexes with estrogens
competitive formation, with estradiol and estriol, 12–15
competitive inhibition by antiestrogens, 18–24
correlation with uterine growth, 2–4
relation to RNA polymerase activity, 4–11
conformational changes caused by urea, 38–39
cytoplasmic
abundance, 2, 11–12
replenishment, 20–24, 181, 361
vs. nuclear, 2, 5, 18, 34
effect of androgens on, 430
extractable vs. nonextractable: correlation with retention in nucleus, 26–28
general character, 33–35, 54–55
of human mammary tumors
level, as basis for choice of therapy: clinical results, 412–414
properties, 412
of human uterus
physical properties, 51–52
predominance of 5S form in, 52–54
relation to proteases: comparison with animal species, 49–51
various cytoplasmic forms, 47–49
of mammary tumors of rat, 411
measurement in cytosols, 410–411
molecular weights: dimeric nature of 5S form, 39–41, 45, 50, 52, 55
transformation (estradiol-mediated) of 4S to 5S form, 359–360
induced by salt, 36–37, 52–53
induced by warming, 35–36, 52–54

F

Fluorescence
quenching, for determining parameters of steroid binding
by α-acid glycoprotein, 453–455, 467
by progesterone-binding protein, 451–455
for various steroids, 454–460
of retinol and its protein complex, 581–582
Follicle-stimulating hormone (FSH), regulation of androgen-binding protein by, 497–499

G

Gene(s) (*see also* Chromatin transcription)
as basis for developing steroid resistance in lymphoma cells, 282
gur, in regulation of glucuronidase activity, 98–100
mouse tumor virus, *see* Mouse tumor virus
responding to glucocorticoid hormones, 259–261, 299–300
testicular feminization in mice and rats (Tfm), 427–428, 501
for studying androgen action, 90–93, 108–109, 113–114, 374
tyrosine aminotransferase and glutamine synthetase, 315–316
Glucocorticoid hormones (*see also* Steroid hormones)
agonist and antagonist action
in various systems, 262–263
mechanism: allosteric model, 265–268
binding by proteins, 227–232
cellular responses to
induction of enzymes in hepatomas, 258–261
inhibition of lymphomas, 261–262
parallels with cAMP, 288–290
regulation of growth hormone production, 261
control of specific mRNA's by, 238–248, 286
general mode of action, 226–227, 253–254
induction of mammary tumor virus RNA by, 302–304
interrelationships with progesterone, 423

lymphoma cell strains resisting, 279–283
mineralocorticoid activity, 334, 336
stimulation of gluconeogenesis, 238
structure–activity relationships, 263–265
use in tumor therapy, 426–427
Glucocorticoid receptors, 227–232, 425
  distribution in tissues, 258, 426
  evidence for involvement, 254
    in hepatomas, 245
  identity verification
    by dexamethasone binding, 228–230, 302
    by protease digestion, 229
  localization within the cell, 255
  physical properties, 229, 256
  purification, 236–237
  replenishment in cytoplasm, 270–272
Glucocorticoid–receptor complexes
  acceptors for, in nucleus, 246–247
  activation for nuclear binding by warming or salt
    involvement of Ca^{2+}, 233
    mechanism, 234–235, 268–270
    rate, 232–233
  binding to DNA, 232–237
    comparison to binding of cAMP, 289
    double-stranded vs. single-stranded, 237
  formation
    correlation with responses of sell cultures, 256–257
    dependence on steroid structure, 227–228, 230–232
    thermodynamic parameters, 230, 255–256
β-Glucuronidase of mouse kidney, regulation of synthesis and excretion, 97–100, 114
Glutamine synthetase, effect of mammary tumor virus on induction, 315–316
Gonadal steroids, effect on brain and pituitary tissue, 354–355; *see also* Androgens; Estrogens; Testosterone; etc.)
Growth hormone, regulation via mRNA and glucocorticoids, 261, 283–285

H

Hepatomas
  glucocorticoid control
    of tryptophan oxygenase in, 243–248
    of tyrosine aminotransferase and other enzymes in, 258–261
  infected with mammary tumor virus, 307–319
Human serum albumin, progesterone binding by, 444
25-Hydroxyvitamin D_3
  binding
    association constants for, in various tissues, 546
    evidence for receptors in, 545
    proteins, 546–550, 552–553
  formation from vitamin D_3, 538–539

L

Lymphoma cells
  killing by glucocorticoid hormones, 261–262
  steroid-resistant strains
    analogies with other steroid-resistant systems, 282–283
    development, 279–280
    phenotypic variants, 280–281
    receptor abnormality in: genetic basis for, 281–282

M

Mammary tumors
  human
    androgen therapy, 428–431
    antiestrogen therapy, 414–416
    estrogen indicators of proper therapy, 413–414
    estrogen receptors in, 412–414
    glucocorticoid therapy, 425–426
    progesterone therapy, 416–418, 422–425
    role of prolactin in, 404–406
    therapy, 413–418, 422–426, 428–431
    uptake of estrogens, 410
Mammary murine tumor virus
  endogenous nature in genome, 300–301
  rat hepatoma cells infected with
    effect of glucocorticoids on, 309–319
    production, 307–309
    stimulation by glucocorticoids, 301–302, 426
Medroxyprogesterone, 95–96, 99–101, 428

Index

Messenger RNA (mRNA)
  for calcium-binding protein, 557–558
  for growth hormone: control by glucocorticoids, 261, 283–285
  induction, assay by hybridization with cDNA, 210, 283–284, 302–303, 305–306
  for mouse tumor virus, induction
    in the mouse, 300–306
    in rat hepatoma, 309–310
  for tryptophan oxygenase
    assay, 240–241
    control by glucocorticoids, 238–248
    purification, 239–240
  for tyrosine aminotransferase, 285–288
    deinduction, 287–288
Mutants, for studying responses to steroid hormones, 113–114, 300

N

Nafoxidine
  as cause of nuclear retention of estrogen receptor, 3, 6, 8–17, 77
  as estrogen agonist-antagonist, 18–24
  for mammary tumor therapy, 414
  progesterone-like effects, 422
  relative affinity for uterine estrogen receptor, 178–180
  as stimulant of RNA polymerase, 8–10, 17
  as uterotropic stimulant, 5, 10, 17–18
Nucleotides
  mono-, reaction with androgen receptors and cations, 144–146
  poly-, reaction with androgen receptors, 146–148

P

Pregnane-3,20-dione
  for displacing progestins from receptors, 455–460, 487–488
  as progesterone metabolite, 159
Pregnenolone, 159, 455–456
Progestin(s) (*see also* Progesterone)
  binding to androgen receptors in mouse kidney, 94–96
  occurrence, 157–158
  receptors, 159
Progesterone (*see also* Steroid hormones)
  accumulation in tissues, 380–381
  binding
    by corticosteroid-binding globulin, 474–475
    by progesterone-binding globulin: kinetics, 459–463
  effects on mammary tumors, 417–418
  in the hamster as test animal, 159–160
  metabolites, 159, 379–381, 418–420
    effects of estrogens on, 419, 422
    effects on sexual behavior, 380
  model of action in uterus, 182
  reduction of testosterone uptake by, 370, 383
  as regulator of progesterone receptor, 179–184
  uptake and retention *in vivo*, 160–161
Progesterone-binding globulin (PBG)
  binding ability after chemical modification of amino acid residues
    lysine, 468–469
    tryptophan, 468
  conformational change induced by steroids
    from circular dichroism, 449–450
    from fluorescence quenching analysis, 451–458
    from ultraviolet spectra, 450–451
  kinetics of formation and dissociation of steroid complexes
    with other steroids, 461–464
    with progesterone, 459–463
    stopped-flow fluorometry for measuring, 458–459
  properties
    affinity for progesterone, 444, 446, 460–461, 477
    composition: monosaccharides and amino acids, 446–447, 475–477
    molecular weight: polydispersity, 446–448, 477
  purification, 445–446
Progesterone receptors
  assay
    competitive, 168
    nuclear, 183–184
    by sucrose-glycerol gradient centrifugation, 163–164
    using synthetic progestin R5020, 480–482

biosynthesis
  inhibition by cycloheximide and actinomycin D, 185
  stimulation by estradiol, 184
  by uterine tissue *in vitro*, 184–185
complexes, effect *in vitro* on chromatin transcription, 210–218, 275, 381–384
distribution
  in deciduoma, 169–171
  in endometrium and myometrium, 169, 420–421, 482–483
  in mammary gland, 173, 421–422
  in pituitary and hypothalamus, 171–173
  in vagina, 171, 483
as indicators of endocrine responsiveness in mammary tumors, 424–425
preservation by buffering and chiling, 161–162
properties, 420–421
regulation
  by estrogen priming action, 176–179, 181, 476–477
  in estrous cycle, 173–175, 479–483
  in pregnancy, 175–176, 483–485
  by progesterone itself, 179–184, 421, 478–479
Scatchard assay
  for small samples, 167–168
  technique, 164–165
  use in presence of CBG-like protein, 167–168
  validation, 165–166
Prolactin
  human mammary tumor dependence on, 404–406
  rat mammary tumor stimulation by, 403–404, 429
  receptors in tumors, occurrence and significance, 406–409
Protein(s)
  binding retinol and related compounds, 583–589
  binding vitamin D_3
    distribution in tissue, 546–548
    effect of environmental factors, 549–550
    properties, 548–549
    selectivity among analogs and homologs, 549, 552–553
  binding $1\alpha,25\text{-}(OH)_2$vitamin D_3, selectivity among analogs and homologs, 559

fetoneonatal estrogen-binding (fEBP), 386–389
glucocorticoid-binding, *see* Glucocorticoid hormone
receptors for hormones, *see* Androgens; Estrogens; Progesterone.
synthesis, stimulation by androgens, 151–152

R

Retinoic acid
  -binding protein
    distribution in tissues, 583, 586–587
    in experimental tumors, 587–589
    isolation and properties, 580–584
    specificity for vitamin A-active compounds, 585–586
  structure, 576
Retinol
  -binding protein
    in experimental tumors, 587–589
    distribution in tissues, 580, 583, 586–587
    isolation and properties, 579–584
    specificity for vitamin A-active compounds, 584–585
  formation, 577
  structure, 573–574
Ribonucleoprotein (RNP) particles
  function, 150–151
  interaction with androgen-receptor complex, 147–148
Rifampicin, assay for RNA polymerase initiation sites, 208–209, 211–212
RNA, *see* Messenger RNA
RNA polymerase I, stimulation
  by androgens, 92, 94, 149–150
  by estrogens, 5, 7–11
  by medroxyprogesterone, 95–96
RNA polymerase II
  stimulation
    by androgens, 92–94, 149–150
    by estrogen, 4–11
  for study of RNA initiation sites, 211–214

S

Spirolactone, Spironolactone, as competitive inhibitor of aldosterone, 268, 335, 341, 344–345

Index

Steroid hormone(s) (see also names of individual hormones)
  competitive binding
    by androgen-binding protein, 496–497
    by uteroglobulin and progesterone receptor, 486–487
  comparison of accumulations by target organs, 556
  proteins acting as acceptors, 443–444
    function and mechanism of action, 488–489
    kinetics of association and dissociation with steroids, 462–464
  regulation of transcription: model, 567
    for cytoplasmic events, 218–219
    for nuclear events, 219–221, 298–299
    stoichiometry, 221–222

T

Testosterone (see also Androgens; Steroid hormones)
  binding in various tissues compared to dihydrotestosterone, 374–376, 523, 525
  competition for binding
    with estradiol, 370–371, 384
    with progestins, 94–96
  complexes with receptors, 125–129
  conversion
    to 5α-dihydrotestosterone, 85, 90, 106–107, 158, 374, 376–377, 427, 508–509
    to estradiol, 370–371, 378, 384
  distribution in animal tissues, 369–370
    compared to dihydrotestosterone, 374–376
  kinetics of binding by progesterone-binding globulin, 461
  levels as evidence for androgen-binding protein 9S, 502
  metabolites, distribution in brain, 376
  receptor, see Androgen receptor
  regulation of androgen-binding protein, 499–501
  restoration of lordosis response, 379
  retention by cell nuclei, 371–372, 508
  stimulation
    of β-glucuronidase, 97–99

of RNA polymerases and renal chromatin, 92–94
synergistic action with prolactin, 109–110
uptake by tissues of injected, 85–86, 370–371

Tryptophan oxygenase, glucocorticoid control of mRNA coding for
  in hepatomas, 243–248
  in rat liver, 238–243

Tyrosine aminotransferase
  induction
    alteration by mammary tumor virus, 315–316
    by glucocorticoids, 256–258, 285–286, 423
  posttranscriptional control, 287–288

U

Ultraviolet difference spectra, 450–451
Uterus
  growth stimulation by retention of estrogen-receptor complexes, 2–5, 9–21
  refractory state induced by repeated doses of estrogens, 76–78
Uteroglobulin (blastokinin) binding of steroids
  affinity for various steroids in, 486–487
  compared to progesterone receptor, 487
  dependence on mercapto groups, 485–486

V

Vitamin A see also Retinol)
  acid, see Retinoic acid
  deficiency in animals, 574–576
    as cause of cancer, 587
  as stimulant of cell differentiation, 578–579
  in tumor therapy, 587–589
Vitamin D
  activation in kidney as endocrine organ, 538–540
  binding in various tissues, 541–542
  biologically active metabolites, see 1,25-Dihydroxyvitamin D_3; 25-Hydroxyvitamin D_3

chemical structure
  and of its analogs, 551
  as a secosteroid, 534–536
  stereochemical aspects: equilibration of conformers, 536–537

history of discovery, 533–534
plasma proteins binding
  properties, 544–545
  purification, 543
as regulator of calcium metabolism, 534